ANNALS OF THE NEW YORK ACADEMY OF SCIENCES

Volume 559

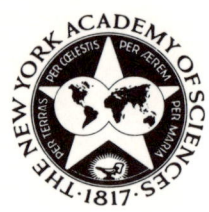

EDITORIAL STAFF
Executive Editor
BILL BOLAND
Managing Editor
JUSTINE CULLINAN
Associate Editor
RICHARD STIEFEL

The New York Academy of Sciences
2 East 63rd Street
New York, New York 10021

THE NEW YORK ACADEMY OF SCIENCES
(Founded in 1817)

BOARD OF GOVERNORS, 1989

WILLIAM T. GOLDEN, *Chairman of the Board*
LEWIS THOMAS, *President*
CHARLES A. SANDERS, *President-Elect*

Honorary Life Governors

SERGE A. KORFF   H. CHRISTINE REILLY   IRVING J. SELIKOFF

Vice-Presidents

MARVIN L. GOLDBERGER   DAVID A. HAMBURG   CYRIL M. HARRIS
DENNIS D. KELLY   PETER D. LAX

HENRY A. LICHSTEIN, *Secretary-Treasurer*

Elected Governors-at-Large

GERALD D. LAUBACH   JOHN D. MACOMBER   NEAL E. MILLER
LLOYD N. MORRISETT   GERARD PIEL   JOSEPH F. TRAUB

FLEUR L. STRAND, *Honorary Past Chair*   HELENE L. KAPLAN, *General Counsel*

OAKES AMES, *Executive Director*

ARACHIDONIC ACID METABOLISM IN THE NERVOUS SYSTEM

PHYSIOLOGICAL AND PATHOLOGICAL SIGNIFICANCE

ANNALS OF THE NEW YORK ACADEMY OF SCIENCES
Volume 559

ARACHIDONIC ACID METABOLISM IN THE NERVOUS SYSTEM

PHYSIOLOGICAL AND PATHOLOGICAL SIGNIFICANCE

Edited by Amiram I. Barkai and Nicolas G. Bazan

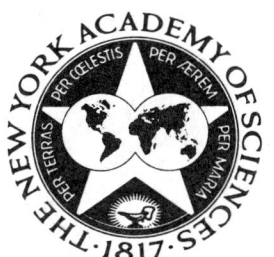

The New York Academy of Sciences
New York, New York
1989

Copyright © 1989 by the New York Academy of Sciences. All rights reserved. Under the provisions of the United States Copyright Act of 1976, individual readers of Annals are permitted to make fair use of the material in them for teaching or research. Permission is granted to quote from the Annals provided that the customary acknowledgement is made of the source. Material in the Annals may be republished only by permission of the Academy. Address inquiries to the Executive Editor at the New York Academy of Sciences.

Copying fees: *For each copy of an article made beyond the free copying permitted under Section 107 or 108 of the 1976 Copyright Act, a fee should be paid through the Copyright Clearance Center, 21 Congress Street, Salem, MA 01970. For articles of more than 3 pages, the copying fee is $1.75.*

∞ The paper used in this publication meets the minimum requirements of American National Standard for Information Sciences—Permanence of Paper for Printed Library Materials, ANSI Z39.48-1984.

Library of Congress Cataloging-in-Publication Data

Arachidonic acid metabolism in the nervous system.

(Annals of the New York Academy of Sciences, ISSN 0077-8923; v. 559)
Papers presented at a conference held by the New York Academy of Sciences in Bethesda, Md. on Apr. 14–16, 1988.
Bibliography: p.
Includes index.
  1. Arachidonic acid—Metabolism—Congresses.
2. Arachidonic acid—Pathophysiology—Congresses.
3. Nervous system—Metabolism—Congresses. 4. Nervous system—Pathophysiology—Congresses. I. Barkai, Amiram I. II. Bazán, Nicholás G. III. New York Academy of Sciences. IV. Series.
Q11.N5 vol. 559 [QP752.A7]   500 s [616.8'0471] 89-8263
ISBN 0-89766-502-3
ISBN 0-89766-503-1 (pbk.)

SP
Printed in the United States of America
ISBN 0-89766-502-3 (cloth)
ISBN 0-89766-503-1 (paper)
ISSN 0077-8923

ANNALS OF THE NEW YORK ACADEMY OF SCIENCES

Volume 559
July 5, 1989

ARACHIDONIC ACID METABOLISM IN THE NERVOUS SYSTEM
PHYSIOLOGICAL AND PATHOLOGICAL SIGNIFICANCE[a]

Editors and Conference Organizers
AMIRAM I. BARKAI AND NICOLAS G. BAZAN

CONTENTS

Preface. *By* AMIRAM I. BARKAI and NICOLAS G. BAZAN	xi
Arachidonic Acid in the Modulation of Excitable Membrane Function and at the Onset of Brain Damage. *By* NICOLAS G. BAZAN	1

Part I. Modulation of Arachidonic Acid Release and Metabolism in the Nervous System

Sources for Brain Arachidonic Acid Uptake and Turnover in Glycerophospholipids. *By* LLOYD A. HORROCKS	17
Isolation, Characterization, and Regulation of Diacylglycerol Lipases from the Bovine Brain. *By* AKHLAQ A. FAROOQUI, KOTTIL W. RAMMOHAN, and LLOYD A. HORROCKS	25
Deacylation-Reacylation of Arachidonoyl Groups in Cerebral Phospholipids. *By* GRACE Y. SUN and RONALD A. MACQUARRIE	37
Modulation of Arachidonate Turnover in Cerebral Phospholipids. *By* AMIRAM I. BARKAI and LEELAVATI R. MURTHY	56
Arachidonic Acid Metabolites in the Rat and Human Brain: New Findings on the Metabolism of Prostaglandin D_2 and Lipoxygenase Products. *By* L. S. WOLFE and L. PELLERIN	74

Part II. The Arachidonic Acid Cascade in the Nervous System

Formation and Function of Eicosanoids in the Central Nervous System. *By* GEORG HERTTING and ANDRÁS SEREGI	84
Prostaglandin E_2, Leukotriene C_4, and Platelet-Activating Factor Receptor Sites in the Brain: Binding Parameters and Pharmacological Studies. *By* F. DRAY, A. WISNER, M. C. BOMMELAER-BAYET, C. TIBERGHIEN, K. GEROZISSIS, M. SAADI, M. P. JUNIER, and C. ROUGEOT	100
Role of Brain Microvessels and Choroid Plexus in the Cerebral Metabolism of Leukotrienes. *By* JAN ÅKE LINDGREN, IRINA KARNUSHINA, and HANS-ERIK CLAESSON	112

[a]The papers in this volume were presented at a conference entitled Arachidonic Acid Metabolism in the Nervous System: Physiological and Pathological Significance, which was held by the New York Academy of Sciences in Bethesda, Maryland on April 14–16, 1988.

Biologically Active Metabolites of the 12-Lipoxygenase Pathway Are Formed by *Aplysia* Nervous Tissue. *By* STEVEN J. FEINMARK, DANIELE PIOMELLI, ELI SHAPIRO, and JAMES H. SCHWARTZ 121

Cerebrospinal Fluid Eicosanoids as an Index of Cerebrovascular Status. *By* RICHARD P. WHITE 131

Eicosanoids and the Blood-Brain Barrier. *By* REYNOLD SPECTOR 146

Part III. Arachidonic Acid and Its Metabolites in Signal Transduction

The Relationship between Phospholipases A_2 and C in Signal Transduction. *By* EDUARDO G. LAPETINA and MICHAEL F. CROUCH 153

Regulation of Phospholipase A_2 and Phospholipase C in Rod Outer Segments of Bovine Retina Involves a Common GTP-binding Protein but Different Mechanisms of Action. *By* CAROLE L. JELSEMA 158

Mechanisms Involved in the Action of Prostaglandins as Modulators of Neurotransmission. *By* LARS E. GUSTAFSSON 178

The Role of Arachidonic Acid and Its Metabolites in the Release of Neuropeptides. *By* SERGIO R. OJEDA, HENRYK F. URBANSKI, MARIE-PIERRE JUNIER, and JORGE CAPDEVILA 192

12-Keto-Eicosatetraenoic Acid: A Biologically Active Eicosanoid in the Nervous System of *Aplysia*. *By* DANIELE PIOMELLI, STEVEN J. FEINMARK, ELI SHAPIRO, and JAMES H. SCHWARTZ 208

Antagonistic Modulation of S-K^+ Channel Activity by Cyclic AMP and Arachidonic Acid Metabolites: Role for Two G Proteins. *By* ANDREA VOLTERRA and STEVEN A. SIEGELBAUM 219

Part IV. The Role of Cerebral Blood Flow and Arachidonic Acid Metabolism in Brain Injury and Ischemic Damage

The Role of Arachidonic Acid and Oxygen Radical Metabolites in the Pathogenesis of Vasogenic Brain Edema and Astrocytic Swelling. *By* PAK H. CHAN, SUSAN LONGAR, SYLVIA CHEN, ALBERT C. H. YU, LARS HILLERED, LILLIAN CHU, SHIGEKI IMAIZUMI, BRYAN PEREIRA, KI MOORE, VICKI WOOLWORTH, and ROBERT A. FISHMAN 237

Ischemia Stress and Arachidonic Acid Metabolites in the Fetal Brain. *By* E. YAVIN, E. GOLDIN, E. MAGAL, A. TOMER, and S. HAREL 248

Arachidonic Acid Metabolism in Ischemic Neuronal Damage *By* KOJI ABE, MIKIO YOSHIDOMI, and KYUYA KOGURE 259

Ischemic Injury in the Brain: Role of Oxygen Radical-Mediated Processes. *By* BRANT D. WATSON and MYRON D. GINSBERG 269

Arachidonic Acid and Its Metabolites in Cerebral Ischemia. *By* C. Y. HSU, T. H. LIU, J. XU, E. L. HOGAN, J. CHAO, G. SUN, H. H. TAI, J. S. BECKMAN, and B. A. FREEMAN 282

The Role of Platelet-Activating Factor in Cerebral Ischemia and Related Disorders. *By* P. BRAQUET, B. SPINNEWYN, C. DEMERLE, D. HOSFORD, V. MARCHESELLI, M. ROSSOWSKA, and N. G. BAZAN 296

Eicosanoids in Deteriorating Stroke: Review of Studies on the Rabbit Spinal Cord Ischemia and Reperfusion Model. *By* GIORA FEUERSTEIN 313

Part V. Arachidonic Acid Metabolism and Convulsive Disorders

Arachidonic Acid Metabolism in Seizures. *By* BO K. SIESJÖ, CARL-DAVID AGARDH, FINN BENGTSSON, and MAJ-LIS SMITH 323

Arachidonic Acid Metabolism and Cerebral Blood Flow in the Normal, Ischemic, and Reperfused Gerbil Brain: Inhibition of Ischemia-Reperfusion–Induced Cerebral Injury by a Platelet-Activating Factor Antagonist (BN 52021). *By* THOMAS PANETTA, VICTOR L. MARCHESELLI, PIERRE BRAQUET, and NICOLAS G. BAZAN 340

Arachidonic Acid and Its Metabolites during Cerebral Ischemia and Recirculation: Pharmacological Interventions. *By* CLAUDIO GALLI, ANNA PETRONI, ANTONELLA BERTAZZO, and SILVIA SARTI 352

Part VI. Arachidonic Acid and Its Metabolites in Normal and Abnormal Brain Functions: Sleep, Temperature Regulation, Alcohol Effects, and Mental Disorders

The Aging Brain: A Normal Phenomenon with Not-So-Normal Arachidonic Acid Metabolism. *By* ALBERTO GAITI 365

Prostaglandin D_2 and Sleep. *By* OSAMU HAYAISHI 374

The Role of Arachidonic Acid Metabolites in Mediating Ethanol Self-Administration and Intoxication. *By* FRANK R. GEORGE 382

Thermoregulatory Actions of Eicosanoids in the Central Nervous System with Particular Regard to the Pathogenesis of Fever. *By* A. S. MILTON 392

Polyunsaturated Fatty Acids, Prostaglandins, and Schizophrenia. *By* DANIEL P. VAN KAMMEN, JEFFREY K. YAO, and KENNETH GOETZ 411

Part VII. Poster Papers

Regenerative Arachidonic Acid Oxygenation Waves as Back-Propagating Neural Signals. *By* STEPHEN C. BAER 424

Platelet-Activating Factor Receptor Blockade Decreases Early Posttraumatic Cerebral Edema in Rats. *By* D. C. BUCHANAN, P. M. KOCHANEK, E. M. NEMOTO, J. A. MELICK, and R. J. SCHOETTLE 427

Nerve Growth Factor Stimulates PC12 Cell Eicosanoid Synthesis: A Role in Nerve Fiber Growth. *By* J. J. DEGEORGE, R. WALENGA, and S. T. CARBONETTO 429

Effects of Traumatic Brain Injury on Arachidonic Acid Metabolism and Brain Water Content in the Rat. *By* PAUL DEMEDIUK, ALAN I. FADEN, ROBERT VINK, ROBERT ROMHANYI, and TRACY K. MCINTOSH 431

Eicosanoid Production after Traumatic Spinal Cord Injury in the Rat: Inhibition by BW755c and Potentiation by Hypomagnesia, *By* PAUL DEMEDIUK and ALAN I. FADEN 433

Prostanoids and Ischemic Brain Edema: Human and Animal Study. *By* BOGDAN M. DJURIČIĆ, VLADIMIR S. KOSTIĆ, and BOGOMIR B. MRŠULJA ... 435

The Role of Arachidonic Acid and Prostaglandins in Neurotransmitter Release from Isolated Cerebellar Glomeruli. *By* ROBERT V. DORMAN and DAVID M. TERRIAN 438

Indomethacin Posttreatment Antagonizes Ethanol-induced Sleep Time. *By* GREGORY I. ELMER and FRANK R. GEORGE 441

Release of Arachidonic Acid Metabolites after Experimental Subarachnoid Hemorrhage. *By* PAOLO GAETANI, FULVIO MARZATICO, DANIELA LOMBARDI, ILARIA FULLE, VITTORIO SILVANI, and RICCARDO RODRIGUEZ Y BAENA 444

Prostaglandin Synthetase Inhibitors Specifically Modulate Ethanol Self-Administration. *By* FRANK R. GEORGE 449

Prostaglandin E_2 Administered Intravenously Crosses the Blood-Brain Barrier and Induces Hyperthermia as a Central Action. *By* HIDEYA HAYASHI, NAOMI EGUCHI, YOSHIHIRO URADE, SEIJI ITO, and OSAMU HAYAISHI 451

The Role and New Action Mechanism of Prostaglandin E_2 in Neurotransmission. *By* SEIJI ITO, MANABU NEGISHI, HIDEYA HAYASHI, and OSAMU HAYAISHI 453

Endothelium-derived Relaxing Factor Release from Cultured Endothelial Cells Does Not Require Phospholipase Activation or Arachidonate Mobilization. *By* ROGER A. JOHNS, PETER J. MILNER, NICHOLAS J. IZZO, JOANNE SAYE, ALEX L. LOEB, and MICHAEL J. PEACH............................ 455

Smooth Muscle Pharmacology of Hydroxylated Docosanoids. *By* JOHN W. KARANIAN, HEE-YONG KIM, TADASHI SHINGU, JAMES YERGEY, and NORMAN SALEM, JR. 457

Structural Analysis of Oxygenated Metabolites of Polyunsaturated Fatty Acids Using Thermospray Liquid Chromatography/Mass Spectroscopy and Gas Chromatography/Mass Spectroscopy. *By* HEE-YONG KIM, J. W. KARANIAN, and N. SALEM, JR. 459

Formation of Lipoxins by the Brain: Ischemia Enhances Production of Lipoxins. *By* SANG JOO KIM AND TEIJI TOMINAGA 461

Cerebral Ischemia in Gerbils: Effect of Postischemic Treatment with Oligoprostaglandin B1. *By* D. V. LUBITZ, S. L. COHAN, D. J. REDMOND, and M. SHERIDAN 465

Effects of Platelet-Activating Factor Antagonist BN 52021 on Cerebral Lipid Metabolism following Ischemia Reperfusion in the Gerbil. *By* VICTOR L. MARCHESELLI, THOMAS PANETTA, PIERRE BRAQUET, KERRY T. THIBODEAUX, and NICOLAS G. BAZAN 468

Eicosanoid Production by Isolated Cerebral Microvessels and Cultured Cerebral Endothelium. *By* STEVEN A. MOORE, PAUL H. FIGARD, ARTHUR A. SPECTOR, and MICHAEL N. HART 471

Arachidonic Acid Metabolism in Glutamate Neurotoxicity. *By* TIM MURPHY, ASHISH PARIKH, RONALD SCHNAAR, and JOSEPH COYLE 474

Selective Inhibition of Thromboxane Synthase Enhances Reperfusion and Metabolism of the Ischemic Brain. *By* L. C. PETTIGREW, L. K. MISRA, J. C. GROTTA, P. A. NARAYANA, and K. K. WU 478

Differential Regulation of Two Types of Cation Channel in BC3H-1 Muscle Cells by Arachidonate. *By* R. E. SHERIDAN and R. MCGEE 480

Increased Peroxidation of Docosahexaenoic Acid in the Rat Brain *in Vitro* and *in Vivo* during Cerebral Ischemia. *By* TADASHI SHINGU, JOHN W. KARANIAN, HEE-YONG KIM, and NORMAN SALEM, JR............................ 482

Increased 5-HETE Production in the Brain following Head Injury. *By* E. SHOHAMI, Y. SHAPIRA, G. YADID, S. COTEV, and G. FEUERSTEIN 485

The Early Effect of Steroidal and Nonsteroidal Antiinflammatory Agents on Neoplastic Epidural Cord Compression. *By* T. SIEGAL, TZ. SIEGAL, Y. SHAPIRA, and E. SHOHAMI 488

Primary Structure of Rat Brain Prostaglandin D Synthetase Deduced from the cDNA Sequence. *By* YOSHIHIRO URADE, AKIHISA NAGATA, YASUHIKO SUZUKI, YUTAKA FUJII, and OSAMU HAYAISHI.. 491

Functional-Site Study of Prostaglandins in the Monkey Brain Using Quantitative Autoradiography and Positron Emission Tomography. *By* Y. WATANABE, B. LÅNGSTRÖM, Y. WATANABE, K. HAMADA, P-G. GILLBERG, C-G. STÅLNACKE, M. HATANAKA, H. HAYASHI, and O. HAYAISHI 494

Prostaglandins in Human Cerebrospinal Fluid? *By* JAMES A. YERGEY, NORMAN SALEM, JR., JOHN W. KARANIAN, MARKKU LINNOILA, and MELVYN P. HEYES.. 497

Inhibition of [1-^{14}C]Arachidonate Incorporation into Synaptosomal Phospholipids by Lipid Peroxides. *By* MALGORZATA M. ZALESKA and DAVID F. WILSON 500

Index of Contributors.. 503

Financial assistance was received from:
- BURROUGHS WELLCOME COMPANY
- CIBA-GEIGY CORPORATION
- GLAXO INCORPORATED
- ICI PHARMACEUTICAL GROUP
- LILLY RESEARCH LABORATORIES
- MERCK SHARP & DOHME RESEARCH LABORATORIES
- MILES INCORPORATED
- NATIONAL INSTITUTE OF MENTAL HEALTH/NIH
- NATIONAL INSTITUTE OF NEUROLOGICAL AND COMMUNICATIVE DISORDERS AND STROKE/NIH
- NATIONAL SCIENCE FOUNDATION
- OFFICE OF NAVAL RESEARCH
- PARKE-DAVIS PHARMACEUTICAL RESEARCH DIVISION
- PFIZER CENTRAL RESEARCH
- SEARLE RESEARCH AND DEVELOPMENT
- UNITED STATES AIR FORCE OFFICE OF SCIENTIFIC RESEARCH
- THE UPJOHN COMPANY

The New York Academy of Sciences believes it has a responsibility to provide an open forum for discussion of scientific questions. The positions taken by the participants in the reported conferences are their own and not necessarily those of the Academy. The Academy has no intent to influence legislation by providing such forums.

Preface

Arachidonic acid (AA) is an essential polyunsaturated fatty acid that is stored in tissue phospholipids. It serves as a precursor for a variety of products conveniently termed "the AA cascade" or "the eicosanoids." Many of these compounds are biologically active and are composed of prostaglandins, thromboxanes, and leukotrienes. The rate-limiting step in the formation of such compounds is the release of AA from membrane phospholipids through the activation of phospholipase A enzymes. Research, which was conducted mostly with tissues other than the nervous system, has indicated that the release of AA from phospholipids occurs following activation of various receptors. Cell types may differ in their phospholipid pools and in the mechanisms that modulate the release of AA and the subsequent formation of eicosanoids. Research on the modulation of AA release and metabolism in the nervous system has increased in volume during recent years; it encompasses studies on the turnover of phospholipids that serve as sources of brain AA, the activity of brain phospholipases, the processes of acylation and deacylation of arachidonyl groups in cerebral phospholipids, and neurotransmitter-mediated changes of arachidonate turnover in cerebral phospholipids.

The study of the formation and function of eicosanoids has been a subject of extensive investigation in a variety of tissues and has been reviewed in the *Annual Review of Biochemistry* in 1975, 1978, 1983, and 1986. Only recently has the metabolic fate of AA oxidation been investigated systematically in nervous tissue. The formation and function of prostaglandins and leukotrienes in the central nervous system (CNS) and the demonstration of corresponding receptors in neuronal membranes have been reported recently. Efforts have also been directed to analyze eicosanoids in the cerebrospinal fluid (CSF). The presence of these compounds in the CSF may serve as important indicators of changes in cerebrovascular function in certain pathological situations.

The role of AA and its metabolites in signal transduction is a subject of investigation in an increasing number of laboratories. Basic research on the mechanisms of signal transduction is developing rapidly, and much attention has been directed to the role of phosphoinositides as precursors of second messengers. Since phosphoinositides are rich in AA, each of the many AA cascade products may potentially serve as a second messenger in the process of neuronal transmission. Although the possibility that eicosanoids could serve as second messengers has not been fully investigated, there is information that AA and its metabolites play an important role in regulating neurotransmitter-synthesizing enzymes and in modulating the release of neuropeptides and hormones. In addition, recent studies indicate that eicosanoids serve as modulators of neurotransmission in the marine mollusk *Aplysia*.

The involvement of AA and its metabolites in the regulation of cerebral blood flow and in the complex pathophysiology of cerebral ischemia, stroke, and brain trauma has been a subject of increasing interest. These problems are of great clinical importance and are attracting very active research groups in the fields of neurology and neurochemistry. Research in these areas addresses issues of cerebrovascular permeability, cerebral edema, ischemic stress in the developing brain, delayed neuronal damage, and the role of oxygen radicals and of eicosanoids in cerebral infarction or brain injury.

AA and its metabolites also play an important role in the neurobiology of brain seizures. Release of AA in the brain is activated during convulsions, and the formation of eicosanoids is increased. Alterations of membrane phospholipids, the formation of

AA and its metabolites, and the receptor-mediated processes underlying these events open new avenues of investigation into the neurobiology of convulsive disorders.

Finally, AA and its metabolic products may play a role in the aging process, the regulation of certain behaviors such as sleep, the neurobiology of pain, and the development of certain psychiatric disorders. Research in these areas has been conducted in several laboratories.

The present volume is a product of an international conference sponsored by the New York Academy of Sciences. The conference was aimed at providing a forum for the review and discussion of recent developments in the research of the neurobiology of AA and its metabolic products, including prostaglandins, thromboxanes, and leukotrienes, in relation to their formation and function in the nervous system. The conference addressed basic and clinical research issues and was inherently interdisciplinary. The major areas of discussion concerned the biochemical, physiological, and pathological aspects of AA and its metabolites in the nervous system. We hope that this conference has filled the gap between the extensively researched field of eicosanoid formation and function in systems other than the nervous system and the rapidly developing fields of basic research on signal transduction, modulation of neuronal function, and clinical research on cerebral ischemia, brain injury, convulsive disorders, and other neurological or psychiatric disorders. We also hope that this conference has helped to stimulate a fruitful interdisciplinary exchange.

We wish to express our gratitude and appreciation to the organizations that provided the financial support necessary to hold this conference and to the many organizers, speakers, and other participants who contributed time and effort to make the conference worthwhile.

AMIRAM I. BARKAI
NICOLAS G. BAZAN

Arachidonic Acid in the Modulation of Excitable Membrane Function and at the Onset of Brain Damage[a]

NICOLAS G. BAZAN[b]

Louisiana State University Medical School
Louisiana State University
Eye Center and Neuroscience Center
New Orleans, Louisiana 70112

INTRODUCTION

Phospholipids of excitable membranes are a heterogeneous group of fatty acyl-glycerophosphate derivatives divided into classes on the basis of their polar head groups (phosphatidylcholine, phosphatidylethanolamine, phosphatidylserine, phosphatidylinositol, and others). These classes comprise many different molecular species defined by the individual fatty acyl substituents present at C_1 and C_2 of the glycerol backbone. Most of the fatty acyl chains at C_1 are saturated or lower unsaturated, and most at C_2 are unsaturated. Thus, stearic (18:0), palmitic (16:0), and oleic (18:1) acids are found most frequently at C_1, while arachidonic acid (20:4, n-6) and docosahexaenoic acid (22:6, n-3) are the main fatty acids found at C_2. Excitable membranes, like other membranes, contain different proportions of molecular species of phospholipids; they are unique, however, because of their very high content of polyunsaturated acyl groups, such as arachidonic (tetraenoic molecular species) and docosahexaenoic (hexaenoic molecular species) acids. In fact, retinal photoreceptors contain docosahexaenoic acid esterified at both carbons of the glycerol backbone; these didocosahexaenoyl molecular species of phospholipids have been called "supraenoic."[1,2]

Polyunsaturated phospholipids are critical for the function of excitable membranes and are protected from reactive oxygen radicals by various endogenous oxidant defenses. One of the major functions of phospholipids is to serve as a source of second messengers. The release of the messengers is triggered by receptor-mediated events. These messengers in turn play an important role in the modulation of cellular responses.[3-9] Electroconvulsive shock (ECS), several other forms of convulsions, and brief ischemia result in the accumulation of free arachidonic acid (AA) and diacylglycerol (DAG) enriched with stearate and arachidonate in the brain.[10-12] The degradation of inositol lipids is thought to be the source of DAG under these conditions.[11-14] Also, the degradation of other phospholipids, such as phosphatidylcholine, may contribute to the accumulating free arachidonic acid.[15] Free arachidonic acid accumulates in the retina, used as an *in vitro* "ready-made brain slice" preparation, when incubated with high K^+ concentrations, or in the presence of dibutyryl cAMP, or in anoxia.[16]

---

[a]This work was supported in part by N.I.H. Grants EY05121, EY02377, and NS 23002. The author is holder of a Jacob Javitz Neuroscience Investigator Award from the National Institute of Neurological and Communicative Disorders and Stroke, National Institutes of Health, United States Public Health Service.

[b]Address for correspondence: LSU Eye Center, 2020 Gravier Street, Suite B, New Orleans, Louisiana 70112.

This opening paper focuses on the release of arachidonic acid and its oxygenated metabolites in the central nervous system, and on their pathophysiological role at the onset of ischemic or epileptic brain damage. The use of *in vivo* experimental approaches is emphasized, including studies on the physiological significance of arachidonoyl-phospholipids and free arachidonic acid in the modulation of excitable membrane function. An overview of the studies carried out in the author's laboratory comprises most of this paper. Many other researchers, particularly the authors of the papers in this volume, have contributed greatly to this field. Due to space limitations, not every primary reference is quoted; however, several review articles have been included.

TIGHT REGULATION OF THE FREE ARACHIDONIC ACID POOL IN THE CENTRAL NERVOUS SYSTEM

In both the retina[17,18] and the brain,[19] free AA is undetectable under resting conditions. This is due to tight metabolic control of the enzymatic steps involved in the activation, acylation, and deacylation of arachidonoyl chains of membrane phospholipids. The activation is catalyzed by arachidonoyl–coenzyme A (CoA) synthetase, which displays a low K_m for arachidonic acid and is found in microsomes[20] and in synaptic membranes.[14,20] This enzyme actively contributes to the retention of arachidonic acid within cells, either upon arrival of the fatty acid to the cell or when free arachidonic acid is released under basal lipid turnover or after receptor-mediated activation of phospholipase A_2. Arachidonoyl coenzyme A synthetase can play a central role in the regulation of eicosanoid synthesis by removing the precursor, free arachidonic acid, and also its oxidized metabolites, hydroxyeicosatetraenoic acids (HETE). The products of this activating enzyme, arachidonoyl CoA and HETE-CoA, do not accumulate because they are rapidly esterified into lipids, most often phospholipids, by acyltransferases. This coupling may occur in the nervous system,[5,21,22] as is discussed below, and as a result may limit the availability of the fatty acid for arachidonoyl–coenzyme A synthetase.

Free AA can be generated by three main reactions (FIG. 1). First, free AA can result from the deacylation of arachidonoyl chains of phospholipids by membrane phospholipase (PL) A_2. This reaction is modulated by G proteins coupled to receptors.[3,23] Calcium stimulates phospholipases A; and, therefore, either through calcium channel activation or intracellular mobilization (e.g., inositol trisphosphate, IP_3), free calcium ions can promote the release of free arachidonic acid. Second, free AA may be released through the sequential degradation of inositol lipids by phospholipase C–diacylglycerol lipase. Phospholipase C activation is triggered by a receptor-mediated mechanism that also is coupled to a G protein and results in the phosphodiesteratic cleavage of phosphatidylinositol 4,5-bisphosphate (PIP_2). Agonists such as beta-adrenergics, muscarinics, cholinergics, and certain peptides activate this system.[3] Despite the fact that the inositol lipids are a quantitatively small pool of phospholipids, their high content of arachidonoyl chains and turnover make them important sources of free AA. A third route for the generation of free AA is the first step in the synthesis of platelet-activating factor (PAF). The precursor of PAF is the phospholipid 1-alkyl-2-acyl-glycerol phosphorylcholine, shown to be enriched in arachidonoyl groups in several tissues. The relationship of PAF synthesis to the generation of free AA is not well understood. However, this first metabolic step in the synthesis of PAF has been shown in macrophages[24] and also, after injury, in the cornea, where PAF accumulation and lipoxygenation of AA take place, presumably after phospholipase A_2 has released AA from its precursor.[25] Increased synthesis of PAF in the rat brain during drug- and ECS-induced convulsions also has been reported.[26]

REGULATION OF PHOSPHOLIPASE A_2

The fatty acid composition of the accumulated endogenous free fatty acids (FFA) in the brain during ischemia shows a predominance of unsaturated fatty acids, with only slight changes in the triacylglycerol (TAG) content.[10] This leads to the proposal that brief ischemia activates brain phospholipases, predominately A_2.[10,27-29]

To assess the possibility that the ischemia-induced activation of phospholipase A_2 was not a postmortem phenomenon but rather the result of overstimulation of an enzyme linked to the function of excitable membranes, the effect of convulsions was

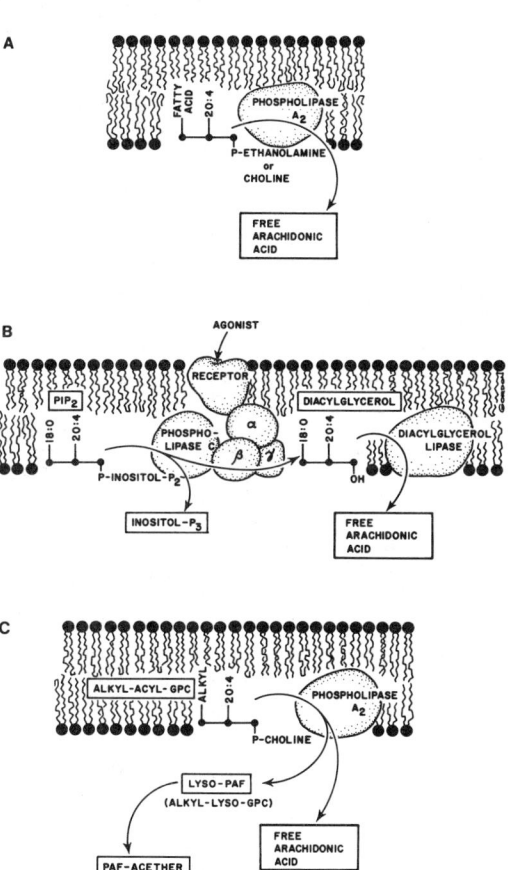

FIGURE 1. Metabolic steps controlling free arachidonic acid release from membrane phospholipids. **A:** Phospholipase A_2 hydrolyzing phosphatidylethanolamine or phosphatidylcholine leads to release of arachidonic acid and the corresponding monoacylated derivative (1-acyl glycerophosphoryl derivative or lysophospholipids, not shown); **B:** Sequential degradation of phosphatidylinositol 4,5 bisphosphate (PIP_2) by phospholipase C (activated by an agonist-receptor-G protein) followed by diacylglycerol lipase; **C:** Phospholipase A_2 hydrolyzing alkyl acyl glycerol phosphorylcholine, releasing free arachidonic acid and lyso PAF (platelet-activating factor), then acetylated to generate PAF. (From N. G. Bazan.[64] Reprinted by permission from Alan R. Liss, Inc.)

studied. This approach was selected because overactivation of the nervous system under *in vivo* conditions makes it possible to follow neurochemical changes during and after convulsions. Moreover, the possibility that in epilepsy enhanced deacylation of membrane phospholipids occurs was explored. In fact, reversible changes in the endogenous content of free fatty acids and of arachidonic acid do occur following 1 second of electrical stimulation, resulting in convulsions. These convulsions are tonic, clonic, and last for about 8-10 seconds. An increase in phospholipase A activating protein (PAAP) synthesis has been reported to regulate AA release and eicosanoid synthesis in endothelial cells upon tumor necrosis factor stimulation.[30,31] A number of modulators may contribute to controlling the release of free arachidonic acid. Lipocortin (lipomodulin or renocortin), a glucocorticoid-inducible phospholipase A_2 inhibitory protein, has been described.[32] Since lipocortin may comprise a group of phospholipid-binding proteins, their effect as modulators may involve a decrease in phospholipase A_2 activity due to substrate removal rather than a specific inhibitory effect on the enzyme.

Receptor-mediated phospholipase A_2 activation through G-proteins has been shown in rod outer segments[23] and in other cells. Transducin, a G-protein, was found to stimulate release of arachidonic acid and thus may lead to the synthesis of eicosanoids that could function as second messengers.[3]

It is widely assumed that phospholipase A_2 is activated by calcium ions. No clear evidence in the nervous tissue is available, however, of the possible modulatory role of this divalent cation. One alternative that deserves consideration is that receptor-activated phospholipase C may lead, through IP_3-mediated Ca^{2+} mobilization from intracellular stores, to increased cytosolic calcium concentration. This could result in the activation of phospholipase A_2 under certain conditions or in certain synaptic circuits.

Another modulatory mechanism is the Na^+-H^+ antiport.[33] This transporter has been shown to promote activation of phospholipase A_2 in platelets as a result of localized cytoplasmic alkalinization resulting from cell proton efflux. Exposure of rat retinas to light also has been shown to increase the release of AA; this effect was greater after 15 minutes of light stimulation.[34]

IN VITRO STUDIES USING THE RETINA AS A MODEL SHOW THAT K^+-INDUCED DEPOLARIZATION SELECTIVELY STIMULATES LIPOXYGENATION OF ARACHIDONIC ACID

Arachidonic acid is metabolized to prostaglandins and hydroxyeicosatetraenoic acids (HETE) in the rat retina.[21] Rat retinas prelabeled by intravitreal injection of [^{14}C]-arachidonic acid and then incubated *in vitro* showed a loss of radioactivity from phospholipids and neutral lipids.[21] Though prostaglandin synthesis was not increased during the incubation period, a 12-fold increase in the level of HETEs was detected, with 12-HETE as the major detected product. Incubation of the prelabeled retinas in a depolarizing medium (45 mM K^+) resulted in a selective increase in HETEs, an effect that was blocked by lipoxygenase inhibitors. This study demonstrated the stimulation of lipoxygenase activity in the central nervous system by membrane depolarization.

INOSITOL PHOSPHOLIPIDS IN CELL SIGNALING: ACCUMULATION OF ARACHIDONIC ACID AND DIACYLGLYCEROL AND DEGRADATION OF PHOSPHATIDYLINOSITOL 4,5-BISPHOSPHATE IN THE CEREBRUM DURING CONVULSIONS

Inositol phospholipids are involved in neuronal responsiveness through the generation of second messengers. The phosphodiesteratic cleavage of inositol phospholipids, mediated by phospholipase C, is activated by neurotransmitters, hormones, growth factors, or other agonists, resulting in the formation of diacylglycerol and water-soluble inositol phosphates as reaction products and then leading to intracellular ionization of Ca^{2+}. Since increased formation of diacylglycerol and inositol 1,4,5-

trisphosphate occurs in the brain during convulsions,[14,35] an enhanced phosphodiesteratic cleavage of polyphosphoinositides occurs. Ischemia also triggers similar neurochemical changes,[12,13] suggesting that the vulnerability of the brain at synapses under these conditions may involve inositol phospholipid degradation.[12]

Diacylglycerol, while it is a reaction product of phospholipase C–mediated degradation of phosphoinositides, is also a substrate for lipases that release arachidonic acid for the synthesis of eicosanoids. In addition, diacylglycerol is a key intermediate in the biosynthesis of other phospholipids and neutral lipids. Free arachidonic and stearic acids may result from the deacylation of diacylglycerol by lipases, following the activation of phospholipase C stimulated by convulsions. Diacylglycerol is an intracellular messenger for the activation of a calcium- and phospholipid-sensitive protein kinase.[36] The water-soluble product of phosphatidylinositol 4,5-bisphosphate hydrolysis, inositol 1,4,5-trisphosphate, acts as a second messenger for the release of calcium from nonmitochondrial intracellular stores (calciosomes) through a specific receptor. Other phosphorylated derivatives of inositol phospholipids (e.g., inositol tetraphosphate) have been described in the brain; their role is as yet unknown.

Inositol lipids are enriched in stearoyl-arachidonoyl molecular species,[37] and they have an increased turnover rate during stimulation.[35] Thus, the endogenous FFA and DAG, with mainly stearic and arachidonic acids that accumulate rapidly upon stimulation in the brain, may result from the breakdown of inositol lipids.[12,38] In platelets, the transient accumulation of stearoyl-arachidonoyl glycerol after thrombin stimulation arises from the breakdown of the three inositol phospholipids.[39] Similarly, the loss of phosphatidylinositol (PI) in stimulated human neutrophils has been correlated with the accumulation of stearoyl-arachidonoyl glycerol.

To assess the changes in the content and fatty acid composition of inositol lipids in the rat cerebrum after electroconvulsive shock, a time-dependent analysis was carried out. Fatty acyl groups of PI, phosphatidylinositol 4-phosphate (PIP), PIP_2, DAG, and FFA present were assessed.[14] The experimental approach used was the rapid inactivation of brain enzymes by high-power head-focused microwave irradiation to measure lipid changes as early as 2 seconds after electroconvulsive shock. This rapid inactivation of brain enzymes was important because inositol phospholipids are rapidly hydrolyzed postmortem[40] and because FFA and DAG increase at the onset of ischemia.

The results of this study demonstrate that within 5 seconds after electroshock, the amount of PIP_2 decreased in the rat cerebrum. Most of this change was due to the loss of arachidonoyl and stearoyl chains. During this same period, the accumulation of stearic acid and AA in the DAG and FFA was consistent with the loss of PIP_2. This accumulation may proceed via the phosphodiesteraic cleavage (by phospholipase C) of PIP_2 and via further partial hydrolysis of DAG by diacylglycerol lipase and monoacylglycerol lipase. The accumulation of FFA, both saturated and unsaturated, within 2 seconds after stimulation and prior to a detectable change in inositol lipid acyl group content suggests that these fatty acids may be released by the action of phospholipases A_1 and A_2 on other phospholipids. Moreover, the accumulation of free docosahexaenoic and palmitic acids in the cerebrum cannot be accounted for by PIP_2 degradation.

In summary, these results suggest that most of the stearic and arachidonic acids of brain FFA and DAG after electroconvulsive shock arise specifically from PIP_2. The remaining arachidonic acid and other fatty acids accumulated are likely derived from other phospholipids. The transient accumulation of DAG is presumably due to the activation of DAG and monoacylglyceride lipases that release stearic acid and arachidonic acid. The earliest event during convulsion-enhanced neurotransmitter release may be the activation of phospholipase A_2 at the presynaptic membrane level, related to events leading to neurotransmitter release. This, in turn, results in subsequent PIP_2 hydrolysis at the postsynaptic membrane level. Since one of the consequences of repeated convulsions is brain damage, and because such conditions enhance operation of the inositol phospholipid cycle,[35] sustained neuronal stimulation may deplete the stores of receptor-linked PIP_2, with accumulation of polyunsaturated fatty acids and oxygenated metabolites ultimately resulting in brain damage.

SYNAPTOSOMES ISOLATED DURING BICUCULLINE-INDUCED STATUS EPILEPTICUS SHOW THAT EXCITABLE MEMBRANES ACCUMULATE FREE ARACHIDONIC ACID AND PREDOMINANTLY GENERATE LIPOXYGENASE METABOLITES DURING CONVULSIONS

A primary event following electroshock and drug-induced seizures is free fatty acid release and accumulation in the brain.[38,41-43] One model that has been used to study the changes in lipid metabolism that accompany seizures is that of bicuculline-induced status epilepticus.[42,44,45] Arachidonic acid is the major fatty acid that accumulates during seizures. Increased synthesis of oxygenated metabolites of arachidonic acid, the eicosanoids (prostaglandins [PGs] and leukotrienes [LTs]), appears to be a consequence of epileptic and other cerebral pathology. Accordingly, studies designed to pinpoint specific alterations in arachidonic acid metabolism to a subcellular location have been carried out. In synaptosomes from bicuculline-treated rats,[22] total free fatty acid levels increased by 14%. Palmitic acid (16:0), 20:4, and 22:6 increased by 25%, 25%, and 23%, respectively, while other fatty acid levels remained fairly constant. When synaptosomes from untreated and bicuculline-treated rats were incubated for one hour, the difference in free fatty acid levels between the two groups was lost. This may be due to higher postconvulsion acyltransferase levels.[46]

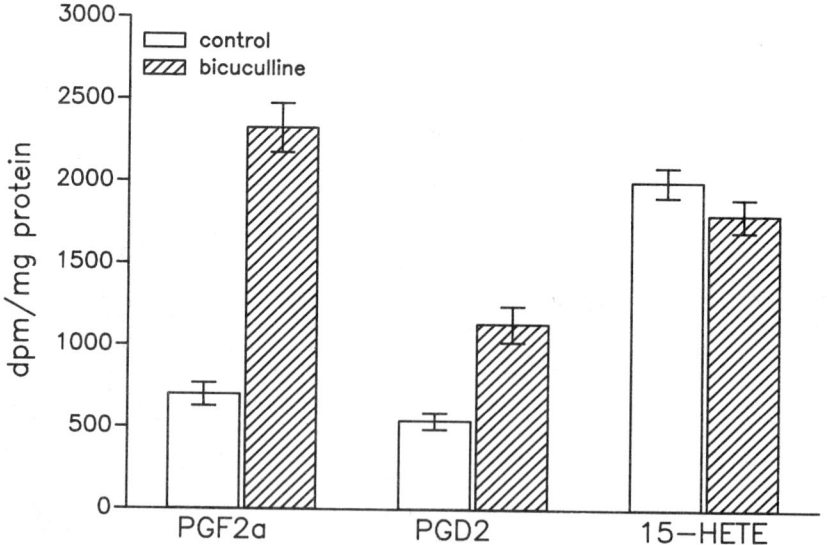

FIGURE 2. Bicuculline-induced status epilepticus stimulates PG synthesis in rat brain microsomes. (Data recalculated from results contained in Birkle & Bazan.[22])

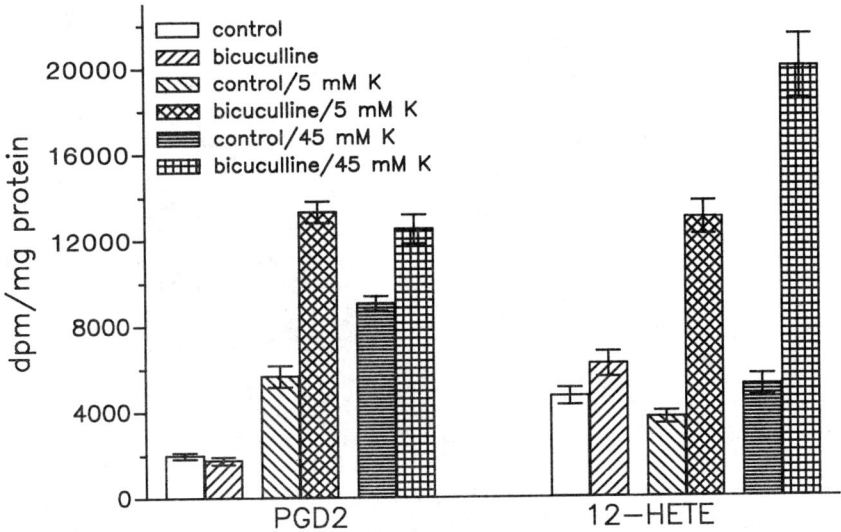

FIGURE 3. Bicuculline-induced status epilepticus stimulates PG and HETE synthesis in rat brain synaptosomes. (Data recalculated from results in Birkle & Bazan.[22])

The distribution of eicosanoid synthesis products at different subcellular levels (i.e., microsomes, synaptosomes, cytosol) was studied using rat cerebrum prelabeled *in vivo* with [1−^{14}C]20:4. The synaptosomal fraction showed the highest activity with regard to eicosanoid synthesis. The synthesis of HETEs, with LTB$_4$, 5-HETE, and 15-HETE as the major lipoxygenase products, was greater than that of PGs in all fractions. In synaptosomes extracted from bicuculline-treated rats immediately upon isolation, an overall tendency toward decreased cyclooxygenase activity was observed. However, 12-lipoxygenase activity in synaptosomes from the treated rats was increased by 50%.

Comparable studies in brain microsomes, a fraction not enriched in excitable membranes, were carried out to help evaluate the specificity of bicuculline-induced changes in synaptosomal 20:4 metabolism. In microsomes from treated rats, there was a 24–30% decrease in labeling of all glycerolipids. Reductions in free [1−^{14}C]20:4 and [1−^{14}C]20:4 in glycerolipids are reflected in increases in PGs (FIG. 2) in this fraction. The effects of *in vitro* depolarization at 5 mM K$^+$ and 45 mM K$^+$ in microsomes and synaptosomes in both untreated and bicuculline-treated rats were studied. Stimulation of lipoxygenase activity only in the synaptosomes was observed (FIG. 3). These results establish that lipoxygenase activity is present in the synaptosomal fraction of the rat brain, and that both seizures and K$^+$ depolarization induce an increase in synaptosomal lipoxygenase activity. It also can be inferred from data on incubated synaptosomes and microsomes that the effects of bicuculline-induced status epilepticus are long-lasting. In summary, this study has demonstrated that bicuculline-induced FFA accumulation is localized mainly in the nerve ending, or synaptosomal, fraction but not at the microsomal level of the brain. The similarities in modifications in arachidonic acid metabolism and lipoxygenase activity between bicuculline-induced status epilepticus and K$^+$ depolarization are supportive of the hypothesis that bicuculline-induced alterations in membrane lipids are mediated through enhanced neuronal activity.

Moreover, bicuculline induces stimulation of lipoxygenase activity in the nerve ending subsequent to neuronal stimulation.

SYNAPTIC VULNERABILITY DUE TO SPECIFIC BREAKDOWN OF MEMBRANE PHOSPHOLIPIDS IN ISCHEMIA AND SEIZURES

Excitation, inhibition, and other membrane-mediated information transfers are intimately related to biochemical events taking place within the neuronal plasma membrane. The synapse, which is the main locus of cell-to-cell communication in the neural tissue, may be the key location at which significant subtle changes in membrane constituents occur. This is, in fact, one of the reasons why great emphasis has been placed on searching for membrane modifications in abnormal experiences such as ischemia, seizure, and epilepsy.

Phospholipids are present in relatively large quantities in a wide variety of classes and molecular species in neuronal membranes. The highly unsaturated long acyl chains facing away from the membrane surfaces create a fluid environment in the membrane. Different regions of the same membrane may actually vary in chemical composition; lipid molecules and proteins may move both laterally and in the transverse plane of the membrane. Thus the neuronal membrane is a highly dynamic structure in which metabolic transformations of membrane components provide increased plasticity and additional means of modifying chemical structure.

The onset of ischemia, certain drug-induced convulsions, and electroconvulsive shock trigger the release of free fatty acids in the brain at a rate similar to that which occurs in adipose tissue under maximal stimulation by lipolytic hormones. As mentioned earlier, arachidonic acid is the main fatty acid liberated, and the convulsion-induced change in this fatty acid is the first change seen in an endogenous component of membranes stimulated within physiological limits *in vivo*.[10,27,41] Because ischemia and convulsions also trigger the accumulation of endogenous DAG, mainly stearoyl-arachidonoyl-glycerol, it can be assumed that the activation of phospholipases A_2 and C must occur.[11]

This effect of brain ischemia has been documented in several laboratory animals.[47] It also is known that newborns and animals resistant to anoxic damage accumulate brain free fatty acids at slower rates than those that are more sensitive to anoxic damage.[11,48] Therefore, ischemia-induced brain lipid changes may be involved in the transition between the reversible and irreversible phases of brain damage.[29,47]

These lipid effects are compatible with brain survival, and not merely a postmortem phenomenon, since brief, nondamaging stimulation of the brain in intact animals produces a transient accumulation of brain free fatty acids.[41,48] Free arachidonic and other free fatty acids are accumulated, as in ischemia, but are then removed from the free pool and reesterified, mainly into phospholipids of excitable membranes.

The rapid impairment of the energy state at the onset of brain ischemia is a consequence of decreased oxygen and glucose delivery, and is accompanied by membrane depolarization, accumulation of free fatty acids and diacylglycerols (reflecting phospholipase A_2 and C activation), reduced Na^+-K^+ ATPase, neurotransmitter release, and increased intracellular ionized calcium concentration. To explain the simultaneity and speed of these events, we have suggested that neurotransmitter receptor interactions are impaired, producing an overstimulation of receptor-mediated events the target of which is the synaptic membrane. More specifically, membrane perturbation of certain domains may occur. Membrane perturbation of presynaptic domains may likely result in an abnormally large release of neurotransmitters and will in turn overstimulate receptors and cause an abnormal generation of second messengers in the presynaptic membrane. The release of free fatty acids with appreciable amounts of arachidonic acid at the onset of ischemia and transiently during convulsions may be the result of such membrane perturbation. This may result in stimulation of the arachidonic acid cascade, leading to the synthesis of second messengers. An overabundance of second messengers is a likely factor involved in brain damage, and may directly influence the reacylation processes that normally occur in the brain.

MOLECULAR BASIS FOR FUNCTIONAL FAILURE OF EXCITABLE MEMBRANES DURING ISCHEMIC INJURY: PHOSPHOLIPID DEGRADATION BY PHOSPHOLIPASE A_2

A strikingly active production of FFA is one of the rapid neurochemical reactions triggered in the mammalian brain at the onset of ischemia; this has been demonstrated in the rat, monkey, and mouse brain and is attributed to polar lipid deacylation by phospholipase A_2.[29] This phenomenon was found to be unique to the mature homeothermic brain[11] and is accompanied by a partial acyl TAG breakdown.

TAG can contribute only partially to the increased DAG or FFA levels exhibited during early brain ischemia.[12] Within a short interval after decapitation, there occurs in the mouse brain rapid and concomitant production of DAG and FFA, both surpassing in magnitude the decreases in TAG. Moreover, TAG are not the sources of free AA or of DAG-arachidonate. The rapid and uneven changes that DAG and FFA undergo in a very short interval after decapitation are indicative of a high turnover rate of arachidonate-containing lipids in vivo. FFA have been found to be greatly increased in synaptosomes from ischemic Mongolian gerbil brains, concomitantly with a 20–35% decrease in the ^{14}C-AA labeling of PI and phosphatidylcholine (PC).[49] Moreover, perturbations in GABA (γ-aminobutyric acid) uptake may result from 20:4 and 22:6 accumulation at this level.[49]

Brain phosphoinositides are uniquely enriched in arachidonate and stearate, which are in almost 1:1 proportion and account for more than 80% of their acyl groups.[37] Brain diacylglycerols consist mainly of 1-stearoyl-2-arachidonoyl molecular species; they are also the major product of phosphoinositide breakdown. It has thus been proposed that the arachidonoyl-diacylglyceride pool of the rat brain may be related to the inositides and may be derived in part from the activity of phosphoinositide-phosphodiesterases. The findings discussed here are consistent with this idea and suggest that part of the diacylglycerols increased during early ischemia, mainly those containing arachidonate and stearate, may originate in these phospholipids.[12]

THE REACYLATION OF PHOSPHOLIPIDS IS INHIBITED IN IRREVERSIBLE BRAIN DAMAGE

The mechanisms resulting in irreversible brain damage during ischemia are not well understood. During the initial period of oxygen deficiency, activation of phospholipases A_2, A_1, and C and of diacylglycerol lipase takes place, resulting in an accumulation of free fatty acids, especially arachidonic acid. These events are an important factor in giving rise to irreversible brain damage. During ischemia-reperfusion, the phospholipids are reacylated, and the free fatty acids removed.

During this transition, the accumulated free fatty acids are exposed to oxygen and may undergo peroxidation.[29,44,50] Moreover, the resulting fatty acid hydroperoxides increase the damage by causing further free radical generation and peroxidation.[29,50,52]

The acylation and deacylation of long-chain fatty acids contribute to the preservation of the functional integrity of membranes.[51] The observation that postischemic neuronal tissue has a decreased ability to reacylate phospholipids constitutes one of the best-documented functional lesions evoked by ischemia and has been reported for both *in vivo* and *in vitro* experimental conditions.[51]

A recent study shows that relatively low levels of lipid hydroperoxides decrease reacylation of synaptic phospholipids.[52] It is suggested that this inhibitory action would be expected to impair postischemic recovery of excitable membranes and could contribute to irreversible injury to neuronal function. Much of the work discussed in this chapter supports this idea.

For example, increased levels of 5-hydroxyeicosatetraenoic acid follow ischemic insult in the gerbil brain[53] and in human cerebrospinal fluid (CSF) after subarachnoid hemorrhage.[54] Lipid peroxidation is initiated during the reperfusion phase after ischemia; this could occur in the hydrophobic moieties of the membranes, where oxygen is most soluble.

Phospholipases A_2 and C are activated by ischemia,[12] and these enzymes are more active on peroxidized than on nonperoxidized lipids.[55,56] Therefore, phospholipase A_2 may, through the release of peroxidized free fatty acids, lead to a progression of free-radical–initiated peroxidation, which results in a further alteration in the reacylation mechanisms that exist in membranes. Such alterations in the reacylation of synaptic phospholipids may be a key factor in the irreversible damage to neuronal function brought on by ischemia and sustained convulsions. The enhanced activity of phospholipases in removing peroxidized fatty acids may also play a protective role, since peroxidized acyl chains of phospholipids may interfere with membrane function.

PLATELET-ACTIVATING FACTOR ANTAGONISTS DECREASE THE ACCUMULATION OF FREE ARACHIDONIC ACID INDUCED BY BRIEF ISCHEMIA AND CONVULSIONS

Platelet-activating factor is a potent lipid mediator formed from 1-0-alkyl-2-arachidonoyl-glycero-3-phosphocholine through a phospholipase A_2 that releases arachidonic acid (FIG. 4) followed by an acetyltransferase. We decided to evaluate if in ischemia or convulsions the accumulated arachidonic acid arises at least in part through the first step of the PAF cycle. Moreover, if this is the case, perhaps brain damage may be linked to the accumulation in the brain of PAF and of arachidonic acid, particularly during ischemia followed by reperfusion.

Accordingly, the effects of a platelet-activating factor antagonist—BN52021, a terpene extracted from *Ginkgo biloba*—on cerebral ischemia-reperfusion in the gerbil has been studied. Following ten minutes of bilateral carotid artery ligation, gerbils were reperfused and injected intraperitoneally with either BN52021 or vehicle (dimethylsulfoxide). Cerebral blood flow and systemic arterial pressure were monitored until 90 minutes of reperfusion; then free fatty acids, diacylglycerols, and polyphosphoinositides were analyzed in forebrains and midbrains. Our results show that BN52021 inhibited the maturation of ischemic injury. Cerebral blood flow increased following 60 to 90 minutes of reperfusion. Free fatty acid levels were reduced, possibly as a result of an inhibition of phospholipase A activation. Slight increases in DAG and PIP$_2$ suggest the possible coinhibition of phospholipase C activity.[57]

The possible role of PAF in mediating the changes in membrane lipids induced by electroconvulsive shock (ECS) and ischemia, using the platelet-activating factor antagonist BN52021 as a pharmacological tool was also explored.[58] BN52021 given to

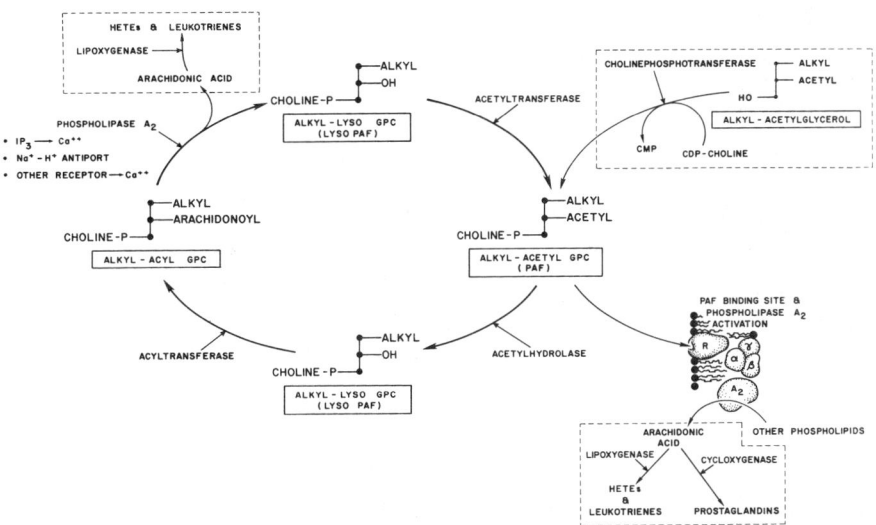

FIGURE 4. Platelet-activating factor (PAF) cycle. Synthesis involves two routes. One route originates with the inactive precursor alkyl-acyl-glycero-phosphocholine (alkyl-acyl GPC) (1-0-alkyl-2-lyso-*sn*-glycero-3-phosphocholine), a minor component of the phosphatidylcholine fraction from cellular membranes. One distinctive feature of alkyl-acyl GPC is that it is enriched in arachidonoyl chains. The first step in PAF synthesis is the deacylation of alkyl-acyl GPC by phospholipase A$_2$ to lyso PAF, a biologically inactive compound, and the subsequent release of arachidonic acid. After the introduction of an acetyl group to lyso PAF, PAF is formed. Three effector systems may modulate the activity of phospholipase A$_2$. They are IP$_3$-induced calcium ionization, the Na$^+$-H$^+$ antiport, or other receptor-mediated events that may enhance intracellular calcium concentration. The second route for PAF synthesis involves the transfer of phosphorylcholine from CDP-choline to alkyl acetylglycerol. After its formation, PAF appears to interact with specific membrane binding sites, resulting in an increase in intracellular calcium level, activation of phospholipases, and activation of other second messenger systems. (From N. G. Bazan.[64] Reprinted by permission from Alan R. Liss, Inc.)

mice 30 minutes before electroconvulsive shock decreased the accumulation of free palmitic (16:0), stearic (18:0), 20:4, and docosahexaenoic (22:6) acids, with no effect on the fatty acids in DAG or the loss of PIP$_2$. These data indicate that BN52021 reduces the injury-induced activation of phospholipases that mediate the accumulation of FFA in the brain, but has a negligible effect on phospholipase C–mediated degradation of PIP$_2$. PAF accumulation in the brain during convulsions has been detected.[26]

IRREVERSIBLE REPRESSION OF GENE EXPRESSION IN ISCHEMIC BRAIN DAMAGE

Among the consequences of brain injury is an impairment in the ability of nerve cells to recover. Many nerve cells, however, even when damaged, are able to survive due to activation of repair mechanisms. Current knowledge in this area is scarce. The drastic changes in arachidonic acid, diacylglycerol, and lipoxygenase metabolites in the early phases after injury (e.g., ischemia or overstimulation, such as in status epilepticus) show large concentration changes in several of the second messengers.[60] These biologically active mediators may be linked to neuronal pathways of cell signal transduction that in turn lead to transcriptional activation or repression of certain genes. In fact c-*fos* mRNA has been shown to be increased in the brain after seizures.[61,62] Arachidonic acid has been reported also to activate c-*fos* expression by a pathway independent of phorbol-ester–sensitive protein kinase C in Swiss 3T3 cells.[63] Moreover, PAF increases c-*fos* transcription in human neuroblastoma cells, suggesting that this lipid mediator may be linked in a signal transduction pathway in neuronal cells.[65] The role of arachidonic acid, stearoyl-arachidonoyl-glycerol, or of oxygenated metabolites of arachidonic acid in the nervous system in relation to gene expression should be explored. This will lead to a better understanding of how signal transduction–derived messengers generated at the plasma membrane of the cell are coupled with gene expression under normal conditions and in such pathophysiological circumstances as those described here.

CONCLUSIONS

The modulation of arachidonic acid metabolism plays a central role in neuronal communication and in the events leading to impaired brain function due to stroke, convulsions, epileptic brain damage, aging, and neurodegenerative disorders. Neuronal signal transduction and neuromodulation are involved in the accumulation of free arachidonic acid, which occurs as a transient phenomenon after electroconvulsive shock. Arachidonic acid accumulation reflects the action of neurotransmitters on phospholipase A_2 linked to receptors. After arachidonic acid accumulation, second messengers are formed, such as lipoxygenase products of AA that could regulate synaptic functions—for example, neurotransmitter release. PLA_2 activation may also alter membrane permeability at the postsynapse. In *Aplysia* sensory neurons, lipoxygenase metabolites of arachidonic acid act as second messengers for presynaptic inhibition.[4,8] Impairment of Ca^{2+} homeostasis and perturbation of excitable membrane domains that contain certain ionic channels, receptors, and lipids engaged in signal transduction (e.g., inositol lipids), as occurs in brain ischemia, result in rapid accumulation of free arachidonic acid. Thus, overstimulation of receptors that control PLA_2 and PLC may lead to derangement of neuronal communication due to degradation of essential phospholipids. In addition to free fatty acid increases, diacylglycerol also accumulates in the brain after seizures; inositol lipids are a likely source of both. These results may reflect ECS-induced release of neurotransmitters associated with stimulation of PLA_1 and PLA_2 at the presynapse, and a receptor-linked PLC-mediated cleavage of PIP_2 at the postsynapse. An influx of Ca^{2+} resulting from depolarization may activate the deacylation of 1-stearoyl-2-arachidonoyl-glycerol.

Excitable membrane lipids are a major target of convulsions, and the activation of phospholipase A_2 is mainly followed by lipoxygenation of arachidonic acid. Moreover, the main targets of seizures may be domains containing phospholipids enriched in polyunsaturated fatty acids, phospholipase A_2, lipoxygenases, and also ionic channels, receptors, and other components of cell signal transduction. These may function in neuronal and glial cell transduction events and may be the primary targets during convulsions and seizures.

Knowledge of the role of excitable membrane lipids in neuronal responsiveness is still in its early stages. In this chapter we have focused on the role of arachidonic acid in the modulation of excitable membrane function at the onset of brain damage. In the normal neuronal membrane, the process of acylation and deacylation of free fatty acids goes on constantly, resulting in the presence of only trace levels of free fatty acids in the cells. In general, the activation of arachidonic acid metabolism is believed to be a common response to injury and inflammation. Specifically, brain ischemia increases phospholipase A_2 and C activity, resulting in an imbalance in membrane metabolism experimentally evidenced by the accumulation of arachidonic acid, peroxidized forms of arachidonic acid, and other fatty acids. This accumulation may be enhanced further as a result of alterations in the reacylation mechanism of free fatty acids into phospholipids of neuronal membranes. Peroxidized derivatives of arachidonic acid have been shown to inhibit these reacylation reactions. These events constitute an important mechanism contributing to irreversible brain damage.

REFERENCES

1. AVELDANO DE CALDIRONI, M. I. & N. G. BAZAN. 1977. Acyl groups, molecular species and labeling by ^{14}C-glycerol and ^{3}H-arachidonic acid of vertebrate retina glycerolipids. Adv. Exp. Med. Biol. **83**: 397–404.
2. AVELDANO DE CALDIRONI, M. I. & N. G. BAZAN. 1980. Composition and biosynthesis of molecular species of retina phosphoglycerides. Neurochem Int. **1**: 381–392.
3. AXELROD, J., R. M. BURCH & C. J. JELSEMA. 1988. Receptor-mediated activation of phospholipase A_2 via GTP-binding proteins: Arachidonic acid and its metabolites as second messengers. Trends Neurosci. **11**: 117–123.
4. PIOMELLI, D., A. VOLTERRA, N. DALE, S. A. SIEGELBAUM, E. R. KANDEL, J. H. SCHWARTZ & F. BELARDETTI. 1987. Lipoxygenase metabolites of arachidonic acid as second messengers for presynaptic inhibition of Aplysia sensory cells. Nature **328**: 38–43.
5. BAZAN, N. G. & D. L. BIRKLE. 1987. Polyunsaturated fatty acids and inositol phospholipids at the synapse in neuronal responsiveness. In Molecular Mechanisms of Neuronal Responsiveness. Y. Ehrlich, R. Lenox, E. Kornecki & W. Berry, Eds.: 45–68. Plenum Press. New York, NY.
6. BURCH, R. M., J. R. CONNOR & J. AXELROD. 1988. Interleukin 1 amplifies receptor-mediated activation of phospholipase A_2 in 3T3 fibroblasts. Proc. Natl. Acad. Sci. USA **85**: 6306–6309.
7. BERRIDGE, M. J. & R. F. IRVINE. 1984. Inositol trisphosphate, a novel second messenger in cellular signal transduction. Nature **312**: 315–321.
8. PIOMELLI, D., E. SHAPIRO, S. J. FEINMARK & J. H. SCHWARTZ. 1987. Metabolites of arachidonic acid in the nervous system of Aplysia: Possible mediators of synaptic modulation. J. Neurosci. **7**: 3675–3686.
9. BRAQUET, P., L. TOUQUI, T. Y. SHEN & B. B. VARGAFTIG. 1987. Perspectives in platelet activating factor research. Pharmacol. Rev. **39**: 97–145.
10. BAZAN, N. G. 1970. Effects of ischemia and electroconvulsive shock on free fatty acid pool in the brain. Biochim. Biophys. Acta. **218**: 1–10.
11. AVELDANO, M. I. & N. G. BAZAN. 1975. Differential lipid deacylation during brain ischemia in a homeotherm and a poikilotherm. Content and composition of free fatty acids and triacylglycerols. Brain Res. **100**: 99–110.
12. AVELDANO, M. I. & N. G. BAZAN. 1975. Rapid production of diacylglycerols enriched in arachidonate and stearate during early brain ischemia. J. Neurochem. **25**: 919–920.
13. IKEDA, M., S. YOSHIDA, R. BUSTO, M. SANTISO & M. GINSBERG. 1986. Polyphospho-

inositides as a probable source of brain free fatty acid accumulated at the onset of ischemia. J. Neurochem. **47:** 123.
14. REDDY, T. S. & N. G. BAZAN. 1987. Arachidonic acid, stearic acid, and diacylglycerol accumulation correlates with the loss of phosphatidylinositol 4,5-bisphosphate in cerebrum 2 seconds after electroconvulsive shock: Complete reversion of changes 5 minutes after stimulation. J. Neurosci. Res. **18:** 449–455.
15. MARION, J. & L. S. WOLFE. 1979. Origin of the arachidonic acid release post mortem in the rat forebrain. Biochim. Biophys. Acta **547:** 25–32.
16. AVELDANO DE CALDIRONI, M. I., N. M. GIUSTO & N. G. BAZAN. 1981. Polyunsaturated fatty acids of the retina. Prog. Lipid Res. **20:** 49–57.
17. AVELDANO, M. I. & N. G. BAZAN. 1974. Displacement into incubation medium by albumin of highly unsaturated retina free fatty acids arising from membrane lipids. FEBS Lett. **40:** 53–56.
18. AVELDANO, M. I. & N. G. BAZAN. 1974. Free fatty acids, diacyl- and triacylglycerols and total phospholipids in vertebrate retina: Comparison with brain, choroid and plasma. J. Neurochem. **23:** 1127–1135.
19. CENNEDELLA, R., C. GALLI & R. PAOLETTI. 1975. Brain free fatty acid levels in rats sacrificed by decapitation versus focused microwave irradiation. Lipids **10:** 290–293.
20. REDDY, T. S. & N. G. BAZAN. 1985. Synthesis of arachidonoyl coenzyme A and docosahexaenoyl coenzyme A in synaptic plasma membranes of cerebrum, cerebellum and brain stem of rat brain. J. Neurosci. Res. **13:** 381–390.
21. BIRKLE, D. L. & N. G. BAZAN. 1984. Effects of K^+ depolarization on the synthesis of prostaglandins and hydroxyeicosatetra(5,8,11,14)enoic acids (HETE) in the rat retina. Evidence for esterification of 12-HETE in lipids. Biochim. Biophys. Acta **795:** 564–573.
22. BIRKLE, D. L. & N. G. BAZAN. 1987. Effect of bicuculline-induced status epilepticus on prostaglandins and hydroxyeicosatetraenoic acids in rat brain subcellular fractions. J. Neurochem. **48:** 1768–1778.
23. JELSEMA, C. 1987. Light activation of phospholipase A_2 in rod outer segments of bovine retina and its modulations by GTP-binding proteins. J. Biol. Chem. **262:** 163–168.
24. CHILTON, F. H., J. M. ELLIS, S. C. OLSON & R. L. WYKLE. 1984. A common source of PAF and arachidonate in human polymorphonuclear leukocytes. J. Biol. Chem. **259:** 12019–12024.
25. BAZAN, H. E. P., S. T. K. REDDY, J. M. WOODLAND & N. G. BAZAN. 1987. The accumulation of platelet activating factor in the injured cornea may be interrelated with the synthesis of lipoxygenase products. Biochem. Biophys. Res. Comm. **149:** 915–920.
26. KUMAR, R., S. A. K. HARVEY, M. KESTER, D. J. HANAHAN & M. S. OLSON. 1988. Production and effects of platelet-activating factor in the rat brain. Biochim. Biophys. Acta **963:** 375–383.
27. BAZAN, N. G. 1971. Changes in free fatty acids of brain by drug-induced convulsions, electroshock and anesthesia. J. Neurochem. **18:** 1379–1385.
28. BAZAN, N. G. 1971. Phospholipases A_1 and A_2 in brain subcellular fractions. Acta Physiol. Lat. Am. **21:** 101–106.
29. BAZAN, N. G. 1976. Free arachidonic acid and other lipids in the nervous system during early ischemia and after electroshock. Adv. Exp. Med. Biol. **72:** 317–335.
30. CLARK, M. A. 1986. Islet-activating protein inhibits leukotriene D_4- and leukotriene C_4- but not bradykinin– or calcium ionophore– induced prostaglandin synthesis in bovine endothelial cells. Proc. Natl. Acad. Sci. USA **83:** 7320–7324.
31. CLARK, M. A., M. J. CHEN, S. T. CROOKE & J. S. BOMALASKI. 1988. Tumour necrosis factor (cachectin) induces phospholipase A_2 activity and synthesis of phospholipase A_2–activating protein in endothelial cells. Biochem. J. **250:** 125–132.
32. FLOWER, L. J. 1988. Lipocortin and the mechanism of action of the glucocorticoids. Brit. J. Pharmacol. **94:** 987–1015.
33. SWEATT, J. D., I. A. BLAIR, E. J. CRAGOE & L. L. LIMBIRD. 1986. Inhibitors of Na^+/H^+ exchange block epinephrine- and ADP-induced stimulation of human platelet phospholipase C by blockade of arachidonic acid release at a prior step. J. Biol. Chem. **261:** 8660–8666.
34. BIRKLE, D. L. & N. G. BAZAN. 1989. Light exposure stimulates arachidonic acid turnover

in glycerolipids in the rat retina and eicosanoids synthesis in intact retina and isolated outer segments. Neurochem. Res. **14:** 185–190.
35. VAN ROOIJEN, L. L. A., R. E. VADNAL, P. DOBARD & N. G. BAZAN. 1986. Enhanced inositol turnover during bicuculline-induced status epilepticus. Biochem. Biophys. Res. Commun. **134:** 378–385.
36. KIKKAWA, U., Y. TAKAI, R. MIYAKE & Y. NISHIZUKA. 1982. Protein kinase C as a possible receptor protein of tumor-promoting phorbol esters. J. Biol. Chem. **257:** 7841.
37. BAKER, R. R. & W. THOMPSON. 1972. Positional distribution and turnover of fatty acids in phosphatidylcholine and phosphatidylethanolamine in rat brain in vivo. Biochim. Biophys. Acta **270:** 489.
38. AVELDANO DE CALDIRONI, M. I. & N. G. BAZAN. 1979. Alpha-Methyl-p-Tyrosine inhibits the production of free arachidonic acid and diacylglycerols in brain after a single electroconvulsive shock. Neurochem. Res. **4:** 213–221.
39. MAUCO, G., C. A. DANGELMAIER & J. B. SMITH. 1984. Inositol lipids, phosphatidate and diacylglycerol share stearoyl arachidonoyl glycerol as common backbone in thrombin stimulated human platelets. Biochem. J. **224:** 933–940.
40. NISHIHARA, M. & R. W. KEENAN. 1985. Inositol phospholipid levels of rat forebrain obtained by free-blowing method. Biochim. Biophys. Acta **835:** 415–418.
41. BAZAN, N. G. & H. RAKOWSKI. 1970. Increased levels of brain free fatty acids after electroconvulsive shock. Life Sci. **9:** 501–507.
42. BAZAN, N. G., S. M. MORELLI DE LIBERTI & E. B. RODRIQUEZ DE TURCO. 1982. Arachidonic acid and arachidonoyl-diglycerides increase in rat cerebrum during bicuculline-induced status epilepticus. Neurochem. Res. **7:** 839–843.
43. BAZAN, N. G., S. G. MORELLI DE LIBERTI, E. B. RODRIQUEZ DE TURCO & M. F. PEDICONI. 1983. Free arachidonic and docosahexaenoic acid accumulation in the central nervous system during stimulation. *In* Neural Membranes. G. Y. Sun, N. G. Bazan, J. Wu, G. Porcellati & A. Y. Sun, Eds.: 123–140. Humana Press. Clifton, NJ.
44. SIESJO, B. K., M. INGVAR & Z. WESTERBERG. 1982. The influence of bicuculline-induced seizures on free fatty acid concentrations in cerebral cortex, hippocampus and cerebellum. J. Neurochem. **39:** 796–802.
45. BAZAN, N. G., D. L. BIRKLE, W. TANG & T. S. REDDY. 1986. The accumulation of free arachidonic acid, diacylglycerols, prostaglandins, and lipoxygenase reaction products in the brain during experimental epilepsy. Adv. Neurol. **44:** 879–902.
46. GINOBILI DE MARTINEZ, M. S., E. B. RODRIGUEZ DE TURCO & F. J. BARRANTES. 1985. Endogenous asymmetry of rat brain lipids and dominance of the right cerebral hemisphere in free fatty acid response to electroconvulsive shock. Brain Res. **339:** 315–321.
47. SIESJO, B. K. 1981. Cell damage in the brain: A speculative synthesis. J. Cereb. Blood Flow Metab. **1:** 155–158.
48. BAZAN, N. G., D. L. BIRKLE, T. S. REDDY & R. E. VADNAL. 1986. Diacylglycerols and arachidonic acid in the molecular pathogenesis of brain injury. *In* Phospholipid Research and the Nervous System. Biochemical and Molecular Pharmacology. L. Horrocks, L. Freysz & G. Toffano, Eds.: 169–180. Liviana Press. Padova.
49. NOREMBERG, K. & J. STROSZNAJDER. 1986. Modifications of GABA and calcium uptake by lipids in synaptosomes from normoxic and ischemic brain. Neurochem. Int. **8:** 59–66.
50. BAZAN, N. G. & E. B. RODRIGUEZ DE TURCO. 1980. Membrane lipids in the pathogenesis of brain edema: Phospholipids and arachidonic acid, the earliest membrane components changed at the onset of ischemia. Adv. Neurol. **28:** 197–205.
51. SUN, G. Y. & R. A. MACQUARRIE. 1989. Deacylation-reacylation of arachidonoyl groups in cerebral phospholipids. Ann. N. Y. Acad. Sci. This volume.
52. ZALESKA, M. M. & D. F. WILSON. 1989. Lipid hydroperoxides inhibit reacylation of phospholipids in neuronal membranes. J. Neurochem. **52:** 255–260.
53. SPAGNUOLO, D., L. SAUTEBIN, G. GALLI, G. RACEGUI, C. GALLI, D. MAZZANI & M. GINESSO. 1979. PGF_{2a}, thromboxane B_2, and HETE levels in gerbil brain after ligation of common carotid arteries and decapitation. Prostaglandins **18:** 53–61.
54. SUZUKI, N., T. NAKAMURA, S. IMABAYASHI, Y. ISHIKAWA, T. SASAKI & T. ASANO. 1983. Identification of 5-hydroxyeicosatetraenoic acid in cerebrospinal fluid after subarachnoid hemorrhage. J. Neurochem. **41:** 1186–1189.

55. SEVANIAN, A., R. A. STEIN & J. F. MEAD. 1981. Metabolism of epoxidized phosphatidylcholine by PLA_2 and epoxide hydrolase. Lipids **16:** 781–789.
56. BECKMAN, J. K., S. M. BOROWITZ & I. M. BURR. 1987. The role of phospholipase A activity in rat microsomal lipid peroxidation. J. Biol. Chem. **262:** 1479–1484.
57. PANETTA, T., V. L. MARCHESELLI, P. BRAQUET, B. SPINNEWYN & N. G. BAZAN. 1987. Effects of a platelet activating factor antagonist (BN52021) on free fatty acids, diacylglycerols, polyphosphoinositides and blood flow in the gerbil brain: Inhibition of ischemia-reperfusion induced cerebral flow. Biochem. Biophys. Res. Commun. **149:** 580–587.
58. BIRKLE, D. L., P. KURIAN, P. BRAQUET & N. G. BAZAN. 1988. Platelet-activating factor antagonist BN52021 decreases accumulation of free polyunsaturated fatty acid in mouse brain during ischemia and electroconvulsive shock. J. Neurochem. **51:** 1900–1905.
60. HORROCKS, L. A. & H. W. HARDER. 1983. Fatty acids and cholesterol. *In* Handbook on Neurochemistry, Vol. 3. A. Lajtha, Ed.: 1–16. Plenum. New York, NY.
61. MORGAN, J. I., D. R. COHEN, J. L. HEMPSTEAD & T. CURRAN. 1987. Mapping patterns of c-fos expression in the central nervous system after seizure. Science **237:** 192–197.
62. POPOVICI, T., G. BARBIN & Y. BEN ARI. 1988. Kainic acid-induced seizures increase c-fos-like protein in the hippocampus. Eur. J. Pharmacol. **150:** 405–406.
63. KACICH, R. L., L. T. WILLIAMS & S. R. COUGHLIN. 1988. Arachidonic acid and cyclic adenosine monophosphate stimulation of c-fos expression by a pathway independent of phorbol ester–sensitive protein kinase C. Molecular Endocrinol. **2:** 73–77.
64. BAZAN, N. G. 1989. Lipid-derived metabolites as possible retina messengers: Arachidonic acid, leukotrienes, docosanoids, and platelet activating factor. *In* Extracellular and Intracellular Messengers in the Vertebrate Retina. D. Redburn & H. Pasantes-Morales, Eds.: 269–300. Alan R. Liss. New York, NY.
65. SQUINTO, S. P. & N. G. BAZAN. 1989. Induction of c-fos transcription by PAF in human neuroblastoma cells. Trans. Amer. Soc. Neurochem. **20:** 101.

PART I. *MODULATION OF ARACHIDONIC ACID RELEASE AND METABOLISM IN THE NERVOUS SYSTEM*

Sources for Brain Arachidonic Acid Uptake and Turnover in Glycerophospholipids[a]

LLOYD A. HORROCKS[b]

Department of Physiological Chemistry
The Ohio State University
Columbus, Ohio 43210

UPTAKE OF FATTY ACIDS INTO THE BRAIN

The glycerophospholipids of the nervous system contain high concentrations of the polyunsaturated fatty acids of the (n-6) and (n-3) series. These polyunsaturated fatty acids may be obtained from the diet and transported to the brain, synthesized in the liver and transported to the brain, or synthesized in the brain from the essential fatty acids, linoleic and linolenic acids. Either the polyunsaturated fatty acids themselves or the precursor essential fatty acids must be transported from the blood into the brain. Most of the fatty acids in brain glycerophospholipids are taken up from the circulation.[1,2] Free fatty acids are taken up more quickly than other lipids. The free fatty acids in the blood stream are mostly bound to serum albumin. The albumin has a number of binding sites for the fatty acids. One popular text book even states that there is no uptake because the fatty acids are bound to the serum albumin. This is not correct. There is an equilibrium between the bound and unbound forms even though the unbound form constitutes less than one percent of the total. The unbound free fatty acids penetrate into the brain very easily because fatty acids, of course, are lipid soluble. Pardridge and Mietus[3] have estimated that about 5% of the palmitate in the plasma is cleared by the brain in a single pass and is incorporated into phospholipids within 15 seconds.

The uptake of intravenous [^{14}C]palmitate into the brain was studied in rats by Miller *et al.*[4] The total radioactivity showed a peak between 15 minutes and 1 hour and then declined. The label was found both in lipids and in proteins. The aqueous fraction of the brain contained radioactivity in glutamate and glutamine that accounted for 48% of the total brain radioactivity at 45 minutes after injection. Apparently this radioactivity entered the aqueous compartment after β-oxidation. The remainder of the labeled palmitate was present in relatively stable protein and lipid compartments. The protein label was mainly from glutamate.

The flux of palmitate into the brain of rats was evaluated by Kimes *et al.*[5] on the basis of autoradiographs of the rat brain at 4 hours after intravenous injection. The flux in the rat was generally in the range of 3 to 6 μmol/g $\cdot$ s $\times$ 10^5 in gray matter areas. The corresponding values for white matter were in the range of 2.0 to 2.8. The

---

[a]This work was supported in part by NIH Research Grants NS-08291 and NS-10165 and by Training Grant NS-07091.
[b]Address for correspondence: Lloyd A. Horrocks, Ph.D., Department of Physiological Chemistry, The Ohio State University, Columbus, Ohio 43210.

autoradiograms showed a good correlation of the flux of palmitate with the flux of 2-deoxyglucose.

Increased resolution and fewer problems with aqueous radioactivity were found with [9, 10-^{3}H]palmitic acid.[6] With this precursor, the maximum incorporation into lipid was found by 15 minutes and then was stable up to 4 hours. The label in the dry brain was 85% in lipids. A majority of the label in the lipids was in the choline glycerophospholipids.

The uptake of [^{3}H]palmitic acid has also been studied by Reddy and Drewes.[7] They infused the labeled palmitic acid for five minutes into the carotid arteries of an isolated canine brain preparation. The radioactivity levels were measured in different brain regions. The transfer constants and net uptake rates were determined. The net uptake rates in cortical gray matter varied between 0.48 and 0.68 nmol/g · min. The net uptake of palmitic acid into cerebral white matter was about 0.2 nmol/g · min. About 80% of the radioactivity was associated with phospholipids, and among the phospholipids 65 to 70% of the label was in phosphatidylcholine. Reddy and Drewes[7] suggest that the blood-brain transfer of palmitic acid occurs at a slow but significant rate and that most of the palmitic acid entering the brain is rapidly esterified into phosphatidylcholine.

The uptake of the saturated fatty acid [^{14}C]octanoic acid was compared with that of [^{14}C]linoleic acid by Spector.[8] The octanoic acid enters the brain by a probenecid-sensitive mechanism. The linoleic acid enters the brain as readily as the octanoic acid from the perfusate but was not inhibited by probenecid or by octanoic acid.

The first study of this type with labeled arachidonic acid was done by DeGeorge et al.[9] [1-^{14}C]Arachidonic acid was administered intravenously in a saline solution with bovine serum albumin into rats. The radioactivity in the brain reached a peak at about 15 minutes and then slowly declined by 15% at four hours. At four hours 5% of the radioactivity was in the aqueous fraction, 6% in the protein pellet, and the remainder in the lipids. Nearly all of the lipid radioactivity was esterified in glycerolipids. At 5 min 41% of the lipid radioactivity was in phosphatidylinositol. This value was only 24% at 4 hours, suggesting a redistribution of radioactivity. Brain slices were used for quantitative autoradiography and showed nonhomogeneous incorporation into brain structures (FIG. 1).

In the adult animal there is no net uptake of free fatty acids; thus there must be an equal degree of efflux from the brain into the blood. In other words, there is a rapid exchange of free fatty acids across the blood-brain barrier.

UPTAKE OF ARACHIDONIC ACID INTO BRAIN GLYCEROLIPIDS

This section describes the results of injection of [^{3}H]arachidonic acid and [^{14}C]adrenic acid as the complexes with bovine serum albumin into the left lateral ventricles of C3H mice (H. W. Harder, P. Demediuk, and L. A. Horrocks, manuscript in preparation). The mice were two months old and received the injection through a cannula. The molar ratio of fatty acid to albumin was 4:1. The injections were done at 6 days after cannulation without anesthesia. Mice were killed at 4, 8, 15, 30, and 60 minutes and 24 hours after injection. The lipids were extracted and analyzed for incorporation of radioactivity into diacylglycerols and the molecular species of ethanolamine, choline and inositol glycerophospholipids. Preparative thin layer chromatography (TLC) was used to separate the diacylglycerols, triacylglycerols, ethanolamine glycerophospholipids, choline glycerophospholipids, and inositol glycerophospholipids. The glycerophospholipids were converted to the diradylglycerol acetates as described by Nakagawa and Horrocks.[10] These were separated with reverse-phase

HPLC, also as described by Nakagawa and Horrocks.[10] The specific radioactivities were determined by making methyl esters of the fatty acids from each fraction and quantitating the amount of arachidonic acid or adrenic acid by gas-liquid chromatography (GLC). The amount of radioactivity was determined by counting another aliquot of the separated molecular species or of the diacylglycerol or triacylglycerol. The radioactivity in the free fatty acid pool declined rapidly between 0 and 15 minutes and then more slowly between 15 minutes and 24 hours. A much greater amount of adrenic acid was injected, and thus a greater proportion of adrenic acid was incorporated into the triacylglycerols.

Previous investigations of the metabolism of arachidonic acid in the brain have been based on specific radioactivity values determined for all of the label, regardless of what fatty acid contained the label. In the present investigation, the specific radioactiv-

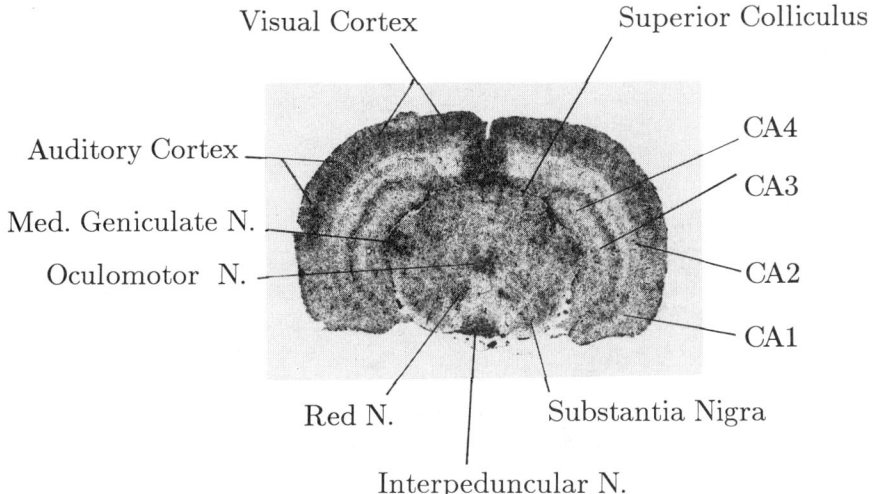

FIGURE 1. Audioradiograph of a brain slice from a rat at 4 hours after the intravenous injection of [1-^{14}C]arachidonic acid.[9] This figure was supplied by Dr. J. J. DeGeorge, Laboratory of Neurosciences, National Institute of Aging.

ity was determined for individual fatty acids. A substantial amount of the arachidonate was elongated to adrenate.

The triacylglycerols had the highest specific radioactivity in their arachidonic acid. The specific radioactivity was also high in the diaclyglycerols. Both had higher specific radioactivities at 8 minutes than at either 4 or 15 minutes. These peak values, dpm/nmol, were 17750 for triacylglycerols and 1250 for diacylglycerols.

The phosphatidylinositol incorporated considerable arachidonic acid (FIG. 2). The specific radioactivities of the molecular species with 18:1 and 16:0 were nearly the same and had a parabolic shape with time. The species with 18:0 had specific radioactivity values less than half those found for 18:1 and 16:0. All three of the major molecular species had specific radioactivity values that were highest at 30 or 60 minutes. The species with 18:1 and 16:0 showed a rapid turnover between 60 minutes and 24 hours. The values decreased to 36% of the 60 minute value at 24 hours for the 18:1 species.

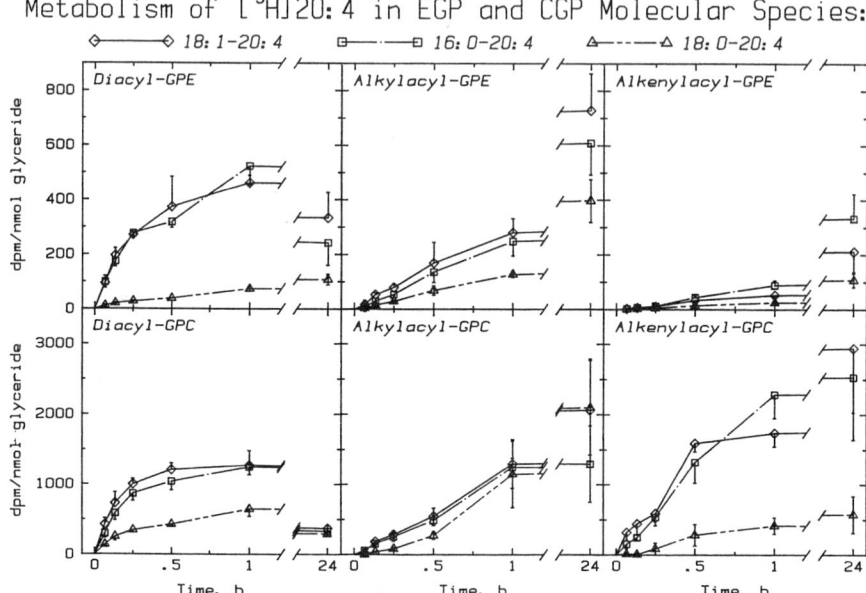

FIGURE 2. Specific radioactivities of molecular species containing arachidonic acid in phosphatidylinositol (*left*), phosphatidylcholine (*center*), and phosphatidylethanolamine (*right*). Only the diacyl types are included.

The incorporation of arachidonate into the phosphatidylcholine was similar to that into the phosphatidylinositol, but the specific radioactivity values were even higher for the phosphatidylcholine. The peak values were at 60 minutes for all three major molecular species. The values for the 18:0 species were less than half of those for the 18:1 and 16:0 species. The turnover of the 18:1 and 16:0 species was even faster for the phosphatidylcholine than it was for the phosphatidylinositol. The 24-hour values for 18:1 and 16:0 were 29% and 27%, respectively, of the 60-minute radioactivity values. If these were homogeneous pools, the half-lives would be about 8 hours.

For the phosphatidylethanolamine, the specific radioactivity values for the arachidonate were much less than for the other two major diacylglycerol types of diacyl glycerophospholipids. The uptake was also slower, with the values still rising at 60 minutes, especially for the 18:0 species, which increased from 38 to 242 dpm/nmol between 30 and 60 minutes. At 60 minutes after injection, the specific radioactivities of the phosphatidylethanolamine species were less than half of the specific radioactivities of the same species in the phosphatidylcholine. The turnover rate for the phosphatidylethanolamine species was less than that for the phosphatidylcholine betwen 1 and 24 hours.

The shapes of the labeling curves for the phosphatidylinositol and the phosphatidylcholine indicate a pulse labeling of these glycerophospholipids. Perhaps this takes place by acylation of the lysoglycerophospholipids with direct incorporation of the arachidonic acid into the *sn*-2 position. The ether types of the glycerophospholipids of the choline and ethanolamine glycerophospholipids showed a different shape of curve for the specific radioactivity values. The lag in uptake indicates a lack of pulse labeling.

The alkylacyl-glycerophosphoethanolamine (GroPEtn) increased in specific radioactivity from 2- to 3-fold over the period of 1 to 24 hours (FIG. 3). Again the 18:1 and 16:0 species had higher specific radioactivity values than did the 18:0 species. The specific radioactivity values for the alkenylacyl-GroPEtn increased even more precipitously. From 15 to 60 minutes there were 5-fold increases, followed by approximately 4-fold increases from 1 to 24 hours. The values for the alkylacyl-GroPEtn were substantially higher than for the alkenylacyl-GroPEtn at all time periods. This is in agreement with the precursor-product relationship that was observed previously.

The amounts of the alkylacyl-glycerophosphocholine(GroPCho) and alkenylacyl-GroPCho were very small. These two lipid classes showed considerable metabolic activity, as indicated by their specific radioactivity values. The alkylacyl-GroPCho had values much greater than the specific radioactivity values for the alkylacyl-GroPEtn. The differences were even greater for the alkenylacyl-GroPCho and the alkenylacyl-GroPEtn. At 60 minutes after injection, the specific radioactivities of the three major molecular species of the alkylacyl-GroPCho were similar to those for the diacyl-GroPCho, except that the value for the 18:0 species was higher in the case of the alkylacyl type. Between 1 and 24 hours after injection, the specific radioactivity values for the 18:0 and the 18:1 species of the alkenylacyl-GroPCho increased considerably and were nearly equal at both times. The 16:0 species did not increase during that time period. The 16:0 species were the major species for both the alkylacyl-GroPCho and alkenylacyl-GroPCho. The specific radioactivities of the 16:0 and 18:1 species of the alkenylacyl-GroPCho were already greater than the specific radioactivities of the corresponding phosphatidylcholine species at 30 minutes. The specific radioactivities of these two species of the alkenylacyl-GroPCho increased even more at 1 and 24 hours. The highest specific radioactivities observed for any molecular species of the glycerophospholipids were in the 18:1 and 16:0 species of the alkenylacyl-GroPCho. In contrast, the radioactivity in the 18:0 species of the alkenylacyl-GroPCho was not detectable.

METABOLIC PATHWAYS

It has been suggested previously that triacylglycerols may serve as an initial reservoir for fatty acids during periods of increased accumulation of lipid in different

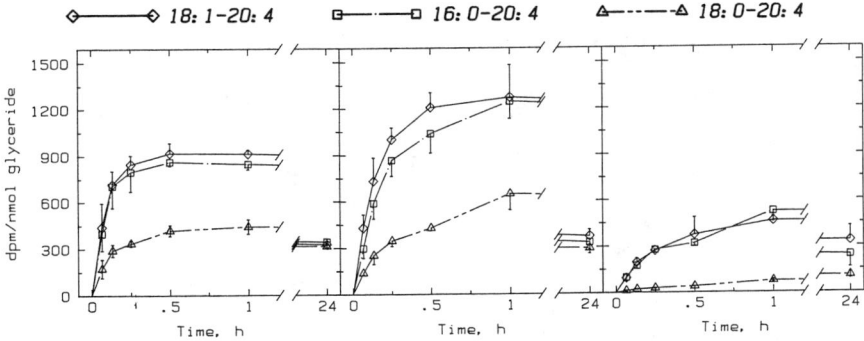

FIGURE 3. Specific radioactivities of molecular species containing arachidonic acid in diacyl (left), alkylacyl (center), and alkenylacyl (right) types of ethanolamine and choline glycerophospholipids.

tissues, including the brain.[11] The possibility should be considered that there might be a possible direct transfer from triacylglycerol to lysoglycerophospholipid.[12] The apparent turnover of the arachidonate in the triacylglycerol is very rapid, as has been previously reported for other fatty acids.[13-17] The triacylglycerol localization could be in the choroid plexus[18] or in neuronal nuclei.[16]

The molecular species with 18:0 attained much lower specific radioactivity values for nearly all of the glycerophospholipid types. The 18:0–20:4 species account for the bulk of the arachidonate in the phosphatidylethanolamine and for a large portion of the alkenylacyl-GroPEtn. The relatively less active metabolism of the 18:0 species cannot be ascribed to the myelin fraction because myelin is enriched in the 18:1 species. The relatively high specific radioactivity values for the 18:1 species, which are higher than those for 18:0 and close to those for the 16:0 species, show that the metabolism of myelin must proceed comparably with the metabolism of glycerophospholipids in other membranes.

Receptor-mediated turnover of alkylacyl-GroPCho and alkenylacyl-GroPCho has been suggested for several tissues, including the brain.[19,20] This turnover may be mediated by phospholipase A_2 with specificity for these glycerophospholipid types or by plasmalogenase in the case of the alkenylacyl-GroPCho. Eicosanoid second messengers can be formed from the arachidonate that is released from the sn-2 position of the glycerophospholipids. Another product, alkyl-2-lyso-GroPCho, lyso PAF, can be acetylated to form platelet activating factor, another potent second messenger. The lack of pulse labeling of these ether types of choline glycerophospholipids and the very high specific radioactivity values suggest that the hydrolyzed arachidonate is replaced by transacylation with arachidonate from the sn-2 position of diacyl-GroPCho by an energy- and coenzyme A–independent mechanism as described in some other tissues.[21-26] This possibility complicates the interpretation of labeling experiments in which the release of labeled arachidonate is examined. In some instances, the specific radioactivity of the ether type of glycerophospholipids increases after stimulation, because the reacylated arachidonate has a higher specific radioactivity than the arachidonate that was released. The net result for the diacyl type of the choline glycerophospholipids is the decrease of radioactivity. However, it must then be determined whether this loss of radioactivity has been by direct release or by transfer to the ether glycerophospholipids.

SUMMARY

Brain arachidonic acid comes from linoleic acid and arachidonic acid in the blood. Part of the brain arachidonic acid is elongated to adrenic acid, 22:4 (n = 6), especially in higher animals. With labeled arachidonic acid injected into cerebral ventricles of mice, the highest specific radioactivity was in triacylglycerols. The highest labeling in PtdCho and PtdIns was found at 15 to 60 minutes. Labeling of PtdEtn was much less. The molecular species with 16:0 and 18:1 were labeled better than those with 18:0. Adrenic acid was preferred by alkylacyl-GroPEtn. The highest level of labeling by arachidonic acid was found in the choline plasmalogens and the alkylacyl-GroPCho at 24 hours after injection. The PtdCho arachidonic acid turned over several times within 24 hours. Part of this turnover probably represents the transfer of labeled arachidonic acid to unlabeled ether-linked choline glycerophospholipids, including 1-alkyl-2-lyso-GroPCho, also known as lyso platelet activating factor. The energy-independent transfer of arachidonic acid from PtdCho to ether-linked choline glycerophospholipids may follow removal of their arachidonic acid by phospholipase A_2 due to receptor activation. The lack of pulse labeling of ether-linked choline glycerophospholipids complicates the study of their function.

REFERENCES

1. BOURRE, J. M. 1982. Biochimie des lipides cérébraux (plus particulièrement des acides gras). Synthèse in situ et origine exogène au cours du développement. Quelques aspects de l'influence de la nutrition. Reprod. Nutr. Dévelop. **22**: 179–191.
2. DHOPESHWARKAR, G. A. & J. F. MEAD. 1973. Uptake and transport of fatty acids into the brain and the role of the blood-brain barrier system. Adv. Lipid Res. **11**: 109–142.
3. PARDRIDGE, W. M. & L. J. MIETUS. 1980. Palmitate and cholesterol transport through the blood-brain barrier. J. Neurochem. **34**: 463–466.
4. MILLER, J. S., J. M. GNAEDINGER & S. I. RAPOPORT. 1987. Utilization of plasma fatty acid in rat brain: Distribution of [^{14}C]palmitate between oxidative and synthetic pathways. J. Neurochem. **49**: 1507–1514.
5. KIMES, A. S., D. SWEENEY, E. D. LONDON & S. I. RAPOPORT. 1983. Palmitate incorporation into different brain regions in the awake rat. Brain Res. **274**: 291–301.
6. NORONHA, J. G., S. YAMAZAKI & S. I. RAPOPORT. 1988. [9,10-^{3}H]palmitic acid as a probe for membrane structure in brain autoradiography. Trans. Am. Soc. Neurochem. **19**: 186.
7. REDDY, P. V. & L. R. DREWES. 1988. Transport of palmitate from blood to brain and its incorporation into lipids. FASEB J. **2**: A1790.
8. SPECTOR, J. 1988. Fatty acid transport through the blood-brain barrier. J. Neurochem. **50**: 639–643.
9. DEGEORGE, J. J., J. G. NORONHA, S. I. RAPOPORT & E. G. LAPETINA. 1988. Incorporation of intravascular 1-^{14}C arachidonate into rat brain. Trans. Am. Soc. Neurochem. **19**: 108.
10. NAKAGAWA, Y. & L. A. HORROCKS. 1983. Separation of alkenylacyl, alkylacyl, and diacyl analogues and their molecular species by high performance liquid chromatography. J. Lipid Res. **24**: 1268–1275.
11. HORROCKS, L. A. 1985. Metabolism and function of fatty acids in brain. In Phospholipids in Nervous Tissues. J. Eichberg, Ed.: 173–199. John Wiley and Sons. New York, NY.
12. DWYER, B. & J. BERNSOHN. 1979. The incorporation of [1-^{14}C]linolenate into lipids of developing rat brain during essential fatty acid deprivation. J. Neurochem. **32**: 833–838.
13. SUN, G. Y. & L. A. HORROCKS. 1971. The incorporation of (^{14}C)-palmitic acid into the lipids of mouse brain in vivo. J. Neurochem. **18**: 1963–1970.
14. YAU, T. M. & G. Y. SUN. 1974. The metabolism of [1-^{14}C]arachidonic acid in the neutral glycerides and phosphoglycerides of mouse brain. J. Neurochem. **23**: 99–104.
15. BAKER, R. R. & H. Y. CHANG. 1980. The incorporation of radioactive fatty acids into the phospholipids of nerve-cell body membranes in vivo. Biochem. J. **188**: 153–161.
16. BAKER, R. R. & H. Y. CHANG. 1983. The rapid incorporation of radioactive fatty acid into triacylglycerols during the in vitro acylation of native lipids of neuronal nuclei. Biochim. Biophys. Acta **752**: 1–9.
17. COOK, H. W. 1981. Metabolism of triacylglycerol in developing rat brain. Neurochem. Res. **6**: 1217–1229.
18. MARINETTI, G. V., A. WEINDL & J. KELLY. 1971. Lipid metabolism in the rabbit choroid plexus. J. Neurochem. **18**: 2003–2006.
19. HORROCKS, L. A., Y. K. YEO, H. W. HARDER, R. MOZZI & G. GORACCI. 1986. Choline plasmalogens, glycerophospholipid methylation, and receptor-mediated activation of adenylate cyclase. Adv. Cyclic Nucleotide Protein Phosphorylation Res. **20**: 263–292.
20. HORROCKS, L. A., H. W. HARDER, R. MOZZI, G. GORACCI, E. FRANCESCANGELI, S. PORCELLATI & G. G. NENCI. 1986. Receptor-mediated degradation of choline plasmalogens and glycerophospholipid methylation: A new hypothesis. In Enzymes of Lipid Metabolism, Vol. 2. L. Freysz, H. Dreyfus, R. Massarelli & S. Gatt, Eds.: 707–711. Plenum Press. New York, NY.
21. SUGIURA, T. & K. WAKU. 1985. CoA independent transfer of arachidonic acid from 1,2-diacyl-sn-glycero-3-phosphocholine to 1-0-alkyl-sn-glycero-3-phosphocholine (lyso

platelet-activating factor) by macrophage microsomes. Biochem. Biophys. Res. Commun. **127:** 384.
22. SUGIURA, T., N. SEKIGUCHI, Y. NAKAGAWA & K. WAKU. 1987. Formation of diacyl and alkylacyl glycerophosphocholine in rabbit alveolar macrophages. Lipids **22:** 589–595.
23. KRAMER, R. M., G. M. PATTON, C. R. PRITZKER & D. DEYKIN. 1984. Metabolism of platelet activating factor in human platelets: Transacylase mediated synthesis of 1-0-alkyl-2-arachidonoyl-sn-glycero-3-phosphocholine. J. Biol. Chem. **259:** 13316–13320.
24. ROBINSON, M., M. L. BLANK & F. SNYDER. 1985. Acylation of lysophospholipids by rabbit alveolar macrophages. Specificities of CoA dependent and CoA independent reactions. J. Biol. Chem. **260:** 7889–7895.
25. REDDY, P. V. & H. H. O. SCHMID. 1985. Selectivity of acyl transfer between phospholipids: Arachidonoyl transacylase in dog heart membranes. Biochem. Biophys. Res. Commun. **129:** 381–388.
26. CHILTON, F. H. & R. C. MURPHY. 1986. Remodeling of arachidonate-containing phosphoglycerides within the human neutrophil. J. Biol. Chem. **261:** 7771–7777.

Isolation, Characterization, and Regulation of Diacylglycerol Lipases from the Bovine Brain[a]

AKHLAQ A. FAROOQUI,[b,c] KOTTIL W. RAMMOHAN,[d]
AND LLOYD A. HORROCKS[b]

Departments of [b]Physiological Chemistry and [d]Neurology
The Ohio State University
Columbus, Ohio 43210

Phospholipids constitute a biologically important group of molecules that form the backbone of cellular membranes.[1] They are asymmetrically distributed between both layers of the plasma membrane; phosphatidylcholine and sphingomyelin face the outside, whereas arachidonate-rich phosphatidylethanolamine, phosphatidylserine and phosphatidylinositol (PI) are located in the inner half of the lipid bilayers. The phospholipid bilayer is penetrated by receptors, enzymes, and ion channels, which protrude through the membrane. Different phospholipids turn over at different rates with respect to their structure and localization in different cells and membranes.[1,2] These membranes are highly interactive and dynamic. The interactions of agonists with receptor-linked enzymes markedly affect membrane lipid metabolism, which in turn regulates the microenvironments of membrane-bound enzymes and ion channels.[1,2]

In mammalian membranes arachidonate, which is almost exclusively located in the sn-2 position of membrane phospholipids, is released by several different pathways. A direct pathway involves the stimulation of phospholipase A_2 (EC 3.1.1.4).[3,4] An indirect pathway requires the action of phospholipase C (EC 3.1.4.3) followed by diacylglycerol and monoacylglycerol lipases (EC 3.1.1.3).[5,6] Another pathway cleaves arachidonate by utilizing a lysophospholipase (EC 3.1.1.5) preceded by a phospholipase A_1.[7,8] Plasmalogenase (EC. 3.2.2.-) and lysophospholipase liberate arachidonate from plasmalogens.[9,10] Although the relative contribution of these pathways to release of arachidonate is still not known, the importance of phospholipase A_2 and diacylglycerol and monoacylglycerol lipases preceded by phospholipase C has been clearly demonstrated in several studies.[3,11,12] The diacylglycerol lipase is rate-controlling for arachidonate release by this pathway, but little information is available on the regulation and characterization of diacylglycerol lipases in mammalian tissues.

DIACYLGLYCEROL AND ITS METABOLIC IMPORTANCE

The receptor-mediated hydrolysis of phosphatidylinositol and the polyphosphoinositides plays an important role in signal transduction.[13-16] The diacylglycerol (DAG)

---

[a]This work was supported in part by Research Grant NS-10165 from the U.S. Public Health Service.
[c]Address for correspondence: A.A. Farooqui, Department of Physiological Chemistry, 1645 Neil Avenue, Room 214, Columbus, Ohio 43210.

TABLE 1. Direct Effects of Diacylglycerols on Activities of Various Enzymes

Enzyme	Effect on Activity
Protein kinase C	Stimulated
Phospholipase A_2	Stimulated
Glycogen synthetase	Inhibited
Tyrosine aminotransferase	Stimulated
Ornithine decarboxylase	Stimulated
Na^+, K^+-ATPase	Inhibited
β-Glucosaminidase	Stimulated
Cytidylyltransferase	Stimulated
Lysophospholipid acyltransferase	Inhibited

^aModified from Farooqui et al.[16]

generated by the phosphoinositide-specific phospholipase C can activate protein kinase C, an enzyme that may play an important role in cell division, differentiation, and signal transduction. The metabolism of released DAG results in the termination of this signal. The other product of phosphoinositol-specific phospholipase C, inositol 1,4,5-trisphosphate, mobilizes Ca^{2+} from intracellular stores.[13-16] In addition to the formation of DAG by the PI cycle, agonist-induced generation of cellular DAG also occurs from phosphatidylcholine.[17,18] The discovery of this pathway for DAG formation is of potential importance in the regulation of cell growth as phosphatidylcholine degradation in fibroblasts is induced by certain agonists.[18,19]

Diacylglycerols are emerging as a new and important class of bioactive molecules that regulate cellular function, growth, and behavior by affecting the activity of a number of important enzymes (TABLE 1). In the brain DAG is either phosphorylated to form phosphatidic acid by a DAG kinase or hydrolyzed to 2-monoacylglycerol (MAG) and fatty acid by a DAG lipase (FIG. 1). MAG is then hydrolyzed to glycerol and fatty acid by MAG lipase. DAG can also be converted to triacylglycerol (TAG) by an acyltransferase, which is quite active in some cultured cells.[20] In the brain diacylglyc-

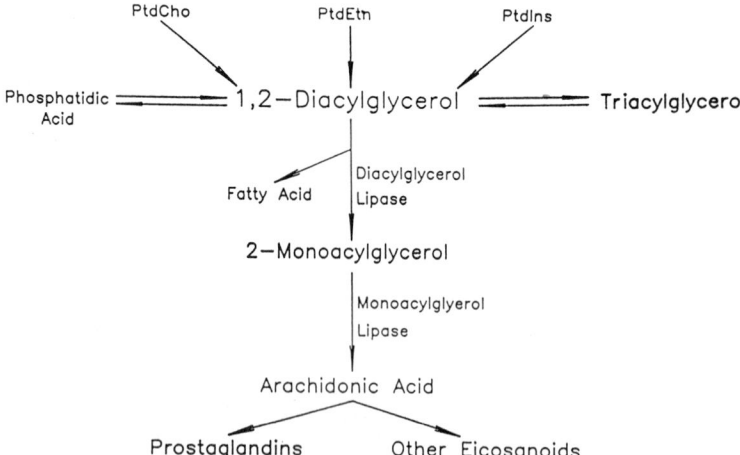

FIGURE 1. Metabolism of diacylglycerol in neural membranes.

erols are generated by the action of phospholipase C on the polar head group of phospholipids,[11-16] by the deacylation of triacylglycerol by triacylglycerol lipase,[21] and by the back reaction of the choline and ethanolamine phosphotransferases.[22,23]

Increased levels of diacylglycerol have been reported to occur in spinal cord trauma, ischemia, and seizures, and after electroconvulsive shock.[24-26] Elevated levels of DAG may affect physiological processes by altering membrane structure and fluidity.[24] In the above pathological situations diacylglycerol may act as the source for the massive release of free fatty acids and prostaglandins. The latter at low concentrations regulate cell growth and function but at high levels produce a variety of toxic effects at the cellular level.[26,27]

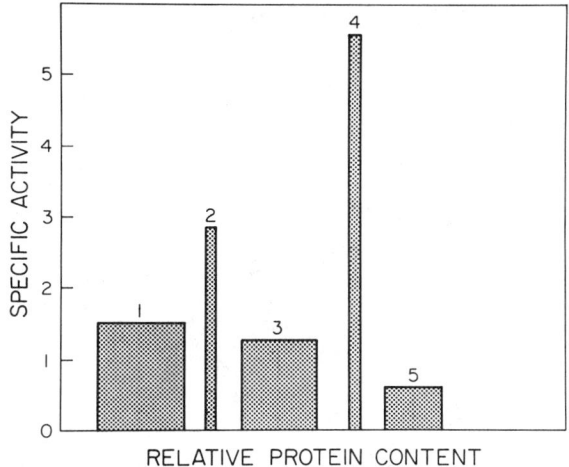

FIGURE 2. Diacylglycerol lipase activity in subcellular fractions of bovine brain. Subcellular fractions were: (1) 12,000 × g supernatant; (2) 48,000 × g pellet (plasma membrane fraction); (3) 48,000 × g supernatant; (4) 105,000 × g pellet (microsomal fraction), and (5) 105,000 × g supernatant (cytosol). One unit is the amount of enzyme hydrolyzing 1 nmol of substrate per min.

PURIFICATION AND PROPERTIES OF DIACYLGLYCEROL LIPASES

Bovine brain contains two diacylglycerol lipases. One is localized in microsomes and the other is found in plasma membranes (FIG. 2). Diacylglycerol lipase in microsomal membranes is stimulated by Triton X-100, whereas the plasma membrane enzyme is inhibited by this detergent.[28] Cabot and Gatt[29] and Stam et al.[30] also found that diacylglycerol lipase activity of the rat brain and heart is strongly inhibited by Triton X-100. Both diacylglycerol lipases can be solubilized with 0.25% Triton and are optimally active at pH 7.4. The occurrence of two forms of diacylglycerol lipase is also indicated by gel filtration studies. Sephadex G-75 chromatography of a detergent extract derived from a bovine brain preparation containing plasma membrane and microsomes shows the separation of two forms of diacylglycerol lipases (FIG. 3). The kinetic parameters and heat inactivation profiles of the two diacylglycerol lipases are quite similar.[31,32] Both lipases are markedly inhibited by RHC80267,[33] a recently described inhibitor of lipases and phospholipases.[31,34]

Heparin, a highly sulfated glycosaminoglycan with anticoagulant and antilipemic properties, markedly inhibits both diacylglycerol lipases but has no effect on monoacylglycerol lipase. Mono- and diacylglycerol lipases can be separated with heparin-Sepharose chromatography (FIG. 4). Diacylglycerol lipases are completely retained on a heparin-Sepharose column and can be eluted with 0.5 M sodium chloride or 2–5 mg/ml heparin, whereas monoacylglycerol lipase is not retained on the column.[35] Chondroitin sulfate and hyaluronic acid have no effect on lipase activities. Adenosine phosphates markedly affect the diacylglycerol lipases in a concentration-dependent manner. ATP is the most potent inhibitor followed by ADP. AMP has no effect, and cyclic AMP slightly stimulates diacylglycerol lipase.[35] Using a multiple column chromatographic procedure, microsomal and plasma membrane diacylglycerol lipases were purified 400-fold. (TABLES 2, 3). Triton X-100–solubilized extracts from microsomes and plasma membranes were subjected to ammonium sulfate fractionation

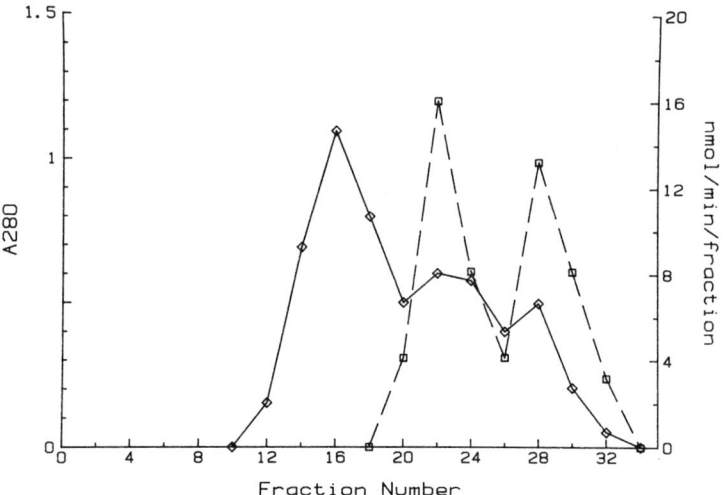

FIGURE 3. Elution profile of diacylglycerol lipases through Sephadex G-75 column. Triton X-100 extract of 12,000 × g supernatant was applied to a Sephadex G-75 column packed in 50 mM MOPS buffer, pH 7.4. A_{280} (—) and Diacylglycerol lipase activity (---).

(0–30%). The pellet containing diacylglycerol lipase activity was applied to a Sephadex G-75 column. The elution profiles were similar to that shown in FIGURE 3. Heparin Sepharose chromatography gave 4-fold purification with 75% recovery over the previous step. Diacylglycerol lipases are completely retained on an octyl-Sepharose column, and 60–65% of the protein is washed out. They can be eluted as a sharp peak when the column is washed with 0.8% sodium taurocholate. Polyacrylamide gel electrophoresis of an octyl-Sepharose fraction showed the presence of three protein bands, one major and two minor. The minor protein bands were separated by FPLC on Superose 12 HR. The final enzyme preparations were homogeneous (FIG. 5), as judged by polyacrylamide gel electrophoresis.

Bovine brain diacylglycerol lipases require no metal ions for their activity. Homogeneous preparations of microsomal and plasma membrane diacylglycerol lipases are not affected by $CaCl_2$. However, in the membrane-bound state the

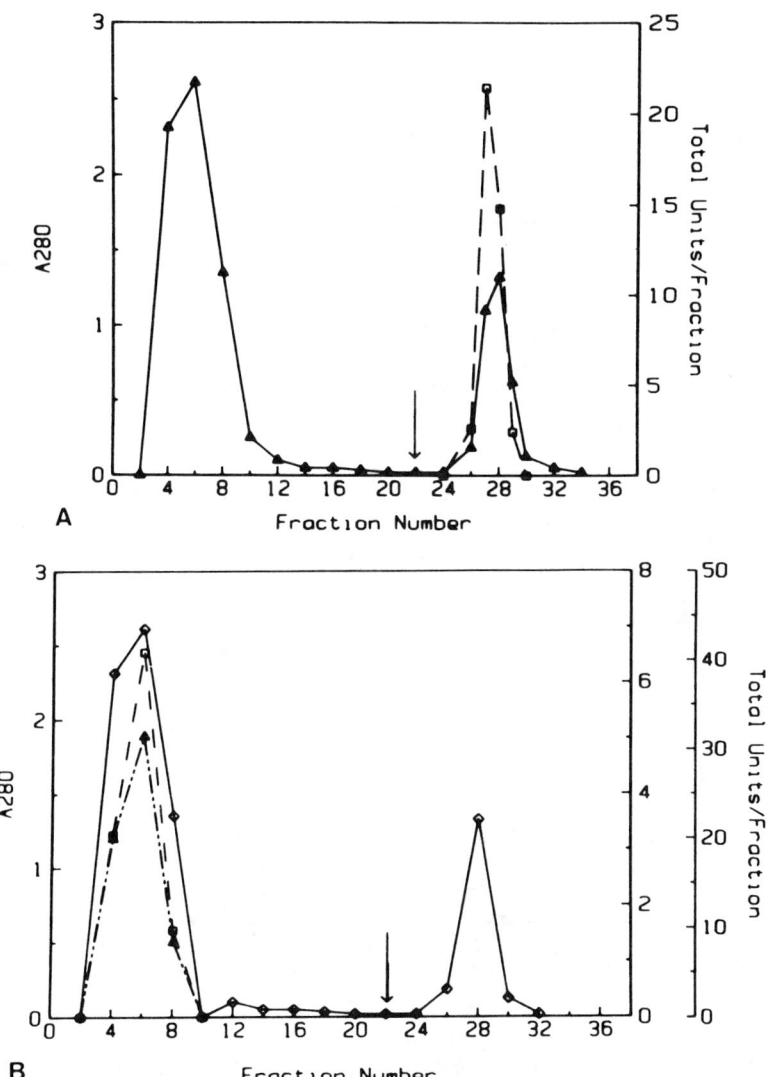

FIGURE 4. Elution profile of microsomal diacylglycerol lipase through heparin Sepharose column. (**A**) Diacylglycerol lipase (□) *right ordinate* and A_{280} (▲) *left ordinate*. (**B**) 2-Monoacylglycerol lipase (□) *far right ordinate*, lysophospholipase (▲) *right ordinate*, and A_{280} (◊) *left ordinate*.

TABLE 2. Purification of Bovine Brain Microsomal Diacylglycerol Lipase

Fraction	Total Protein (mg)	Total Units (nmol/min)	Specific Activity (nmol/min/mg)	Yield %
Solubilized microsomes	1078	2400	2.2	100
0–30% $(NH_4)_2SO_4$	539	1849	3.4	77
Sephadex G-75	150	1560	10.4	65
Heparin-Sepharose	30	1170	39.0	49
Octyl-Sepharose	6	860	143.3	36
Superose 12HR	4.5	820	182	34

microsomal diacylglycerol lipase activity is stimulated by a high concentration of $CaCl_2$, whereas the enzyme activity in plasma membrane is not affected by $CaCl_2$. The differential response of diacylglycerol lipases in the membrane-bound state may be due to differences in the membrane lipid composition of the two membranes. Diacylglycerol lipases are not affected by calmodulin in the presence or absence of $CaCl_2$. Sodium chloride and sodium azide (up to 150 mM) have no effect, but sodium fluoride at 75 mM produced 50% inhibition of microsomal and plasma membrane diacylglycerol lipases. Rat heart diacylglycerol lipase is also inhibited by sodium fluoride.[30] Polyamines such as spermine and tetracaine, inhibitors of phospholipase A_2,[36] stimulated the purified preparations of microsomal and plasma membrane diacylglycerol lipase. The stimulation of diacylglycerol lipase by spermine and tetracaine was similar to the stimulatory effect of polyamines on calcium-dependent phosphatidylinositol phosphodiesterase.[37]

Polyclonal antibodies against microsomal diacylglycerol lipases were prepared by injecting homogeneous enzyme preparations into rabbits. An Ouchterlony plate showing the precipitin line for microsomal diacylglycerol lipase is shown in FIGURE 6. These antibodies cross-react with homogeneous preparations of plasma membrane diacylglycerol lipase. The antiserum raised against microsomal diacylglycerol lipase inhibits both diacylglycerol lipases in a concentration-dependent manner.

The purified microsomal and plasma membrane diacylglycerol lipases are glycoproteins with molecular weights of 27,000 and 52,000, respectively. The treatment of purified diacylglycerol lipases with bacterial neuraminidase does not affect their enzymatic activities; thus N-acetylneuraminyl groups are not involved in the diacylglycerol lipase catalyzed reaction.

The retention of microsomal and plasma membrane diacylglycerol lipases on a concanavalin-A Sepharose column and their elution with methyl α-D-mannoside shows that the binding of these enzymes to concanavalin-A Sepharose is through the carbohydrate moiety. Concanavalin-A Sepharose chromatography of a detergent extract prepared from a bovine brain preparation containing plasma membranes and

TABLE 3. Purification of Bovine Brain Microsomal Diacylglycerol Lipase

Fraction	Total Protein (mg)	Total Units (nmol/min)	Specific Activity (nmol/min/mg)	Yield %
Solubilized plasma membrane	1382	3595	2.6	100
0–30% $(NH_4)_2SO_4$	570	3135	5.5	87
Sephadex G-75	192	2485	13.0	69
Heparin-Sepharose	35	1890	54.0	52
Octyl-Sepharose	7	1253	179.0	35
Superose 12HR	6	1200	200.0	33

microsomes indicates that the two diacylglycerol lipases can be partially separated (FIG. 7) by washing the concanavalin-A Sepharose column with a 0 to 1-M gradient of methyl α-D-mannoside. This shows that microsomal and plasma membrane diacylglycerol lipases differ from each other in their carbohydrate composition.

REGULATION AND ROLE OF DIACYLGLYCEROL LIPASES

Like phospholipase A_2, the regulation of diacylglycerol lipases is complex. The enzyme activity may be regulated by free fatty acids that are an end product of the diacylglycerol lipase reaction. *In vitro* this inhibition can be reversed by fatty acid–free

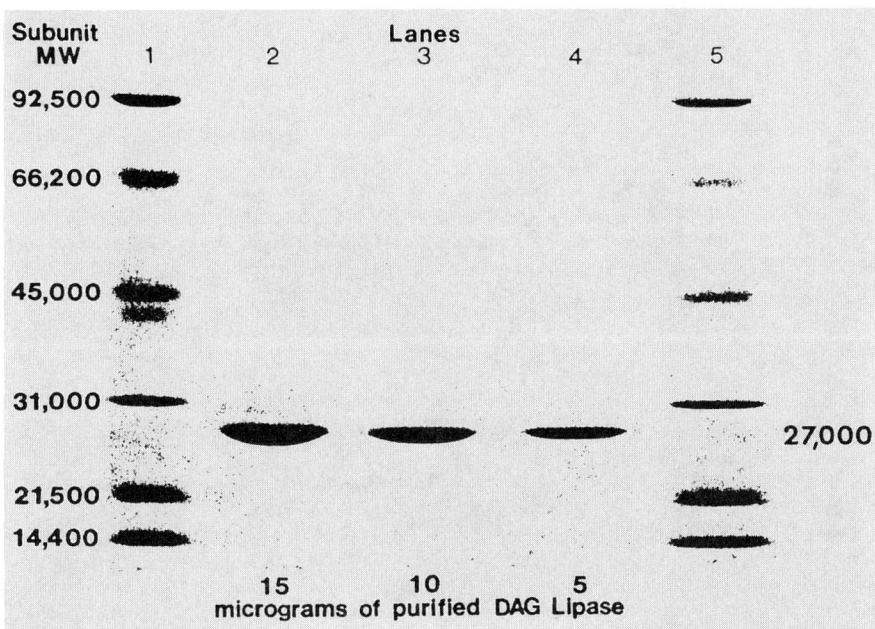

FIGURE 5. SDS-polyacrylamide gel electrophoresis of purified microsomal diacylglycerol lipase. *Lanes* 1 and 5 are molecular weight standards. *Lanes* 2, 3, and 4 contain the specified amounts of diacylglycerol lipase. The apparent molecular weight of diacylglycerol lipase is 27,000.

bovine serum albumin.[38] Recent studies have indicated that C-MT peptide, the C-terminus of the middle-sized tumor antigen of polyoma virus, inhibits the activities of various phospholipases, including A_2, C, D, and phosphatidylinositol-specific phospholipase C.[39] This peptide has an amino acid sequence similar to a portion of lipocortin I, an endogenous phospholipase regulatory protein.[40] Both microsomal and plasma membrane diacylglycerol lipases are strongly inhibited by C-MT peptide (FIG. 8). The degree of C-MT inhibition was several-fold higher for diacylglycerol lipases than for phospholipases. The effect of lipocortin on diacylglycerol lipases is not known.

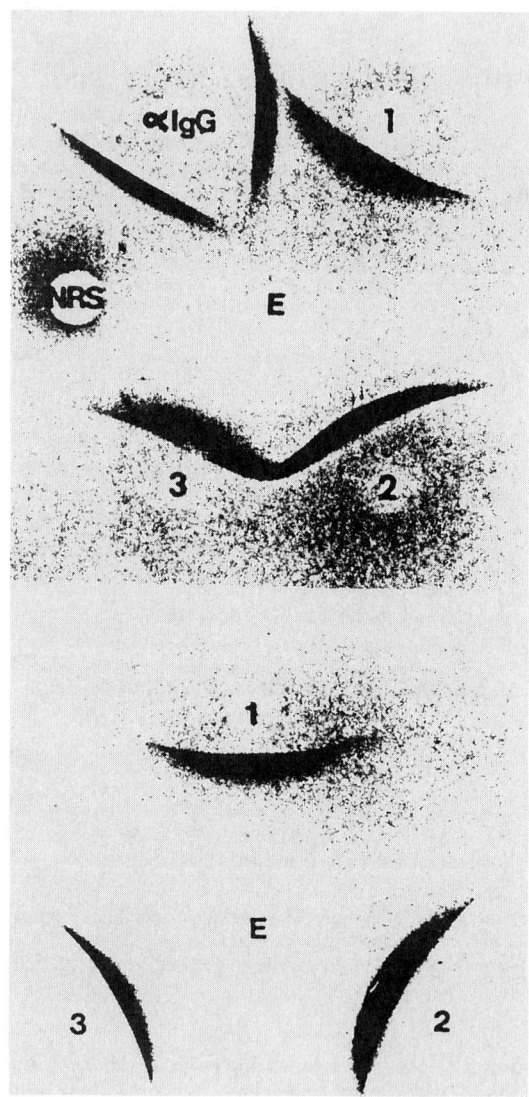

FIGURE 6. Ouchterlony double immunodiffusion of immunized rabbit serum and purified microsomal diacylglycerol lipase. E is the central well containing diacylglycerol lipase; 1, 2, and 3 are rabbit numbers; NRS is normal rabbit serum, and αIgG is antirabbit IgG.

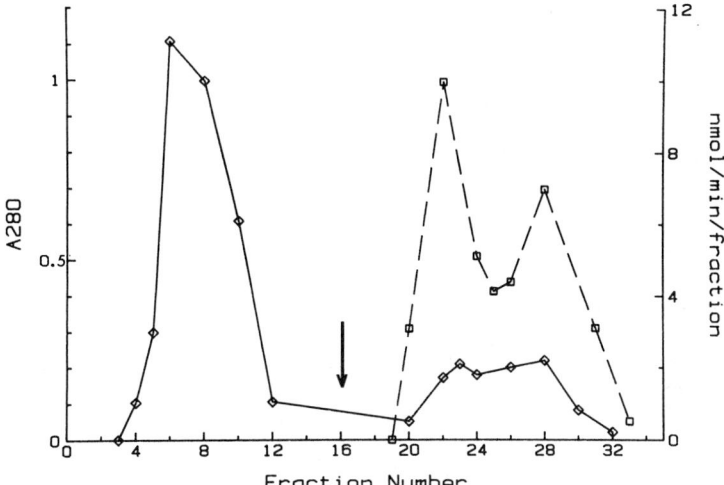

FIGURE 7. Elution profile of diacylglycerol lipases through a concanavalin A-Sepharose column. A_{280} (—) *left ordinate* and diacylglycerol lipase activity (---) *right ordinate*. The methyl α-D mannoside gradient (0–1 M) was applied at the *arrow*.

The role of the lipases in the brain is not fully understood. The low levels and rapid turnover of acylglycerols in neural membranes and the relatively high activity of their lipases suggest that the lipases have an important function in the central nervous system. Under normal conditions lipases maintain low levels of acylglycerols in neural membranes. However, under pathological situations such as ischemia, spinal cord trauma, and viral infections, the lipases may be involved in the massive release of free

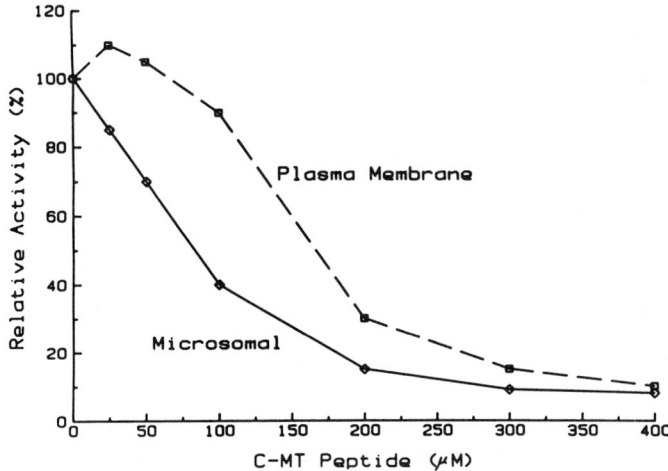

FIGURE 8. Effect of C-MT peptide on microsomal (—) and plasma membrane (---) diacylglycerol lipases.

fatty acids and prostaglandins, which may cause serious cell damage.[41] Furthermore, recent studies[42,43] have also shown markedly increased activities of lipolytic enzymes (including diacylglycerol lipases) in membrane fractions obtained from nucleus basalis and hippocampal regions of patients with Alzheimer's disease. The enhanced activities of these enzymes may be due to alterations in levels of neuropeptides. For example, activities of lipases may be increased by β-endorphin and bradykinin,[44,45] in view of the fact that these neuropeptides are known to induce lipolysis.[46,47]

CONCLUSION

Diacylglycerol lipases from bovine brain microsomes and plasma membranes have been purified to homogeneity using multiple-column chromatographic procedures. The two lipases resemble each other in kinetic properties, glycoprotein nature, and response to certain inhibitors. The antibodies raised against microsomal diacylglycerol lipase can cross-react with the plasma membrane enzyme. They differ in subcellular localization response to detergents, molecular weights, and carbohydrate composition. Activities of neural membrane diacylglycerol lipases may be regulated by free fatty acids, lipocortins, and neuropeptides.

REFERENCES

1. PORCELLATI, G. 1983. Phospholipid metabolism in neural membranes. *In* Neural Membranes. G. Y. Sun, N. Bazan, J. Y. Wu, G. Porcellati & A. Y. Sun, Eds.: 3–35. Humana Press. New York, NY.
2. FAROOQUI, A. A. & L. A. HORROCKS. 1985. Metabolic and functional aspects of neural membrane phospholipids. *In* Phospholipids in the Nervous System, Vol. II: Physiological Role. L. A. Horrocks, J. N. Kanfer & G. Porcellati, Eds.: 341–348. Raven Press. New York, NY.
3. CHANG, J., J. H. MUSSER & H. MCGREGOR. 1987. Phospholipase A_2: Function and pharmacological regulation. Biochem. Pharmacol. **36**: 2429–2436.
4. BALSINDE, J., E. DIEZ, A. SCHULLER & F. MOLLINEDO. 1988. Phospholipase A_2 activity in resting and activated human neutrophils. J. Biol. Chem. **263**: 1929–1936.
5. BELL, R. L., D. A. KENNERLY, N. STANDFORD & P. W. MAJERUS. 1979. Diglyceride lipase: A pathway for arachidonic release from human platelets. Proc. Natl. Acad. Sci. USA **76**: 3238–3241.
6. MAUCO, G., J. FAUVEL, H. CHAP & L. DOUSTE-BLAZY. 1984. Studies on enzymes related to diacylglycerol production in activated platelets: Subcellular distribution, enzymatic properties and positional specificity of diacylglycerol and monoacylglycerol lipases. Biochim. Biophys. Acta **796**: 169–177.
7. VAN DEN BOSCH, H. 1980. Intracellular phospholipases A. Biochim. Biophys. Acta **604**: 191–246.
8. VAN DEN BOSCH, H. 1982. Phospholipases. *In* Phospholipids. J. N. Hawthorne & G. B. Ansell, Eds.: 313–357. Elsevier Biomedical. Amsterdam.
9. HORROCKS, L. A., H. W. HARDER, R. MOZZI, G. GORACCI, E. FRANCESCANGELI, S. PORCELLATI & G. G. NENCI. 1986. Receptor-mediated degradation of choline plasmalogens and glycerophospholipid methylation: A new hypothesis. *In* Enzymes of Lipid Metabolism, Vol. 2. L. Freysz, H. Dreyfus, R. Massarelli & S. Gatt, Eds.: 707–711. Plenum Press. New York, NY.
10. HORROCKS, L. A., Y. K. YEO, H. W. HARDER, R. MOZZI & G. GORACCI. 1986. Choline plasmalogens, glycerophospholipid methylation, and receptor-mediated activation of adenylate cyclase. Adv. Cyclic Nucleotide Protein Phosphorylation Res. **20**: 263–292.
11. BERRIDGE, M. J. 1984. Inositol trisphosphate and diacylglycerol as second messengers. Biochem. J. **220**: 345–360.

12. NISHIZUKA, Y. 1983. Phospholipid degradation and signal translation for protein phosphorylation. Trends Biochem. Sci. **8:** 13–16.
13. NISHIZUKA, Y. 1986. Studies and perspectives of protein kinase C. Science **233:** 305–312.
14. SEKAR, M. C. & L. E. HOKIN. 1986. The role of phosphoinositides in signal transduction. J. Membrane Biol. **89:** 193–210.
15. ABDEL-LATIF, A. A. 1986. Calcium-mobilizing receptor polyphosphoinositides and the generation of second messenger. Pharm. Rev. **38:** 227–272.
16. FAROOQUI, A. A., T. FAROOQUI, A. J. YATES & L. A. HORROCKS. 1988. Regulation of protein kinase C activity by various lipids. Neurochem. Res. **13:** 499–511.
17. DANIEL, L. W., M. WAITE & R. L. WYKLE. 1986. A novel mechanism of diglyceride formation: 12-0-tetradecanoylphorbol-13-acetate stimulates the cyclic breakdown and resynthesis of phosphatidylcholine. J. Biol. Chem. **261:** 9128–9132.
18. BESTERMAN, J. M., V. DURONIO & P. CUATRECASAS. 1986. Rapid formation of diacylglycerol from phosphatidylcholine: A pathway for generation of a second messenger. Proc. Natl. Acad. Sci. USA **83:** 6785–6789.
19. MAIR, J. G. & A. W. MURRAY. 1987. Bombesin and phorbol ester stimulate phosphatidylcholine hydrolysis by phospholipase C. J. Cell Physiol. **130:** 382–391.
20. CABOT, M. C., C. J. WELSH, Z. C. ZHANG & H. CHABBOTT. 1987. Assays and substrate preparation for the enzymatic hydrolysis of diacylglycerol and phorbol diester. Methods Enzymol. **141:** 301–313.
21. MIZOBUCHI, M., K. SHIRAE, N. MATSUOKA, Y. SAITO & A. KUMAGAI. 1981. Studies on lipase in rat brain. J. Neurochem. **36:** 301–303.
22. GORACCI, G., L. A. HORROCKS & G. PORCELLATI. 1977. Reversibility of ethanolamine and choline phosphotransferases (EC 2.7.8.1 and EC 2.7.8.2) in rat brain microsomes with labeled alkylacylglycerols. FEBS Lett. **80:** 41–44.
23. GORACCI, G., E. FRANCESCANGELI, L. A. HORROCKS & G. PORCELLATI. 1981. The reverse reaction of cholinephosphotransferase in rat brain microsomes: A new pathway for degradation of phosphatidyl choline. Biochim. Biophys. Acta. **664:** 373–379.
24. DEMEDIUK, P. P., R. D. SAUNDERS, N. R. CLENDENON, E. D. MEANS, D. K. ANDERSON & L. A. HORROCKS. 1985. Changes in lipid metabolism in traumatized spinal cord. Prog. Brain Res. **63:** 211–226.
25. HORROCKS, L. A., R. V. DORMAN & G. PORCELLATI. 1984. Fatty acids and phospholipids in brain during ischemia. *In* Cerebral Ischemia. A. Bes, P. Braquet, R. Paoletti & B. K. Siesjö, Eds.: 211–222. Excerpta Medica, Congress Series 654. Elsevier. Amsterdam.
26. BAZAN, N. G., D. L. BIRKLE, W. TANG & T. S. REDDY. 1986. The accumulation of free arachidonic acid, diacylglycerol, prostaglandins, and lipoxygenase reaction products in the brain during experimental epilepsy. Adv. Neurol. **44:** 879–902.
27. NEEDLEMAN, P., T. TURK, B. A. JAKSCHIK, A. R. MORRISON & J. B. LEFKOWITH. 1986. Arachidonic acid metabolism. Ann. Rev. Biochem. **55:** 69–102.
28. FAROOQUI, A. A., W. A. TAYLOR & L. A. HORROCKS. 1986. Characterization and solubilization of membrane bound diacylglycerol lipases from bovine brain. Int. J. Biochem. **18:** 991–997.
29. CABOT, M. C. & S. GATT. 1976. Hydrolysis of neutral glycerides by lipases of rat brain microsomes. Biochim. Biophys. Acta **431:** 105–115.
30. STAM, H., S. BROEKHOVEN-SCHOKKER & W. C. HULSMANN. 1986. Characterization of mono-, di- and triacylglycerol lipase activities in the isolated rat heart. Biochim. Biophys. Acta **875:** 76–86.
31. FAROOQUI, A. A., C. E. PENDLEY, II, W. A. TAYLOR & L. A. HORROCKS. 1985. Studies on diacylglycerol lipases and lysophospholipases of bovine brain. *In* Phospholipids in the Nervous System, Vol. II: Physiological Role. L. A. Horrocks, J. N. Kanfer & G. Porcellati, Eds.: 179–192. Raven Press. New York, NY.
32. FAROOQUI, A. A., W. A. TAYLOR & L. A. HORROCKS. 1986. Membrane bound diacylglycerol lipases in bovine brain: Purification and characterization. *In* Phospholipid Research and the Nervous System: Biochemical and Molecular Pharmacology. L. A. Horrocks, L. Freysz & G. Toffano, Eds.: 181–190. Liviana Press. Padova, Italy.
33. SUTHERLAND, C. A. & D. AMIN. 1982. Relative activities of rat and dog platelet phospholipase A_2 and diglyceride lipase: Selective inhibition of diglyceride lipase by RHC80267. J. Biol. Chem. **257:** 14006–14010.

34. OGLESBY, T. D. & R. R. GORMAN. 1984. The inhibition of arachidonic acid metabolism in human platelets by RHC80267, A diacylglycerol lipase inhibitor. Biochim. Biophys. Acta **793:** 269–277.
35. FAROOQUI, A. A., W. A. TAYLOR & L. A. HORROCKS. 1984. Separation of bovine brain mono- and diacylglycerol lipases by heparin Sepharose affinity chromatography. Biochem. Biophys. Res. Commun. **122:** 1241–1246.
36. CHEAH, K. S. & A. M. CHEAH. 1981. Mitochondrial calcium transport and calcium-activated phospholipase in porcine malignant hyperthermia. Biochim. Biophys. Acta **634:** 70–84.
37. EICHBERG, J., W. J. ZETUSKY, M. E. BELL & E. CAVANAGH. 1981. Effect of polyamines on calcium-dependent rat brain phosphatidylinositol-phosphodiesterase. J. Neurochem. **36:** 1868–1871.
38. FAROOQUI, A. A., W. A. TAYLOR & L. A. HORROCKS. 1986. Membrane bound diacylglycerol lipases of bovine brain. *In* Proceedings of the Membrane Protein Symposium. S. C. Goheen, Ed.: 729–746. Bio-Rad Laboratories. Richmond, CA.
39. NOTSU, Y., S. NAMIUCHI, T. HATTORI, K. MATSUDA & F. HIRATA. 1985. Inhibition of phospholipases by Met-Leu-Ile-Leu-Ile-Lys-Arg-Ser-Arg-His-Phe-, C Terminus of middle-sized tumor antigen. Arch. Biochem. Biophys. **236:** 195–204.
40. DENNIS, E. A. 1987. Regulation of eicosanoid production: Role of phospholipases and inhibitors. Bio/Technology **5:** 1294–1300.
41. FAROOQUI, A. A., W. A. TAYLOR & L. A. HORROCKS. 1988. Phospholipases, lysophospholipases and lipases and their involvement in various diseases. Neurochem. Path. **7:** 99–128.
42. FAROOQUI, A. A., L. LISS & L. A. HORROCKS. 1988. Stimulation of lipolytic enzymes in Alzheimer's disease. Ann. Neurol. **23:** 306–308.
43. FAROOQUI, A. A., L. LISS & L. A. HORROCKS. 1988. Neurochemical aspects of Alzheimer's disease. Involvement of membrane phospholipids. Metabolic Brain Dis. **3:** 19–35.
44. FAROOQUI, A. A., L. LISS, G. A. TEJWANI, S. H. HANISSIAN & L. A. HORROCKS. 1988. Lipases and phospholipases in different regions of brain in Alzheimer's disease. Trans. Am. Soc. Neurochem. **19:** 225.
45. FAROOQUI, A. A., C. J. FLYNN, E. BRADEL, D. ANDERSON, G. MEANS & L. A. HORROCKS. 1988. Mono- and diacylglycerol lipases in cultured neuronal and glial cells. Trans. Am. Soc. Neurochem. **19:** 205.
46. RICHTER, W. O., P. KERSCHER & P. SCHWANDT. 1983. β-Endorphin stimulates in vivo lipolysis in the rabbit. Life Sci. (suppl I) **33:** 743–746.
47. GECSE, A., A. MEZEI & G. TELEGDY. 1987. Neuropeptides and arachidonate cascade in the central nervous system. Front. Horm. Res. **15:** 299–323.

Deacylation-Reacylation of Arachidonoyl Groups in Cerebral Phospholipids[a]

GRACE Y. SUN

Sinclair Comparative Medicine Research Farm and
Department of Biochemistry
University of Missouri
Columbia, Missouri 65203

RONALD A. MacQUARRIE

School of Basic Life Sciences
University of Missouri–Kansas City
Kansas City, Missouri 64110

Due to its role as a precursor in the biosynthesis of eicosanoids, arachidonic acid (20:4) is one of the most important polyunsaturated fatty acids in the brain. Under normal conditions, 20:4 is stored in esterified form among glycerolipids with only trace amounts present in the free form. It has been known for several years that 20:4 and other free fatty acids (FFA) are released during cerebral ischemia, electroconvulsive shock, as well as other forms of brain injury.[1-6] More recently, FFA release has been linked to neurotransmitters and receptor-mediated events.[7-9] Nevertheless, the exact mechanism for FFA release from the brain is not yet completely understood. Since arachidonic acid in the brain is maintained in a dynamic equilibrium between the free and esterified forms, factors perturbing this equilibrium are of importance in the release mechanism.[10]

The deacylation-reacylation cycle is probably one of the most important events for controlling the metabolic activity of 20:4 in the brain. Besides 20:4 release, activation of this cyclic event would generate lysophospholipids, which may be important in regulating neuronal membrane functions.[11] In order to gain better understanding of the metabolism of 20:4 in the brain, factors regulating enzymes involved in the deacylation-reacylation cycle are discussed in this chapter.

DISTRIBUTION OF ARACHIDONIC ACID IN BRAIN GLYCEROLIPIDS

Arachidonic acid is uniquely distributed among different glycerolipids in the brain. Our previous studies on the fatty acid profile of phospholipids in brain synaptosomes indicated the following proportions for 20:4: 6% in phosphatidylcholines (PC), 14.2% in phosphatidylethanolamines (PE), 16.6% in ethanolamine plasmalogens (PEpl), 2.3% in phosphatidylserines (PS) and 31.5% in phosphatidylinositols (PI).[12] The predominance of stearoyl-arachidonoyl species in PI was observed earlier by Baker and Thompson.[13] Since polyphosphoinositides (poly-PI) are phosphorylated derivatives of PI, it is not surprising that the proportion of 20:4 in poly-PI is similar to that for PI.[14] The diacylglycerols (DG) in the brain also contain a high proportion (29%) of their

---

[a]This work was supported in part by research grant BNS 84-19063 from the National Science Foundation.

acyl groups as 20:4.[15,16] The high content of 20:4 in DG suggested a metabolic relationship between phosphoinositides and DG in the brain.[17] The phosphatidic acid (PA) in the brain is comprised of 12–14% of the acyl groups as 20:4.[15] Although there are only trace amounts of triacylglycerols (TG) in the brain, analysis of their acyl group composition revealed the presence of a small proportion (6%) of 20:4.[15,16] In many instances, information on acyl group profiles of brain glycerolipids has been useful towards understanding the metabolism of specific lipid pools within the membrane.

OVERVIEW OF ENZYMES INVOLVED IN THE DEACYLATION-REACYLATION REACTIONS IN THE BRAIN

The enzymic pathways for biosynthesis of phospholipids are known to involve a number of acyltransfer reactions. Theoretically, 20:4 in its activated form (i.e.,

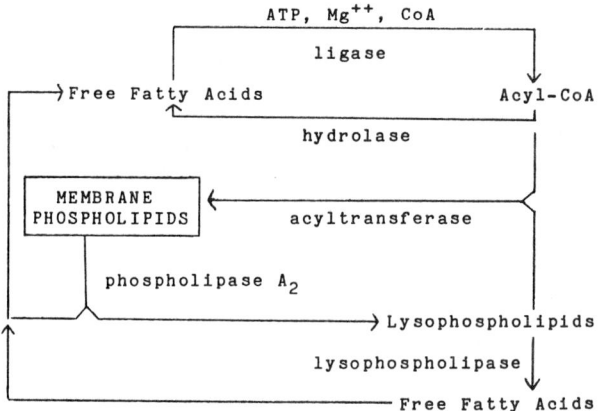

FIGURE 1. A scheme depicting the enzymic reactions involved in the deacylation-reacylation mechanism. (From Sun et al.[11] Reprinted by permission from Humana Press.)

20:4-CoA) may participate in all of the acyltransfer reactions for *de novo* biosynthesis of phospholipids. In addition, 20:4 in the brain also participates in deacylation-reacylation activity, as described by Lands and Crawford.[18] Involvement of 20:4 in this cyclic event may be related to several important cellular functions: (1) to control the amount of 20:4 for eicosanoid synthesis, (2) to regulate the level of acyl-CoA and lysophospholipids, and (3) to enrich specific phospholipids (e.g., PI) with 20:4. As shown in FIGURE 1, phospholipase A_2 and acyl-CoA:lysophospholipid acyltransferase are the two key enzymes mediating the deacylation and reacylation events, respectively. Under normal conditions, this cyclic event is probably maintained in a dynamic equilibrium under stringent regulation.[10,11] The completion of this cyclic event also requires the participation of other enzymes.

Phospholipase A_2 acting on specific pools of membrane phospholipids can be the initiation point of activation, resulting in the generation of FFA and lysophospholipids (FIG. 1). The FFA formed can diffuse freely within the membrane or be transported to the cytoplasm in the presence of acyl carrier proteins. Therefore, this product is probably not accumulated at the site of the reaction. However, in order to reutilize the FFA, it is necessary to activate the FFA to their acyl-CoA by the ATP-dependent fatty acid ligase.

The lysophospholipids generated from phospholipase A_2 action may either return to the membrane through acyl-CoA:lysophospholipid acyltransferases or undergo hydrolysis through the action of lysophospholipases. Since these lipid intermediates generated through the deacylation-reacylation cycle are implicated in a role in modulating neuronal membrane function, it is important to understand the properties of the enzymes and the factors controlling the metabolism of these lipids.

ACYL-CoA:LYSOPHOSPHOLIPID ACYLTRANSFERASES

Activity towards Different Lysophospholipids

Acyl-CoA:lysophospholipid acyltransferase is the key enzyme for recycling the lysophospholipids generated in membranes.[18] Frequently, *in vitro* assays of the acyltransferase activity produce higher activity when acyl-CoA is generated *in situ* rather than added exogenously. This is probably due to the potent detergent effects of acyl-CoA, which may inhibit the acyltransferase activity if it is present in excess quantity. The ATP-dependent fatty acid ligase is widely distributed in brain membranes.[19,20] In the presence of ATP, Mg^{2+}, and CoASH, brain synaptosomes were active in transferring labeled 20:4 to 1-acyl-glycerophosphocholine (GPC) and 1-acyl-glycerophosphoinositol (GPI), whereas other lyso-compounds (e.g., 1-acyl-glycerophosphoethanolamine, GPE) were poor acceptors.[12] Similar results were obtained by Baker and Thompson[21] for the transfer of arachidonoyl groups to 1-acyl-GPI. With this assay system, the transfer of 20:4 to 1-acyl-GPI and 1-acyl-GPC was greatly dependent on the amount of substrate present in the assay system (FIG. 2).[12] In fact, inhibition of the reaction rate was observed at high concentrations of both acyl-CoA and lysophospholipids.[12,22] Therefore, substrate concentration appears to be an important form of regulation for this type of enzyme.

Whether or not specific enzymes are present for the transfer of acyl groups to different lyso-substrates has been the subject of discussion for a number of years. Recent studies have provided evidence suggesting that different acyltransferases are present for different lyso-substrates. Therefore, acyl-CoA:1-acyl-GPC acyltransferase purified from brain microsomes was shown to react only with 1-acyl-GPC as acyl acceptor.[23] The purified enzyme showed a clear preference for the transfer of arachidonoyl-CoA with little or no activity towards saturated acyl-CoA (TABLE 1).[23] Working with heart microsomes, Sanjanwala[24] was able to separate the acyl-CoA:1-acyl-GPI acyltransferase from acyl-CoA:1-acyl-GPC acyltransferase by affinity column chromatography. Both enzymes were specific in their lysoacceptors, although broader specificity was exhibited for the acyl donor.

Acylation Activity among Brain Subcellular Fractions

Although controversies exist regarding the subcellular localization of the acyl-CoA:lysophospholipid acyltransferases in the brain, it is generally recognized that enzyme activity is highest in the microsomal fraction. However, acyltransferase activity was found in cell plasma membranes, for instance, rabbit thymocytes,[25] and activity in this membrane fraction was correlated to concanavallin A stimulation as

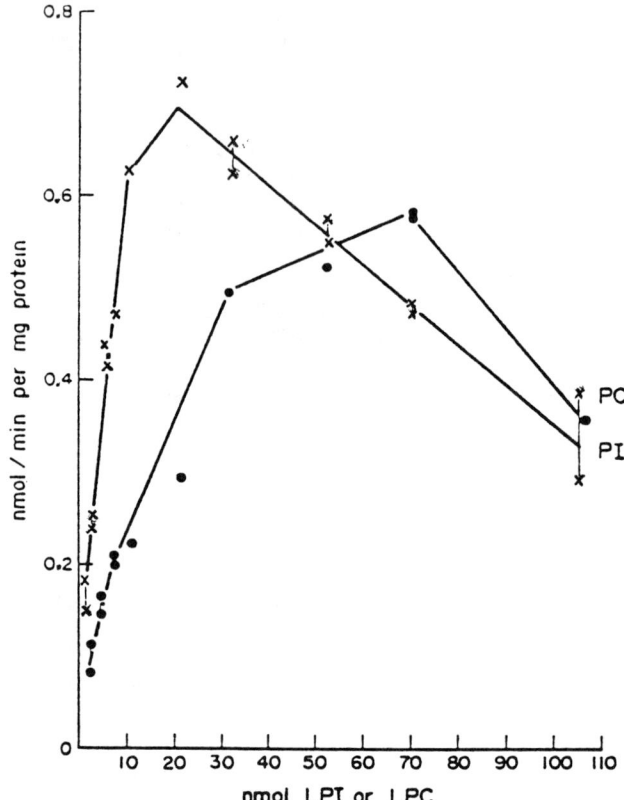

FIGURE 2. Transfer of [^{14}C]-20:4 to 1-acyl-glycerophosphatidylinositol and 1-acyl-glycerophosphatidylcholine as a function of lyso-substrate concentration. Rat brain synaptosomes were incubated in a system containing labeled 20:4, ATP, Mg^{2+}, CoASH, and the specified lysophospholipid. Enzymic activity is expressed as nmol of 20:4 incorporated into the respective phosphoglycerides/min/mg of synaptosomal protein. (From Corbin and Sun.[12] Reprinted by permission from *Journal of Neurochemistry*.)

well as activation of (Na$^+$ + K$^+$)-ATPase activity.[25,26] Acyltransferase activity was present in synaptosomes and subsynaptic membranes.[12] One problem that may have precluded accurate measurement of the acyltransferase activity in intact synaptosomes is the difficulty of acyl-CoA or ATP crossing the synaptic membrane. This phenomenon was tested by comparing the synaptosomal acyltransferase activity prior to or after permeabilizing synaptosomes with saponin. Indeed, the permeabilized synaptosomes showed a two-fold increase in acyltransferase activity.[27] Although different subcellular membrane fractions exhibited different patterns for the transfer of labeled 20:4 to individual phospholipids, most membrane fractions indicated a higher uptake of 20:4 by PI than by PC.[27] In addition, labeled 20:4 was also incorporated into TG. Since no exogenous lysophospholipids were added to the membranes during incubation, the acyltransfer activity may reflect the amount of endogenous lysophospholipids or DG present in the membrane.

Effects of Membrane Perturbing Agents

The membrane-bound nature of acyl-CoA:lysophospholipid acyltransferases suggests that these enzymes are sensitive to agents perturbing the membrane. In general, these enzymes are more sensitive to inhibition by nonionic detergents than ionic detergents.[22] On the other hand, serum albumin seems to exert a specific effect on enhancing 20:4 incorporation into synaptosomal PI but not PC (FIG. 3).[27,28] The reason for this effect is not clearly understood. It is possible that 20:4 transfer to 1-acyl-GPI is more sensitive to oxidative metabolites that can be removed by albumin. Acyltransferase activity is unstable at elevated temperatures.[27] Whether the instability is related to an enhanced formation of these metabolites remains to be further investigated.

DEACYLATION OF ARACHIDONOYL PHOSPHOLIPIDS

Release of Arachidonic Acid from Prelabeled Phospholipids in Brain Synaptosomes due to K^+-Depolarization

In the past, studies of phospholipase A_2-mediated deacylation of phospholipids in the brain have been limited, because both enzyme and substrates are integral parts of the membrane. Using acetone powder preparations, researchers have reported the presence of phospholipase A_2 activity in brain subcellular membranes.[29,30] However, assay of phospholipase A_2 activity using acetone powder as the enzyme source required the presence of detergents. Thus, little information is available on the ability of brain synaptosomes to metabolize exogenous phospholipids. Using labeled phospholipids incubated with synaptosomes, we observed that labeled PI was susceptible to hydrolysis by both phospholipase A_2 and phospholipase C in the fraction, resulting in the release of FFA and DG, respectively.[31] On the other hand, labeled PC was only degraded by phospholipase A_2 to release FFA (TABLE 2).[31]

TABLE 1. Specificity of Purified LPC Acyltransferase toward Acyl-CoA Derivatives

Substrate[a]	Relative Acyltransferase Activity[b]
Arachidonoyl-CoA (20:4)	100
Eicosatrienoyl-CoA (20:3)	20
cis-11-Eicosaenoyl-CoA (20:1)	13
Linolenoyl-CoA (18:3)	8
Linoleoyl-CoA (18:2)	13
Oleoyl-CoA (18:1)	13
Palmitoyl-CoA (16:0)	0
Stearoyl-CoA (18:0)	0
Decanoyl-CoA (10:0)	58
Myristoyl-CoA (14:0)	41

NOTE: Acyl-CoA:1-acyl-GPC acyltransferase was isolated from bovine brain microsomes by column chromatography as described in Reference 23. The purified enzyme used only 1-acyl-GPC (LPC) as substrate.

[a]All acyl-CoA derivatives were used at a concentration of 4 μM. LPC was used as an acyl acceptor at a concentration of 50 μm.

[b]All activities were relative to that obtained with arachidonoyl-CoA (580 nmol/min/mg), which is set at 100. The activity was measured in terms of nmol/min of [^{14}C]LPC incorporated into PC with different acyl-CoA derivatives as acyl donors. (Data taken from Reference 23.)

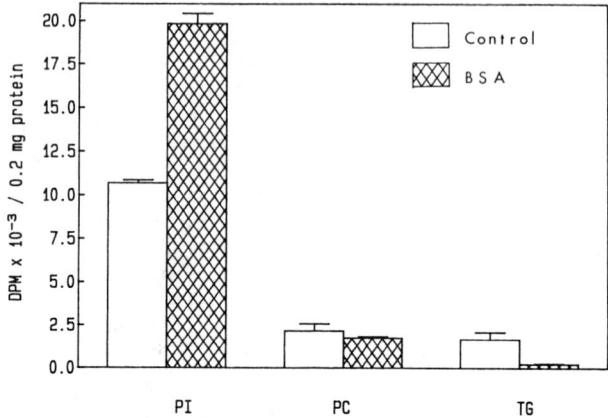

FIGURE 3. Effect of bovine serum albumin (BSA) treatment on [^{14}C]-20:4 incorporation into phospholipids and triacylglycerols (TG) of rat brain plasma membranes. Two equal aliquots of brain homogenate were subjected to isolation of brain plasma membranes. At the last centrifugation step, one of the samples was treated with BSA prior to obtaining the membrane pellets. Samples (0.2 mg of protein) were incubated with [^{14}C]-20:4 (0.1 μCi), ATP (2.5 mM), MgCl$_2$ (10 mM), and CoASH (0.1 mM) at 37°C for 10 min. Results depict the amount of radioactivity incorporated into PI, PC, and TG in control and BSA-washed samples.

TABLE 2. Enzymatic Hydrolysis of Labeled Phosphoglycerides by Brain Synaptosomes

Types of Labeled Phosphoglycerides	Product of Degradation	Time (min)			
		0	10	30	60
1-acyl-2-[^{14}C]-arachidonoyl-GPI	DG	1.0	5.0	13.6	15.5
(52,000 cpm, 6 μm)	FFA	2.8	3.4	5.7	6.8
	PA	0.2	0.2	0.2	0.2
1-acyl-2-[^{14}C]-arachidonoyl-GPC	DG	0.4	0.4	0.5	0.5
(45,000 cpm, 20 μm)	FFA	3.4	4.4	7.8	8.9
	PA	0.4	0.4	0.4	0.4
1-acyl-2-[^{14}C]-oleoyl-GPC (35,000	DG	0.6	0.6	—	0.7
cpm, 20 μm)	FFA	0.2	—	—	4.7
	PA	0.3	—	—	0.3
1,2-[^{14}C]-palmitoyl-GPC (750,000	DG	0.4	—	—	0.8
cpm, 20 μm)	FFA	0.6	—	—	2.3
	PA	1.0	—	—	0.2

NOTE: Labeled phospholipids, either synthesized by our own laboratory or purchased from a commercial source were incubated at 37°C with rat brain synaptosomes (0.5 mg protein/ml) and sodium deoxycholate (2 mg/ml) for the time period indicated. Reaction was terminated by adding 4 volumes of chloroform/methanol (2:1, v/v) to the incubation mixture. Radioactivity of diacylglycerols (DG), free fatty acids (FFA), and phosphatidic acids (PA) were determined after separating the lipid extract by TLC. Results are expressed as percent of labeled products formed. (Data taken from Reference 31.)

Incubation of albumin-washed synaptosomes at 37°C resulted in a time-dependent increase in both saturated and unsaturated fatty acids (FIG. 4). Under this condition, the release of 20:4 was linear with time up to 60 min. To further elucidate the type of phospholipid contributing to the FFA release, synaptosomes prelabeled with 20:4 were incubated at 37°C in the presence and absence of Ca^{2+}. Under this condition, the increase in labeled 20:4 was marked by a decrease in labeled PC, PI, and PS (FIG. 5).[32]

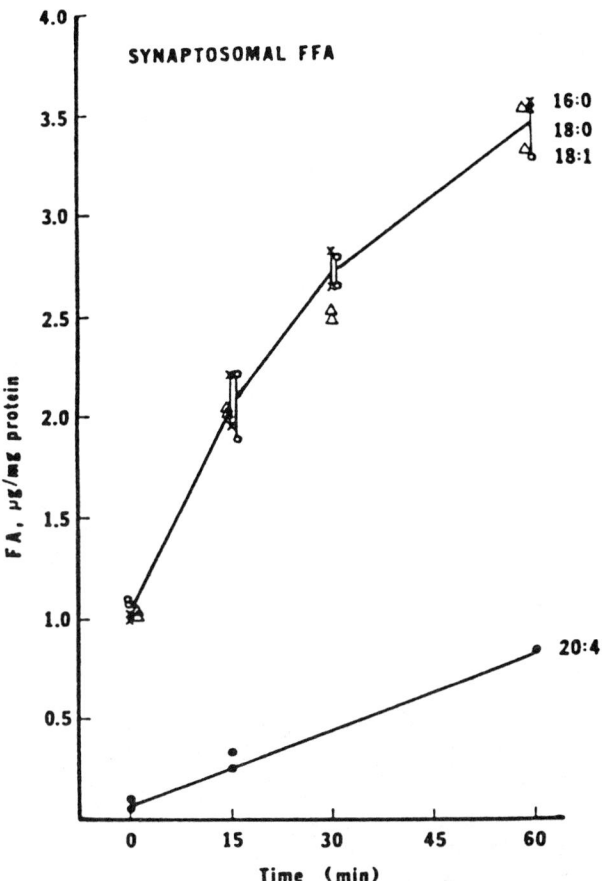

FIGURE 4. Release of free fatty acids (FFA) from synaptosomes due to incubation at 37°C. Synaptosomes were washed with bovine serum albumin prior to incubation. FFA (μg/mg protein) were converted to their methylesters and subsequently analyzed by gas-liquid chromatography. (From Sun et al.[11] Reprinted by permission from Humana Press.)

Interestingly, there was no change in labeled DG due to the incubation. Degradation of PI was completely dependent on Ca^{2+}, whereas that for PC was only partially dependent on Ca^{2+} (FIG. 5).[32] We also observed that synaptosomes isolated from ischemic brain samples had the tendency to show a higher rate of 20:4 release, as compared to synaptosomes from nonischemic samples.[33]

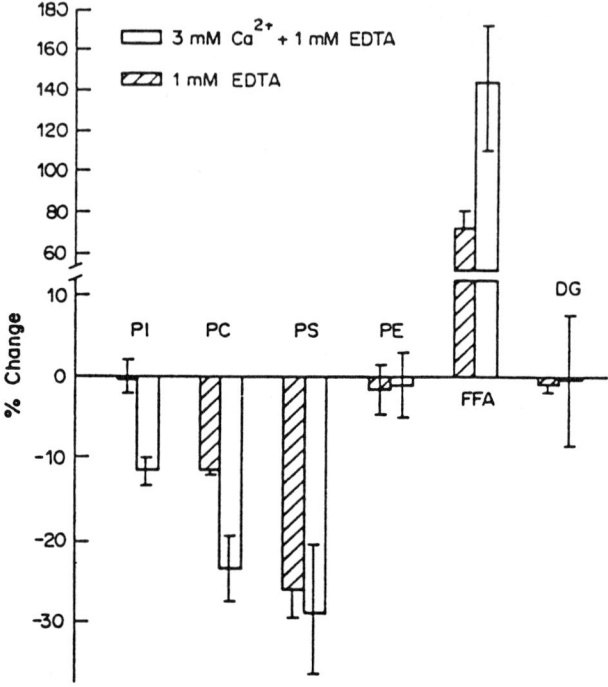

FIGURE 5. Percent change in radioactivity of phospholipids, free fatty acids (FFA), and diacylglycerols (DG) in 20:4-labeled synaptosomes after incubation in the absence (1 mM EDTA) or presence (2 mM) of Ca^{2+} for 60 min at 37°C. Each value is the mean ± SD of six separate experiments done in duplicate or triplicate. PI = phosphatidylinositol; PC = phosphatidylcholine; PS = phosphatidylserines; PE = phosphatidylethanolamine. (From Kelleher and Sun.[32] Reprinted by permission from *Neurochemistry International*.)

When synaptosomes prelabeled with [^{14}C]-20:4 were placed in a chamber and superfused with Krebs-Ringer-bicarbonate buffer containing 0.2% bovine serum albumin, subsequent depolarization of the synaptosomes by elevating the K^+ concentration in the superfusion medium from 5 to 55 mM resulted in a Ca^{2+}-dependent release of 20:4 (Fig. 6).[34] Under similar conditions, synaptosomes preloaded with [^{3}H]-norepinephrine (NE) also responded to K^+ depolarization in the release of NE in a Ca^{2+}-dependent manner. Results of these experiments suggested that stimulation of synaptosomes to elicit neurotransmitter release is associated with activation of phospholipase A_2. On examination of the prelabled phospholipids after K^+ depolarization, there was an indication that 20:4 release was derived from labeled PI and PC in the membrane fraction (Fig. 7).[35]

Release of Arachidonic Acid in the Rat Brain due to Ischemic Insult

An increase in the FFA pool in the brain is known to occur due to electroconvulsive shock and ischemia.[1-6] FFA release is apparently enzyme-mediated, since this process can be arrested after inactivation by microwave irradiation.[36] In the brain excited due to electroconvulsive shock, the increase in FFA and DG could be detected within 2 sec after shock, and these changes returned to normal within 5 min after stimulation.[37] In the decapitative ischemic model, we observed a biphasic mode of increase in FFA in the rat brain cortex.[6] The initial rapid phase (within 1 min) involved a three-fold increase in stearic acid (18:0) and 20:4. Since phosphoinositides are known to contain a high proportion of 18:0 and 20:4, the initial release of these fatty acids seems to suggest that these phospholipids may contribute to the FFA release through the DG-lipase action.[38,39] Indeed, rapid degradation of poly-PI with a concomitant increase in DG and inositol phosphates was observed in the brain due to convulsions and during the first minute of ischemic treatment.[40–44] Nevertheless, these results did not provide strong evidence for a precursor-product relationship between DG and FFA. Besides, Bazan and Birkle[45] showed that FFA increase due to electroconvulsive shock was more rapid than poly-PI breakdown and DG accumulation, further suggesting that FFA release and poly-PI breakdown may be mediated by two different mechanisms.

To further explore the source of 20:4 release due to ischemic insult, an experiment was carried out in our laboratory in which rats were injected intraventricularly with [^{14}C]-20:4. Labeled 20:4 rapidly taken up by the glycerolipids in the brain.[46] After 5 min of post-decapitative ischemic treatment, there was an increase in radioactivity in FFA and DG fractions, and a decrease in poly-PI and PC fractions (FIG. 8).[44] Based on the amount of labeled poly-PI degraded, we conclude that this decrease is not sufficient

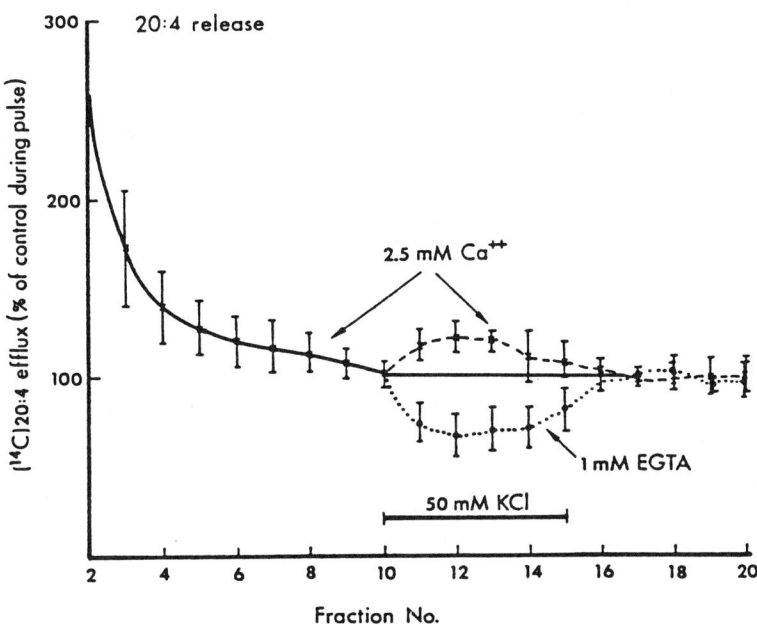

FIGURE 6. Ca^{2+}-dependent K^+-induced release of [^{14}C]-20:4 from rat brain synaptosomes. Prelabeled synaptosomes were placed in a superfusion chamber and 1 ml fractions were collected. Results depict the amount of radioactivity released during the washout period (10 min) and during the pulse, which contained either 50 mM of K^+ plus 2.5 mM of Ca^{2+} or 50 mM of K^+ plus 1 mM of EGTA. After 5 min of superfusion with the pulse media, a 5 min superfusion with the standard medium was continued. Results are expressed as percent change in radioactivity using the steady state level as 100%. Results are mean ± SD from four to six experiments in each condition. (From Lazarewicz et al.[34] Reprinted by permission from Neurochemistry International.)

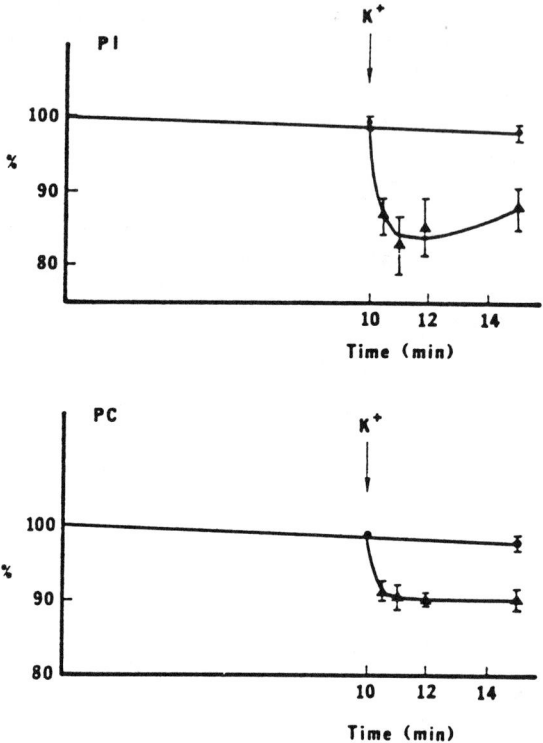

FIGURE 7. Effect of K$^+$ stimulation on synaptosomal phospholipids prelabeled with [^{14}C]-20:4. Results are expressed as percent of control values (mean ± SEM) from five experiments. (●) represents percent radioactivity of phospholipids during incubation with Krebs-Ringer-bicarbonate medium. (▲) represents values obtained after raising the K$^+$ concentration of the medium to 55 mM. (From Majewska and Sun.[35] Reprinted by permission from *Neurochemistry International*.)

to account for the amount of labeled FFA increase. On the other hand, FFA increase may be derived from the arachidonoyl-PC pool, which showed a decrease due to the ischemic treatment. The involvement of phospholipase A$_2$ acting on a specific pool of PC would also explain our earlier observation of a transient increase in lysophosphatidylcholines in the brain during the first 2 min of ischemic treatment.[47] Apparently, more studies are needed to further elucidate this mechanism.

REGULATION OF DEACYLATION-REACYLATION ACTIVITY IN THE BRAIN

Cooperativity between Fatty Acid Activation and Transfer to Phospholipids

Due to generation of lipid intermediates that possess potent detergent properties, enzymes involved in the metabolic turnover of 20:4 through the deacylation-reacylation mechanism must be stringently controlled.[10,11] The lipid intermediates, especially the acyl-CoA and lysophospholipids, are known for their membrane-perturbing properties.[48-52] Under normal conditions, only trace amounts of these compounds are present in the cell.

Since brain microsomes contain enzymes for fatty acid activation as well as the transfer of fatty acids to the lysophospholipids, there is evidence that these two enzymic processes are operated in a cooperative manner.[53,54] Thus, in the presence of 1-acyl-GPC or 1-acyl-GPI, the conversion of labeled 20:4 to its acyl-CoA is enhanced, and acyl-CoA is transferred to the lysophospholipid to form the respective phospholipids (FIG. 9).[54] This coupling effect seems to pertain mainly to the type of lysophospholipids that are good substrates of the acyltransferase, since other lyso-compounds were either not effective or inhibitory. These results further suggest that fatty acid ligase and acyltransferase are located in close proximity within the membrane, so that the newly synthesized acyl-CoA can be effectively utilized (see FIG. 12). Thus, the cooperative mechanism is important in regulating cellular levels of acyl-CoA and lysophospholipids so that these compounds would not accumulate in localized areas of the membrane.

Futile Cycle for Acyl-CoA Synthesis and Hydrolysis and Its Regulation by Lysophospholipids

It is interesting that in spite of an energy-dependent pathway for the synthesis of acyl-CoA, active acyl-CoA hydrolase is found in the brain as well as in other

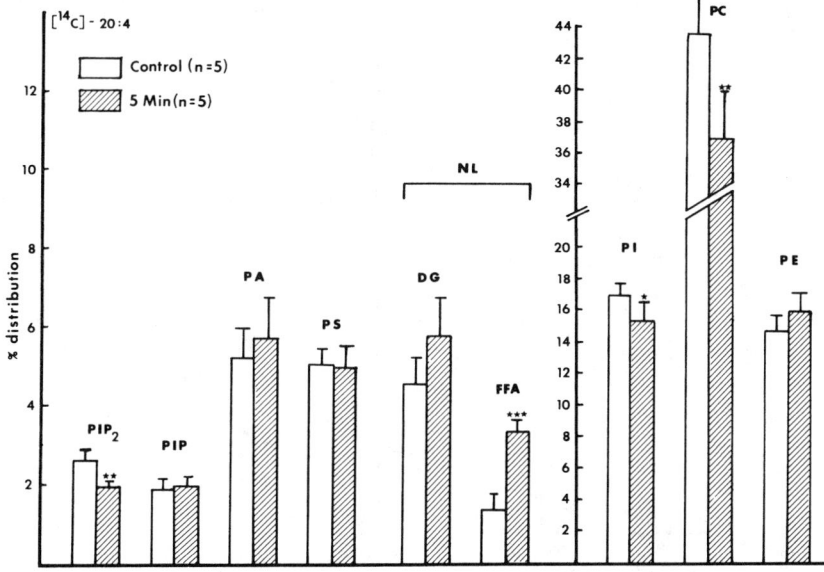

FIGURE 8. Percent distribution (mean ± SD from four to five samples) of radioactivity among individual phospholipids, free fatty acids (FFA), and diacylglycerols (DG) of rat brain cortex after intracerebral injection with [1-^{14}C]-20:4. Animals were injected 2 hr prior to ischemic treatment. Values of the 5 min ischemic samples that are significantly different from controls based on analysis of variance are indicated by *($p < 0.05$), **($p < 0.025$), and ***($p < 0.005$). PIP$_2$ = phosphatidylinositol 4,5-bisphosphate; PIP = phosphatidylinositol monophosphate; PA = phosphatidic acid; PS = phosphatidylserine; DG = diacylglycerol; PI = phosphatidylinositol; PC = phosphatidylcholine; PE = phosphatidylethanolamine; NL = neutral lipid. (From Sun.[44] Reprinted by permission from Liviana Press.)

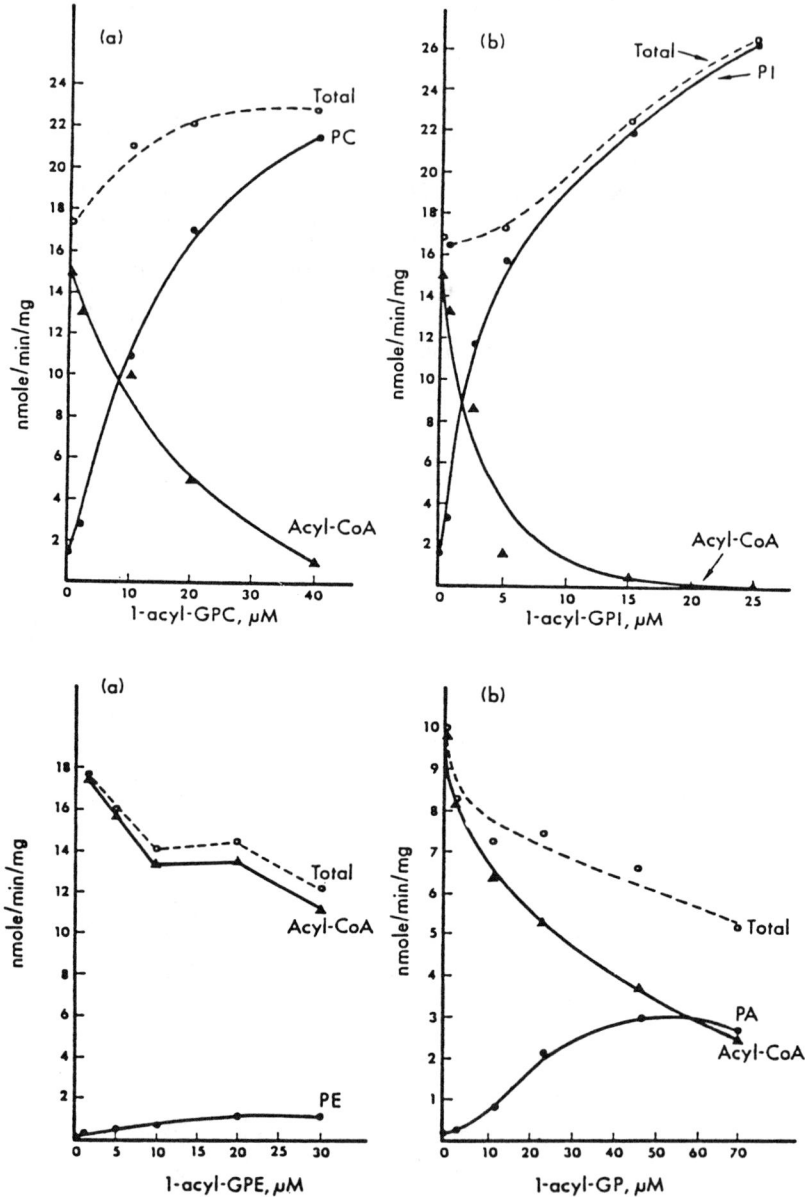

FIGURE 9. Effects of lysophospholipids on 20:4 activation to acyl-CoA and subsequent transfer to phospholipids. *Dotted line* represents total 20:4 activated in the incubation system containing brain microsomes, [^{14}C]-20:4, ATP, Mg^{2+}, CoASH, and lysophospholipids. (▲) denotes the amount of acyl-CoA recovered and (●) the amount of acyl-CoA incorporated into the respective phospholipids. PC = phosphatidylcholine, GPC = glycerophosphatidylcholine; PI = phosphatidylinositol, GPI = glycerophosphatidylinositol; PE = phosphatidylethanolamine, GPE = glycerophosphatidylethanolamine; PA = phosphatidic acid; GP = glycerophosphate. (From Tang and Sung.[54] Reprinted by permission from *Neurochemical Research*.)

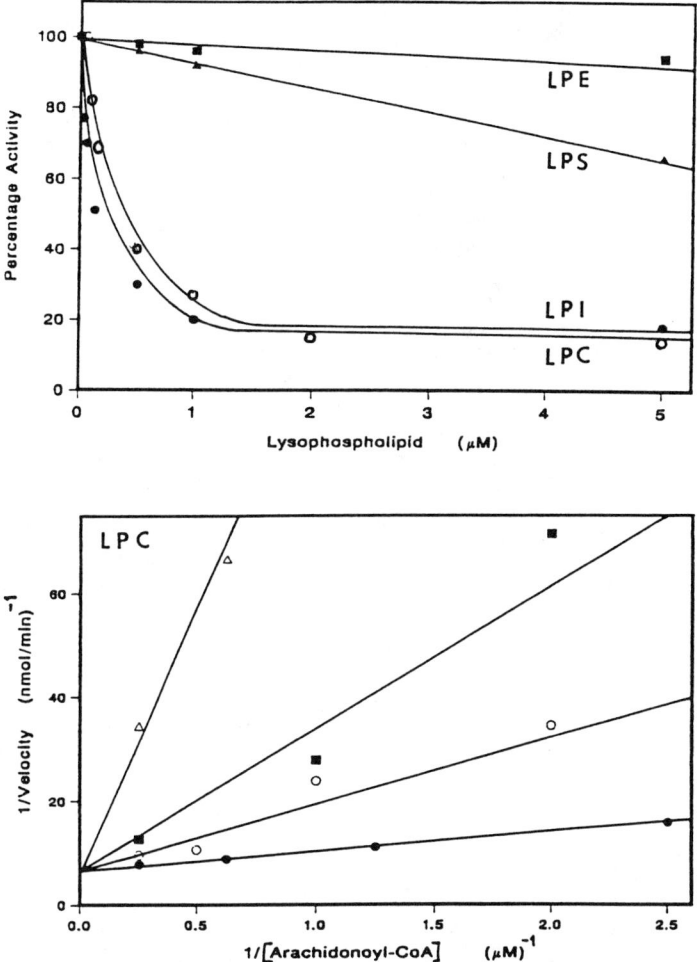

FIGURE 10. Top: Inhibition of the rate of arachidonoyl-CoA hydrolysis by lysophospholipids. Arachidonoyl-CoA concentration was 4 μM, and enzyme assays were performed using the spectrophotometer procedure. Abbreviations: LPE = lysophosphatidylethanolamine; LPS = lysophosphatidylserine; LPI = lysophosphatidylinositol; LPC = lysophosphatidylcholine. **Bottom:** Inhibition of the rate of arachidonoyl-CoA hydrolysis by lysophosphatidylcholine (LPC). Reactions were assayed either in the absence of LPC (●) or in the presence of 0.025 μM (○), 0.1 μM (■), or 0.75 μM (△) of LPC. (From Sanjanwala et al.[60] Reprinted by permission from *Archives of Biochemistry and Biophysics.*)

tissues.[55-58] Studies with long-chain acyl-CoA hydrolases purified from rat brain cytosol and bovine heart muscle microsomes indicated that this type of enzyme showed a wide degree of specificity towards long-chain acyl-CoA with little dependency on either the acyl chain length or the degree of unsaturation of the acyl group.[59,60] The presence of active acyl-CoA hydrolase strongly suggests that the accumulation of acyl-CoA is deleterious to the cellular system. Studies with acyl-CoA hydrolase in liver microsomes,[61] as well as the purified enzyme from bovine heart microsomes, indicated potent inhibition by lysophospholipids (FIG. 10).[60] Interestingly, the inhibitory effect of lysophospholipids pertains only to those that are substrates of the acyltransferase. Therefore, it is reasonable to conclude that lysophospholipids are important *in vivo* regulators of this futile cyclic event mediating the conversion of FFA to acyl-CoA.

Existence of a Distinct Membrane Pool for Enzymes in the Deacylation-Reacylation Cycle

There is increasing evidence that enzymes involved in the deacylation-reacylation cycle (including fatty acid ligase and acyl-CoA hydrolase) are present in a cluster within the same membrane domain (see Fig. 12). This enzyme cluster is probably distal from other phospholipid metabolizing enzymes, for example, lysophospholipase and phospholipase C. The existence of such domains could be demonstrated by generating 20:4-labeled PI in plasma membranes (via the acyltransferase route) and further incubating the prelabeled membranes under conditions favorable for phospholipase A_2 or phospholipase C activity. We observed that although a portion of this membrane PI pool was susceptible to hydrolysis by phospholipase A_2 on incubation in the presence of Ca^{2+}, there was no indication of hydrolysis by phospholipase C (TABLE 3).[62] Hydrolysis of the 20:4-labeled PI pool by phospholipase C could occur only if deoxycholate and Ca^{2+} were added to the incubation medium. On the other hand, exogenously added labeled PI was susceptible to hydrolysis by phospholipase C in the presence of Ca^{2+} alone (TABLE 3). These results indicate that this PI pool labeled through the action of acyltransferase is distal to phospholipase C and is probably restricted only to metabolism by enzymes involved in the deacylation-reacylation cycle. Consequently, the heterogeneity in membrane distribution of enzymes and substrates is probably an important form of regulation of the deacylation-reacylation activity *in vivo*.

TABLE 3. Hydrolysis of $[^{14}C]$-20:4-PI by Phospholipase A_2 and Phospholipase C in Rat Brain Synaptosomes: A Comparison of Reactivity between Membrane-Bound and Exogenous Substrates

	% Release			
	Membrane-Bound PI		Exogenous PI	
Incubation Condition	DG	FFA	DG	FFA
None added	trace	3.8	trace	4.5
Ca^{2+} (2 mM)	trace	7.5	15.0	4.5
Deoxycholate (1 mg/ml)	3.0	trace	7.0	trace
Ca^{2+} + deoxycholate	11.0	trace	17.0	trace

NOTE: To generate membrane-bound PI labeled with $[^{14}C]$-20:4, synaptosomes were incubated with $[^{14}C]$-20:4 in the presence of ATP, Mg^{2+}, CoASH, and a small amount of 1-acyl-GPI. Prelabeled synaptosomes were washed with 0.32 M sucrose buffer containing 1% bovine serum albumin prior to further incubation at 37°C for 30 min under the conditions described above. For a comparison, unlabeled synaptosomes were incubated with $[^{14}C]$-20:4-PI (isolated from the membrane), which was added exogenously to the incubation mixture at 37°C for the same time period. Phospholipase C activity is depicted by labeled DG formed and phospholipase A_2 by labeled FFA release. Values represent the percent radioactivity of DG and FFA formed due to incubation under the specified conditions. (Data taken from Reference 62.)

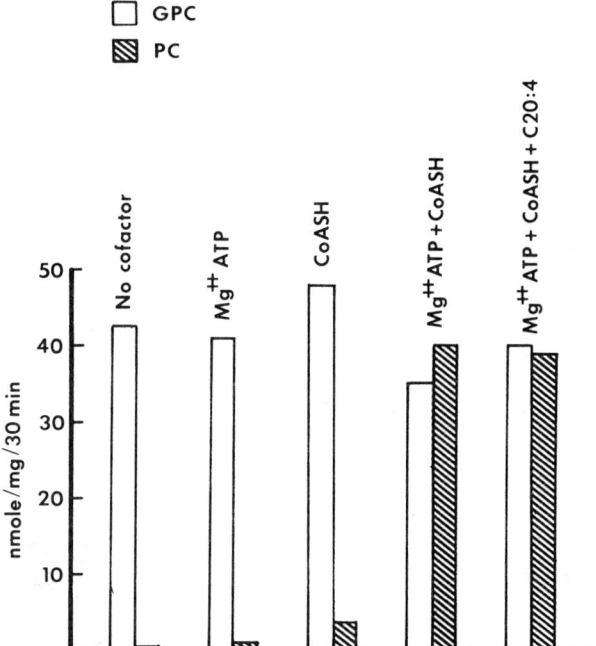

FIGURE 11. Metabolic relationship between lysophospholipase and acyl-CoA:lysophospholipid acyltransferase in the metabolism of lysophosphatidylcholines (LPC) by brain microsomes. ^{32}P-LPC were incubated with brain membranes alone or with specified cofactors added. Lysophospholipase activity is depicted by the release of labeled glycerophosphocholines (GPC) into the aqueous phase, and acyltransferase activity is depicted by the formation of labeled phosphatidylcholines (PC) after incubation with cofactors. Results indicate that lysophospholipase activity is not affected by conditions favoring the acyltransferase reaction.

Physiological Role of Lysophospholipids in Synaptic Transmission

Besides participating in the reacylation process, lysophospholipids are also known to be degraded by lysophospholipases present in the brain as well as in most other tissues.[63-67] In many cellular systems, lysophospholipase activity is found in both particulate and soluble fractions. Unlike lysophospholipid acyltransferases, in which different enzymes are responsible for specific lysophospholipids, lysophospholipase(s) seems to exhibit a rather broad specificity towards lysophospholipids with different polar head groups and acyl chains.[66] The lysophospholipase in rat brain membranes does not require Ca^{2+} for activity, although other divalent cations such as Hg^{2+}, Fe^{2+}, and Zn^{2+} potently inhibit the enzyme.[66] Although enzyme activity is also partially inhibited by both saturated and polyunsaturated fatty acids, the physiological significance of this inhibitory effect is not known. However, it is interesting to note that lysophospholipase activity is not affected by conditions favoring the acyltransferase reaction. Thus, when labeled 1-acyl-GPC was incubated with brain microsomes, lysophospholipid degradation by lysophospholipase occurred regardless of whether a portion of this substrate was reacylated by the acyltransferase (FIG. 11). Consequently, it is reasonable to speculate that lysophospholipases and acyltransferases are located in different domains within the membrane (FIG. 12).

Lysophospholipids at physiological concentrations were shown to promote membrane fusion activity[68] and alter activity of membrane-bound enzymes.[69-72] There is increasing evidence indicating that phospholipase A_2 activity in cell plasma membranes is controlled by a receptor-mediated mechanism involving GTP-binding proteins.[7-9,73,74] Studies with glioma cells further indicated that acetylcholine could simultaneously activate phospholipase C and phospholipase A_2 in the release of inositol phosphates and 20:4, respectively.[8,9] It is possible that the transient release of lysophospholipids during cell stimulation may serve a second messenger role for the

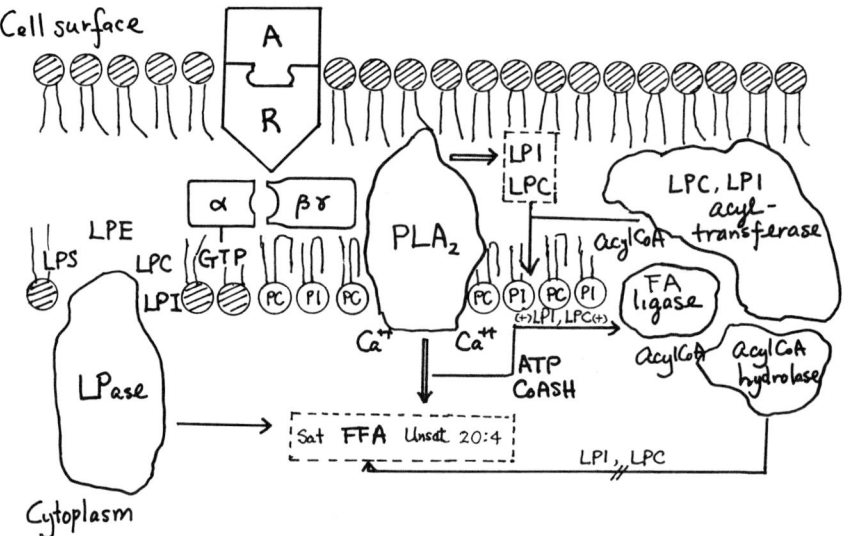

FIGURE 12. A diagram depicting the enzyme cluster involved in the deacylation-reacylation cycle. LPase = lysophospholipase; PLA_2 = phospholipase A_2; FA ligase = fatty acid:CoASH ligase; A = agonist; R = receptor; FFA = free fatty acid; LPC = lysophosphatidylcholine; LPE = lysophosphatidylethanolamine; LPI = lysophosphatidylinositol; LPS = lysophosphatidylserine; PC = phosphatidylcholine; PI = phosphatidylinositol.

secretory process as well as for other ion transport activities. Evidently, more studies are needed towards further elucidating this mechanism.

CONCLUSION

We have presented evidence that 20:4 in the brain is actively engaged in the deacylation-reacylation mechanism. The deacylation-reacylation process is maintained in a dynamic equilibrium, and stimulation of phospholipase A_2 activity is probably the initial point of activation of the cycle. There is evidence that this stimulation can be triggered by specific agonists interacting with their receptors. Arachidonic acid released through this mechanism is important in the regulation of eicosanoid biosynthesis. In addition, the lysophospholipids formed may also serve as second messengers for mediating other membrane processes. Operation of this cyclic event may provide a viable mechanism for reutilization of the lipid intermediates produced. In this regard, the level of lysophospholipids in the system seems to be a key factor for regulating the level of acyl-CoA in the reacylation process (FIG. 12). Consequently, the putative role of lysophospholipids as second messengers in the membrane signaling mechanism should not be underestimated. Future studies should be directed to elucidating the mechanisms for phospholipase A_2 activation as well as the second messenger role of 20:4 and lysophospholipids in synaptic transmission.

ACKNOWLEDGMENT

Thanks are due to Mrs. R. Kite for her help in preparation of the manuscript.

REFERENCES

1. BAZAN, N. G. 1970. Biochim. Biophys. Acta **218**: 1–10.
2. BAZAN, N. G. & H. RAKOWSKI. 1970. Life Sci. **9**: 501–507.
3. BAZAN, N. G., D. L. BIRKLE, T. S. REDDY & R. E. VADNAL. 1986. *In* Phospholipid Research and the Nervous System: Biochemical and Molecular Pharmacology. L. A. Horrocks, L. Freysz & G. Toffano, Eds.: 169–180. Liviana Press. Padova, Italy.
4. DEMEDIO, G. E., G. GORACCI, L. A. HORROCKS, J. W. LAZAREWICZ, S. MAZZARI, G. PORCELLATI, J. STROSZNAJDER & G. TROVARELLI. 1980. Ital. J. Biochem. **29**: 412–432.
5. SHIU, G. K., J. P. NEMMER & E. M. NEMOTO. 1983. J. Neurochem. **40**: 880–884.
6. TANG, W. & G. Y. SUN. 1982. Neurochem. Int. **4**(4): 269–273.
7. AXELROD, J., R. M. BURCH, C. JELSEMA. 1988. TINS **11**(13): 117–123.
8. DEGEORGE, J. J., A. H. OUSLEY, K. D. MCCARTHY, E. G. LAPETINA & P. MORELL. 1987. J. Biol. Chem. **262**: 8077–8083.
9. DEGEORGE, J. J., A. H. OUSLEY, I. D. MCCARTHY, P. MORRELL & E. G. LAPETINA. 1987. J. Biol. Chem. **262**: 9979–9983.
10. SUN, G. Y., K. L. SU, O. M. DER & W. TANG. 1979. Lipids **14**(2): 229–235.
11. SUN, G. Y., W. TANG, M. D. MAJEWSKA, D. W. HALLETT, L. FOUDIN & S. HUANG. 1983. *In* Neural Membranes. (G.Y. Sun, N. Bazan, J.-Y. Wu, G. Porcellati & A.Y. Sun, Eds.: 67–95. Humana Press. Clifton, NJ.
12. CORBIN, D. R. & G. Y. SUN. 1978. J. NEUROCHEM. **30**: 77–82.
13. BAKER, R. & W. THOMPSON. 1972. Biochim. Biophys. Acta **270**: 489–503.
14. SUN, G. Y., H-M. HUANG, J. A. KELLEHER, E. B. STUBBS, JR. & A. Y. SUN. 1988. Neurochem. Int. **12**(1): 69–77.
15. SU, K. L. & G. Y. SUN. 1978. J. Neurochem. **31**: 1043–1047.
16. SUN, G. Y. 1970. J. Neurochem. **17**: 445–446.
17. KEOUGH, K. M. W., G. MACDONALD & W. THOMPSON. 1972. Biochim. Biophys. Acta **270**: 337–347.
18. LANDS, W. E. M. & C. G. CRAWFORD. 1976. *In* The Enzymes of Biological Membranes, Vol. 2. A. Martonosi, Ed.: 3–85. Plenum Press. New York, NY.
19. REDDY, T. S. & N. G. BAZAN. 1983. Arch. Biochem. Biophys. **226**: 125–133.
20. REDDY, T. S. & N. G. BAZAN. 1985. J. Neurosci. Res. **13**: 381–390.
21. BAKER, R. R. & W. THOMPSON. 1973. J. Biol. Chem. **298**: 7060–7065.
22. SUN, G. Y., D. R. CORBIN, R. W. WISE & R. A. MACQUARRIE. 1980. Int. J. Biochem. **10**: 557–563.
23. DEKA, N., G. Y. SUN & R. MACQUARRIE. 1986. Arch. Biochem. Biophys. **246**(2): 554–563.
24. M. SANJANWALA. 1987. Ph.D. Dissertation. Univeristy of Missouri-Kansas City. Kansas City, MO.

25. FERBER, E., C. REILLY & K. RESCH. 1976. Biochim. Biophys. Acta **448:** 143–154.
26. SZAMEL, M., S. SCHNEIDER & K. RESCH. 1981. J. Biol. Chem. **256**(17): 9198–9204.
27. LIN, T.-N., R. MACQUARRIE & G. Y. SUN. 1988. Lipids. Accepted for publication.
28. STROSZNAJDER, J., L. FOUDIN, W. TANG & G. Y. SUN. 1983. J. Neurochem. **40:** 84–90.
29. WEBSTER, G. R. 1973. J. Neurochem. **21:** 873–876.
30. WOELK, H. & G. PORCELLATI. 1973. Hoppe-Seyler's Z. Physiol. Chem. **354:** 90–100.
31. DER, O. M. & G. Y. SUN. 1981. J. Neurochem. **36**(2): 355–362.
32. KELLEHER, J. A. & G. Y. SUN. 1985. Neurochem. Int. **7**(5): 825–831.
33. MAJEWSKA, M. D., R. MANNING & G. Y. SUN. 1981. Neurochem. Res. **6**(5): 567–576.
34. LAZAREWICZ, J. W., V. LEU, G. Y. SUN & A. Y. SUN. 1983. Neurochem. Int. **5:** 471–478.
35. MAJEWSKA, M. D. & G. Y. SUN. 1982. Neurochem. Int. **4**(5): 427–433.
36. SOUKUP, T. S., R. O. FRIEDEL & S. M. SHANBERG. 1978. J. Neurochem. **30:** 635–637.
37. REDDY, T. S. & N. G. BAZAN. 1987. J. Neurosci. Res. **18:** 449–455.
38. ABE, K., K. KOGURE, M. YAMAMOTO, M. IMAZAWA & K. MIYAMOTO. 1987. J. Neurochem. **48:** 503–509.
39. YOSHIDA, S., M. IKED, R. BUSTO, M. SANTISO, E. MARTINEZ & M. D. GINSBERG. 1986. J. Neurochem. **47:** 744–757.
40. BAZAN, N. G., S. A. MORELLI DE LIBERTI & E. B. RODRIGUEZ DE TURCO. 1982. Neurochem. Res. **7**(7): 839–843.
41. SUN, G. Y., H.-M. HUANG & R. CHANDROSEKHAR. 1988. Neurochem. Int. **13:** 63–68.
42. HUANG, S. F.-L. & G. Y. SUN. 1986. Neurochem. Int. **9**(1): 185–190.
43. SUN, G. Y. & S. F.-L. HUANG. 1987. Neurochem. Int. **10**(3): 361–369.
44. SUN, G. Y. 1988. *In* Phospholipids in the Nervous System, Vol. 4. N. Bazan, L. A. Horrocks & G. Toffano, Eds. Liviana Press. Padova, Italy. In press.
45. BAZAN, N. G. & D. L. BIRKLE. 1987. *In* Molecular Mechanisms of Neuronal Responsiveness. Y. H. Ehrlich, R. H. Lenox, E. Kornecki & W. O. Berry, Eds.: 45–68. Plenum. New York, NY.
46. YAU, T. M. & G. Y. SUN. 1974. J. Neurochem. **23:** 99–104.
47. SUN, G. Y. & L. L. FOUDIN. 1984. J. Neurochem. **43:** 1081–1086.
48. WELTZEIN, H. V. 1979. Biochim. Biophys. Acta **559:** 259–287.
49. ASIMAKIS, G. K. & L. A. SORDAHL. 1977. Arch. Biochem. Biophys. **179:** 200–210.
50. KAWAGUCHI, A. & K. BLOCH. 1976. J. Biol. Chem. **251:** 1406–1412.
51. VIGNAIS, P. V. 1976. Biochim. Biophys. Acta. **456:** 1–38.
52. WOOD, J. M., B. BUSH, B. J. R. PITTS & A. SCHWARTZ. 1977. Biochem. Biophys. Res. Commun. **74:** 677–684.
53. AMUR, S. G. & S. G. MURTHY. 1985. Ind. J. Biochem. **22:** 197–203.
54. TANG, W. & G. Y. SUN. 1985. Neurochem. Res. **10**(10): 1343–1353.
55. ANDERSON, A. D. & V. G. ERWIN. 1971. J. Neurochem. **18:** 1179–1186.
56. BERGE, R. K. & M. FARSTAD. 1979. Eur. J. Biochem. **95:** 89–97.
57. KNAUER, T. E. 1979. Biochem. J. **179:** 515–523.
58. SRERE, P. A., N. SEUBERT & F. LYNIN. 1959. Biochim. Biophys. Acta. **33:** 313–319.
59. LIN, A. Y., G. Y. SUN & R. MACQUARRIE. 1984. Neurochem. Res. **9**(11): 1571–1591.
60. SANJANWALA, M., G. Y. SUN & R. A. MACQUARRIE. 1987. Arch. Biochem. Biophys. **258**(2): 299–306.
61. SUN, G. Y., R. E. SMITH, K. CHAN & R. MACQUARRIE. 1980. Biochem. Biophys. Res. Commun. **94**(4): 1278–1284.
62. NAVIDI, M., R. MACQUARRIE & G. Y. SUN. 1987. Soc. Neurosci. (Abstr.) **13**(II): 1416.
63. DE JONG, J. G. N., H. VAN DEN BOSCH, D. REJKEN, & L. L. M. VAN DEENEN. 1974. Biochim. Biophys. Acta **369:** 50–63.
64. LEIBOVITZ-BENGERSHON, Z. & S. GATT. 1974. J. Biol. Chem. **249:** 1525–1529.
65. LEIBOVITZ-BENGERSHON, Z., I. KOBILER & S. GATT. 1972. J. Biol. Chem. **247:** 6840–6847.
66. SUN, G., W. TANG, S. F.-L. HUANG & R. A. MACQUARRIE. 1987. Neurochem. Res. **12:** 451–458.
67. VAN DEN BOSCH, H. & J. G. N. DE JONG. 1975. Biochim. Biophys. Acta **398:** 244–257.
68. LUCY, J. A. 1970. Nature **227:** 815–817.
69. GRAHAM, A. B. & G. C. WOOD. 1974. Biochim. Biophys. Acta **370:** 431–440.
70. HUNG, S. A. & G. MELNYKOCK. 1976. Biochim. Biophys. Acta **429:** 409–420.

71. SHIER, W. T. & J. T. TROOTER. 1976. FEBS Lett. **62:** 165–168.
72. SHIER, W. T., J. H. BALWIN, R. NILSEN-HAMILTON & N. M. THANASSI. 1976. Proc. Natl. Acad. Sci. USA **73:** 1586–1593.
73. JELSEMA, C. L. 1987. J. Biol. Chem. **262:** 163–168.
74. OKANO, Y., K. YAMADA, K. YANO & Y. NOZAWA. 1987. Biochem. Biophys. Res. Commun. **145:** 1267–1275.

Modulation of Arachidonate Turnover in Cerebral Phospholipids[a]

AMIRAM I. BARKAI AND LEELAVATI R. MURTHY

Department of Psychiatry
Columbia University College of Physicians and Surgeons and
New York State Psychiatric Institute
New York, New York 10032

INTRODUCTION

The metabolic turnover of membrane phospholipids (PL) has been shown to be closely related to the regulation of membrane functions that are linked to neuronal transmission (for reviews see References 1–5). Receptor-mediated processes that are involved in the metabolic breakdown of phosphoinositides have been studied extensively in recent years, and much attention has been given to the activation of the phospholipase C pathway that results in the formation of second messengers such as inositol-3-phosphate (IP3), which acts to mobilize intracellular calcium, and diacylglycerol (DAG), which activates protein kinase C.[4-6] However, the phospholipase C pathway is only one of several enzymatic pathways that are involved in PL degradation. FIGURE 1 illustrates the major enzymes acting on a typical phosphoinositide molecule and their metabolic by-products. There are not many studies that address the question of whether or not receptor-mediated processes also affect the turnover of the acyl moieties of membrane phospholipids. The activation of phospholipase A-1 or A-2 enzymes could enhance the formation of lyso-PL and free fatty acids (FFA). These products are very effective in modifying the activity of membrane-bound enzymes,[7-11] and their levels in the membrane are extremely important for membrane functions.[12-13] The levels of FFA and lyso-PL in the membrane are controlled, to a large extent, by processes of deacylation and reacylation of PL (FIG. 2). Reacylation is an ATP-dependent process that is initiated by the conversion of the FFA to its acyl-CoA derivative prior to reincorporation into lyso-PL.[14,15] The deacylation-reacylation processes that involve arachidonic acid (AA) are of major interest in neuronal tissue, since the release of AA leads to the formation of prostaglandins and other eicosanoids that act as modulators of neurotransmission.[16-20] Incorporation studies of labeled AA into brain PL have shown preferential uptake into phosphatidylinositol (PI) and phosphatidylcholine (PC),[21-23] indicating that these PL serve as metabolically active sources for AA and its metabolites in cerebral tissue.

The mechanisms responsible for the modulation of deacylation-reacylation processes have not been thoroughly investigated. Several neurotransmitters have been shown previously to be capable of stimulating AA release in neuronal preparations,[24-26] but their effects on deacylation and reacylation of AA-containing PL have not been investigated in detail. A previous study from our laboratory[27] has demonstrated that AA incorporation into PI can be enhanced in the presence of norepinephrine (NE) or serotonin (5HT), while its incorporation into other PL was significantly reduced. This

---

[a]This work was supported in part by National Institute of Mental Health Grant No. 33690 to A.I.B.

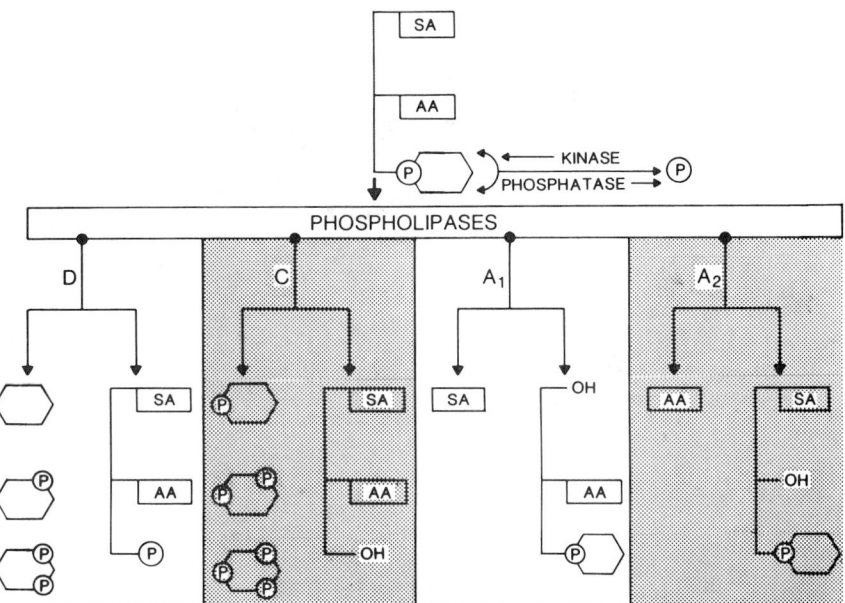

FIGURE 1. Major enzymes that may act on a phosphatidylinositol (PI) molecule. Kinase and phosphatase activities regulate the formation of polyphosphoinositides, which may be acted upon by a specific phospholipase C to produce the second messengers IP-3 and DAG. Only three species of inositol phosphates are depicted here, although the formation of more is possible. The phospholipases A-1 and A-2 act to form FFA and lyso-PI. Since cerebral PI is enriched in AA at the 2 position, the activation of phospholipase A-2 would result in enhanced release of AA and the formation of eicosanoids. At least some of the products of the AA cascade may act as second messengers or modulators of signal transduction. Both phospholipase C and A-2 may be activated by neurotransmitter-receptor interactions. SA = stearic acid, AA = arachidonic acid.

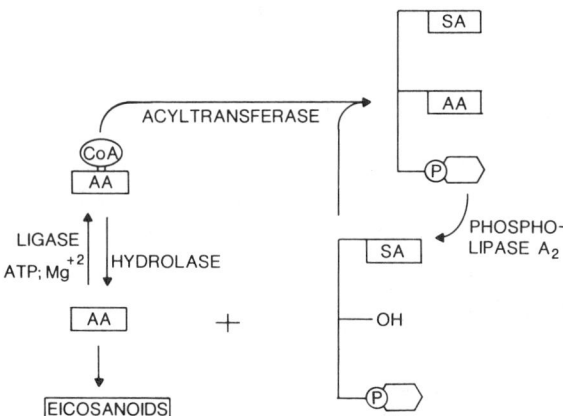

FIGURE 2. A deacylation-reacylation cycle involving a phosphatidylinositol (PI) molecule. The activities of phospholipase A and acyltransferase regulate the amount of free arachidonic acid (AA) and lyso-PI in the membrane. Higher levels of AA would result in enhanced formation of eicosanoids. There is evidence that specific acyltransferases exist for individual phospholipids species.

observation was made with rat cerebral cortex slices, in which cell integrity was largely preserved. The increased AA incorporation into PI was not seen, however, when cortical membranes were used instead of the slice preparation. We describe here experiments that were designed to extend our original observations and examine the dose-effect relationship of both NE and 5HT. We have also addressed the questions of whether or not the observed effects were mediated by neurotransmitter receptors and whether or not these effects require a functionally intact system for the reuptake of NE or 5HT by presynaptic nerve terminals. In addition, we investigated the possible involvement of hydrogen peroxide that is formed by the action of monoamine oxidase (MAO) on the neurotransmitter. We examined the structure-activity relationships of other related compounds, and we conducted experiments aimed at investigating whether the neurotransmitter acts on enzymes that enhance acylation, on enzymes that enhance deacylation, or on both types of enzymes.

METHODS

Materials

[5,6,8,9,11,12,14,15,-3H] Arachidonic acid (sp. act. 84 Ci/mmole) was obtained from New England Nuclear Corporation (Boston, MA). NE, 5HT, carbamylcholine (CCH), propranolol, isoproterenol, clonidine, phenylephrine, pargyline, mepacrine, and ATP were obtained from Sigma (St. Louis, MO). Coenzyme A (CoA) was obtained from Calbiochem (San Diego, CA). Phospholipid standards were obtained from Supelco (Bellefonte, PA). Ketanserin was obtained from Janssen Pharmaceutical Company (Piscataway, NJ). Methysergide was obtained from Sandoz (Hanover, NJ). High performance thin layer chromatography plates (HPTLC), precoated with Silica Gel 60, were purchased from VWR Scientific (South Plainfield, NJ). Reagents used for buffer preparations, protein determination, scintillation counting, and other purposes were obtained from commercial sources. Prazosin was a kind gift from Pfizer (Groton, CT), and delta-9-tetrahydrocannabinol (THC) was a kind gift of Dr. Michael Kogan of the New York State Psychiatric Institute Neurotoxicology Division.

Preparation of Brain Slices

Adult male Sprague-Dawley rats (250–300 g) were decapitated and their brains removed rapidly. Cerebral cortex tissue was dissected over ice and cross-chopped (350 × 350 μm) with a McIlwain tissue slicer. The slices were placed in a glass vial containing 3 ml Krebs Ringer (KRB) and gassed with a mixture of oxygen (95%) and carbon dioxide (5%). The slices were allowed to settle, and the supernatant was discarded. Aliquots of the slices' slurry (25 μl; 1 mg protein) were transferred to individual vials for assaying the incorporation of 3[H]-AA into PL.

Assay of 3[H]-AA Incorporation

Each assay tube contained slices representing 1 mg protein in a final volume of 0.45 ml KRB. The slices were preincubated for 30 min at 37°C under 95% oxygen and 5% carbon dioxide in the presence and absence of tested neurotransmitters, or drugs, or combinations of both. The incorporation of 3[H]-AA was initiated by the addition of

50 μl KRB solution containing 0.25 μCi 3[H]-AA and ATP, CoA, and Mg^{++} to produce final concentrations of 2.5 mM, 0.1 mM, and 10 mM, respectively. The incubation was continued for 5 additional minutes (or for longer periods of time when kinetics were studied) and the reaction terminated by adding 1.5 ml mixture of chloroform:methanol (1:2) followed by the addition of 1 ml chloroform and 0.5 ml water. After separation of the lower phase, aliquots were taken for determination of total radioactivity and for the separation of individual PL on potassium-oxalate-impregnated HPTLC plates that were heat-activated at 110°C for 15 minutes. The chromatography system used was according to Jolles et al.[28] Individual PL were detected by iodine vapor, and PL spots were scraped off the plate into scintillation vials for radioactivity determinations. The results were expressed as percent of total radioactivity in the incubation system that was incorporated into a given PL representing 1 mg of tissue protein as determined by the method of Lowry et al.[29]

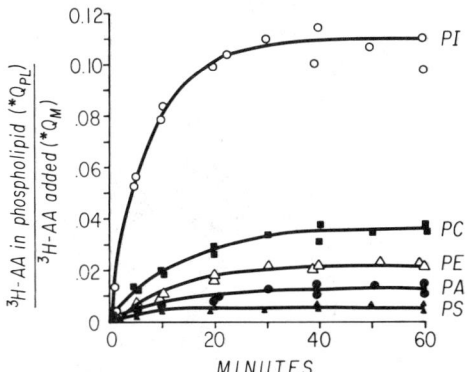

FIGURE 3. Incorporation of 3[H]-AA with time into various phospholipids (PL) during incubation of cortical slices with 0.25 μCi 3[H]-AA, 2.5 mM ATP, 0.1 mM CoA, and 10 mM Mg^{+2}. *Qpl denotes the amount of PL-bound 3[H]-AA, and *Qm denotes the amount of free 3[H]-AA added at 0 time (0.25 μCi). The curves representing 3[H]-AA accumulation in individual PL were analyzed according to a closed two-compartmental model (see FIG. 4) to obtain the kinetic parameters presented in TABLE 1.

RESULTS AND DISCUSSION

Kinetics of 3[H]-AA Incorporation into Phospholipids

When cortical slices were incubated with 3[H]-AA in the presence of ATP, Mg^{+2}, and CoA and the accumulation of 3[H]-AA in the PL was measured as a function of time, it was found that the labeling of individual PL increased in accordance with an exponential function of time and reached an apparent asymptotic value. In control experiments the highest asymptotic value was obtained for PI, whereas the lowest value was obtained for phosphatidylserine (PS). The curves representing change of radioactivity with time are presented in FIGURE 3. These curves were analyzed according to a closed two-compartmental model.[30] One compartment represented free 3[H]-AA in the incubation system (*Qf), and the other compartment represented PL-bound 3[H]-AA (*Qb). The model and the equation used for the fitting of the experimental data are presented in FIGURE 4. The values for Kfb and Kbf were obtained by nonlinear regression analysis of the experimental data using a PC NONLIN computer program (Statistical Consultants Inc., Lexington, KY). This analysis revealed that in cortical slices the values for Kfb varied from 0.011 per min for PI to 0.0006 per min for PS, whereas the values for Kbf remained within a relatively narrow range (from 0.067 for PC to 0.098 for PS). In this model, under steady state conditions, the ratio Kfb/Kbf is equal to the ratio Qb/Qf, where Qb represents the metabolically active pool of PL-bound AA. Thus, when Kfb and Kbf are known, estimation of Qf could provide information about the size of the PL-bound pool, Qb. An example of data analysis according to this model is presented in FIGURE 5 for the PI-bound metabolically active AA pool. This analysis reveals that the size of the

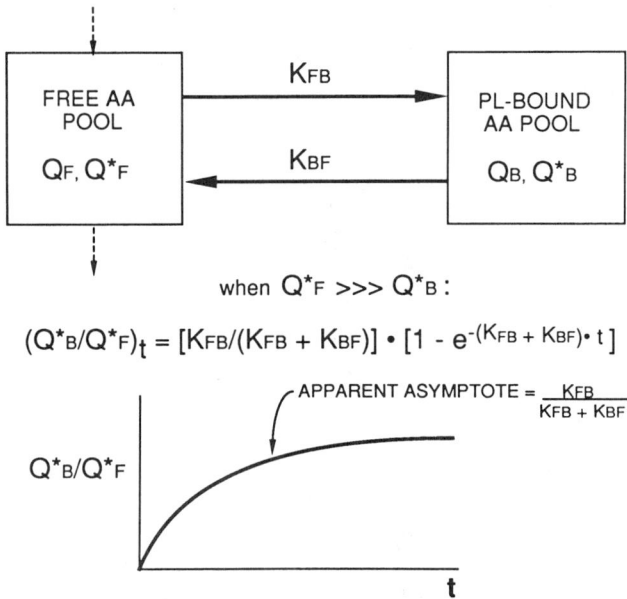

FIGURE 4. The closed two compartmental model used for analysis of the data presented in FIGURE 3. The experimental data were fitted to the exponential function shown, and the estimates of the rate constants were obtained by nonlinear regression analysis using the PC NONLIN computer program.

PI-bound AA pool that turns over rapidly to provide free AA and lyso-PI within a relatively short time was 0.36 nmols, or 0.75% of the total amount of 48 nmols PI available in the system (rat cortex tissue was found to contain 48 nmoles PI per mg protein). The Kbf value determines the half-life (T1/2) of the metabolically active PI-bound AA pool, which in the case of PI was calculated as 7.7 min. Values for the pool size and T1/2 obtained for other PL are presented in TABLE 1.

The finding that Kfb values for individual PL varied markedly whereas Kbf values remained within a relatively narrow range indicates that the differences in accumulation of 3[H]-AA in the slice PL with time probably stem from differences in the rates of acylation of individual PL, while the rates of deacylation are not appreciably different. The possibility that individual PL are acylated at different rates is supported

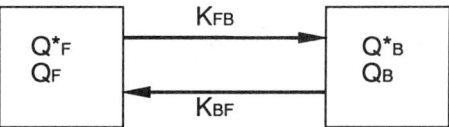

AT A STEADY STATE: $Q_B/Q_F = K_{FB}/K_{BF}$
EXAMPLE FOR PI-AA:

$K_{FB} = 0.011 \cdot \text{min}^{-1}$
$K_{BF} = 0.090 \cdot \text{min}^{-1}$

$Q_F = 3.3$ nmol (measured by GC)
$Q_B = 0.36$ nmol (total PI in incubation = 48 nmol)

$T_{1/2}(Q_B) = 0.693/K_{BF} = 7.7$ min

FIGURE 5. An example of data analysis according to the compartmental model. Data obtained for 3[H]-AA accumulation in PI with time were analyzed as explained in FIGURE 4, and the rate constants Kfb and Kbf were found. The amount of free AA, Qf, in the incubation system was estimated by gas chromatography analysis, and the Qb value was then derived. The value of 0.36 nmols found for Qb represents the size of the PI-bound AA pool that is readily exchangeable with the pool of free AA in the system. This metabolically active PI-bound AA pool represents only 0.75% of the total PI in the incubation system. The T1/2 value for this pool was calculated as 7.7 minutes.

by the findings of Corbin and Sun,[22] which indicated that separate acyl transferase enzymes exist for the acylation of individual lyso-PL in cerebral tissue.

The compartmental analysis also revealed that the pool of PL-bound AA that is active in deacylation-reacylation processes is distributed differentially among the various PL. Thus more than 50% of this pool is located in PI, but only 0.75% of the total PI molecules in the slice preparation appear to be active in deacylation-reacylation processes involving AA. The percentage of active molecules among other PL was found to be much smaller. The small fraction of PL molecules that appear to be active in the deacylation and reacylation of AA might represent only molecules that are located on membrane surface. Alternatively, the present system represents exchange of PL-bound

TABLE 1. Pool Size, Rate Constants, and Half-Life Values for the Metabolically Active PL-Bound AA Pool in Rat Brain Slices

PL[a]	PL Content[b] (Nmol/Incubation)	Rate Constants (Per Minute)		Metabolically Active pL-Bound AA Pool (Nmol/Incubation)	T1/2 (minutes)
		Kfb	Kbf		
PI	48	0.0121	0.096	0.36	7.7
PC	350	0.0032	0.067	0.17	10.3
PE	420	0.0023	0.091	0.07	8.2
PA	64	0.0010	0.069	0.03	10.0
PS	92	0.0006	0.098	0.02	7.1

[a]PL = phospholipid; PI = phosphatidylinositol; PC = phosphatidylcholine; PE = phosphatidylethanolamine; PA = phosphatidic acid; PS = phosphatidylserine.
[b]Based on estimation in cortex tissue containing 1 mg protein.

AA with a distinct AA pool that is readily accessible to exogenously added AA but may not be readily exchangeable with other intracellular pools of free AA.

Effects of Neurotransmitters

The effects of NE and 5HT on the incorporation of 3[H]-AA into individual PL were investigated after preincubation of the slice preparation for 30 min in the presence of the neurotransmitter, followed by additional 5-min incubation in the presence of 3[H]-AA, ATP, Mg^{+2}, and CoA. Initial experiments that were conducted with relatively high concentrations of NE (1 mM) or 5HT (2.5 mM) resulted in a marked increase in 3[H]-AA incorporation into PI, accompanied by a significant decrease of the 3[H]-AA incorporation into other PL (FIG. 6). In subsequent experiments it was demonstrated that the changes observed with both NE and 5HT were concentration-dependent. In the case of PI, the enhanced incorporation of 3[H]-AA reached a maximal value that was 2–3 fold higher than the level observed with the absence of the neurotransmitter. The concentration-effect relationships indicate that the processes that determine the rate of 3[H]-AA incorporation into PI in rat cortical slices are more sensitive to NE than to 5HT (FIG. 7).

The effects of NE and 5HT are mediated in part by activation of phospholipase A-2 and the formation of lyso-PL prior to reacylation by acyl-transferase enzymes. Previous investigators have demonstrated that neurotransmitters stimulate AA release from membrane PL,[4,24–26] most probably by enhancing phospholipase A-2 activity. It is not clear, however, if the enhanced AA release by neurotransmitters is receptor-mediated. If the process is receptor-mediated, it is possible that the activation of phospholipase A-2 enzymes could be linked to the interaction of the neurotransmitter with its own receptor; or, alternatively, the AA release may be secondary to the

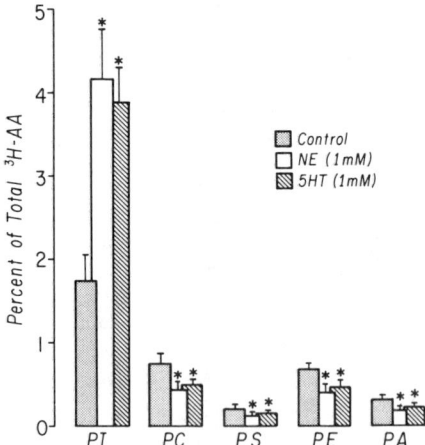

FIGURE 6. Effects of norepinephrine (NE) and serotonin (5HT) on the incorporation of 3[H]-AA into individual phospholipids in rat cortical slices. Slices (1 mg protein) were incubated for 30 min in the absence (control) or presence of the neurotransmitter. Then 3[H]-AA, ATP, CoA, and Mg^{+2} were added and the incubation continued for an additional 5 min. Phospholipids were separated and analyzed for radioactivity, as described in the test. * = significantly different from controls, $p < 0.01$.

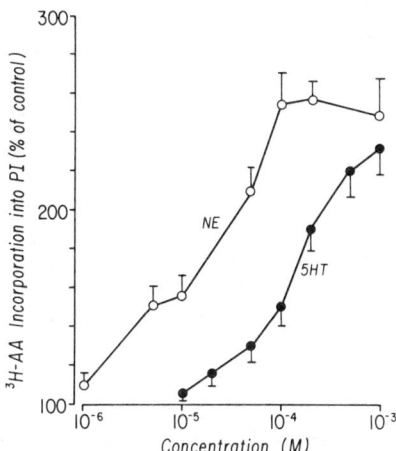

FIGURE 7. Dose-related changes in 3[H]-AA incorporation into phosphatidylinositol (PI). Each *point* represents a mean of 4–8 experiments. Note that the system is more sensitive to norepinephrine (NE) than to serotonin (5HT).

activation of phospholipase C and the formation of DAG, which is then deacylated by a specific DAG lipase. The latter pathway has been demonstrated in other cell types (for review see References 4, 5, and 18). To investigate whether the NE- or 5HT-induced changes in 3[H]-AA incorporation into PI and other PL were mediated by NE or 5HT receptors, the slices were incubated in the presence of various pharmacological agents known for their effects on NE or 5HT receptors. When the beta-adrenergic agonist isoproterenol was applied at a concentration of 100 μM, it had an effect similar to that seen in the presence of NE, whereas the application of the alpha-1 agonist phenylephrine (100 μM), or the alpha-2 agonist clonidine (100 μM) did not produce significant changes in 3[H]-AA incorporation into any of the examined PL. The application of the beta-adrenergic blocker propranolol (100 μM) or the alpha-1 blocker prazosin in the presence of NE failed, however, to antagonize the NE-induced changes. In a similarly designed experiment application of the 5HT receptor blockers methysergide or ketanserin did not produce a significant antagonistic effect on the 5HT-induced changes in the incorporation of 3[H]-AA into PL (TABLE 2).

The results obtained by pharmacological manipulations of NE or 5HT receptors did not support the hypothesis that the changes induced by the neurotransmitter in 3[H]-AA incorporation into PL were receptor-mediated. Although the beta-adrenergic agonist isoproterenol produced effects similar to those produced by NE, these effects were not antagonized by the beta blocker propranolol. However, the pharmacological manipulations of NE or 5HT receptors in testing effects on deacylation and reacylation processes of membrane PL encounter some difficulties that are related to the cationic amphiphilic nature of many of the drugs used for this purpose. Cationic amphiphilic drugs are likely to affect PL metabolism in cerebral tissue.[31] We found that propranolol at concentrations higher than 0.5 mM reduced substantially the incorporation of 3[H]-AA into PI. Thus, the significance of testing the effects of higher concentrations of this drug on the isoproterenol-induced increase in 3[H]-AA incorporation into PI was questionable. Clearly, the question of whether or not the neurotransmitter-induced effects are receptor-mediated needs further research. The

TABLE 2. Effects of Agonists and Antagonists of Norepinophrine (NE) and Serotonin (5HT) Receptors on the Incorporation of ³H-AA into Phospholipids in the Cerebral Cortex Slice of the Rat

Treatment	³H-AA Incorporation: % of Control					Comments[a]
	PI	PC	PS	PE	PA	
NE (50 µM)	217 ± 18	73 ± 6	82 ± 4	68 ± 11	76 ± 8	a
NE (100 µM)	247 ± 15	53 ± 4	76 ± 5	52 ± 6	48 ± 7	a
Isoproterenol (100 µM)	265 ± 20	54 ± 4	58 ± 4	39 ± 4	37 ± 9	a
Clonidine (100 µM)	108 ± 3	86 ± 8	103 ± 5	105 ± 7	94 ± 12	b
Phenylephrine (100 µM)	105 ± 7	100 ± 4	106 ± 5	108 ± 14	79 ± 11*	b
Propranolol (100 µM)	101 ± 8	80 ± 7*	80 ± 7*	78 ± 6*	102 ± 6	b
+ NE (50 µM)	207 ± 3	55 ± 8	54 ± 10	50 ± 12	57 ± 8	a, c
+ Isoproterenol (100 µM)	262 ± 18	53 ± 6	51 ± 8	40 ± 11	38 ± 9	a, c
Prazosin (100 µM)	113 ± 17	95 ± 8	116 ± 16	115 ± 14	89 ± 12	b
+ NE (100 µM)	265 ± 30	56 ± 6	66 ± 8	54 ± 9	59 ± 7	a, c
5HT (100 µM)	158 ± 2	99 ± 3	61 ± 4	48 ± 5	48 ± 6	a
Ketanserin (100 µM)	120 ± 5*	96 ± 4	91 ± 6	86 ± 2*	82 ± 4*	b
+ 5HT (100 µM)	180 ± 12	105 ± 3	68 ± 1	39 ± 6	62 ± 8	a, d
Methysergide (100 µM)	122 ± 6*	113 ± 12	95 ± 7	102 ± 8	88 ± 9	b
+ 5HT (100 µM)	168 ± 3	N.D.	69 ± 2	38 ± 6	39 ± 9	a, d

NOTE: Abbreviations as in TABLE 1.

[a] a = Values are significantly different from controls ($p > 0.01$), Student's t-test. b = Values are not significantly different from controls except when marked by *, which indicates $p < 0.05$ compared to control. c = Value for blocker + agonist (NE or isoproterenol) are not significantly different from values obtained with agonist alone, except when marked with *. d = Values for 5HT + blocker are not different from values obtained with 5HT alone.

use of stereoisomers of NE or isoproterenol as well as the application of more hydrophilic beta-receptor blockers such as atenolol or timolol, may provide additional information regarding the mode of action of NE on the deacylation-reacylation processes.

Is the Presynaptic Uptake System Involved?

Since pharmacological manipulations of established NE or 5HT receptors did not appear to modify significantly the neurotransmitter-induced changes in 3[H]-AA incorporation into PL, it was of interest to investigate the possibility that the observed effects are presynaptic in nature. It is possible that presynaptic uptake of NE or 5HT and the subsequent storage of these compounds in presynaptic vesicles involve changes in deacylation-reacylation processes within presynaptic membranes. To examine

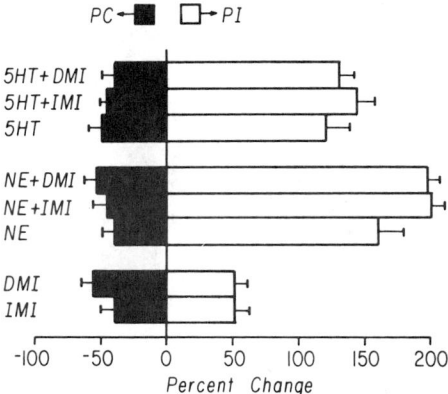

FIGURE 8. Effects of imipramine (IMI), desipramine (DMI) (100 μM each) and their application in combination with norepinephrine (NE) (100 μM) and serotonin (5HT) (500 μM) on the incorporation of 3[H]-AA into phosphatidylinositol (PI) and phosphatidylcholine (PC). Note the slight additive effect obtained when the drug and neurotransmitter were applied together.

whether or not a functional reuptake system for NE or 5HT was required for the neurotransmitter-induced changes in 3[H]-AA incorporation, the two tricyclic antidepressants imipramine (IMI) and desipramine (DMI) were used. These drugs are active in blocking the reuptake of 5HT or NE by presynaptic nerve terminals.[32] When cortical slices were preincubated with either IMI or DMI in the absence of the neurotransmitters, it was found that both drugs increased the incorporation of 3[H]-AA into PI while decreasing the 3[H]-AA incorporation into PC (FIG. 8). Preincubation of slices with IMI or DMI in the presence of the neurotransmitter resulted in an apparent additive effect on the increase of 3[H]-AA incorporation into PI (FIG. 8). The finding that both IMI and DMI had no antagonistic effect on neurotransmitter-induced changes in 3[H]-AA incorporation indicates that reuptake of the neurotransmitter does not play an important role in producing the neurotransmitter effect. The observation that the combined application of the drug and the neurotransmitter produced additive effects indicates that the drug effects probably

TABLE 3. Relationship between Compound Structure and Its Activity in Modifying 3[H]-AA Incorporation into Phosphatidylinositol (PI) and Phosphatidylcholine (PC)

Compound (100 μM)	Ring Structure	Side Chain	^{3}[H]-AA Incorporation (% of Control)	
			PI	PC
	Phenyl ring			
Norepinephrine	3—,4—,OH	CHOHCH$_2$NH$_2$	226 + 18^a	58 + 3^a
Isoproterenol	3—,4—,OH	CHOHCH$_2$NHCH(CH$_3$)$_2$	243 + 23^a	60 + 3^a
Dopamine	3—,4—,OH	CH$_2$CH$_2$NH$_2$	124 + 6^b	75 + 7^b
L-Dopa	3—,4—,OH	CH$_2$CH(NH$_2$)COOH	114 + 5	72 + 6^b
DOPAC	3—,4—,OH	CH$_2$COOH	116 + 10	103 + 8
DHPG	3—,4—,OH	CHOHCH$_2$OH	139 + 6^a	67 + 3^a
Normetaneph.	4—OH, 3—OCH$_3$	CHOHCH$_2$NH$_2$	101 + 8	93 + 6
Caffeic acid	3—,4—,OH	CH=CHCOOH	37 + 5^a	53 + 3^a
Dimethoxycinnamic acid	3—,4—,OCH$_3$	CH=CHCOOH	112 + 8	116 + 7
Homogentisic acid	2—,5—,OH	CH$_2$COOH	26 + 3^a	55 + 5^a
Tyramine	4—OH	CH$_2$CH$_2$NH$_2$	114 + 5	78 + 9^b
	Indole ring			
5HT	5—OH indole	CH$_2$CH$_2$NH$_2$	148 + 6^a	63 + 3^a
5HTP	5—OH indole	CH$_2$CH(NH$_2$)COOH	88 + 5	72 + 6^b
5HIAA	5—OH indole	CH$_2$COOH	93 + 11	98 + 3

^{a}Significantly different from control, $p < 0.01$.
^{b}Significantly different from control, $p < 0.05$.

were mediated by mechanisms that are different from those producing the neurotransmitter effect. The effects of IMI or DMI may be attributed, in part, to their cationic amphiphilic characteristics. Prolonged administration of DMI to fibroblast cultures has been shown to produce a significant increase in the concentration of PI, suggesting that this drug inhibits PI-specific phospholipase C.[33] It is possible that IMI and DMI also inhibit PI-specific phospholipase A-2 in a manner similar to that observed after adding cationic amphiphilic drugs to rat liver lysosomes.[34] Clearly, more research is needed to investigate the mode of action of these drugs on deacylation-reacylation processes of cerebral PL.

Structure-Activity Studies

Catecholamines have been reported to stimulate the biosynthesis of prostaglandins in a variety of tissues, probably by enhancing the release of AA from tissue PL (for review see Reference 35). It has been suggested that the observed effects on this metabolic pathway of AA required a catechol nucleus and an ethylamine side chain.[36] These observations prompted our interest in examining whether or not similar structure-activity requirements exist for the observed effects on 3[H]-AA incorporation into PL. Compounds containing a catechol nucleus, hydroxyl groups in other ring positions, deaminated or methoxy- metabolites of such compounds, and compounds with side chains of other natures, as well as 5HT related compounds were investigated. The results are presented in TABLE 3. While these results should be regarded as preliminary observations of possible structure-activity relationships, they indicate that the structural requirements for stimulating 3[H]-AA incorporation into PI differ from those required for attenuating 3[H]-AA incorporation into PC. As mentioned previously, the enhanced incorporation into PI was probably due to activation of a lyso-PI specific arachidonyl transferase, whereas the decreased rate of incorporation into PC was probably a result of enhanced release of AA due to activation of deacylation processes. Decreased 3[H]-AA incorporation, which was most probably associated with enhancement of PC deacylation, required the presence of two hydroxyl groups in the aromatic ring. The nature of the side chain or a presence of an amine group did not appear to be critical. Thus, except for DOPAC, all the tested compounds containing two hydroxyl groups in the aromatic ring were effective in attenuating 3[H]-AA incorporation into PC. DOPAC and 5HIAA, both acetic acid derivatives, had no significant effect on 3[H]AA incorporation, but homogentisic acid, also a derivative of acetic acid, was very potent in attenuating 3[H]-AA incorporation into both PC and PI. Formation of methyl ethers of one or both of the hydroxyl groups completely abolished these effects. Thus, while norepinephrine stimulated 3[H]-AA incorporation into PI and attenuated its incorporation into PC, norepinephrine's methylated metabolite, normetanephrine, had no significant effect on 3[H]-AA incorporation to either PI or PC. Similarly, caffeic acid (3,4,dihydroxy cinnamic acid) was very potent in reducing 3[H]-AA incorporation into both PC and PI, whereas its dimethyl ether (dimethoxy cinnamic acid) was ineffective.

The results also indicated that compounds that acted to increase 3[H]-AA incorporation into PI had a catechol nucleus and an additional hydroxyl group at the beta position on the side chain. Thus, compounds such as NE, isoproterenol, and DHPG were effective in producing this stimulatory effect. It is possible that this molecular configuration may be effective in stimulating a lyso-PI specific arachidonyl transferase. On the other hand, the observation that caffeic acid and homogentisic acid both acted to decrease substantially the 3[H]-AA incorporation into PI indicates that these compounds may act as inhibitors of a lyso-PI–specific arachidonyl transferase. Further studies are clearly needed to determine whether or not specific structural requirements exist for stimulating PL deacylation and whether or not other molecular configurations are preferred for stimulating reacylation.

Is the Neurotransmitter Effect Related to H_2O_2 Formation?

Polgar and Taylor[37] have shown that hydrogen peroxide (H_2O_2) is a strong stimulator of AA release and prostaglandin synthesis in intact cells. Since hydrogen peroxide is a by-product of MAO activity, it was of interest to examine the effects of both hydrogen peroxide and MAO inhibitors on NE- or 5HT-induced changes in 3[H]-AA incorporation into PL.

Slices were preincubated in the presence or absence of NE, with or without the addition of H_2O_2, catalase, and the MAO inhibitor pargyline or tranylcypromine, and the incorporation of 3[H]-AA into PL was assayed as described previously. The results of these experiments are summarized in TABLE 4. The presence of 100 μM H_2O_2 in the incubation medium reduced significantly the incorporation of 3[H]-AA into both PI and PC. This effect was found to be concentration-dependent and was abolished by the addition of catalase. The attenuation of 3[H]-AA incorporation into both PI and PC in these experiments may be explained by stimulated AA release in the presence of H_2O_2 as described by Polgar and Taylor.[37] However, addition of catalase or MAO inhibitors had no significant effect on the NE-induced changes in 3[H]-AA incorporation into PL (TABLE 4). These results indicate that the observed effects of NE on 3[H]-AA incorporation into PL are not closely associated with MAO activity and were probably mediated by mechanisms other than the formation of H_2O_2.

Seregi et al.[38] studied the mechanism of the involvement of MAO in catecholamine-stimulated biosynthesis of prostaglandins in the rat brain and the apparent role of H_2O_2. They found that pargyline abolished the stimulatory effect of catecholamines on the formation of prostaglandins and concluded that the observed stimulatory effect was due, in part, to the formation of H_2O_2 during catecholamine metabolism. It should be noted, however, that relatively large concentrations of catecholamines are necessary to stimulate prostaglandin biosynthesis in rat brain slices or homogenates.[38–41]

TABLE 4. H_2O_2-Catalase and NE-Pargyline Interactions on the Incorporation of 3[H]-AA into Phosphatidylinositol (PI) and Phosphatidylcholine (PC)

H_2O_2 (100μM)	Catalase (5μG)	NE (100μM)	Pargyline (100μM)	3[H]-AA Incorporation (% of control)	
				PI	PC
+	−	−	−	73 + 4[a]	71 + 6[a]
+	+	−	−	112 + 9	92 + 7
−	−	+	−	256 + 22[a]	58 + 4[a]
−	+	+	−	224 + 18[a]	51 + 4[a]
−	−	+	+	231 + 16[a]	66 + 6[a]
−	−	−	+	96 + 6	103 + 8

NOTE: NE = norepinephrine.
[a]Significantly different from control experiments, $p < 0.01$.

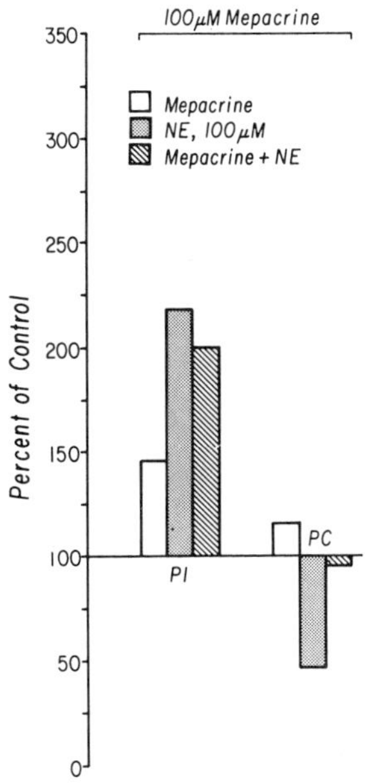

FIGURE 9. Effect of mepacrine on the norepinephrine (NE)–produced change in 3[H]-AA incorporation into phosphatidylinositol (PI) and phosphatidylcholine (PC). This phospholipase A-2 inhibitor abolished the NE-produced decrease in 3[H]-AA incorporation into PC without having a significant effect on the NE-produced increase in 3[H]-AA incorporation into PI.

Interactions of the Neurotransmitter with Deacylation and Reacylation

In an attempt to elucidate the mode of action of the neurotransmitters on the incorporation of 3[H]-AA into PL, we initiated a number of experiments aimed at investigating whether the observed effects were due to changes in deacylation, reacylation, or both processes. These experiments were conducted with the phospholipase A-2 inhibitor mepacrine[42] and the acyl-transferase inhibitor delta-9-tetrahydrocannabinol.[43] It was found that mepacrine (100 μM) had no significant effect on the NE-produced increase in 3[H]-AA incorporation into PI, but that this drug antagonized the NE-produced decrease in the incorporation of 3[H]-AA into PC (FIG. 9). Application of THC at a low concentration of 10 μM resulted in a substantial reduction of the NE-produced increase in the incorporation of 3[H]-AA into PI without an apparent effect on the NE-produced decrease in 3[H]-AA incorporation into PC (FIG. 10). The findings of the mepacrine studies suggest that the NE-produced decrease in 3[H]-AA incorporation into PC was largely due to activation of phospholipase A-2 by the neurotransmitter. The finding that THC was very potent in attenuating the NE-produced increase in the incorporation of 3[H]-AA into PI without appreciably influencing the NE-produced decrease of 3[H]-AA incorporation into PC suggests that NE may enhance the reacylation of lyso-PI by activating a lyso-PI–specific arachidonyl transferase.

The neurotransmitter effects on deacylation and reacylation of cerebral PL may play an important role in controlling the levels of membrane lyso-PL and FFA. The acyl transferase enzymes that are involved in PI reacylation are of particular importance in regulating the membrane content of polyenoic fatty acids, such as AA. The membrane levels of the polyenoic fatty acids are important not only for the

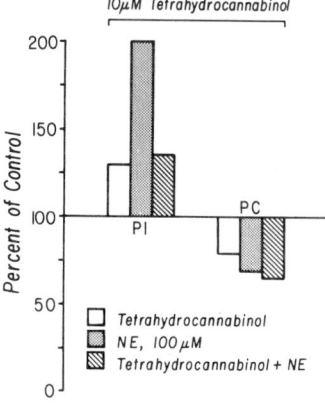

FIGURE 10. Effect of delta-9-THC on the norepinephrine (NE)–produced changes in 3[H]-AA incorporation into phosphatidylinositol (PI) and phosphatidylcholine (PC). This acyltransferase inhibitor markedly reduced the NE-produced increase in 3[H]-AA incorporation into PI without an appreciable effect on the NE-produced change in 3[H]-AA incorporation into PC.

formation of various eicosanoids but also for modulating the activities of membrane enzymes that play a key role in neuronal transmission, such as Na^+ K^+ ATP-ase.[44]

In addition, the reacylation of lyso-PI is important for replenishing the pool of PI that is depleted rapidly during the transduction of signals across excitable membranes. FIGURE 11 depicts major pathways of PI metabolism that may be influenced by NE. The activation of PIP_2-specific phospholipase C by NE is known to be mediated by alpha-1-adrenergic receptors.[45] There is also an increasing amount of evidence that the stimulation of AA release by NE results from activation of phospholipase A-2 through alpha-1 receptors.[4] Thus, the interaction of NE with alpha-1-adrenergic receptors might initiate processes aimed at increasing the production of the second messengers DAG and IP3, with a concomitant increase in AA release and eicosanoid formation. The activation of these processes would enhance the depletion of the relatively small pool of PI that is accessible to PI kinases for PIP_2 formation and to phospholipase A-2 for AA release. An effective way to replenish this metabolically active PI pool would be to enhance reacylation processes involving lyso-PI (FIG. 11). Our studies suggest that in addition to activating PIP_2-specific phospholipase C and phospholipase A-2 via alpha-1-adrenergic receptors, NE may stimulate a lyso-PI–specific arachidonyl transferase via mechanisms that have not yet been elucidated. This action of NE is directed to prevent the rapid depletion of the relatively small pool of PI that serves as a major source for both PIP_2 and AA.

SUMMARY

The effects of the neurotransmitters NE and 5HT on the turnover of AA in cerebral PL were investigated in slices of rat brain cortex. Incorporation of 3[H]-AA into individual PL was first analyzed in accordance with a closed two-compartmental model. Apparent rates of deacylation and reacylation as well as sizes of the metabolically active PL-bound AA pools were calculated. It was found that rates of reacylation of individual PL varied markedly, while deacylation rates remained within a relatively narrow range. The rate of PI acylation was found to be the most rapid, while the rate of PS acylation was the slowest observed. The pool of PL-bound AA that is readily accessible to deacylation-reacylation processes was distributed differentially among the various PL, with more than 50% of this pool in PI; but only 0.75% of the PI content was associated with this pool. Both NE and 5HT enhanced the incorporation of 3[H]-AA into PI in a dose-related manner, while they attenuated its incorporation into other PL. Pharmacological studies indicated that the neurotransmitter effects were not mediated by known NE or 5HT receptors and that a functional presynaptic reuptake system was not required for these effects. The observed effects did not appear to be related to the formation of hydrogen peroxide by the action of MAO on the neurotransmitter. Examination of the structure-activity relationships indicated that the presence of two hydroxyl groups in the aromatic ring was needed for attenuating 3[H]-AA incorporation into PC, whereas an active catechol nucleus with an additional hydroxyl group in the beta position of the side chain appeared to enhance 3[H]-AA incorporation into PI. Results obtained with the phospholipase A-2 inhibitor mepacrine and the acyltransferase inhibitor THC suggest that NE attenuates PL acylation by activating phospholipase A-2, but it concomitantly enhances PI acylation by selectively stimulating a PI-specific arachidonyl transferase via mechanisms that have not yet been elucidated.

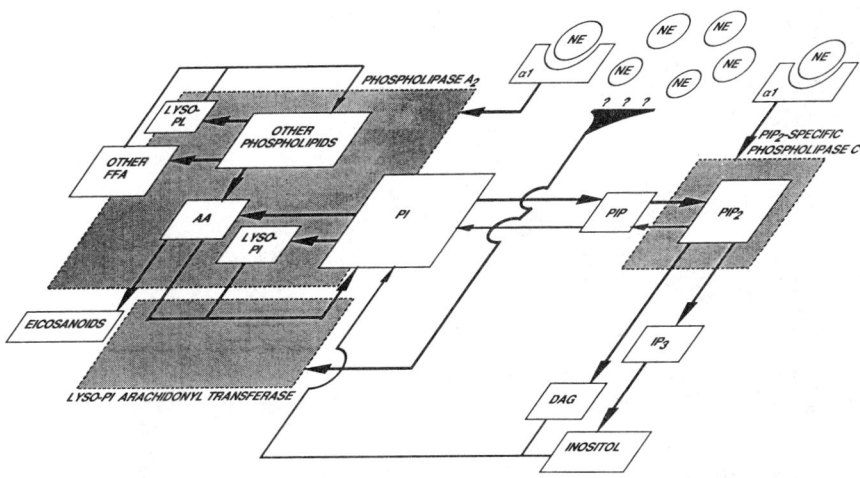

FIGURE 11. Major pathways involved in the turnover of the metabolically active phosphatidylinositol (PI) pool in excitable membranes and possible effects of norepinephrine (NE). The deacylation-reacylation cycle of arachidonic acid (AA)–containing PI is depicted on the *left-hand side*. The conversion of PI to PIP_2 and its subsequent degradation by PIP_2-specific phospholipase C to form the second messengers IP3 and DAG, are depicted on the *right-hand side*. The different enzymic "domains" are shown as *shaded areas*. Free AA is formed from PI and from other phospholipids following the activation of phospholipase A-2. A portion of the newly formed AA is used for the formation of eicosanoids. Another portion is used for the reacylation of lyso-PI by a specific arachidonyl transferase. The simultaneous activation of both phospholipase A-2 and phospholipase C by NE through alpha-1 receptors results in a rapid depletion of the metabolically active PI pool. An increasing amount of PI is converted to lyso-PI, AA, and PIP_2. To compensate for the rapid loss of PI, NE may also act to stimulate lyso-PI–specific arachidonyl transferase through a mechanism that has not yet been elucidated. This stimulation of arachidonyl transferase should increase the reutilization of free AA and provide an efficient pathway for the restoration of the rapidly decreasing PI pool.

REFERENCES

1. MICHELL, R. H. 1975. Biochem. Biophys. Acta **415**: 81–147.
2. HAWTHORNE, J. N. & M. R. PICKARD. 1979. J. Neurochem. **32**: 4–14.
3. ABDEL-LATIF, A. A. 1982. *In* Handbook of Neurochemistry. 2nd edit. A. Lajhta, Ed.: 91–131. Plenum Press. New York, NY.
4. ABDEL-LATIF, A. A. 1986. Pharmacol. Rev. **38**: 227–272.
5. SEKAR, M. C. & L. E. HOKIN. 1986. J. Membrane Biol. **89**: 193–210.
6. NISHIZUKA, Y. 1984. Science **225**: 1365–1370.
7. KIRSCHBAUM, B. B. & H. B. BOSMANN. 1973. FEBS Lett. **34**: 129–132.
8. MOOKERJEE, S. & J. M. W. YOUNG. 1974. Biochem. Biophys. Res. Commun. **57**: 815–822.
9. SHIER, W. T. & J. T. TROTTER. 1976. FEBS Lett. **62**: 165–168.
10. PICARD, A. L. & W. Y. CHEUNG. 1977. J. Biol. Chem. **252**: 4872–4875.
11. O'DOHERTY, P. J. 1978. Lipids **13**: 297–300.
12. MARIKOVSKI, Y., C. S. BROWN, R. S. WEINSTEIN & H. H. WORTIS. 1976. Exp. Cell Res. **98**: 313–324.
13. WELTZEIN, H. V. 1979. Biochim. Biophys. Acta **559**: 259–287.
14. BROPHY, P. J. & D. E. VANCE. 1976. Biochem. J. **160**: 247–251.
15. MURPHY, M. G. & M. W. SPENCE. 1982. J. Neurochem. **38**: 675–679.
16. BERGSTROM, S., L. D. FARMIBO & K. FUXE. 1973. Europ. J. Pharmacol. **21**: 362–368.
17. HILLIER, K. & W. W. TEMPLETON. 1980. Br. J. Pharmacol. **70**: 969–973.
18. WOLFE, L. S. 1982. J. Neurochem. **38**: 1–17.
19. HAYAISHI, O. 1983. Prostaglandin Throm. Leukot. Res. **12**: 333–337.
20. DEGEORGE, J. L., P. MORRELL, K. D. MCCARTHY & E. G. LAPETINA. 1986. J. Biol. Chem. **261**: 3928–3933.
21. BAKER, R. R. & W. THOMPSON. 1973. J. Biol. Chem. **298**: 7060–7065.
22. CORBIN, D. R. & G. Y. SUN. 1978. J. Neurochem. **30**: 77–82.
23. STROSZNAJDER, J., L. FOUDIN, W. TANG & G. Y. SUN. 1983. J. Neurochem. **70**: 84–90.
24. LUNT, G. G. & C. E. ROWE. 1971. Brain Res. **35**: 215–220.
25. MALLORGA, P., J. F. TALLMAN, R. C. HENEBERRY, F. HIRATA, W. T. STRITTMATTER & J. AXELROD. 1980. Proc. Natl. Acad. Sci. USA **77**: 1341–1345.
26. SNIDER, R. M., M. MCKUNNY, C. FORRAY & E. RICHELSON. 1984. Proc. Natl. Acad. Sci. USA **81**: 3905–3909.
27. BARKAI, A. I. & L. R. MURTHY. 1988. Neurochem. Int. In press.
28. JOLLES, J., L. H. SCHRAMA & W. H. GIPSEN. 1981. Biochim. Biophys. Acta **666**: 90–98.
29. LOWRY, O. H., N. J. ROSENBROUGH, A. L. FARR & R. J. RANDALL. 1951. J. Biol. Chem. **193**: 265–275.
30. RIGGS, D. S. 1963. The Mathematical Approach to Physiological Problems. Wilkins and Sons, Baltimore, MD.
31. HAUSER, G. & A. S. PAPPU. 1982. *In* Phospholipids in the Nervous System, Vol. 1: Metabolism. L. A. Horrocks, J. N. Kanfer & G. Porcellati, Eds.: 283–300. Raven Press. New York, NY.
32. JAVAID, J. I., J. M. PEREL, & J. M. DAVIS. 1979. Life Sci. **24**: 21–28.
33. FAUSTER, R., U. HONEGGER & U. WEISMANN. 1983. Biochem. Pharmacol. **32**: 1737–1744.
34. MATSUZAWA, Y. & K. Y. HOSTETLER. 1980. J. Biol. Chem. **255**: 5190–5194.
35. ABDEL-LATIF, A. A., J. P. SMITH, S. Y. K. YOUSOFZAI & R. K. DOVER. 1983. *In* Neural Membranes. G. Y. Sun, N. Bazan, J.-Y. Wu, G. Porcellati & A. Y. Sun, Eds.: 97–122. Humana Press. Clifton, NJ.
36. ABDEL-LATIF, A. A., J. P. SMITH & R. K. DOVER. 1983. Biochem. Pharmacol. **32**: 729–732.
37. POLGAR, P. & L. TAYLOR. 1980. Prostaglandins **19**: 693–700.
38. SEREGI, A., P. SERFOZO, Z. MERGL & A. SCHAEFER. J. Neurochem. **38**: 20–27.
39. LESLIE, C. A. 1976. Res. Comm. Chem. Pathol. Pharmac. **27**: 213–218.
40. WOLFE, L. S., K. ROSTOZOWSKI & H. M. PAPPIUS. 1976. Canad. J. Biochem. **54**: 629–640.

41. SCHAEFER, A., M. KOMLOS & A. SEREGI. 1978. Biochem. Pharmacol. **27:** 213–218.
42. WALLACH, D. P. & J. R. BROWN. 1981. Biochem. Pharmacol. **30:** 1315–1329.
43. GREENBERG, J. H. & A. MELLORS. 1978. Biochem. Pharmacol. **27:** 329–333.
44. BLOJ, B., R. D. MORERO, R. N. FARIAS & R. E. TRUCCO. 1973. Biochim. Biophys. Acta **311:** 67–79.
45. BROWN, E., D. A. KENDALL & S. R. NAHORSKI. 1984. J. Neurochem. **42:** 1379–1387.

Arachidonic Acid Metabolites in the Rat and Human Brain

New Findings on the Metabolism of Prostaglandin D_2 and Lipoxygenase Products[a]

L. S. WOLFE AND L. PELLERIN

Donner Laboratory of Experimental Neurochemistry
Montreal Neurological Institute
McGill University
Montréal, Québec, Canada H3A 2B4

INTRODUCTION

A wide range of stimuli activate arachidonic acid release from tissues, including the brain, and initiate the enzymatic synthesis of many oxygenated metabolites: neurotransmitters, peptides, growth factors, calcium ionophores, electrical stimulation, seizures, trauma, hypoxia and ischemia, and tumor promoters, such as 4-β-12-0-tetradecanoyl phorbol-13-acetate (TPA), to name only a few.[1-7] Eicosanoids themselves—for example, leukotriene C_4 (LTC_4)—can promote the synthesis of prostaglandins.[8] An important step in the initiation of arachidonic acid release after activation of membrane receptors is stimulation of phospholipase C acting on 1-stearoyl-2-arachidonyl phosphatidylinositol bisphosphate and activation of a phospholipase A_2, which release arachidonic acid from phosphatidylinositol and phosphatidyl choline.[9] In the brain the biosynthesis of prostaglandins (PGE_2, PGD_2, PGI_2, and $PGF_{2\alpha}$) and thromboxane A_2 (TxA_2) is now well documented.[1] More recently, besides fatty acid cyclooxygenase products, lipoxygenase metabolites—particularly leukotriene C_4, leukotriene B_4, and 12-hydroxyeicosatetraenoic acid (12-HETE)—have been shown to be synthesized in the brain[10-14] and are increased after brain injury and ischemia.[15-17] At the hypothalamic level LTC_4 can mediate the specific release of luteinizing hormone.[18]

The present study addresses two aspects of eicosanoid formation in the brain. First, prostaglandin D_2 (PGD_2) was found to be metabolized by an NADPH-dependent 11-ketoreductase in the human but not the rat brain. In the rat brain the extensive studies of Professor Hayaishi's group in Japan have shown that PGD_2 has important physiological and pharmacological effects, inducing sedation, sleep, and hypothermia, and has anticonvulsant properties.[19-21] Prostaglandin D_2 synthetase is very active in the rat brain,[22] and PGD_2 is known to increase serotonin content and turnover.[23,24] However, only very low synthesis of PGD_2 could be detected in the human cerebral cortex in contrast to that of the rat. This difference can now be interpreted as due to the active conversion of PGD_2 into $9\alpha, 11\beta$ prostaglandin F_2 (11-epi-PGF_2) in the human cerebral cortex, as has been reported in other human tissues[25-28] but not in the rat.[29] Second, the formation of lipoxygenase products—particularly 12-HETE in the rat

---

[a]This work was supported by a grant from the Medical Research Council of Canada. L. S. W. is a career investigator of the MRC, and L. P. is an NSERC Scholar.

pineal gland, retina, and brain—has been previously reported.[13,30-33] Of considerable interest in the present report is that under specific conditions in intact rat brain cerebral cortical slices, activation of specific glutamate and alpha-adrenergic receptors stimulates 12-hydroxyeicosatetraenoic acid (12-HETE) formation.

EXPERIMENTAL PROCEDURES

Measurement of Prostaglandin D_2 and Its Metabolism

Prostaglandins, including PGD_2, were extracted and purified from incubations of brain tissue homogenates in phosphate buffer at pH 7.4 by the method of Powell[34] and as previously reported.[35] Tetradeuterated $PGF_{2\alpha}$ (1 μg) was added to the initial extracting solvents, and PGD_2 was quantified by gas chromatography electron impact mass fragmentography, after reduction with sodium borohydride, on a VG-Micromass ZAB mass spectrometer linked to a cross-linked methyl silicone capillary column.[36] The ions monitored for the methyl ester trimethylsilyl ether derivatives of $PGF_{2\alpha}$ and 11-epi-PGF_2 were m/z 423 and 427. The n-butylboronate derivatives were formed by the method of Pace-Asciak and Wolfe,[37] and the ions of the methyl ester and trimethylsilyl ether derivatives were monitored at m/z 435 and 439.

Biopsy pieces of human brain cerebral cortex were made available by Dr. Allan Sherwin and neurosurgeons of the Montreal Neurological Institute after surgical treatment of patients for epilepsy. Prostaglandin D_2 11-ketoreductase activity was measured after incubation of the cortex homogenates (100–200 mg) at 37° for various times in 0.1-M phsophate buffer at pH 7.4 with addition of PGD_2 (1–10 μg) and an NADPH-generating system.[26] Extraction, purification on ODS Sep-Pak cartridges, and silicic acid chromatographic separations of the prostaglandins were as described above. The quantification of the amount of $9\alpha\,11\beta\,PGF_2$ formed was calculated by subtracting the amount of $9\alpha\,11\alpha\,PGF_2$ ($PGF_{2\alpha}$) as its n-butylboronate derivative from the total PGF_2 ($9\alpha\,11\alpha$ and $9\alpha\,11\beta$) determined by mass spectrometry of the methyl ester and trimethylsilyl ether derivatives monitored at m/z 423. The relative intensities to the base peak, m/z 191, of the 423 ion in the two PGF_2 isomers did not differ by more than 5 percent.

Measurement of 12-Hydroxyeicosatetraenoic Acid Formation

Intact pieces of rat fronto-parietal cerebral cortex of 2–3 mm diameter and 0.5 mm thick were sliced at 4°C, placed in cold pH 7.4 phosphate-buffered saline containing 5.5 mM glucose but without calcium or magnesium, and preincubated for 5 minutes at 37°C. Calcium (2 mM), calcium ionophore A 23187 (10 μM), arachidonic acid (75 μM), and TPA (100 ng/ml) or the neurotransmitters or their agonists were added to incubation flasks, and the reaction was continued for various times. The reaction was stopped by adding 1 volume of cold methanol. Lipoxygenase products were purified on Sep-Pak ODS cartridges and separated by reversed-phase high performance liquid chromatography on a 5 μm Spherisorb column with a mobile phase of methanol-water-acetic acid (75:25:01) at a flow rate of 1.0 ml/minute. Identification of the compounds absorbing at 280 and 235 nm was done by retention time using pure standards and quantification by interface with an IBM computer. After collection of the HETE peaks and removal of solvents, the HETEs were rapidly hydrogenated with activated platinum oxide, under conditions to avoid hydrogenolysis, and analyzed by capillary gas chromatography mass spectrometry. Hydrogenation of the HETEs was

TABLE 1. Synthesis of Prostaglandins and Thromboxanes by Brain Tissue Pieces

Tissue	$PGF_{2\alpha}$	PGE_2	PGD_2	6-keto-$PGF_{1\alpha}$	TxB_2
Rat neocortex	141	45	720	9	365
Rat hypothalamus	262	70	320	—	—
Cat neocortex	660	203	N.D.	12	420
Human temporal cortex (biopsy)	81	38	11	7	70
Human hypothalamus (autopsy)	102	22	5	9	—

NOTE: Results are in ng/g tissue/15 min. They are the means of at least three tissue samples and were quantified by gas chromatography–mass fragmentography methods. N.D. = not detectable.

absolutely essential, because during gas chromatography, the unhydrogenated compounds are rapidly degraded.

RESULTS AND DISCUSSION

Prostaglandin D_2 Formation and Metabolism by an NADPH-Dependent 11-Ketoreductase Enzyme in the Human Cerebral Cortex

TABLE 1 shows the relative amounts of the different prostaglandins and thromboxane B_2 formed by incubation of brain tissue pieces from various species. Prostaglandin D_2 is the major endoperoxide metabolite formed in the rat brain, as many investigators have found previously. However, its synthesis in the cat cortex was not detectable and was very low in the human cerebral cortex and hypothalamus.

In preliminary experiments [^{3}H] PGD_2 was added to high-speed supernatant fractions prepared from rat and human cerebral cortex. After 10-minute incubations

TABLE 2. C-Values and Relative Retention Times of Fatty Acids, PGF_2 Isomers, LTB_4, and HETEs

Compounds[a]	C-Values	Relative Retention Times[c]
18:1 (ω9)	17.37	0.96
18:0	18.00	1.00
20:4 (ω6)	19.33	1.22
12-OH 18:1 (ω9)	19.85	1.33
20:0	20.00	1.36
9-OH 18:0	20.09	1.38
22:0	22.00	1.78
24:0	24.00	2.23
9β11α-PGF_2	23.41	2.09
9α11β-PGF_2	23.92	2.20
9α11α-PGF_2	23.95	2.22
12(S)-HETE[b]	22.01	1.78
5(S)-HETE[b]	22.09	1.80
15(S)-HETE[b]	22.18	1.82
LTB_4[b]	23.90	2.20

[a]Methyl esters and trimethylsilyl ether derivatives when applicable.
[b]Hydrogenated.
[c]Cross-linked methyl silicone (Ultra 1) capillary column, 50 m, film 0.17 μM 200–285 °C at 4° per minute.

FIGURE 1. Formation with time of 9α11β-PGF$_2$ in human temporal cortex homogenates after addition of 5 μg PGD$_2$ and an NADPH-generating system. Values (means of three separate brain biopsy samples) were determined by capillary column mass spectrometry. In boiled homogenates or in the absence of NADPH, less than 15 ng/g of the PGF$_2$ isomer were detected.

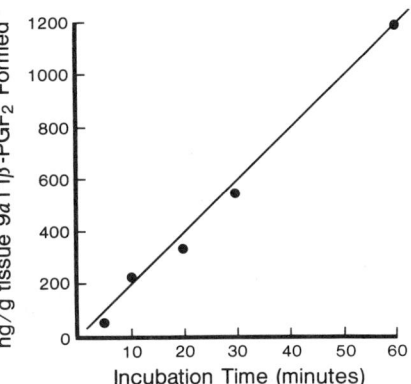

with addition of NADPH (1 mM), the prostaglandins were extracted, purified, and separated by thin layer chromatography, and the radioactivity in regions corresponding to PGD$_2$ and PGF$_2$ zones were determined. It was found that 18 percent of the radioactivity was present in the PGF$_2$ region in the human cortex and less than 1 percent in the rat cortex or in heat-inactivated human supernatant fractions. At this time it became known that PGD$_2$ was the principal cyclooxygenase product formed by human mast cells and in patients with mastocytosis[38,39] and was also a bronchoconstrictor potentiating the effect of histamine.[40-42] Later it was found that PGD$_2$ was metabolized in the human liver and lung, and probably in other tissues as well, by a 11-ketoreductase pathway to form (5Z,13E)-(15S)-9α 11β, 15-trihydroxyprosta-5-13-dien-1-oic acid (9α 11β-PGF$_2$) by a cytosolic NADPH-dependent enzyme, as previously mentioned. Further, in human lung tissue with the endoperoxide PGH$_2$ as

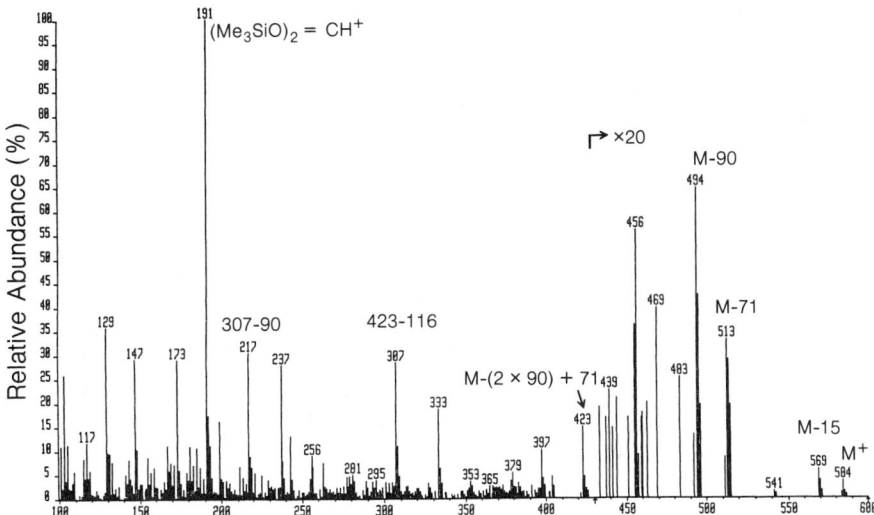

FIGURE 2. Electron impact mass spectrum of 9α11β-PGF$_2$ formed from PGD$_2$ by human temporal cortex homogenates.

TABLE 3. Formation of PGF_2 Isomers by Human and Rat Cerebral Cortex

Conditions	$9\alpha11\alpha$-PGF_2 (from PGH_2)	$9\alpha11\beta$-PGF_2 (from PGD_2)
Human temporal cortex	81	413
Human temporal cortex without NADPH generating system	65	86
Human temporal cortex boiled	3	13
Rat fronto-parietal cortex	138	0

NOTE: Results are in ng/g tissue/30 min. They are the means of three experiments. $9\alpha11\alpha$-PGF_2 determined as the n-butylboronate trimethylsilyl ether methyl ester derivative, ions monitored m/z 435 and 439 from the tetradeuterated internal standard. See EXPERIMENTAL PROCEDURES for assay of $9\alpha11\beta$-PGF_2 after addition of 5 µg PGD_2 and an NADPH-generating system.

substrate, only $9\alpha 11\alpha$ PGF_2($PGF_{2\alpha}$) was formed. In rat tissues, including the brain, the conversion of PGD_2 to $9\alpha, 11\beta$-prostaglandin F_2 could not be detected. These studies led us to examine the metabolism of PGD_2 in the human cerebral cortex.

The capillary column gas chromatographic retention times of the PGF_2 isomers relative to several fatty acids and hydroxyeicosatetraenoic acids are shown in TABLE 2. These results form the basis for the GC-MS studies. The formation of $9\alpha 11\beta$ PGF_2

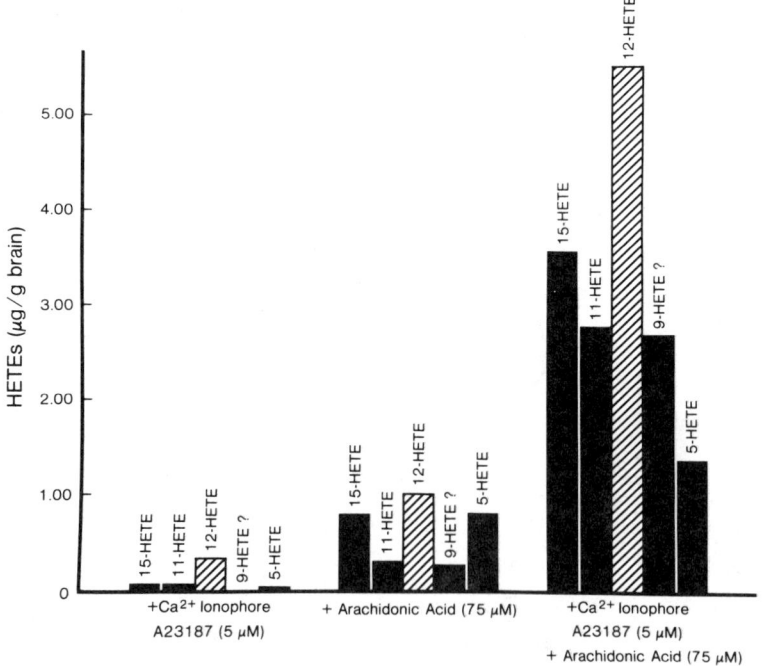

FIGURE 3. The formation by rat brain slices of hydroxyeicosatetraenoic acids (15-, 11-, 12- and 5-HETEs) after 20-min incubation. The 9-HETE has not been positively identified. The *hatched columns* highlight the 12-lipoxygenase metabolite.

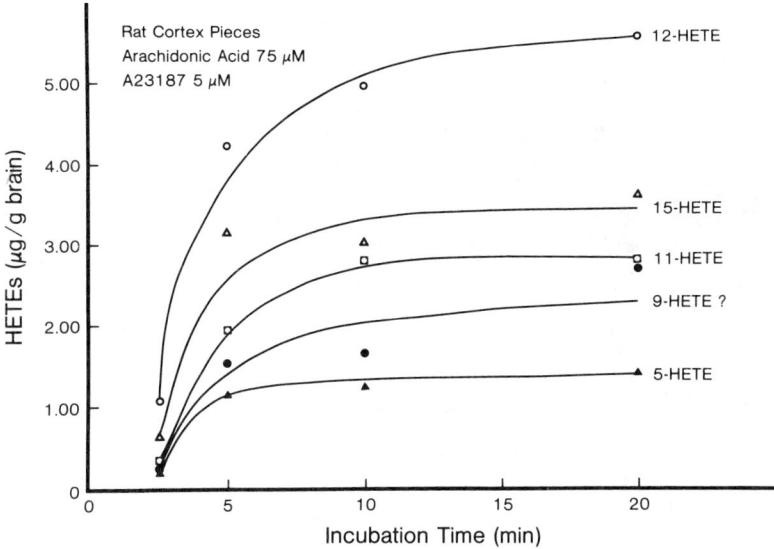

FIGURE 4. Time course of formation of HETEs by rat brain pieces in the presence of calcium ionophore and arachidonic acid.

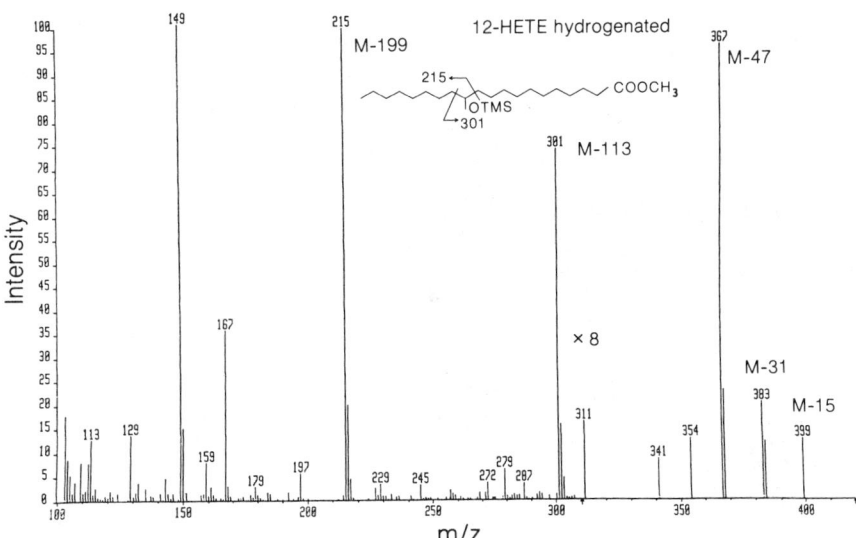

FIGURE 5. Electron impact mass spectrum of hydrogenated 12-HETE formed by rat cerebral cortex pieces.

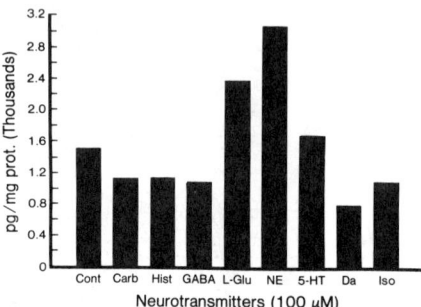

FIGURE 6. The effect of neurotransmitters on 12-HETE formation by rat cerebral cortex. Cont = control, Carb = carbachol, Hist = Histamine GABA = γ-amino butyric acid, L-Glu = L-glutamate, NE = norepinephrine 5-HT = 5-hydroxytryptamine, DA = dopamine, and Iso = isoproterenol.

when human temporal cortex homogenates were incubated with 5 μg or PGD_2 in the presence of a NADPH-generating system is shown in FIGURE 1. The mass spectrum of the 11-epi-PGF_2 isomer formed in the brain is shown in FIGURE 2. The spectrum shows all the ions characteristic of pure standards of the isomeric forms of PGF_2. Mass spectrometry evidence also indicated the presence of other isomers, some with a shift in the Δ^{13} double bond to the Δ^{12} position. Comparison of the formation of PGF_2 isomers from human brain tissue is shown in TABLE 3.

We conclude that PGD_2 is formed in the human brain but is rapidly metabolized to $9\alpha\,11\beta$-PGF_2 by an 11-ketoreductase. Since this isomer has biological activities, such as inhibition of platelet aggregation, vasoconstriction, and elevation of blood pressure,[25] it must be considered along with other eicosanoids when it is formed in pathophysiological situations, such as brain injury and ischemia.

Formation of 12-Hydroxyeicosatetraenoic Acid by Rat Cerebral Cortex Pieces and Factors that Affect Its Synthesis

Neurons, like many other cell types, possess biochemical mechanisms for receptor-mediated signal transduction, and the sequelae involve calcium ion movement and mobilization and phosphorylation of specific proteins by second messengers, which initiate the physiological responses.[43] Arachidonic acid metabolites are important in the mediation and bioregulation of synaptic responses.[44,45] The studies reported here concentrate on the lipoxygenase pathways in intact, physiologically responsive rat brain cortical slices. FIGURE 3 shows the stimulation of synthesis of various hydroxyeicosatetraenoic acids by the calcium ionophore A23187 alone and in the presence of

FIGURE 7. The effect of L-glutamate (L-Glu), N-Methyl-D-aspartate (NMDA), and kainate on 12-HETE synthesis by rat cerebral cortex. Cont = control.

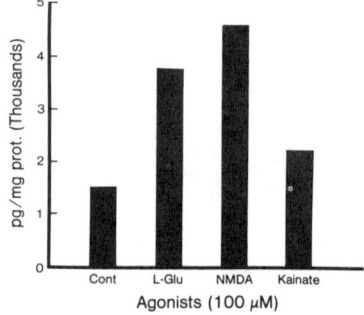

added arachidonic acid. What came as a surprise was the 12-hydroxyeicosatetraenoic acid (12-HETE) was quantitatively the most important lipoxygenase product formed in this situation. The time course of formation in the rat brain showed that maximum formation occurred within 10 minutes of incubation (FIG. 4). The amount formed was in order of one microgram per gram of tissue, considerably higher than any of the prostaglandins (see TABLE 1). The precise identity of each of the HETEs was determined by mass spectrometry; the spectrum of the hydrogenated 12-HETE after elution from reversed phase HPLC analysis is shown in FIGURE 5. We then examined the effect of neurotransmitters or their agonists on 12-HETE formation and found that only L-glutamate and norepinephrine increased 12-HETE formation (FIG. 6). The action of norepinephrine was likely through alpha-receptors, since isoproterenol had no effect. Since there are several types of glutamate receptors in the brain, we next examined the effect of N-methyl-D-aspartate (NMDA) in the absence of magnesium (FIG. 7). NMDA, but not kainic acid, was an even more potent stimulator of 12-HETE synthesis. These studies open up new directions in the understanding of the regulatory roles of eicosanoids on neurotransmitter pathways and modulation of synaptic plasticity in the brain. Of particular interest is the possibility that the 12-hydroperoxy precursor of 12-HETE may be involved in the regulation of activity-dependent enhancement of synaptic efficiency (long-term potentiation, LTP) both in the cerebral cortex and the hippocampus.[46] It is also important to consider the role of 12-HETE formation on the activation of guanylate cyclase in the presence of extracellular calcium.[47] Research on these interesting problems is in progress. A preliminary abstract of this research has appeared.[48]

ACKNOWLEDGMENTS

We thank Klara Rostworowski for her excellent technical help and Dr. Orval Mamer for assistance in the mass spectrometry. Marie Clark expertly prepared the manuscript.

REFERENCES

1. WOLFE, L. S. 1982. Eicosanoids: prostaglandins, thromboxanes, leukotrienes and other derivatives of carbon-20 unsaturated fatty acids. J. Neurochem. **38:** 1–14.
2. NISHIZUKA, Y. 1984. Turnover of inositol phospholipids and signal transduction. Science **225:** 1365–1367.
3. ASHENDEL, C. L. 1985. Tumor promoting phorbol esters may affect cell membrane signal transmission and arachidonate metabolism by modulating calcium-activated, phospholipid-dependent protein kinase. *In* Arachidonic Acid Tumor Promotion. S. M. Fisher & J. J. Slaga, Eds.: 102–129. Martinus Nijhoff. Boston, MA.
4. HALENDA, S. P., G. B. ZAVOICO & M. B. FEINSTEIN. 1985. Phorbol esters and oleoylglycerol enhance release of arachidonic acid in platelets stimulated by Ca^{2+} ionophore A23187. J. Biol. Chem. **260:** 12484–12491.
5. PAPPIUS, H. M. & L. S. WOLFE. 1983. Functional disturbances in brain following injury: search for underlying mechanisms. Neurochem. Res. **8:** 63–72.
6. SAUNDERS, R. & L. A. HORROCKS. 1987. Eicosanoids, plasma membranes, and molecular mechanisms of spinal cord injury. Neurochem. Path. **7:** 1–22.
7. BAZAN, N. G., M. I. AVELDANO DE CALDIRONI & E. B. RODRIQUEZ DE TURCO. 1981. Rapid release of free arachidonic acid in the central nervous system due to stimulation. Prog. Lipid Res. **20:** 523–529.
8. CRAMER, E. G., L. POLOGE, N. A. PAWLOWSKI, Z. A. COHN & W. A. SCOTT. 1983.

Leukotriene C promotes prostacyclin synthesis by human endothelial cells. Proc. Natl. Acad. Sci. USA **80:** 4109–4113.

9. MAJERUS, P. W., D. B. WILSON, T. M. CONNOLLY, T. E. BROSS & E. J. NEUFELD. 1985. Phosphoinositide turnover provides a link in stimulus-response coupling. Trends Biochem. Sc. **10:** 168–171.
10. LINDGREN, J. A., T. HOKFELT, S.-E. DAHLEN, C. PATRONO & B. SAMUELSSON. 1984. Leukotrienes in the rat central nervous system. Proc. Natl. Acad. Sci. USA **81:** 6212–6216.
11. DEMBINSKA-KIEC, A., T. SIMMET & B. A. PESKAR. 1984. Formation of leukotrien C_4-like material by rat brain tissue. Eur. J. Pharmacol. **99:** 57–62.
12. BAZAN, N. G. & D. L. BIRKLE. 1985. Depolarization or convulsions increase the formation of HETE and prostaglandins in the central nervous system. Adv. Prostaglandin Thormboxane Leukotriene Res. **15:** 569–571.
13. WOLFE, L. S., H. M. PAPPIUS, R. POKRUPA & A. HAKIM. 1985. Involvement of arachidonic acid metabolites in experimental brain injury. Identification of lipoxygenase products in brain. Adv. Prostaglandin Thromboxane Leukotriene Res. **15:** 585–588.
14. ADESUYI, S. A., C. S. COCKRELL, D. A. GAMACHE & E. F. ELLIS. 1985. Lipoxygenase metabolism of arachidonic acid in brain. J. Neurochem. **45:** 770–776.
15. MOSKOWITZ, M. A., K. J. KIWAK, K. HEKIMIAN & L. LEVINE. 1984. Synthesis of compounds with properties of leukotrienes C_4 and D_4 in gerbil brains after ischemia and reperfusion. Science **224:** 886–889.
16. KIWAK, K. J., M. A. MOSKOWITZ & L. LEVINE. 1985. Leukotriene production in gerbil brain after ischemic insult, subarachnoid hemorrhage, and concussive injury. J. Neurosurg. **62:** 865–869.
17. DEMPSEY, R. J., M. W. ROY, K. MEYER, D. E. COWEN & H. H. TAI. 1986. Development of cyclooxygenase and lipoxygenase metabolites of arachidonic acid after transient cerebral ischemia. J. Neurosurg. **64:** 118–124.
18. HULTING, A. L., J. A. LINDGREN, T. HOKFELT, P. ENERROTH, S. WERNER, C. PATRONO & B. SAMUELSSON. 1985. Leukotriene C_4 as a mediator of luteinizing hormone release from rat anterior pituitary cells. Proc. Natl. Acad. Sci. USA **82:** 3834–3838.
19. SHIMIZU, T., N. MIZUNO, T. AMANO & O. HAYAISHI. 1979. Prostaglandin D_2, a neuromodulator. Proc. Natl. Acad. Sci. USA **76:** 6231–6234.
20. UENO, R., S. NARUMIYA, T. OGOROCHI, T. NAKAYAMA, Y. ISHIKAWA & O. HAYAISHI. 1982. Role of prostaglandin D_2 in the hypothermia of rats caused by bacterial liposaccharide. Proc. Natl. Acad. Sci. USA **79:** 6093–6097.
21. UENO, R., K. HONDA, S. INOUE & O. HAYAISHI. 1983. Prostaglandin D_2 a cerebral sleep-inducing substance in rats. Proc. Natl. Acad. Sci. USA **80:** 735–737.
22. SHIMIZU, T., S. YAMAMOTO & O. HAYAISHI. 1979. Purification and properties of prostaglandin D synthetase from rat brain. J. Biol. Chem. **254:** 5222–5228.
23. HOLLINGSWORTH, E. G. & G. A. PATRICK. 1985. The effects produced by prostaglandin D_2 on serotonin turnover and release and tryptophan uptake. Pharm. biochem. Behav. **22:** 371–375.
24. BHATTACHARYA, S. K. & P. J. R. MOHAN RAO. 1987. Prostaglandin D_2 induced catalepsy in rats: role of 5-hydroxy tryptamine. J. Pharm. Pharmacol. **39:** 743–745.
25. PUGLIESE, G., E. G. SPOKAS, E. MARCINKIEWICZ & P. Y.-K. WONG. 1985. Hepatic transformation of prostaglandin D_2 to a new prostanoid, 9α 11β-prostaglandin F_2, that inhibits platelet aggregation and constricts blood vessels. J. Biol. Chem. **260:** 14621–14625.
26. WATANABE, K., Y. IGUCHI, S. IGUCHI, Y. ARAI, O. HAYAISHI & L. J. ROBERTS, II. 1986. Stereospecific conversion of prostaglandin D_2 to (5Z,13E)-9α,-11β,15-trihydroxy-prosta-5,13-dien-1-oic acid ($9\alpha,11\beta$-prostaglandin F_2) and of prostaglandin H_2 to prostaglandin $F_{2\alpha}$ by bovine lung prostaglandin F synthase. Proc. Natl. Acad. Sci. USA **83:** 1583–1587.
27. SEIBERT, K., J. R. SHELLER & J. ROBERTS, II. 1987. ((5Z,13E)-(15S)-$9\alpha,11\beta,15$-Trihydroxyprosta-5,13-dien-1-oic acid ($9\alpha,11\beta$-prostaglandin F_2): Formation and metabolism by human lung and contractile effects on human bronchial smooth muscle. Proc. Natl. Acad. Sci. USA **84:** 256–260.
28. WENDELBORN, D. F., K. SEIBERT & L. J. ROBERTS, II. 1988. Isomeric prostaglandin F_2

compounds arising from prostaglandin D_2: A family of icosanoids produced in vivo in humans. Proc. Natl. Acad. Sci. USA **85**: 304–308.
29. HAYAISHI, H., S. ITO, T. TANAKA, M. NEGISHI, H. KAWABE, H. YOKOHAMA, K. WATANABE & O. HAYAISHI. 1987. Determination of $9\alpha,11\beta$-prostaglandin F_2 by stereospecific antibody in various rat tissues. Prostaglandins **33**: 517–530.
30. MIYAMOTO, T. J. A. LINDGREN & B. SAMUELSSON. 1987. Isolation and identification of lipoxygenase products from the rat central nervous system. Biochim. Biophys. Acta **922**: 372–378.
31. YOSHIMOTO, T., M. KUSAKA, F. SHINJO & S. YAMAMOTO. 1984. 12- and 15-lipoxygenases in rat pineal gland. Prostaglandins **28**: 279–285.
32. BIRKLE, D. L. & N. G. BAZAN. 1984. The effect of K^+ depolarization on the synthesis of prostaglandins and hydroxyeicosatetraenoic acids in the rat retina: Evidence for esterification of 12-HETE in lipids. Biochem. Biophys. Acta **795**: 564–573.
33. PREUD'HOMME, Y., D. DEMOLLE & J. M. BOEYNAEMS. 1985. Metabolism of arachidonic acid in rabbit iris and retina. Invest. Ophthal. Vis. Sci. **26**: 1336–1342.
34. POWELL, W. S. 1980. Rapid extraction of oxygenated metabolites of arachidonic acid from biological samples using octadecylsilyl silica. Prostaglandins **20**: 947–957.
35. PAPPIUS, H. M. & L. S. WOLFE. 1983. Effects of indomethacin and ibuprofen on cerebral metabolism and blood flow in traumatized brain. J. Cerebral Blood Flow Metabolism **3**: 448–459.
36. ABDEL-HALIM, M. S., M. HAMBERG, B. SJOQUIST & E. ANGGARD. 1977. Identification of prostaglandin D_2 as a major prostaglandin in homogenates of rat brain. Prostaglandins **14**: 633–643.
37. PACE-ASCIAK, C. & L. S. WOLFE. 1971. N-Butylboronate derivatives of the F prostaglandins. Resolution of prostaglandins of the E and F series by gas-liquid chromatography. J. Chromatogr. **56**: 129–133.
38. ROBERTS, L. J., B. J. SWEETMAN, R. A. LEWIS, K. F. AUSTEN & J. A. OATES. 1980. Increased production of prostaglandin D_2 in patients with systemic mastocytosis. N. Engl. J. Med. **303**: 1400–1404.
39. LEWIS, R. A., N. A. SOTER, P. T. DIAMOND, K. F. AUSTIN, J. A. OATES & L. J. ROBERTS, II. 1982. Prostaglandin D_2 generation after activation of rat and human mast cells with anti-IgE. J. Immunol. **129**: 1627–1631.
40. LISTON, T. E. & L. J. ROBERTS, II. 1985. Transformation of prostaglandin D_2 to $9\alpha 11\beta$-(15S)-trihydroxy-prosta-(5Z,13E)-dien-1-oic acid ($9\alpha\ 11\beta$-prostaglandin F_2): A unique biologically active prostaglandin produced enzymatically in vivo in humans. Proc. Natl. Acad. Sci. USA **82**: 6030–6034.
41. MURRAY, J. J., A. B. TONNEL, A. R. BRASH, L. J. ROBERTS, II, P. GOSSET, R. WORKMAN, A. CAPRON & J. A. OATES. 1986. Release of prostaglandin D_2 into human airways during acute angiten challenge. N. Engl. J. Med. **315**: 800–804.
42. BEASLEY, R., J. VARLEY, C. ROBINSON & S. T. HOLGATE. 1987. Cholinergic-mediated bronchoconstriction induced by prostaglandin D_2, its initial metabolite $9\alpha, 11\beta$-PGF_2, and $PGF_{2\alpha}$ in asthma. Am. Rev. Respir. Dis. **136**: 1140–1144.
43. BERRIDGE, M. J. 1987. Inositol trisphosphate and diacylglycerol: Two interacting second messengers. Ann. Rev. Biochem. **56**: 159–193.
44. PIOMELLI, D., A. VOLTERRA, N. DALE, S. A. SIEGELBAUM, E. R. KANDEL, J. H. SCHWARTZ & F. BELARDETTI. 1987. Lipoxygenase metabolites of arachidonic acid as second messengers for presynaptic inhibition of Aplysia sensory cells. Nature **328**: 38–43.
45. PIOMELLI, D., E. SHAPIRO, S. J. FEINMARK & J. H. SCHWARTZ. 1987. Metabolites of arachidonic acid in the nervous system of Aplysia: Possible mediators of synaptic modulation. J. Neurosci. **7**: 3675–3686.
46. COLLINGRIDGE, G. 1987. The role of NMDA receptors in learning and memory. Nature **330**: 604–605.
47. SNIDER, R. M., M. MCKINNEY, C. FORRAY & E. RICHELSON. 1984. Neurotransmitter receptors mediate cyclic GMP formation by involvement of arachidonic acid and lipoxygenase. Proc. Natl. Acad. Sci. USA **81**: 3905–3909.
48. PELLERIN, L. & L. S. WOLFE. 1988. Glutamate and norepinephrine induce 12-HETE formation in intact peices of rat cerebral cortex. Trans. Amer. Soc. Neurochem. **19**: 106.

PART II. THE ARACHIDONIC ACID CASCADE
IN THE NERVOUS SYSTEM

Formation and Function of Eicosanoids in the Central Nervous System

GEORG HERTTING AND ANDRÁS SEREGI

Department of Pharmacology
University of Freiburg
D-7800 Freiburg, Federal Republic of Germany

INTRODUCTION

Eicosanoids are naturally occurring, biologically active enzymatic oxidation products of arachidonic acid. They involve prostanoids (prostaglandins and thromboxane) synthesized by the cyclooxygenase pathway, hydro|per|oxy fatty acids (H|P|ETE), and leukotrienes (LT), which are formed via the lipoxygenase pathway.[1]

The presence of prostaglandins (PG) in the central nervous system was first described by Samuelsson in 1964.[2] Their formation in brain tissue has subsequently been demonstrated under *in vitro* and *in vivo* conditions.[3] In the rodent brain prostaglandin PGD_2 is the major cyclooxygenase metabolite formed, followed by lower concentrations of $PGF_{2\alpha}$, PGE_2, thromboxane $(TX)A_2$, and prostacyclin (PGI_2).[4-8] The synthesis of lipoxygenase products, including LTs, by the brain has also been reported.[9-17] Prostaglandins of the E and F series can mediate hyperthermia and fever.[18,19] PGD_2 may be involved in the physiological regulation of sleep[20] and has been proposed to have a neuromodulatory role,[21] as well. Exogenously administered PGs of the E type possess anticonvulsive properties.[3,22] Among lipoxygenase products LTs have been shown to excite Purkinje cells,[23] while HETEs can mediate or modulate neurotransmission.[24]

Under *in vivo* conditions basal eicosanoid levels are very low.[6,7,25] Marked increases in brain eicosanoid synthesis occur during brain hypoxia[9,13,26] and convulsive states.[6,7,25,27-29] During the last years we have characterized convulsion-induced cerebral prostanoid and LT synthesis, and we have investigated whether prostaglandins or LTs modify the induction and propagation of seizures. In order to better understand the central functions of eicosanoids, the cellular site of their origin has also been studied.

CONVULSION-INDUCED EICOSANOID SYNTHESIS IN BRAIN TISSUE

Prostanoids

In all *in vivo* experiments from our laboratory described below post mortem synthesis of cerebral prostaglandins was carefully avoided by immediate deep-freezing of the animals' heads after decapitation. The frozen brains were then homogenized in ice-cold methanol to inactivate synthesizing and metabolizing enzymes and to extract the prostanoids. The methanol extract containing the prostaglandins was evaporated, and the prostaglandins were resuspended in radioimmunoassay buffer. Using specific and sensitive radioimmunoassays developed in our laboratory, PGD_2, $PGF_{2\alpha}$, PGE_2,

6-keto-PGF$_{1\alpha}$ and thromboxane B$_2$ could be determined simultaneously (for detailed description of methods see References 6, 7, 25, 30). Basal prostanoid values estimated under these conditions are very low, in the same range as those measured after microwave irradiation of the brain.[31]

If centrally acting convulsant drugs like pentylenetetrazol (PTZ) and picrotoxin were administered to mice, clonic seizures were induced after a certain time.[7,25,29] The formation of cerebral prostaglandins coincided with the occurrence of clonic convulsions (FIG 1.). Following injection of a lower dose of picrotoxin, clonic seizures started later, and also the prostaglandins increased only after this longer time interval. The same results were obtained with two different doses of PTZ.[7] Already these data indicate a close correlation between increases in neuronal activity and induction of

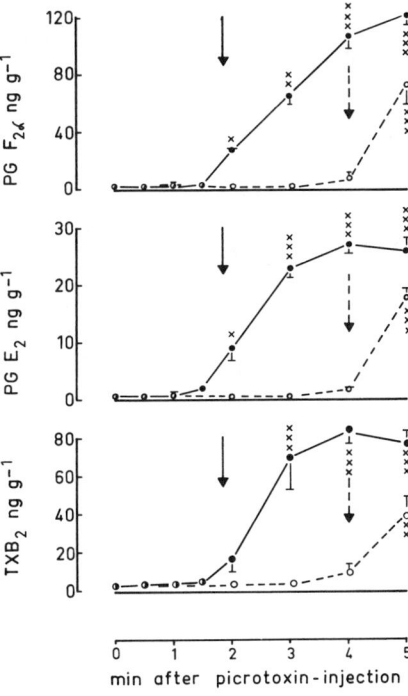

FIGURE 1. The effect of injections of picrotoxin (3.0 mg/kg. i.p. O---O, or 8.0 mg/kg. ip ●——●) on the levels of PGF$_{2\alpha}$, PGE$_2$, and TXB$_2$ in the mouse brain *in vivo*. *Arrows* indicate the onset of clonic seizures. Each point is the mean ± SEM of five determinations.

prostaglandin synthesis. Relatively low doses of anticonvulsive drugs like diazepam and trimethadione reduced chemically induced convulsions and significantly decreased prostaglandin formation. Higher doses of the drugs, which completely abolished convulsions, reduced the prostaglandin formation to almost basal levels.[25]

Neither PTZ (up to 10^{-3} M) nor picrotoxin (10^{-4} M) had any influence on PGF$_{2\alpha}$ synthesis in synaptosomes from mouse brain. This shows that intact, functioning neurons are a prerequisite for the action of these drugs.[25] FIGURE 2 shows the concentrations of five different prostanoids in the mouse brain measured at various times following convulsions induced by maximal electroconvulsive shock (ECS). Following the tonic-clonic convulsions, which lasted less than 1 min, the highest

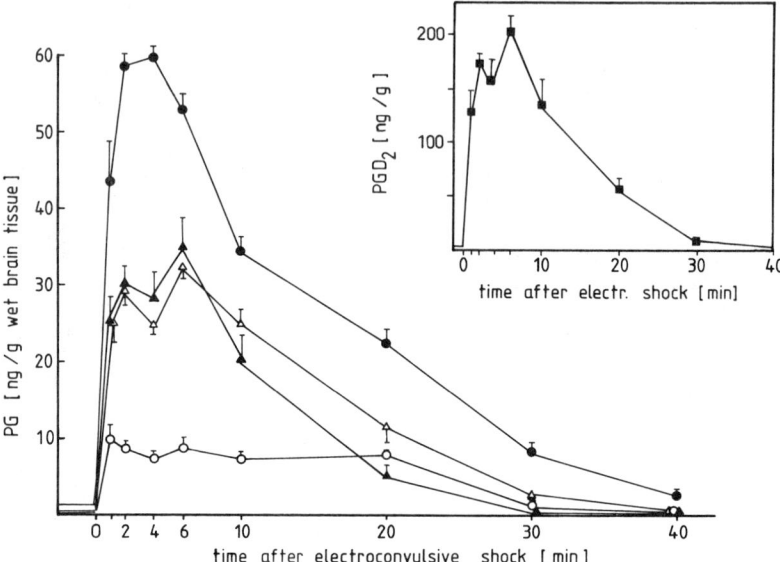

FIGURE 2. Time-dependent changes in content of arachidonic acid metabolites in total mouse brain following administration of electroconvulsive shock ($PGF_{2\alpha}$ ●——●, PGE_2 ▲——▲, TXB_2 △——△, and 6-keto-$PGF_{1\alpha}$ ○——○). Data represent mean ± SEM, $n = 4$. (From Föstermann et al.[7] Reprinted by permission from *Brain Research*.)

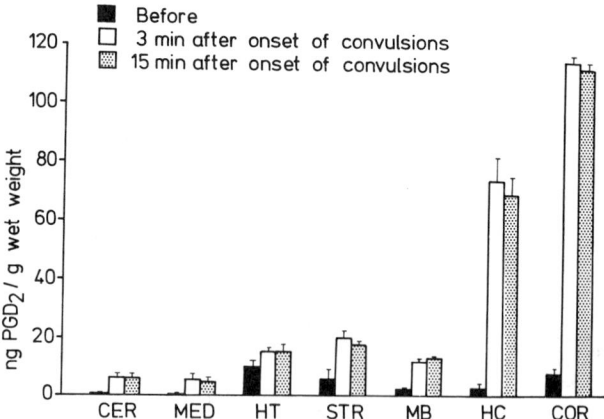

FIGURE 3. Regional distribution of PGD_2 and $PGF_{2\alpha}$ in the brain of convulsion-prone gerbils before and at different times after generalized clonic seizures elicited by environmental stress. Values of each column are derived from 12 animals. The results are the means ± SEM. CER = cerebellum; MED = medulla oblongata; HT = hypothalamus; STR = striatum; MB = midbrain; HC = hippocampus; COR = cerebral cortex. (From Seregi et al.[33] Reprinted by permission from *Brain Research*.)

prostaglandin concentrations were reached between 2–6 min. Prostaglandin D_2 was the major metabolite, followed by $PGF_{2\alpha}$ and lower concentrations of the other prostanoids. After about 50 min, all prostanoids had reached basal levels again.[7] Basically the same time-course and pattern of prostanoid synthesis was obtained following ECS-induced seizures in the rat,[6] or in gerbils, when convulsions were induced by mild environmental stimuli.[32] In all cases brain prostanoid concentrations declined in coincidence with the cessation of convulsions.

When the different prostanoids were measured in seven regions of the rat brain after electroconvulsive shock or administration of PTZ, the highest increments were found in the cerebral cortex and hippocampus. This held true for all prostanoids measured.[6] By analogy,[33] the largest increases in brain prostanoid formation occurred in the cortex and hippocampus of gerbils following spontaneous seizures (FIG. 3). Studies on prostanoid production by homogenates of various regions of the rat brain have shown that the hippocampus and cortex were the most active areas.[34,35] However, the 2–5-fold differences in synthetic capacities of the areas studied cannot explain the extremely high (15–20-fold) convulsion-induced increases in PGD_2 and $PGF_{2\alpha}$ concentrations in the hippocampus and cerebral cortex. This region-specific PG formation seems to correlate rather with the increased neuronal activity occurring in these areas during experimental convulsions.[36,37]

Leukotrienes

More recently, we have also investigated whether or not spontaneous seizures were accompanied by sulphidopeptide-leukotriene (SP-LT) formation in the gerbil brain.[14,38]

Deep-frozen brains were homogenized in ice-cold methanol. High-speed supernatants of the homogenates were subjected to C_{18} SEP-PAK^R extraction, and LTC_4-like material was estimated by radioimmunoassay. In some cases, LTC_4-like material was further analyzed by reversed phase HPLC. We have found, in addition to the increased prostanoid levels, that the concentrations of SP-LTs rapidly rise following tonic-clonic seizures in the brain of spontaneously convulsing gerbils. Maximum tissue levels were reached 6 min after the onset of convulsions both for prostanoids and LTC_4-like material. HPLC analysis combined with radioimmunoassay showed that the immunoreactive LTC_4-like material was LTC_4 and LTD_4.[14,38] At 54 min after the onset of seizures, LTE_4 was detectable as well.[38] At 18 min the ratio between prostanoid and SP-LT levels in the brain was about 40:1, as calculated on a molar basis.[32,38] Complete inhibition of the cyclooxygenase pathway by pretreating of the animals with 5 mg/kg indomethacin two hours before induction of seizures resulted only in a twofold increase of cerebral SP-LT concentrations (FIG. 4).

Triggering Mechanism

One could argue that impaired breathing during seizures may cause cerebral hypoxia. Hypoxia is one of the known stimuli inducing cerebral eicosanoid synthesis.[9,13,14,26] However, seizures of similar duration and intensity provoked by strychnine did not cause any rise in brain prostaglandin formation.[30] Similarly, severe tonic seizures of audiogenic seizure-prone mice are not accompanied by cerebral prostanoid formation.[39] In these two seizure models neuronal discharges are limited to the brain stem and spinal cord,[40] causing motor arrest and respiratory difficulties. In muscle-relaxed mice, where normal ventilation was guaranteed by artificial breathing,

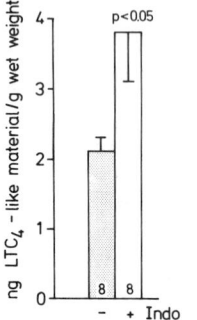 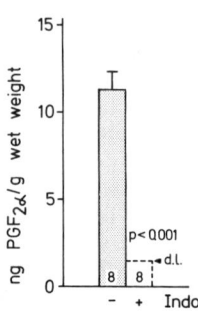

FIGURE 4. The effect of indomethacin (Indo) pretreatment on brain levels of LTC_4-like material and that of $PGF_{2\alpha}$ 18 min after the onset of generalized spontaneous convulsions of the gerbil. Note the different ordinate scales for the two metabolites. Results are the means ± SEM. $n = 8$; d.l. = detection limit.

pentylenetetrazol-induced prostaglandin synthesis was of similar magnitude to that in normal mice.[30] In the gerbil, reperfusion after 5-min bilateral carotid artery ligation induced a rapid rise of brain prostanoid[26] and LT[13,14] levels. The tonic-clonic convulsions of seizure-prone gerbils lasted only 10–20 s. After this period, breathing of the animals recovered to normal. Even if respiration was impaired during this short period of seizures, this impairment was unlikely to cause severe cerebral hypoxia.

Systemic application of kainic acid to rats led to an increase of prostanoid formation in the hippocampus, amygdala/pyriform cortex, and parietal cortex when the first behavioral changes occurred. At this time there was no impairment of breathing or signs of cellular damage.[41]

Taken together, these data strongly suggest that it is not systemic hypoxia but rather increased neuronal activity that triggers eicosanoid formation in the brain during convulsions. However, at the cellular level in the convulsive state, transient local hypoxia cannot be excluded.

ANTICONVULSIVE PROPERTIES OF BRAIN PROSTAGLANDINS

Anticonvulsive properties of administered prostaglandins of the E series have been reported.[3] We investigated the possible role of endogenously formed prostanoids in the convulsive state.[7,42] Treatment of mice with different cyclooxygenase inhibitors, in doses that markedly impaired brain prostaglandin synthesis, significantly shortened the time interval between the injection of the convulsant PTZ and the occurrence of final *tonic* seizures[42] (TABLE 1). In contrast, the latency time of *clonic* seizures was not altered by nonsteroidal antiinflammatory drugs (NSAID).[7] The first clonic seizure occurred about 1 min after administration of the convulsant. At this time cerebral prostaglandins were still very low,[7,25,29,30] (FIG. 1), and no important effects of cyclooxygenase inhibitors could be expected. In contrast, final tonic seizures developed about 4 min after PTZ injection, when prostaglandin levels were markedly elevated.[7] Therefore, the delay in the onset of tonic seizure may be caused by the endogenously formed prostanoids. Inhibition of their synthesis shortened the time until the onset of tonic convulsions.

Since at the dose of PTZ used in these studies (100 mg/kg) the animals generally died in a final tonic seizure, it seemed of interest to investigate whether cyclooxygenase inhibition induced by different NSAIDs had any influence on the acute toxicity of PTZ (evaluated by the LD_{50}). Chemically different cyclooxygenase inhibitors, in doses that inhibited brain prostanoid formation, increased the acute toxic effect of PTZ (decrease in LD_{50}).[7,42] To corroborate these findings further, mice were injected with PTZ, and the time of onset of clonic seizures was measured. If 1 min earlier an electroconvulsive shock was applied to increase cerebral prostaglandin levels (see FIG. 2), there was a marked prolongation of latency time of clonic seizures. Indomethacin almost completely abolished this delay caused by the preceding ECS. ECS was without effect on clonic convulsions if the time interval between the shock and the PTZ injection was long enough (40 min) to restitute low prostaglandin levels (FIG. 5). Concomitantly, LD_{50} values of PTZ were significantly increased by the preceding electroconvulsive shock but lowered by indomethacin pretreatment. If 40 min elapsed between the electrically induced seizure and the PTZ injection, the electroconvulsion had no influence on the LD_{50} of the convulsant drug.[7] All of the above data support the hypothesis that increased cerebral prostaglandin levels have distinct anticonvulsive properties and may attenuate convulsions.

In gerbils (*Meriones unguiculatus*) seizures were induced by taking the animals out of the home cage and putting them onto the palm of the investigator. Prior to the actual experiments, animals were tested five times at 3–6 day intervals for their ability to exert spontaneous convulsions. Gerbils showing no convulsions at any time in these tests were considered nonconvulsive. In convulsion-prone gerbils basal levels of brain prostaglandins were significantly lower than in the nonconvulsive controls. Moreover, if control animals were pretreated with indomethacin, which decreased their cerebral prostaglandin levels, these animals developed seizures with the same frequency as convulsion-prone animals.[43] This also points to a possible anticonvulsant effect of endogenous brain prostaglandins.

When spontaneously convulsing gerbils were tested again 15 min after the first convulsion (time of maximal prostaglandin elevation in total brain), only 3.4% of the animals exhibited a second convulsion, and only moderate seizures were seen. If, however, one week later the same group of animals was pretreated with indomethacin, second convulsions could be induced in 23.3% of these animals. Also, the intensity of these seizures was much higher.[32] These findings strongly suggest that in the gerbil as well as in the rat elevated cerebral prostanoid levels exert protective effects against convulsions.

The following studies were performed to clarify which of the prostaglandins synthesized during convulsions might be responsible for the anticonvulsive effects. Clear anticonvulsive properties are known for prostaglandins of the E series,[3] but these prostaglandins are formed in relatively small amounts during convulsions.[6,7,32] Data

TABLE 1. Effect of Nonsteroidal Antiinflammatory Drugs on the Synthesis of Prostaglandin $F_{2\alpha}$ in the Mouse Brain and on the Latency Time between Pentylenetetrazol Treatment[a] and the Onset of Tonic Seizures

Treatment	Dose (mg/kg)	n	Time until Onset of Seizures (sec ± SE)	$PGF_{2\alpha}$-Synthesis (% of Control ± SE)
Saline		10	243 ± 19	100
Aspirin	100	8	241 ± 23	85 ± 7
Paracetamol	30	8	255 ± 27	98 ± 8
Ibuprofen	10	8	219 ± 31	51 ± 11
Diclofenac	10	9	155 ± 15[b]	8 ± 3
Indomethacin	10	8	174 ± 20[b]	3 ± 1
Flurbiprofen	10	24	180 ± 12[c]	3 ± 1

[a] 100 mg/kg, ip.
[b] $p < 0.01$ as compared to saline treatment.
[c] $p < 0.05$ as compared to saline treatment.

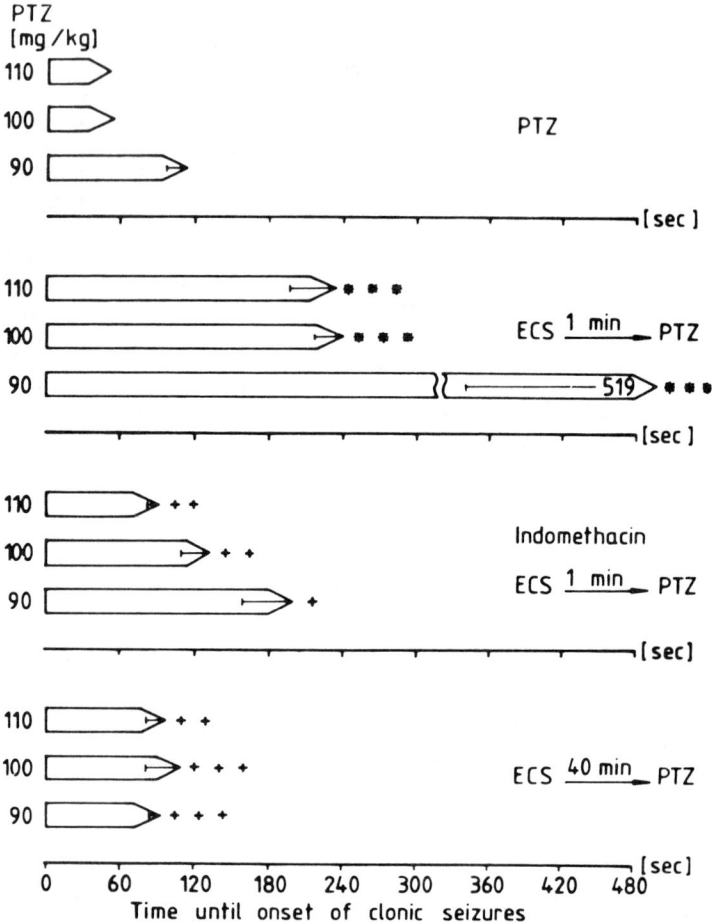

FIGURE 5. Time intervals until the onset of clonic seizures induced by 3 different doses of pentylenetetrazol (PTZ). The intervals are greatly increased if an electroconvulsive shock (ECS) is administered 1 min before PTZ injection (***, $p < 0.001$, compared to PTZ alone). This increase is significantly reduced if the animals are pretreated with 10 mg/kg indomethacin or if the time interval between ECS administration and PTZ injection is prolonged to 40 min (+, $p < 0.05$; ++, $p < 0.025$; +++, $p < 0.01$; all compared to ECS). Each value represents the mean ± SEM of 20 determinations. (From Förstermann et al.[7] Reprinted by permission from *Brain Research*.)

about the actions of $PGF_{2\alpha}$ on convulsions are inconsistent in the literature.[22] Little is known about the effects of PGD_2, although it is the major metabolite formed in brain tissue.[4-8] When 20 μg of PGD_2, $PGF_{2\alpha}$, and PGE_2 was injected intracerebroventricularly into rats and the animals were challenged 4 min later with 80 mg/kg PTZ, the time until the onset of clonic seizures was prolonged, while the incidence of tonic seizures, the intensity of the seizures, and the incidence of deaths following PTZ were significantly diminished.[22] The two other prostaglandins tested also had this effect, but

PGD_2 appeared to be the most potent arachidonic acid metabolite in this respect. It could be argued that these effects are only pharmacological actions of the prostaglandins administered. However, the concentrations reached in the total brain following the intracerebroventricular administration were not substantially higher than those of endogenous prostaglandins after electroconvulsive shock.[22]

It cannot be excluded that the rise of lipoxygenase products following cyclooxygenase inhibition (FIG. 4) is at least partially responsible for the decreased seizure threshold. At present, however, sufficient data to support this possibility are not available.[44]

CELLULAR SITES OF BRAIN EICOSANOID FORMATION

Many of the above findings point to a close correlation of neuronal activity and prostanoid formation. To elucidate the cellular source of brain prostanoids we have studied prostanoid synthesis in primary neuronal cell cultures and astroglial cultures. Cells were characterized by various immunocytochemical procedures. At the time of the experiment, neuronal cell cultures corresponded to the age of newborn rats. Astroglial cultures, however, corresponded to the brains of two-week-old rats. Neuronal cell cultures were contaminated with 2–10% (mainly immature) glia cells. Astroglial cultures contained up to 3% oligodendrocytes and less than 1% fibroblasts.[45] Prostanoid synthesis was stimulated by the Ca^{2+}-ionophor A 23187 in a concentration-dependent manner.[45,46] As shown in TABLE 2, intense prostanoid formation took place in astroglial cells. As in brain tissue, the predominant arachidonic acid metabolite was PGD_2. Surprisingly large amounts of TXB_2 were formed as well. Only relatively small amounts of PGE_2 and $PGF_{2\alpha}$ were found after the 15-min stimulation period. The formation of TXB_2 and PGE_2 has been confirmed by other groups.[47,48] In contrast to the astrocytes, cultured neuronal cells produced only negligible amounts of prostanoids, irrespective of whether homogenates or intact cells were studied.[45,49] Both neuronal and astroglial cells have been shown to incorporate and liberate comparable amounts of arachidonic acid into and from their membrane phospholipids.[45] Therefore, substrate availability cannot be responsible for the differences of prostanoid formation. These differences can rather be explained by the extremely low cyclooxygenase activity of neuronal cells.[49] Even if the properties of the neuronal and astroglial cell cultures cannot be directly compared due to different developmental stages, our results strongly suggest that astroglial cells are a powerful source of prostanoids in brain tissue. Astroglial cultures are also capable of synthesizing lipoxygenase products.[50,51] Due to the close relationship of metabolic processes between neuronal and astroglial cells, eicosanoid synthesis in the latter can be triggered by enhanced neuronal activity.

The motor activity of generalized clonic convulsions following PTZ application to newborn and one-week-old rats is imperfectly coordinated as compared to that of adult animals. At the age of 2 weeks the observed clonic convulsions as well as the electrocorticogram of the convulsing animals already becomes indistinguishable from those of adults. Despite the apparent functional maturity of the cerebral cortex,[52] which is the major site of prostanoid formation during seizures, convulsion-induced prostanoid synthesis typical for adult rodents did not take place by day 14, but first occurred at the end of the third postnatal week (FIG. 6). Also, the prostanoid forming capacity of brain homogenates was low at birth, increased during development, and nearly reached adult values by day 21 (FIG. 7). This time course for the expression of the brain prostanoid forming system seems to correlate with the development of

TABLE 2. Comparison of Prostanoid Formation in Primary Cell Cultures of the Rat Brain after 6 (Neuronal Cell Cultures) and 14 (Astroglial Cell Cultures) Days of Cultivation

	Prostanoid (ng/mg protein/15 min)					
	Neuronal Cell Cultures			Astroglial Cell Cultures		
	Control	A 23187[a]	A 23187[a] + Indomethacin[b]	Control	A 23187[a]	A 23187[a] + Indomethacin[b]
PGD_2	0.38 ± 0.05	2.67 ± 0.20	0.18 ± 0.04	11.05 ± 1.29	55.66 ± 5.92	5.54 ± 0.90
$PGF_{2\alpha}$	0.36 ± 0.05	1.25 ± 0.15	0.30 ± 0.05	2.20 ± 0.10	6.51 ± 0.42	1.21 ± 0.18
PGE_2	0.14 ± 0.03	0.48 ± 0.10	0.15 ± 0.05	1.42 ± 0.15	5.81 ± 0.50	0.56 ± 0.10
TXB_2	0.28 ± 0.04	0.91 ± 0.15	0.24 ± 0.05	6.60 ± 0.99	27.29 ± 2.69	3.78 ± 0.46
Sum of prostanoids formed	1.16 ± 0.17	5.31 ± 0.60[c]	0.87 ± 0.19	21.27 ± 2.53	95.27 ± 9.53[c]	11.09 ± 1.64[d]

NOTE: Results represent the means ± SEM of experiments from 5–7 independent cultivations (incubations were performed in triplicate: $n = 15$–21).
[a] Used in 1-μM concentrations.
[b] Used in 10-μM concentrations.
[c] Significant difference from controls: $p < 0.001$, Student's t-test (two-tailed).
[d] Significant difference from controls: $p < 0.005$, Student's t-test (two-tailed).

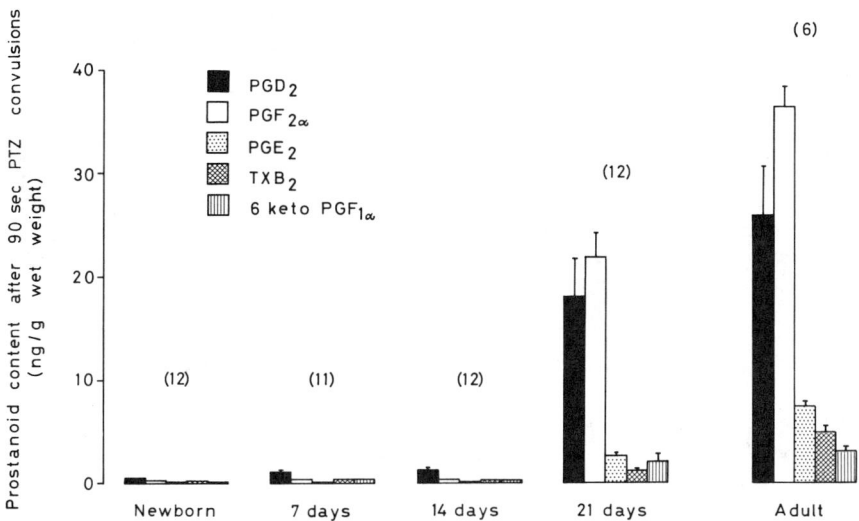

FIGURE 6. Prostanoid formation in the developing rat brain. Clonic convulsions were induced by pentylenetetrazole (PTZ). Results are the means ± SEM. Numbers in brackets represent the number of animals. (From Seregi et al.[52] Reprinted by permission from *Brain Research*.)

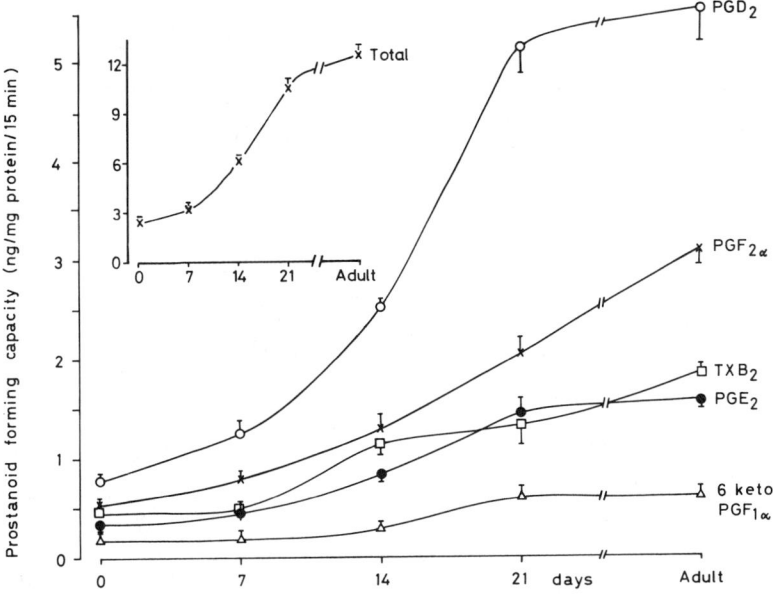

FIGURE 7. Prostanoid forming capacity in homogenates from developing rat brain. *Inset:* changes during postnatal development of the total prostanoid forming capacity (expressed as the sum of prostanoids formed). Results are the means of four experiments performed in triplicate from four independent litters ± SEM. (From Seregi et al.[52] Reprinted by permission from *Brain Research*.)

cellular and functional markers characteristic of mature astrocytes.[52] This view is supported by our *in vitro* results from primary astrocyte cultures. One-week-old cultures, which contain mainly dividing glioblasts and immature astrocytes, produce only negligible amounts of prostanoids. After the second week of cultivation, when most of the cells have become mature-shaped, there was a seven-fold increase in their prostanoid forming capacity (TABLE 3). Homogenates from 2-week-old astrocytes in culture had a specific activity twice that of homogenates from the hemispheres of the adult rat brain (compare TABLE 3 and FIG. 7), demonstrating that the prostanoid synthesizing enzyme complex is enriched in this cell type. Taken together, all these results strongly suggest that the cerebral prostanoid forming system is located predominantly in mature astrocytes.

STIMULI INDUCING ASTROGLIAL EICOSANOID SYNTHESIS

It is generally believed that prostanoid synthesis in cells involves the following sequence of events: increase of intracellular free calcium; activation of phospholipase(s); liberation of arachidonic acid from membrane phospholipids; further transformation of arachidonic acid enzymatically to eicosanoids. The rate-limiting step is supposed to be the free arachidonic acid concentration. In astrocyte cultures prostanoid formation could be induced by the Ca^{2+}-ionophor A 23187, by the phospholipase (PL) A_2 activator melittin, by PLA_2 and by PLC.[46] The effect of these agents was dependent on the availability of free intracellular calcium; no increased prostanoid formation took place in the absence of extracellular calcium[46,47] or in the presence of the intracellular calcium immobilizing agent 3,4,5-trimethoxybenzoicacid-8-(diethylamino)-octylester-HCl.[46] Mepacrine and p-bromphenacylbromide, which are known to inhibit PLA_2 activity, also prevented the PG formation otherwise induced by all the above stimuli.[46] This underlines the key role of Ca^{2+}-dependent PLA_2 in prostanoid formation of astrocytes.

We have further investigated the question of which of the neuronal signals might activate astroglial PLA_2 activity. Neuronal firing is followed by an increase of extracellular K^+, which is known to stimulate the metabolic activity of astrocytes. However, potassium depolarization (up to 40 mM) of cultured astrocytes did not enhance prostanoid formation in these cells.[46] Astroglial cells possess functional receptors for neurotransmitters.[53] Therefore, we also studied the possible effect of different neurotransmitter receptor agonists on astroglial prostanoid synthesis. In the periphery, noradrenaline and ATP act as cotransmitters in the perivascular sympathetic nerves of some arteries[54]; ATP excerts its contractile effects via P_2 receptors. In the central nervous system no P_2 purinoceptors have yet been identified.

TABLE 3. Prostanoid Forming Capacity in Homogenates from Primary Astroglial Cell Cultures as a Function of Cultivation Time

Age	Prostanoid Formed (ng/mg protein/15 min)			
	PGD_2	$PGF_{2\alpha}$	PGE_2	TXB_2
7 days ($n = 5$)	0.78 ± 0.31	0.78 ± 0.19	0.68 ± 0.33	0.44 ± 0.35
14 days ($n = 6$)	10.20 ± 0.61	2.38 ± 0.53	1.31 ± 0.25	3.62 ± 0.53
21 days ($n = 6$)	7.79 ± 1.12	1.74 ± 0.42	1.15 ± 0.17	3.11 ± 0.71

NOTE: Results are the means ± SEM of experiments performed in quadruplicate from independent cultivations (n indicated in parentheses).

TABLE 4. Effect of Phorbol 12-Miristate, 13-Acetate (TPA), and Phorbol 12,13-Dibutyrate (PDB) on Basal and A 23187–Stimulated Prostaglandin D_2 Synthesis by Cultured Astrocytes

	Prostaglandin D_2 (ng/mg protein/15 min)	
	Basal	A 23187 (100 nM)
Control	3.1 ± 0.5	13.0 ± 1.5[a]
TPA (10 nM)	3.7 ± 0.5	41.2 ± 5.2[b]
TPA (100 nM)	17.5 ± 1.1[a]	76.6 ± 6.8[b]
PDB (10 nM)	3.4 ± 0.7	29.9 ± 2.9[b]
PDB (100 nM)	6.8 ± 0.5[a]	39.1 ± 6.2[b]

NOTE: Fourteen-day-old cultures were used. Results are the means ± SEM of experiments performed in triplicate from four independent cultivations.
[a]Significantly different from the corresponding control ($p < 0.001$). ANOVA was used.
[b]Significantly different from the sum of values obtained in the presence of phorbol ester and ionophor alone ($p < 0.001$). ANOVA was used.

Prostaglandin synthesis in cultured astrocytes could be induced by a physiologically relevant ligand, ATP, via a P_2 purinoceptor. ATP and related nucleotide triphosphates (NTP) as well as stable NTP analogs and nucleotide diphosphates stimulated PGD_2 synthesis in a concentration-dependent manner. Nucleotide monophosphates and adenosine were without effect. Pretreatment of astroglia with islet-activating protein (IAP) resulted in a reduction of ATP-stimulated PG synthesis. At least three IAP-sensitive G proteins have been identified as astroglial cells. It is concluded that ATP released into the synaptic cleft from neurons acts via P_2 receptors on the astroglial cells.[55] Neurotransmitters and drugs with affinity to α or β adrenoceptors, or to dopamine, 5-hydroxytryptamine, muscarine, histamine, GABA, glutamate, aspartate, adenosine and opioid receptors failed to stimulate prostanoid biosynthesis. Also, compounds like angiotensin, bradykinin, and thrombin were ineffective in this respect.[46]

Similar results were obtained by De George et al. and Pearce et al.; they, also, have not found increased astroglial eicosanoid synthesis in the presence of noradrenaline,[56,57] acetylcholine, histamine, glutamate, GABA, and serotonin[57] or the muscarinic cholinergic receptor agonist oxotremorine,[56] even if most of these agents stimulated PLC-catalyzed phosphatidylinositol (PI) breakdown.[56,57] There was only a rapid, transient, and moderate accumulation of arachidonic acid following such stimuli,[57] in contrast to the effect of the calcium ionophor, which caused a massive and long-lasting increase of free arachidonic acid concentration and synthesis of cyclooxygenase products.[45-47,56,57] These results suggest that Ca^{2+}-dependent PLA_2 activity, rather than PLC-catalyzed PI breakdown, is the source of arachidonic acid for eicosanoid synthesis in astrocytes. However, receptor-mediated PI hydrolysis seems to be involved as well: diacylglycerol(DAG)-mimetic phorbol esters, which are known to activate protein kinase C (PKC), enhanced PGE_2,[48,58] $PGF_{2\alpha}$, PGI_2, and TXB_2,[58] as well as PGD_2[59] (TABLE 4) synthesis in a concentration-dependent manner. Furthermore, already subthreshold concentrations of phorbol esters (10 nM) potentiated markedly the effect of the calcium ionophor on astroglial prostanoid synthesis (TABLE 4), strongly suggesting a synergism between Ca^{2+}-mediated PLA_2 activation and PI metabolism. This would mean that astroglial free arachidonic acid levels and eicosanoid synthesis could be modulated by neurotransmitters acting on PLC-coupled receptors via eliciting PI hydrolysis, DAG liberation, and PKC activation. One can speculate that PKC may act by opening calcium channels, liberating PLA_2 activity from lipocortin inhibition, inhibiting acyltransferases to reacylate free arachidonic acid into phospholipids, or stimulating directly cyclooxygenase and/or lipoxygenase activity. Further research is required to learn the exact mechanism of the synergistic action of the two pathways on astroglial eicosanoid synthesis.

SUMMARY AND CONCLUSIONS

Neuronal firing during experimental convulsions triggered a large increase in brain eicosanoid synthesis. Mature astrocytes are an important source of cerebral prostanoids. Endogenously formed prostaglandins possess anticonvulsive properties of biological relevance. These conclusions suggest new ideas that might explain the formation and functions of prostanoids in the brain. First, as augmented neuronal discharge is a prerequisite for enhanced prostanoid syntehsis during seizures, a functional coupling between firing neurons and prostanoid-forming astrocytes may be expected. Second, the anticonvulsive effects of endogenous prostanoids suggest that astroglia-derived substances might regulate neuronal activity. The phenomenon of convulsion-induced prostanoid synthesis may, therefore, represent a new example of neuron-glia interaction. Neither K^+-induced membrane depolarization nor receptor activation by drugs with affinity to α or β adrenoceptors, dopamine, serotonin, muscarine, histamine, GABA, glutamate, aspartate, adenosine, and opioid receptors evoked eicosanoid synthesis in astrocytes. The only physiologically relevant ligand that induced prostanoid synthesis concentration dependently in astrocytes was ATP and related nucleotide triphosphates, as well as nucleotide diphosphates. In peripheral nerves ATP serves as a cotransmitter. The effect of the P_2 agonists was reduced by pertussis toxin. The mechanism by which eicosanoids regulate neuronal activity remains to be elucidated.

REFERENCES

1. NEEDLEMAN, PH., J. TURK, B. A. JAKSCHIK, A. R. MORRISON & J. B. LEFKOWITZ. 1986. Arachidonic acid metabolism. Annu. Rev. Biochem. **55:** 69–102.
2. SAMUELSSON, B. 1964. Identification of a smooth muscle-stimulating factor in bovine brain. Biochim. Biophys. Acta **84:** 218–219.
3. WOLFE, L. S. 1982. Eicosanoids: Prostaglandins, thromboxanes, leukotrienes, and other derivatives of carbon-20 unsaturated fatty acids. J. Neurochem. **38:** 1–14.
4. ABDEL-HALIM, M. S., M. HAMBERG, B. SJÖQUIST & E. ANGGARD. 1977. Identification of prostaglandin D_2 as a major prostaglandin in homogenates of rat brain. Prostaglandins **14:** 633–643.
5. ABDEL-HALIM, M. S., I. LUNDÉN, G. CSEH & E. ANGGARD. 1980. Prostaglandin profiles in nervous tissue and blood vessels of the brain of various animals. Prostaglandins **19:** 249–258.
6. BERCHTOLD-KANZ, E., H. ANHUT, R. HELDT, B. NEUFANG & G. HERTTING. 1981. Regional distribution of arachidonic acid metabolites in rat brain following convulsive stimuli. Prostaglandins **22:** 65–78.
7. FÖRSTERMANN, U., R. HELDT, F. KNAPPEN & G. HERTTING. 1982. Potential anticonvulsive properties of endogenous prostaglandins formed in mouse brain. Brain Res. **240:** 303–310.
8. SEREGI, A. & G. HERTTING. 1984. Changes in cyclooxygenase activity and prostaglandin profiles during monoamine metabolism in rat brain homogenates. Prostagland. Leuk. Med. **14:** 113–121.
9. SPAGNUOLO, C., L. SAUTEBIN, G. GALLI, G. RACAGNI, C. GALLI, S. MAZZARI & M. FINESSO. 1979. $PGF_{2\alpha}$, thromboxane B_2 and HETE levels in gerbil brain cortex after ligation of common carotid arteries and decapitation. Prostaglandins **18:** 53–61.

10. ADESUYI, S. A., C. S. COCKRELL, D. A. GAMACHE & E. F. ELLIS. 1985. Lipoxygenase metabolism of arachidonic acid in brain. J. Neurochem. **45**: 775–776.
11. DEMBINSKA-KIEC, A., TH. SIMMET & B. A. PESKAR. 1984. Formation of leukotriene C_4-like material by rat brain tissue. Eur. J. Pharmacol. **99**: 57–62.
12. LINDGREN, J.-A., TH. HÖKFELT, S.-E. DAHLEN, C. PATRONO & B. SAMUELSSON. 1984. Leukotrienes in rat central nervous system. Proc. Natl. Acad. Sci. USA **81**: 6212–6216.
13. MOSKOWITZ, M. A., K. J. KIWAK, K. L. HEKIMIAN & L. LEVINE. 1984. Synthesis of compounds with properties of leukotrienes C_4 and D_4 in gerbil brains after ischemia and reperfusion. Science **224**: 886–889.
14. SIMMET, TH., A. SEREGI & G. HERTTING. 1987. Formation of sulphidopeptide-leukotrienes in brain tissue of spontaneously convulsing gerbils. Neuropharmacology **26**: 107–110.
15. SHIMIZU, T., Y. TAKUSAGAWA, T. IZUMI, N. OHISHI & Y. SEYEMA. 1987. Enzymic synthesis of leukotriene B_4 in guinea pig brain. J. Neurochem. **48**: 1541–1546.
16. MIYAMOTO, T., J.-A. LINDGREN, TH. HÖKFELT & B. SAMUELSSON. 1987. Regional distribution of leukotriene and mono-hydroxyeicosatetraenoic acid production in the rat brain. FEBS Lett. **216**: 123–127.
17. BIRKLE, D. L. & N. G. BAZAN. 1987. Effect of bicuculline-induced status epilepticus on prostaglandins and hydroxyeicosatetraenoic acids in rat brain subcellular fractions. J. Neurochem. **48**: 1768–1778.
18. FELDBERG, W. & A. S. MILTON. 1978. Prostaglandins and body temperature. *In* Handbook of Experimental Pharmacology. J. R. Vane & S. H. Ferreira, Eds.: 615–656. Springer-Verlag. Berlin.
19. LIPTON, J. M. 1980. Fever. Raven Press. New York, NY.
20. UENO, R., K. HONDA, S. INOVE & O. HAYAISHI. 1983. Prostaglandin D_2: A cerebral sleep inducing substance in rats. Proc. Natl. Acad. Sci. **80**: 1735–1737.
21. HAYAISHI, O. 1983. Prostaglandin D_2: A neuromodulator. *In* Advances in Prostaglandin, Thromboxane and Leukotriene Research, Vol. 12. B. Samuelsson, R. Paoletti & P. Ramwell, Eds.: 333–337. Raven Press. New York, NY.
22. FÖRSTERMANN, U., R. HELDT & G. HERTTING. 1983. Effects of intracerebro-ventricular administration of prostaglandin D_2 on behaviour, blood pressure and body temperature as compared to prostaglandin E_2 and $F_{2\alpha}$. Psychopharmacology **80**: 365–370.
23. PALMER, M. R., W. R. MATHEWS, B. J. HOFFER & R. C. MURPHY. 1981. Electrophysiological response of cerebellar Purkinje neurones to leukotriene D_4 and B_4. J. Pharmacol. Exp. Ther. **219**: 91–96.
24. PIOMELLI, D., E. SHAPIRO, S. J. FEINMARK & J. H. SCHWARTZ. 1987. Metabolites of arachidonic acid in the nervous system of Aplysia: Possible mediators of synaptic modulation. J. Neurosci. **7**: 3675–3686.
25. STEINHAUER, H. B., H. ANHUT & G. HERTTING. 1979. The synthesis of prostaglandins and thromboxane in the mouse brain *in vivo*. Naunyn-Schmiedeberg's Arch. Pharmacol. **310**: 53–58.
26. GAUDET, R. J., I. ALAM & L. LEVINE. 1980. Accumulation of cyclooxygenase products of arachidonic acid metabolism in gerbil brain during a reperfusion after bilateral common carotid artery occlusion. J. Neurochem. **35**: 653–658.
27. FOLCO, G. C., D. LONGIAVE & E. BOSISIO. 1977. Relations between prostaglandin E_2, $F_{2\alpha}$, and cyclic nucleotides levels in rat brain and induction of convulsions. Prostaglandins **13**: 892–900.
28. ZATZ, M. & R. H. ROTH. 1975. Electroconvulsive shock raises prostaglandin F in rat cerebral cortex. Biochem. Pharmacol. **4**: 2101–2103.
29. SEREGI, A., G. FOLLY, M. ANTAL, P. SERFÖZÖ & A. SCHAEFER. 1981. Studies on prostaglandin $F_{2\alpha}$ formation caused by pentamethylenetetrazol-induced convulsions in rat brain. Prostaglandins **21**: 217–226.
30. FÖRSTERMANN, U., R. HELDT & G. HERTTING. 1983. Increase in brain prostaglandins during convulsions is due to increased neuronal activity and not to hypoxia. Arch. Int. Pharmacodyn. Ther. **263**: 180–188.
31. GALLI, C. & G. RACAGNI. 1982. Use of microwave techniques to inactivate brain enzymes rapidly. Methods Enzymol. **86**: 635–643.
32. FÖRSTERMANN, U., A. SEREGI & G. HERTTING. 1984. Anticonvulsive effects of endogenous

prostaglandins formed in brain of spontaneously convulsing gerbils. Prostaglandins **27:** 913–923.
33. SEREGI, A., U. FÖRSTERMANN, R. HELDT & G. HERTTING. 1985. The formation and regional distribution of prostaglandins D_2 and $F_{2\alpha}$ in the brain of spontaneously convulsing gerbils. Brain Res. **337:** 171–174.
34. ABDEL-HALIM, S. & E. ANGGARD. 1979. Regional and species differences in endogenous prostaglandin biosynthesis by rat brain homogenates. Prostaglandins **17:** 411–418.
35. GEROZISSIS, K., J. M. SAAVEDRA & F. DRAY. 1983. Prostanoid profile in specific brain areas, pituitary and pineal gland of the male rat. Brain Res. **279:** 133–139.
36. LONGO, V. G. 1962. Electroencephalographic Atlas for Pharmacological Research, Vol. 2: 65–79. Elsevier. Amsterdam.
37. LOSKOTA, W. J. & P. LOMAX. 1975. The mongolian gerbil (*Meriones unguiculatus*) as a model for the study of the epilepsies: EEG records of seizures. Electroencephalogr. Clin. Neurophysiol. **38:** 597–604.
38. SIMMET, TH., A. SEREGI & G. HERTTING. 1988. Characterization of seizure-induced cysteinyl-leukotriene formation in the brain of convulsion-prone gerbils. J. Neurochem. **50:** 1738–1742.
39. SEREGI, A., G. FOLLY, R. HELDT, E. S. VIZI & G. HERTTING. 1988. Differential convulsion-induced prostanoid formation in the brain of mice susceptible (DBA 2/J) and resistant (CFLP) to acoustic stimulation. Epilepsy Res. Submitted for publication.
40. MAXSON, S. C. & J. S. COWEN. 1976. Electroencephalographic correlates of the audiogenic seizure response of inbred mice. Physiol. Behav. **16:** 623–629.
41. BARAN, H., R. HELDT & G. HERTTING. 1987. Increased prostaglandin formation in rat brain following systemic application of kainic acid. Brain Res. **404:** 107–112.
42. STEINHAUER, H. B. & G. HERTTING. 1981. Lowering of the convulsive threshold by non-steroidal anti-inflammatory drugs. Eur. J. Pharmacol. **69:** 199–203.
43. SEREGI, A., U. FÖRSTERMANN & G. HERTTING. 1984. Decreased levels of brain cyclo-oxygenase products as a possible cause of increased seizure susceptibility in convulsion-prone gerbils. Brain Res. **305:** 393–395.
44. FEUERSTEIN, G. & J. M. HALLENBECK. 1987. Leukotrienes in health and disease. FASEB J. **1:** 186–192.
45. KELLER, M., R. JACKISCH, A. SEREGI & G. HERTTING. 1985. Comparison of prostanoid forming capacity of neuronal and astroglial cell in primary cultures. Neurochem. Int. **7:** 655–665.
46. KELLER, M., A. SEREGI, R. JACKISCH & G. HERTTING. 1987. Prostanoid formation in primary astroglial cell cultures: Ca^{2+}-dependency and stimulation by A 23187, melittin and phospholipases A_2 and C. Neurochem. Int. **10:** 433–443.
47. MURPHY, S., J. JEREMY, B. PEARCE & P. DANDONA. 1985. Eicosanoid synthesis and release from primary cultures of rat central nervous system astrocytes and meningeal cells. Neurosci. Lett. **61:** 61–65.
48. HARTUNG, H.-P. & K. V. TOYKA. 1987. Phorbol diester TPA elicits prostaglandin E release from cultured rat astrocytes. Brain Res. **417:** 347–349.
49. SEREGI, A., M. KELLER, R. JACKISCH & G. HERTTING. 1984. Comparison of prostanoid forming capacity in homogenates from primary neuronal and astroglial cell cultures. Biochem. Pharmacol. **33:** 3315–3318.
50. HARTUNG, H.-P. & K. V. TOYKA. 1987. Leukotriene production by cultured astroglial cells. Brain Res. **435:** 367–370.
51. SEREGI, A., TH. SIMMET & G. HERTTING. 1988. Characterization of cysteinyl-leukotriene formation by rat astroglial cells in primary culture. In preparation.
52. SEREGI, A., M. KELLER & G. HERTTING. 1987. Are cerebral prostanoids of astroglial origin? Studies on the prostanoid forming system in developing rat brain and primary cultures of astrocytes. Brain Res. **404:** 113–120.
53. MURPHY, S. & B. PEARCE. 1987. Functional receptors for neurotransmitters on astrocytes. Neurosci. **22:** 381–394.
54. RAMME, D., J. T. REGENOLD, K. STARKE, R. BUSSE & P. ILLES. 1987. Identification of the neuroeffector transmitter in jejunal branches of the rabbit mesenteric artery. Naunyn-Schmiedeberg's Arch. Pharmacol. **336:** 267–273.

55. WURSTER, S., P. J. GEBICKE-HAERTER, A. SCHOBERT & G. HERTTING. 1988. The astroglial P_2-purinoceptor. Paper presented at the Fourth International Congress of Cell Biology, Montréal, August 14–19, 1988. Naunyn-Schmiedeberg's Arch. Pharmakol. In press.
56. PEARCE, B., J. JEREMY, CH. MORROW, S. MURPHY & P. DANDONA. 1987. Inositol phospholipids are probably not the source of arachidonic acid for eicosanoid synthesis in astrocytes. FEBS Lett. **211:** 73–77.
57. DEGEORGE, J. J., P. MORELL, K. D. MCCARTHY & E. G. LAPETINA. 1986. Adrenergic and cholinergic stimulation of arachidonate and phosphatidate metabolism in cultured astroglial cells. Neurochem. Res. **11:** 1061–1071.
58. JEREMY, J., S. MURPHY, CH. MORROW, B. PEARCE & P. DANDONA. 1987. Phorbol ester stimulation of prostanoid synthesis by cultured astrocytes. Brain Res. **419:** 364–368.
59. GEBICKE-HAERTER, P., A. SEREGI, A. BRENNER & G. HERTTING. 1988. Involvement of protein kinase C in prostaglandin D_2 synthesis by cultured astrocytes. Neurochem. Int. In press.

Prostaglandin E_2, Leukotriene C_4, and Platelet-Activating Factor Receptor Sites in the Brain

Binding Parameters and Pharmacological Studies

F. DRAY,[a] A. WISNER, M. C. BOMMELAER-BAYET,
C. TIBERGHIEN, K. GEROZISSIS, M. SAADI,
M. P. JUNIER, AND C. ROUGEOT

Unité de Radioimmunologie Analytique
Institut Pasteur/INSERM
75724 Paris Cedex 15, France

INTRODUCTION

Central neuroendocrine secretions are under the influence of various factors, including hormones and mediators. Hormones secreted by the hypothalamus, hypophysis, epiphysis, and the peripheral glands exert their effects through short and/or long loops integrated into positive or negative feedback mechanisms. The possibility that prostaglandins (PGs) might act within the central nervous system, more precisely within neuroendocrine systems, has been a subject of great interest for more than 15 years and has been reviewed several times.[1]

Whereas the importance in the brain of prostanoids such as PGE_2 or PGD_2 has been emphasized,[2-10] new metabolites of arachidonate originating from the lipoxygenase[11-15] or epoxygenase pathways[16] and the etherophospholipid, platelet-activating factor (PAF), have recently stolen the limelight because of their potent and diversified effects on several neuroendocrine secretions.[17-23]

This study of the specific binding of some of these lipid compounds (PGE_2, 12-HETE (hydroxyeicostetraenoic acid), leukotriene (LT) C_4, LTD_4 and PAF to preparations of hypothalamic membranes was carried out to elucidate the mechanism whereby they are recognized by their target cells. The binding was analyzed in terms of a single neurosecretory process: the secretion of luteinizing hormone-releasing hormone (LHRH).[2,12,13,21]

PROSTAGLANDIN E_2

Pharmacological Effects

Prostaglandin E_2 is a well-known modulator of several central neuroendocrine secretions. Its action varies from one secretory process to another:

(a) *Luteinizing hormone (LH) secretion:* stimulation of the basal and norepinephrine (NE)-stimulated LHRH secretion, but no effect on the basal and LHRH-stimulated LH secretion.[2,7]

---

[a]Address for correspondence: Professor Fernand Dray, Institut Pasteur, Service URIA, 28, rue du Docteur Roux, 75724 Paris Cedex 15, France.

(b) *Growth hormone (GH) secretion:* no effect on growth hormone releasing factor (GRF) and somatostatin (SRIF) release,[24] but stimulation of the basal and GRF-stimulated GH secretion.[25]

(c) *Adrenocorticotropin hormone (ACTH) secretion:* stimulation of corticotrope releasing factor (CRF)-like activities, but stronger inhibition of CRF-induced ACTH secretion.[27]

(d) *Thyreostimulin hormone (TSH) secretion:* no effect on thyreostimulin releasing hormone (TRH) secretion, but stimulation of TRH-induced TSH secretion.[28]

(e) *Prolactin (PRL) secretion:* increase of stimulating hypothalamic activity(ies), through increase of releasing factor(s) or decrease of inhibitory factor(s), but no effect on pituitary PRL secretion.[29]

(f) *Melatonin secretion:* unconfirmed[14,15] stimulation of synthesis and secretion of melatonin.[1]

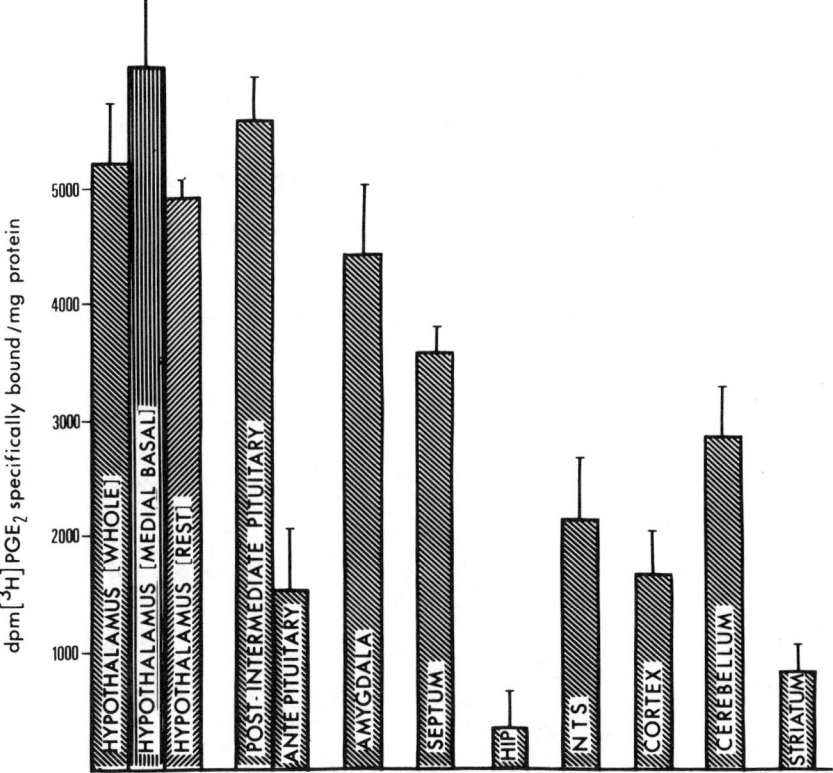

FIGURE 1. [^{3}H]PGE$_2$-specific binding to different rat brain areas and the pituitary gland.[4] Specific binding was determined using membrane fractions P$_2$ of different areas of the rat brain, except for postpituitary, for which we used an homogenate instead of P$_2$. Incubation was performed at 22 °C for 30 min with 10 nM [^{3}H]PGE$_2$, with or without an excess of unlabeled PGE$_2$ (2 μM). Results are expressed as dpm of [^{3}H]PGE$_2$-specific binding per mg protein (mean ± SEM, for groups of 3 different experiments, measured in triplicate). HIP = hippocampus; NTS = nucleus tractus solitarius.

Prostaglandin E_2 Production

PGE_2 is synthesized in various parts of the brain, but its endogenous production is not precisely known because of the rapid *in vitro* formation of other prostanoids such as PGD_2.[30] However, the increase in PGE_2 values observed by us in dynamic experiments requires consideration. Two studies will be discussed. One was of the stimulatory effect of NE on the *in vitro* synthesis of PGE_2 by the median eminence of adult rats. This effect was limited to this prostanoid and was much greater when the median eminence (ME) was separated from the medial basal hypothalamus.[2] The other study to be discussed concerned the stimulatory effects of vasopressin and synthetic ovine CRF[27] and GRF[25] on PGE_2 synthesis by the rat adenohypophysis. The other prostanoids were not formed under these conditions.

Prostaglandin E_2 Binding Sites

Binding Parameters

PGE_2 binding sites have been shown in several structures of the brain in several species, including rat, monkey, pig, and man (postmortem), using biochemical or autoradiographic techniques.[4,5] We observed that this binding was predominantly localized in the hypothalamus and the hypophysis in the rat (FIG. 1). Complementary studies using porcine hypothalamic membrane preparations showed that PGE_2 binding was saturable, reversible, and specific (FIG. 2). Nonlinear regression analysis of the saturation curve revealed the existence of two populations of low-capacity binding sites—one of high affinity (R_H) and the other of low affinity (R_L) (TABLE 1 and Reference 31). Specific binding sites with similar characteristics were found also on porcine pituitary membranes (data not shown). However, studies carried out with porcine cortex also revealed the existence of two PGE_2 binding sites, but only after membrane solubilization.[8]

Correlation between Binding and Pharmacological Effects

There was a good correlation between the relative binding of various PG analogs, their stimulatory effects on LHRH release from the hypothalamus, and their inhibitory effect on [^{3}H]NE (TABLE 2).

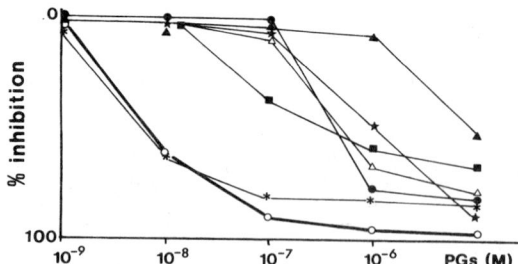

FIGURE 2. [^{3}H]PGE_2 binding specificity. Competition binding experiments were performed using porcine membrane preparations: aliquots of membranes (1 mg protein/tube) were incubated in buffer A with 2 nM radioligand and increasing concentrations of the test substances for determination of the [^{3}H]PGE_2 binding specificity. Incubations were performed at 22 °C for 2 hours with continuous shaking, and bound and free radioactivity were separated by filtration under constant vacuum through Whatman GF/B glass filters, PGE_2 (O); PGE, (*); $PGF_{2\alpha}$ (●); PGD_2 (▲); PGB_2 (★); 15K PGE_2 (△); 13–14 DHE_1 (■).

TABLE 1. [³H]PGE₂ Binding Parameters

	Dissociation Constant (K_D) (10^{-9} M)	Number of Sites (B_{max}) (fmoles/mg of Protein)
R_H	0.87 ± 0.19	6.62 ± 0.67
R_L	13.57 ± 1.18	12.4 ± 1.1

NOTE: Membrane preparations (1 mg protein/tube) were incubated for 2 h in 10 mM Tris buffer pH 7.4 with 10 mM aspirin and 0.1 mM phenylmethylsulfonyl fluoride (buffer A) over a radioligand concentration range of 0.5 nM to 10 nM. Binding parameters were determined using nonlinear regression analysis[57] for cooperative and noncooperative binding studies from the saturation curve. Data are the means ± SE of determined parameters from 3 or 4 separate experiments.

Interrelations between PGE₂ Binding Sites and Adrenoceptors in Rat Hypothalamus

Pharmacological manipulations using noradrenergic agonists and antagonists were used to demonstrate that PGE₂ binding sites were distinct from α_2 presynaptic and α_1 postsynaptic adrenoceptors involved in the NE negative feedback on [³H]NE release and the stimulatory effect of NE on LHRH release.[6,7] However, these results do not completely exclude possible interrelations between the PGE₂ binding sites and these adrenoceptors.

Our results suggest that the first event in the action of PGE₂, inhibition of [³H]NE release and stimulation of LHRH release, involves the binding of the PGE₂ molecule to

TABLE 2. Relationships between Ki Value Displacement of [³H]PGE₂ Binding by Prostaglandin (PG) Analogues and Their Potencies to Enhance Luteinizing Hormone-Releasing Hormone (LHRH) Release or to Decrease K⁺-Evoked [³H]NE Release from Rat Hypothalamus

PG Analogues	Ki Values (nM[a])	LHRH Release[b] (% over Control)	K⁺ Evoked of [³H]NE[c] (% Reduction)
PGE₂	10.2	199 ± 7[d]	36 ± 0.08[d]
PGE₁	14.7	96 ± 6[d]	18 ± 0.06[d]
PGA₂	28.1	58 ± 5[d]	17 ± 0.05[e]
16,16 dimethyl PGE₂	49.2	57 ± 5[d]	7 ± 0.03
11 epi PGE₂	53.3	ND	7 ± 0.02
8 iso PGE₂	422	18 ± 4	5 ± 0.03
PGF₂α	7040	0	—
PGD₂	>10000	0	—

[a]Hypothalamic membranes (500 μg protein/tube) were incubated in the presence of 10 nM [³H]PGE₂ and increasing concentrations of the compound tested at 22 °C for 30 min. Nonspecific binding was determined in the presence of unlabeled PGE₂ (2 μM) and was subtracted from all values. IC₅₀ values were calculated from the concentration response curves of inhibition, and Ki values were calculated according to the formula $IC_{50}/1 + C/Kd$, where C represents the concentration and Kd the dissociation constant determined by Malet et al.[4]

[b]MEs of male rats were preincubated in KRBG for 15 min, followed by a 30-min incubation period in the presence (10^{-6} M) or absence of test substances. LHRH release is expressed as the percentage increase over the control response. Values are the mean ± SEM of six experiments.

[c][³H]NE release was calculated as percentage of the total concentration of tritium in the tissue and expressed as a percentage decrease from the control response. Values are the mean ± SEM of six experiments.

[d]$p < 0.05$.
[e]$p < 0.01$.

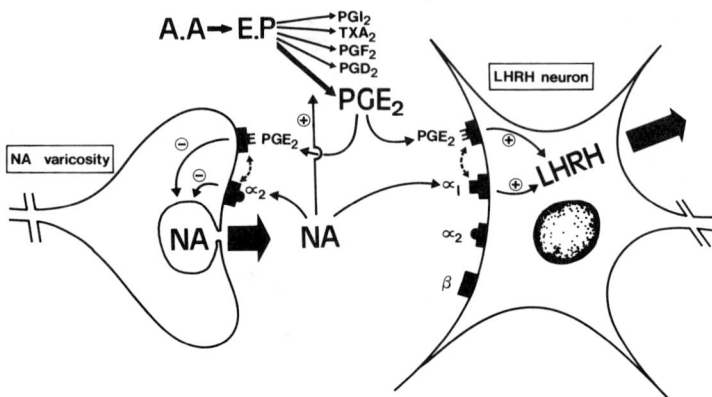

FIGURE 3. Hypothetical schema of the relationships between NE, PGE_2, and LHRH in the median eminence of adult male rats. PGE_2 is specifically bound to pre- and/or postsynaptic membranes and therefore participates in the regulation of LHRH secretion (stimulation of the peptide release and inhibition of NE release). The PGE_2 receptor(s) are independent from α_2 pre- and α_1 postnoradrenergic receptors.

its own receptor(s); and that this synaptic modulation of PGE_2 is carried on PGE_2 pre- and/or postsynaptic receptors, as represented in FIGURE 3.

Coupling to Adenylyl Cyclase System

It has recently been shown in studies on hypothalamic membrane preparations that PGE_2 and cAMP are involved in the release of LHRH.[32,33] Our studies with hypothalamic membranes indicate that the stimulatory effect of PGE_2 on cyclic AMP (cAMP) release is dependent on guanine nucleotides. Moreover, the addition of such unmetabolizable guanine nucleotide analogues as Gpp(NH)p to the incubation mixture blocks the PGE_2 receptor in its reversible state (R_L), thus lowering the proportion of high affinity binding sites (R_H) from 35% to 19% without altering the total number of binding sites.[31] This type of result is typically found when there is interconversion of two states of a receptor coupled to an adenylyl cyclase through an intermediate regulating protein, as previously described in another tissue, the renal medulla.[34]

Another cyclooxygenase metabolite of arachidonic acid, PGD_2, is specifically bound to brain membranes. The complex of PGD_2 with its specific binding sites also triggered an increase in cAMP, as demonstrated using thin slices of rat brain. Moreover, the effect of PGD_2 on neuroblastoma-glioma hybrid cells was accompanied by membrane depolarization. That the PGD_2 binding to these membrane preparations is strongly Na^+ dependent[9,10] suggests a coupling of the PGD_2 receptor to an ionic channel.

LEUKOTRIENES

Pharmacological Studies

Leukotrienes play an important role in numerous biological systems. The observation that LTC_4 and LTD_4 caused a prolonged excitation of cerebellar Purkinje cells[35] was the first indication of a functional involvement of LTs in the brain. In addition, LTs may be involved in vasogenic cerebral edema and cerebral vasospasm.[36,37] It is of particular interest in this context that LTC_4 in the picomolar range stimulated LH release from dispersed anterior pituitary cells of the rat.[11] Recently we reported that LTC_4 and LTD_4, but not LTE_4, specifically stimulated LHRH release from the rat median eminence. These stimulatory effects were observed at low concentrations of LTC_4 and had different dose-response curves: bimodal for LTC_4 (maximum at 10^{-8} M and 10^{-16} M), biphasic for LTD_4 (maximum at 10^{-8} M).[13]

Leukotriene Production in the Brain

Rat and gerbil brain tissue have recently been shown to produce LTC_4, $-D_4$, and $-E_4$.[38,41] The ionophore A23187 causes a dose-dependent stimulation of LTB_4 and LTC_4 synthesis. Regional distribution studies indicated that the highest production of LTC_4 is in the hypothalamus and ME, and the lowest is in the cerebellum and brain cortex.[38,42] Immunohistochemical studies also revealed that LTC_4 and LHRH are localized in the same neurofibers, close to the portal vessels.[38]

Furthermore, there is minimal metabolism of LTC_4 in the cerebro-spinal fluid (CSF) and brain, and active transport of LTC_4 in the choroid plexus, suggesting a protection of CSF from both blood-borne and locally formed LTC_4, which might be deleterious when it is produced in large amounts, as, for instance, in cerebral ischemia or subarachnoid hemorrhage.[36,43]

Leukotriene Binding Sites

Pharmcological studies and binding studies using [^{3}H]leukotrienes provide presumptive evidence for the presence of a heterogeneous receptor population, each selective for individual leukotrienes, which vary from tissue to tissue, and for the

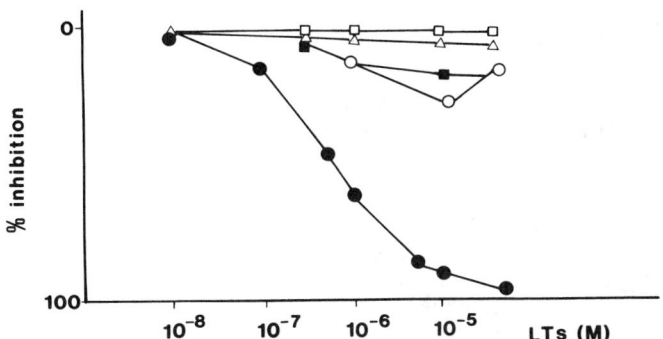

FIGURE 4. [^{3}H]LTC_4 binding specificity. [^{3}H]LTC_4 binding experiments were performed on rat membrane preparations in 10 mM Tris buffer pH 7.4 with 20 mM Ca^{2+} and 0.1 mM phenylmethylsulfonyl fluoride in the presence of 80 mM serine-borate (buffer B). Aliquots of membrane (1 mg protein/tube) were incubated in buffer B with 1 nM radioligand and increasing concentrations of the test substances for determination of the [^{3}H]LTC_4 binding specificity. Incubations were performed at 0 °C for 20 min with continuous shaking, and bound and free radioactivity were separated by filtration under constant vacuum through Whatman GF/C glass filters. LTC_4 (●); LTD_4 (○); LTE_4 (■); FPL 55712 (□); glutathione (△).

presence of multiple receptor subtypes in the same tissue.[44] [^{3}H]LTC$_4$ binding sites were described in the rat and guinea pig brain.[45-47] The highest binding capacity was observed in the brain stem and hippocampus, whereas the binding in the hypothalamus was low. Very low or no binding of LTD$_4$, LTE$_4$, or LTB$_4$ was found. The *in vivo* functional study showed that the ability of LT agonists to produce uterine contraction was in the order of LTC$_4$ > LTD$_4$ > LTE$_4$, which is compatible with their relative effect on inhibition of brain [^{3}H]LTC$_4$ binding.[45] LTC$_4$ binding sites were also localized by autoradiography in the mouse brain.[48]

We have studied binding parameters and neurosecretion in the same part of the brain in order to define a possible role for leukotrienes in the central nervous system. The IC$_{50}$ for the displacement of the [^{3}H]LTC$_4$-specific binding to hypothalamic membrane preparations of adult male rats was 5.10^{-7} M with LTC$_4$ (FIG. 4)—that is, similar to that already obtained with the guinea pig brain.[45] The specificity of [^{3}H]LTC$_4$ binding sites was assessed by measuring the capacity of the SRS-A antagonist FPL 55712, LTD$_4$, LTE$_4$, LTB$_4$, and glutathione to inhibit [^{3}H]LTC$_4$ binding. FIGURE 4 shows that none of these compounds displaced the radioligand. However, a more complete analysis of the competition binding data for LTC$_4$ using low

TABLE 3. Relationships between the Inhibitory Concentration, 50% (IC$_{50}$) Values for Specific Binding of [^{3}H]LTC$_4$ (1 nM) and Leukotrienes or Glutathione and Their Potencies to Stimulate Luteinizing Hormone-Releasing Hormone (LHRH) Release from Incubated ME using 10^{-8} M or 10^{-16} M Test Substances

	IC$_{50}$ (M)	LHRH Release Stimulation (% of Control)	
		10^{-8}-M Test Substances	10^{-16}-M Test Substances
LTC$_4$	5.10^{-7}	$225 \pm 20^*$ ($n = 13$)	$189 \pm 17^*$ ($n = 13$)
LTD$_4$	$>10^{-5}$	$198 \pm 14^*$ ($n = 13$)	110 ± 18 ns ($n = 13$)
LTE$_4$	$>10^{-5}$	109 ± 13 ns ($n = 8$)	102 ± 13 ns ($n = 8$)
LTB$_4$	$>10^{-5}$	115 ± 9 ns ($n = 4$)	97 ± 11 ns ($n = 11$)
Glutathione	$>10^{-5}$	$195 \pm 38^*$ ($n = 8$)	$256 \pm 49^*$ ($n = 6$)

NOTE: * = $p < 0.001$; ns = not significant.

concentrations of [^{3}H]LTC$_4$ (1 to 2 nM) revealed a composite profile (manuscript in preparation) suggesting that several events are involved and indicating the inherent difficulty in evaluating precise affinity constant(s) for LTC$_4$ binding in the brain. This limitation is further emphasized by other peculiar results:

(a) the unusual bimodal pattern of the dose response curve for the stimulatory effect of LTC$_4$ on LHRH release.[13] The two very broad curves observed could be due to the formation of monomeric and dimeric active effector complex with the receptor, as formulated for LTC$_4$-stimulated LH release.[49]

(b) the absence of competition of FPL 55712 (up to 10^{-5} M) with LTC$_4$ binding sites. In our model, FPL 55712 stimulated the basal release of LHRH at 10^{-6} M and did not alter LTC$_4$-induced LHRH release.[13]

(c) the biological role of LTD$_4$ in the brain, where a stimulatory effect on LHRH release was obtained with a biphasic dose-response curve (maximum effect at 10^{-8} M) and no binding of [^{3}H]LTD$_4$. In this case, there may be a higher lability of LTD$_4$ than of LTC$_4$ binding sites, which would require other experimental conditions for their study. In fact, this lability was suspected in the case of longitudinal strips of guinea pig ileum muscle, where LTC_4 and LTD_4 had contractile effects, and only [^{3}H]LTC_4 binding sites were found. There may also be a large degradation of the LTD_4 molecule in the presence of brain membrane preparations in our experimental conditions. This possibility seems unlikely, due to the presence of large amounts of cysteine in the LTD_4 binding studies. This amino acid prevents the LTD_4 molecule from degrading into LTE_4.

(d) the absence of competition with glutathione and glutathionyl PGA_1 at 10^{-5} M, showing the necessity of having both lipid and peptide parts of the LTC_4 molecule for binding activity. However, the glutathione moiety probably contributes to the binding specificity and to the LHRH release activity. Indeed, a modification of the peptide (LTD_4-LTE_4) part of LTC_4 leads to weaker binding and LHRH release activity. The binding site in the brain seems to be specific for LTC_4; however, the LTD_4 stimulates LHRH release at 10^{-8} M, and glutathione alone has maximum stimulatory activity at 10^{-16} M (TABLE 3).

PLATELET-ACTIVATING FACTOR

Pharmacological Effects

PAF, identified as 1-0-alkyl-2-acetyl-*sn*-glyceryl-2-phosphorylcholine, stimulates the release of the granule content from several cell systems[50,51] and acts as a mediator in inflammatory and allergic processes.[52] However, little information is available on its action in the brain. PAF has recently been shown to decrease the amplitude of the electrophysiological response to light stimulation in the rat retina.[53] In our laboratory, we have demonstrated that PAF, incubated with the ME from adult male rats, stimulated CRF and β-endorphin, with a maximum at 10^{-8} M,[20] whereas it inhibited LHRH and SRIF release with a maximum at 10^{-14} M.[21] On the other hand, GRF production was not significantly altered. PAF also strongly counteracted the Ca^{2+} ionophore A 23187-stimulated release of LHRH and SRIF from ME and medio-basal hypothalamus (>50% inhibition).[21] These results suggest the involvement of Ca^{2+}-dependent events in PAF action. This inhibitory effect was specific to the hypothalamus, since such an inhibition was not observed for LH and GH from the rat pituitary gland, where, to the contrary, PAF tended to stimulate LH and GH release.[21] A stimulatory effect of PAF on PRL and GH release from anterior pituitary has been recently demonstrated.[23] There has also been a recent report of a stimulatory effect of PAF on CRF secretion by explants of rat hypothalamus *in vitro* (maximal effect at 10^{-8} M).[22] Interestingly, PAF-induced CRF secretion was not altered by treatment with nordihydroguaiaretic acid, a lipoxygenase inhibitor; whereas indomethacin, a cyclooxygenase inhibitor, completely prevented the PAF stimulatory effect, suggesting the existence of a link between the cyclooxygenase metabolites of arachidonic acid and PAF at the hypothalamic level. Moreover, the trialobenzodiazepin, alprazolam, which is known to inhibit PAF effects on platelets, also inhibited PAF-induced CRF secretion.

Endogenous Production of Platelet-Activating Factor

PAF has been identified in the bovine brain,[54] and an acetyl hydrolase involved in its biosynthesis was found in high amounts in the rat brain.[17] Moreover, neurotransmitters, such as acetylcholine and dopamine and the calcium ionophore A 23187, can all induce PAF production by chick retina.[18]

Platelet-Activating Factor Binding Sites

The biological effects of PAF have been found to be mediated by specific receptors in many tissues.[55,56] Because of the potent effects of PAF on hypothalamic secretion, we looked for a specific binding of this etherolipid on whole brain and hypothalamic membrane preparations. The different binding assays performed revealed the existence of two populations of PAF binding sites of high affinity and low capacity, both in whole brain and in the hypothalamus. However, the binding parameter values were different in the whole brain and the hypothalamus. The affinity (K_D) of each binding class in the whole brain was 0.45 ± 0.16 nM and 13.45 ± 4.4 nM, respectively, with a corresponding capacity of 10.1 ± 1.5 and 70 ± 11 fmol/mg protein. In the same conditions, the binding parameters of the two populations of binding sites in the hypothalamus had affinities of 2.14 ± 0.32 nM and 61.6 ± 16.4 nM, with a binding capacity of 25.4 ± 3.2 and 146.2 ± 47.5 fmol/mg protein, respectively. In both cases, the affinity of the first class of binding sites was close to that reported for the PAF binding sites in human lung, rabbit platelets, and guinea pig smooth muscle.[55,56] However, unlike the binding of PAF to rat brain membranes, only one class of sites was present in these tissues. The fact that different [^{3}H]PAF binding parameters were found in whole brain and in hypothalamus suggests the presence of extrahypothalamic PAF binding site populations. We therefore investigated PAF-specific binding in various parts of the brain. The greatest number of binding sites was found in the telencephalic structures, whereas no detectable binding was found in the pituitary. This last result suggests that the effect of PAF at the pituitary level is not a receptor-mediated process.

Lyso-PAF, a structural derivative of PAF, did not inhibit [^{3}H]PAF binding to hypothalamic membranes, while L-652,731, kadsurenone, and BN52021, all known antagonists of PAF action in platelets, were potent inhibitors of this binding with the same relative effectiveness that they have in the platelets (FIG. 5). Moreover, whereas lyso-PAF was found not to alter neuropeptide release, L-652,731, kadsurenone, and

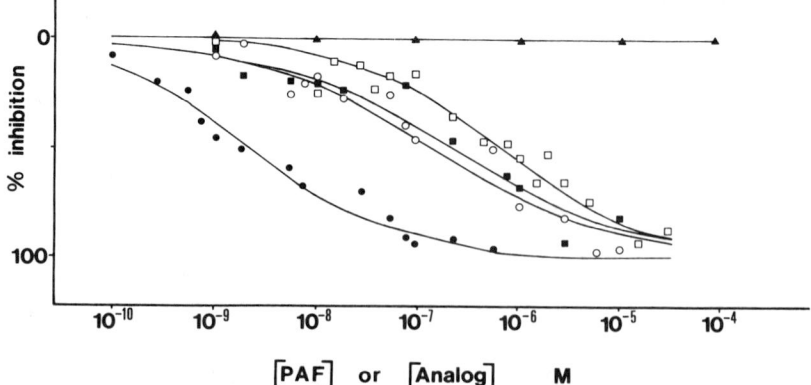

FIGURE 5. Competition of [^{3}H]PAF-acether (1 nM) binding to rat hypothalamic membranes by unlabeled PAF-acether (●); L-652,731 (○); kadsurenone (■); BN52021 (□).

TABLE 4. Comparative Effect of PAF and PAF Related Compounds on the [^{3}H]PAF Binding to Rat Hypothalamic Membranes and on the A 23187 (5 μM)-Stimulated Luteinizing Hormone-Releasing Hormone (LHRH) and Somatostatin (SRIF) Release from Rat Median Eminence

	IC$_{50}$ nM	LHRH Release (%)	SRIF Release (%)
A 23187	—	143 ± 34	55 ± 25
PAF	2.28 ± 0.15	12 ± 14*	−3 ± 9*
L-652,731	138 ± 75	41 ± 8*	−21 ± 7*
Kadsurenone	283 ± 176	51 ± 17*	−15 ± 5*
BN 52021	780 ± 480	59 ± 11*	18 ± 14
Lyso-PAF	>10000	74 ± 19	38 ± 13

NOTE: PAF and related compounds are used at 10^{-14} M. * = $p < 0.05$, significant in front of the A 23187 group.

BN 52021 mimicked the action of PAF on neuropeptide release, with relative effectiveness on LHRH and SRIF secretion similar to that observed in binding experiments (TABLE 4). The relative potency of these three drugs to stimulate CRF and β-endorphin release from ME has not yet been established.

CONCLUSION

Several lipid structures such as hydroxylated derivatives of arachidonic acid and the etherophospholipid PAF, have potent pharmacological actions within the brain. A number of them with differing actions on the secretion of the hypothalamic neuropeptide LHRH were selected for study. One of them, PAF, inhibited LHRH release; whereas the others, PGE$_2$, 12-HETE, LTC$_4$, and LTD$_4$, stimulated it.

It has been shown in several biological models that the first event linked to the recognition of the cell membrane by an active lipid may be a general disturbance of membrane fluidity, a local modification of ionic channels or/and a specific binding to macromolecule component(s).

Rat hypothalamic membranes or synaptosome preparations and tritiated ligands were used to:

(1) demonstrate the existence of specific binding sites for PGE$_2$ and PAF but not for 12-HETE;
(2) confirm the existence of specific binding sites for LTC$_4$ and the absence of such binding sites for LTD$_4$;
(3) establish a good correlation between the potency of various structural analogs of each ligand studied to displace the titriated ligand from its binding sites and to alter the secretion of LHRH.

These results suggest that in the first step in the modulation of LHRH secretion by PGE$_2$, LTC$_4$, and PAF is initiated by their interaction with specific receptors.

The analysis of binding parameters for each active lipid, PGE$_2$, LTC$_4$, and PAF appears to be complex and suggests the existence of multiple types of binding sites in a simple tissue and from one tissue to another. Substantial progress in this field could be made using specific agonists and antagonists of the ligand studied.

The relative participation of each active lipid in the modulation of LHRH secretion remains to be elucidated. However, the physiological role of PGE$_2$ is already clear from the numerous data available. Indeed, PGE_2 appears to be a *synaptic modulator* of norepinephrine-induced LHRH secretion.

REFERENCES

1. CARDINALI, O. P. & M. N. RITTA. 1983. Neuroendocrinology **36**: 152–160.
2. OJEDA, S. R., A. NEGRO-VILAR & S. M. MC CANN. 1979. Endocrinology **104**(3): 617–624.
3. OJEDA, S. R., H. F. URBANSKI, K. H. KATZ, M. E. COSTA & P. M. CONN. 1986. Proc. Natl. Acad. Sci. USA **83**: 4932–4936.
4. MALET, C., H. SCHERRER, J. M. SAAVEDRA & F. DRAY. 1982. Brain Res. **236**: 227–233.
5. WATANABE, Y., A. YAMASHITA, K. TASHIRO & O. HAYAISHI. 1984. Neurochem. Res. **9**: 1136.
6. DRAY, F. & M. HEAULME. 1984. Neuropharmacology **23**(4): 457–462.
7. HEAULME, M. & F. DRAY. 1984. Neuroendocrinology **39**: 403–407.
8. YUMOTO, N., Y. WATANABE, K. WATANABE, Y. WATANABE & O. HAYAISHI. 1986. J. Neurochem. **46**(1): 125–132.
9. SHIMIZU, T., A. YAMASHITA & O. HAYAISHI. 1982. J. Biol. Chem. **257**(22): 13570–13575.
10. WATANABE, Y., A. YAMASHITA, H. TOKUMOTO & O. HAYAISHI. 1983. Proc. Natl. Acad. Sci. USA **80**: 4542–4545.
11. HULTING, A. L., J. A. LINDGREN, T. HOKFELT, P. ENEROTH, S. WERNER, C. PATRONO & B. SAMUELSSON. 1985. Proc. Natl. Acad. Sci. USA **82**: 3834–3838.
12. GEROZISSIS, K., B. VULLIEZ-LE NORMAND, J. M. SAAVEDRA, R. C. MURPHY & F. DRAY. 1985. Neuroendocrinology **40**: 272–276.
13. GEROZISSIS, K., M. SAADI & F. DRAY. 1987. Brain Res. **416**: 54–58.
14. VACAS, M. I., M. I. KELLER-SARMIENTO, G. S. ETCHEGOYEN, E. N. PEYREYRA, M. F. GIMENO & O. P. CARDINALI. 1987. Neuroendocrinology. **46**: 412–416.
15. SAKAI, K., V. FAFEUR, B. VULLIEZ-LE NORMAND & F. DRAY. 1988. Prostaglandins **35**: 969–976.
16. CAPDEVILLA, J., N. CHACOS, J. R. FALCK, S. MANNA, A. NEGRO-VILAR & S. R. OJEDA. 1983. Endocrinology **113**(1): 421–423.
17. BLANK, M. L., T. C. LEE, V. FITZGERALD, F. SNYDER. 1981. J. Biol. Chem. **256**: 175–178.
18. BUSSOLINO, F., F. GREMO, C. TETTA, G. P. PESCARMONA, G. CAMUSSI. 1986. Abstr. 6th Int. Conf. on Prostaglandins and Related Compounds, Florence, June 1986: 333.
19. SPINNEWYN, B., N. BLAVET, F. CLOSTRE, N. BAZAN & P. BRAQUET. 1987. Prostaglandin **34**(3): 337–347.
20. ROUGEOT, C., M. P. JUNIER, S. EVERAERE, P. BRAQUET & F. DRAY. 1988. *In* New Trends in Lipid Mediators Research, Vol. 2. P. Braquet, Ed.: 79–84. Karger AG. Basel.
21. JUNIER, M. P., C. TIBERGHIEN, C. ROUGEOT, V. FAFEUR & F. DRAY. 1988. Endocrinol. **123**: 72–80.
22. BERNARDINI, R., A. E. CALOGERO, G. P. CHROUSOS, C. SAOUTIS & P. W. GOLD. 1987. Abstr. 17th Meeting of the Society for Neurosciences, New Orleans, Louisiana: 1622.
23. GRANDISON, L. 1987. Program of the IPSEN Foundation, Platelet-activating factor in the immune response. Paris. Abstr.: 50.
24. ROUGEOT, C., V. GUILLAUME, M. P. JUNIER, V. FAFEUR, C. OLIVER & F. DRAY. 1986. Abstr. 6th International Conference on Prostaglandins and Related Compounds, Florence, June, 1986: 115.
25. FAFEUR, V., E. GOUIN & F. DRAY. 1985. Biochem. Biophys. Res. Commun. **126**(2): 725–733.
26. HEDGE, G. A. 1977. Life Sci. **20**: 17–34.
27. VLASKOVSKA, M., G. HERTTING & W. KNEPEL. 1984. Endocrinology **115**: 895–903.
28. WRIGHT, K. C. & G. A. HEDGE. 1981. Endocrinology **109**: 637–643.
29. HARMS, P. G., S. R. OJEDA & S. M. MC CANN. 1973. Science **181**: 760–761.
30. GEROZISSIS, K., J. M. SAAVEDRA & F. DRAY. 1983. Brain Res. **279**: 133–139.

31. WISNER, A., M. C. BOMMELAER-BAYET, C. TIBERGHIEN, C. A. RENARD, F. DAVID & F. DRAY. 1988. Eur. J. Pharmacol. Submitted for publication.
32. RAMIREZ, V. D., K. KIM & D. DLUZEN. 1985. Progesterone action on the LHRH and the nigrostriatal dopamine neuronal systems: *In vitro* and *in vivo* studies. Recent Prog. Horm. Res. **41:** 421–472.
33. OJEDA, S. R., K. H. URBANSKI, K. H. KATZ & M. F. COSTA. 1985. Endocrinology **117:** 1175–1178.
34. WATANABE, T., K. UMEGAKI & W. L. SMITH. 1986. J. Biol. Chem. **261:** 13430–13437.
35. PALMER, M. R., R. MATHEWS, B. J. HOFFER & R. C. MURPHY. 1980. J. Pharmacol. Exp. Ther. **219:** 91–96.
36. BLACK, K. L. 1984. Prostagland. Leuk. Med. **14:** 339–340.
37. ROSENBLUM, W. I. 1985. Stroke **16:** 262–263.
38. LINDGREN, J. A., T. HOFKELT, S. E. DAHLEN, C. PATRONO & B. SAMUELSSON. 1984. Proc. Natl. Acad. Sci. USA **81:** 6212–6216.
39. DEMBINSKA-KIEC, A., T. SIMMET & B. A. PESKAR. 1984. Eur. J. Pharmacol. **99:** 57–62.
40. MOSKOWITZ, M. A., K. J. KIWAK, K. HEKIMIAN & L. LEVINE. 1984. Science **224:** 886–888.
41. WOLFE, S., H. M. PAPPIUS, R. POKRUPA, A. HAKIM. 1985. *In* Advances in Prostaglandin, Thromboxane and Leukotriene Research. Proceedings of the Kyoto Conference on Prostaglandins, Vol. 15. O. Hayaishi & S. Yamamoto, Eds.: 585–588. Raven Press. New York, NY.
42. MIYAMOTO, T., J. A. LINDGREN, T. HOKFELT & B. SAMUELSSON. 1987. FEBS Lett. **216:** 123–127.
43. SUZUKI, N., T. NAKAMURA, I. SUKEHIRO, Y. ISHIKAWA, T. SASAKI & A. TAKAO. 1983. J. Neurochem. **41:** 1186–1189.
44. FLEISCH, J. H., L. E. RINKEMA & W. S. MARSHALL. 1984. Biochem. Pharmacol. **33(24):** 3919–3922.
45. CHENG, J. B. & R. G. TOWNLEY. 1984. Biochem. Biophys. Res. Commun. **119:** 612–617.
46. CHENG, J. B., D. LANG, A. BEWTRA & R. G. TOWNLEY. 1985. J. Pharmacol. Exp. Ther. **232:** 80–87.
47. SCHALLING, M., A. NEIL, L. TERENIUS, J. A. LINDGREN, T. MIYAMOTO, T. HOKFELT & B. SAMUELSSON. 1986. Eur. J. Pharmacol. **122:** 251–257.
48. GOFFINET, A. M. 1986. C.R. Acad. Sci. Paris. Ser. III, Vol. 302, **17:** 633–636.
49. LEISER, J., P. M. CONN & J. J. BLUM. 1986. Proc. Natl. Acad. Sci. USA **83:** 5963–5967.
50. BENVENISTE, J., M. TENCE, P. VARENNES, J. BIDAULT, C. BOUILLET, J. POLONSKY. 1979. C.R. Acad. Sci. Paris. Ser. D, Vol. 289d:1037–1040.
51. DEMOPOULOS, C. A., R. N. PINKARD, D. J. HANAHAN. 1979. J. Biol. Chem. **254:** 9355–9358.
52. BENVENISTE, J. & B. B. VARGAFTIG. 1983. *In* Ether-lipids: Biomedical Aspects. H. F. Mangold & F. Paltauf, Eds.: 356–376. Academic Press. New York, NY.
53. DOLY, M., P. BRAQUET, B. BONHOMME & G. MEYNIEL. 1986. Pharmacol. Res. Commun. Vol. 18. Suppl.
54. TOKUMURA, A. & H. TSUKATANI. 1986. Program of the Second International Conference on Platelet-Activating Factor, October 26–29, 1986. Gotlinburg, TN. Abstr.: 37.
55. HWANG, S. B., M. H. LAM & T. Y. SHEN. 1985. Biochem. Biophys. Res. Commun. **128:** 972–979.
56. HWANG, S. B., M. H. LAM & S. S. PONG. 1986. J. Biol. Chem. **261:** 532–537.
57. VINDIMIAN, E., C. ROBERT & G. FILLION. 1983. J. Appl. Biochem. **5:** 261–268.

Role of Brain Microvessels and Choroid Plexus in Cerebral Metabolism of Leukotrienes[a]

JAN ÅKE LINDGREN,[b] IRINA KARNUSHINA,[c] AND
HANS-ERIK CLAESSON

*Department of Physiological Chemistry
Karolinska Institutet
S-104 01 Stockholm, Sweden*

INTRODUCTION

Leukotriene (LT) formation from arachidonic acid proceeds via the unstable epoxide intermediate LTA_4, which can be converted enzymatically by hydration into LTB_4 or by glutathione conjugation to LTC_4.[1] This compound is further metabolized into LTD_4 and LTE_4 by sequential action of gamma-glutamyl transpeptidase (γ-GTP) and dipeptidase, respectively.

Biosynthesis of leukotrienes was originally observed in leukocytes.[1] More recently, the production of cysteinyl-containing leukotrienes (LTC_4, $-D_4$ and $-E_4$) and the dihydroxy acid LTB_4 in brain tissue from various species has been reported.[2-7]

The cysteinyl-containing leukotrienes induce vasoconstriction[8] and plasma leakage[9] in peripheral tissue. Similar effects have been reported in the central nervous system. Thus, leukotrienes B_4, C_4, and D_4 constricted mouse cerebral arteriols.[10] The effect of LTC_4 was inhibited by the slow reacting substance (SRS) antagonist FPL 55712. In addition, leukotrienes increased the blood-brain barrier permeability and caused vasogenic brain edema after intraparenchymal administration in rats.[11] These findings, together with the reported enhanced production of leukotrienes in the gerbil brain after ischemia and reperfusion[4] indicate that leukotrienes may be pathophysiological mediators involved in brain edema and vasospasm.

Since leukotrienes might be potentially harmful in the central nervous system, it can be assumed that the concentrations of these compounds are controlled by eliminating and metabolizing enzymes within the blood-brain and blood–cerebrospinal fluid (CSF) barriers. Active transport of LTC_4 from the cerebrospinal fluid into the blood through the choroid plexus has been reported.[12,13]

The present study shows that both cerebral microvessels and choroid plexus from the rat efficiently transformed LTC_4 into LTD_4 and LTE_4. Furthermore, microvessels converted exogenous LTA_4 into LTC_4. This formation was observed only in the presence of exogenously added glutathione. The results suggest that the blood-brain and blood-CSF barriers constitute important systems for metabolism of leukotrienes in the brain.

---

[a]This work was supported by grants and a fellowship (to Irina Karnushina) from the Swedish Medical Research Council (Project Numbers 03X-06805, 03X-07135, and 03W-08296) and Karolinska Institutets Research Funds.
[b]To whom correspondence should be addressed.
[c]Visiting scientist from Biological Research Center, Szeged, Hungary.

METHODS

Isolation of Brain Microvessels

Brain microvessels from perfused brains of 8–10-week-old rats were purified essentially according to Diglio et al.[14] Extraparenchymal vessels and white matter were carefully removed from the brain tissue, yielding approximately 6 g of cortex from 10 animals. The tissue was homogenized by hand in 60 ml of Hank's Balanced Salt Solution (HBSS) using a teflon-glass Potter homogenizer. In order to remove large vessels, the homogenate was filtered through a nylon sieve (pore size 250 μm), followed by centrifugation at 1000 g for 10 min. The pellet was resuspended in 15% Dextran (Sigma, clinical grade, 77 800 mol wt) in HBSS containing 5% fetal calf serum. After a second centrifugation at 1000 g for 15 min, the obtained small pellet was washed with HBSS and further purified by three successive low-speed centrifugations (200 g, 1 min). The final pellet represented an essentially pure microvessel preparation, which was used for 4–6 incubations.

Isolation of Choroid Plexus

Choroid plexuses were manually dissected from perfused rat brains after opening of the lateral ventricles. The tissue was rinsed and collected in cold HBSS. Five to 10 intact plexuses were used per incubaton.

Incubation Procedure and Leukotriene Analysis

After 5 min preincubation at 37 °C, leukotriene synthesis and metabolism were initiated by addition of synthetic leukotrienes or ionophore A23187. The incubations were terminated by the addition of 3 volumes of cold ethanol, followed by centrifugation and evaporation. Identification and quantitation of the leukotrienes were performed using reversed phase–high performance liquid chromatography (RP-HPLC) and on-line UV spectroscopy.[6]

Tissue Accumulation of Leukotrienes

Accumulation of leukotrienes by the tissue was determined after incubation of intact brain microvessels or choroid plexuses with ^{3}H-LTC$_4$, ^{3}H-LTD$_4$, or ^{3}H-LTE$_4$ (0.5 μM; 100 000 cpm) for various intervals. After vacuum filtration of the samples through glass filters (G/F B, Reeve Angel, Clifton, NJ, USA), followed by 3 washes with cold PBS, filtrates and tissue on filters were extracted with ethanol and evaporated. Thereafter, the samples were analyzed on RP-HPLC and the distribution of radioactivity determined by liquid scintillation counting of collected fractions.

Gamma-Glutamyl Transpeptidase and Protein Assay

Gamma-glutamyl transpeptidase activity was measured spectrophotometrically, using γ-glutamyl-p-nitroanilide as substrate, according to Szasz.[15]

Protein content in the samples was measured by the BCA assay (Pierce Chem. Co., Rockford, IL, USA) using human serum albumin as standard.

RESULTS

Transformation of Leukotriene A_4 by Isolated Brain Microvessels

Incubation of microvessels with LTA_4 (7 μM) in the presence of glutathione (3 mM) for 5 min led to the formation of cysteinyl-containing leukotrienes. FIGURE 1 shows the HPLC chromatogram of the products. Using co-chromatography of the sample with authentic standards, and UV spectroscopy (Fig. 2), peaks I and II were

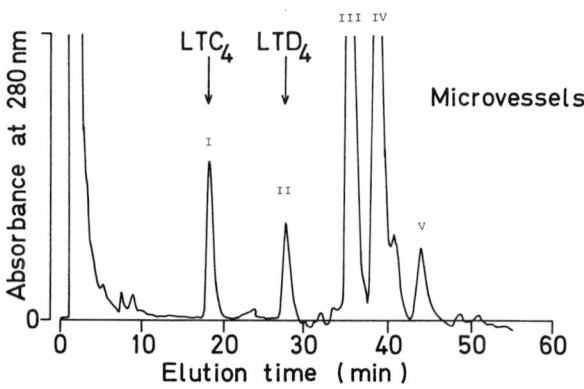

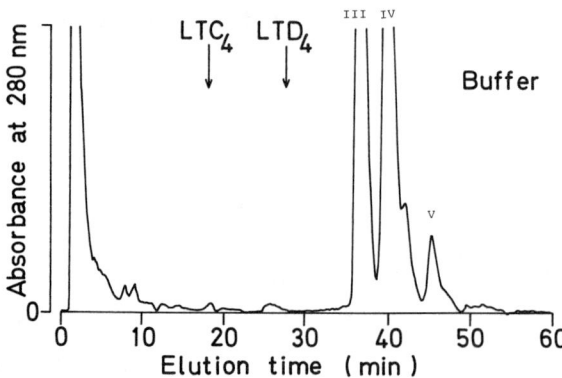

FIGURE 1. RP-HPLC profile of the products formed by rat cerebral microvessels (*upper panel*) or buffer alone (*lower panel*) after incubation with LTA_4 (7 μM) plus glutathione (3 mM) for 5 min.

identified as LTC_4 and LTD_4, respectively. Peaks designated III and IV were identified as the non–enzymatically formed Δ^6-*trans* LTB_4 and 12-*epi*-Δ^6-*trans* LTB_4, respectively. In control experiments with LTA_4, incubated under identical conditions but in the absence of cells, no LTC_4 or LTD_4 could be detected (FIG. 1). Peak V, with a retention time corresponding to that of synthetic LTB_4, was similar in both samples.

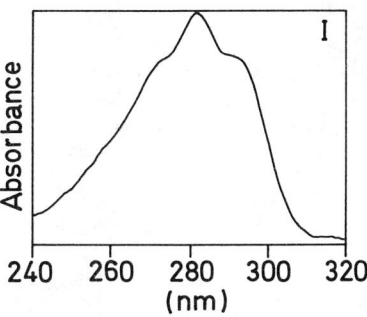
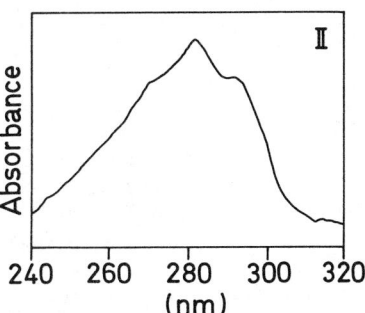

FIGURE 2. UV spectra of the material eluted in peaks I and II of FIGURE 1, respectively.

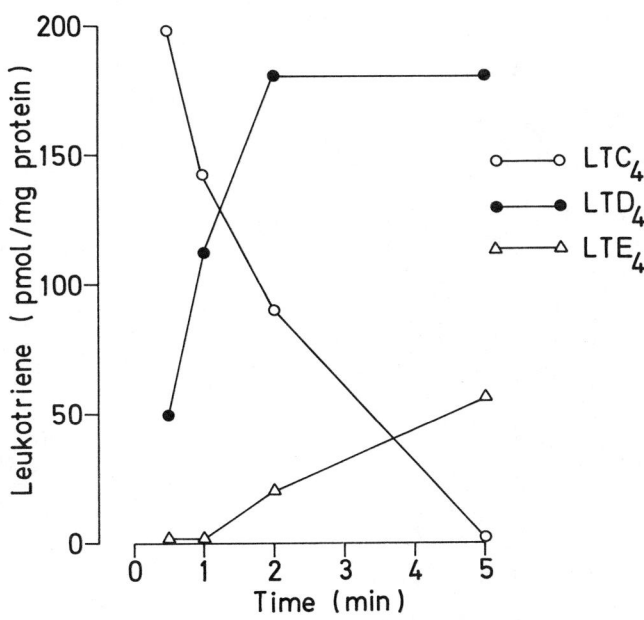

FIGURE 3. Time courses of leukotriene formation by rat cerebral microvessels after addition of LTC_4 (0.5 μM).

In three separate experiments, 40–160 pmoles of cysteinyl-containing leukotrienes/mg of protein were formed after incubation with 5–14 μM LTA$_4$ for 5 min. In the absence of exogenously added glutathione, no formation of LTC$_4$ and LTD$_4$ was observed (data not shown).

Leukotrienes were not formed by isolated brain microvessels after stimulation with ionophore A23187 in the absence or presence of arachidonic acid (data not shown).

Metabolism of Leukotriene C$_4$ by Isolated Brain Microvessels

FIGURE 3 shows that microvessels efficiently converted LTC$_4$ (0.5 μM) to LTD$_4$ and LTE$_4$ during 5 min of incubation. The mean conversion rate of LTC$_4$ to LTD$_4$/LTE$_4$ was 100 pmoles/mg protein × min ($n = 5$). In contrast, further metabolism of LTD$_4$ into LTE$_4$ was much slower than the conversion of LTC$_4$ to LTD$_4$.

Metabolism of Leukotriene C$_4$ by Isolated Choroid Plexuses

Isolated choroid plexuses readily metabolized exogenously added LTC$_4$ into LTD$_4$ and LTE$_4$ (FIG. 4). The identification of the peaks was based on UV spectroscopy and chromatographic properties on RP-HPLC. In the presence of 0.5 μM LTC$_4$, about 40 pmoles of LTC$_4$ were converted to LTD$_4$/LTE$_4$ per mg of protein × min ($n = 3$). In agreement with these results, choroid plexus efficiently transferred the γ-glutamyl residue from synthetic γ-glutamyl-p-nitroanilide to glycyl-glycine, as determined spectrophotometrically (FIG. 5). The γ-GTP activity was not significantly changed in plexuses from perfused rat brain, as compared to tissue from nonperfused brain,

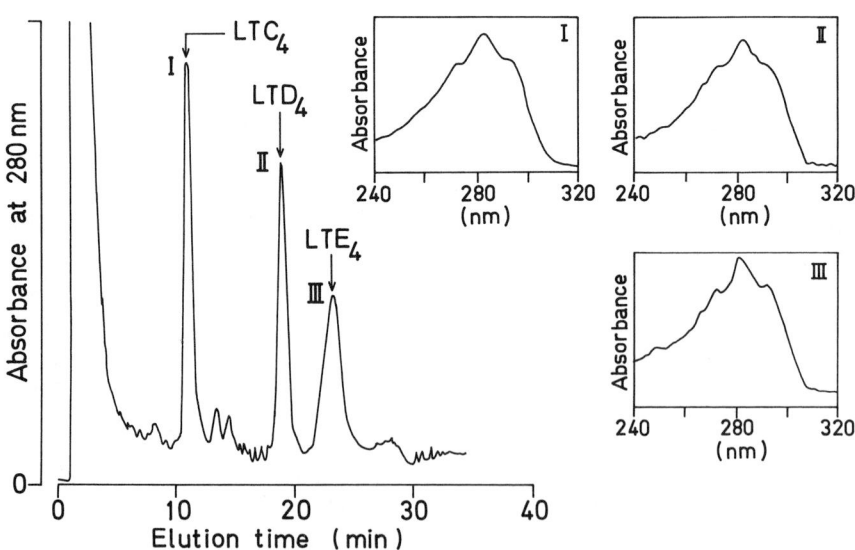

FIGURE 4. RP-HPLC chromatogram and UV spectra of the products formed by rat choroid plexus after incubation with LTC$_4$ (0.5 μM) for 10 min.

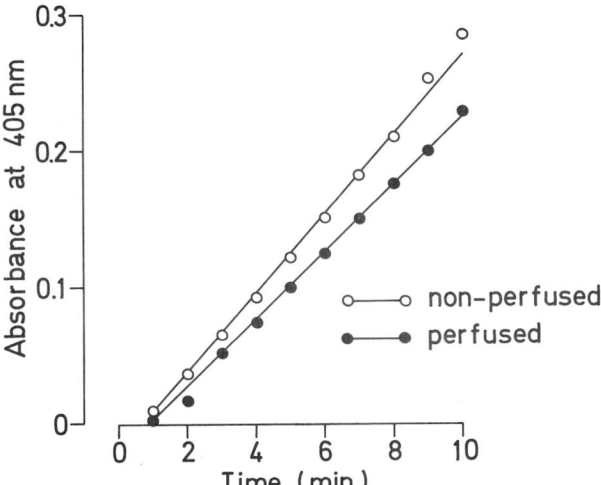

FIGURE 5. Gamma-glutamyl transpeptidase activity by perfused and nonperfused rat choroid plexus, measured spectrophotometrically at 405 nm using γ-glutamyl-p-nitroanilide as substrate.

indicating that the enzyme activity was possessed mainly by the choroid plexus and not by circulating blood cells.

Accumulation of Leukotrienes to Isolated Brain Microvessels or Choroid Plexuses

The possible leukotriene accumulation to brain microvessels or choroid plexuses was investigated. In these experiments, the relative amount of leukotrienes associated with the tissue was compared to the amount of compounds present in the buffer. Microvessels or choroid plexuses were incubated with 0.5 μM of ^{3}H-labeled (100 000 cpm) LTC_4, LTD_4, or LTE_4 for 10 min, and the incubation was terminated by fast vacuum filtration. After three washes with cold PBS, the filters and the filtrated buffer were treated with ethanol prior to RP-HPLC. The distribution of radioactivity was determined in collected HPLC fractions. The results (TABLE 1) suggested a substantial accumulation of LTE_4 to the choroid plexus. After incubation of microvessels with LTC_4, no remaining LTC_4 could be recovered, indicating total degradation of this compound to LTD_4 and LTE_4. In microvessels, the accumulation of leukotrienes to the tissue was much less evident (TABLE 1).

DISCUSSION

The present report indicates that brain microvessels and choroid plexuses efficiently participate in the metabolism of leukotrienes in the central nervous system (FIGS. 1–4). The brain microvessels efficiently transformed LTC_4 to LTD_4 and, more slowly, to LTE_4. In contrast to an earlier report,[13] metabolism of LTC_4 was also observed in the choroid plexus. Our results are in agreement with early findings demonstrating high activity of gamma-glutamyl transpeptidase in the endothelial cells of brain microvessels and the epithelial cells of the choroid plexus.[16,17] In addition, brain microvessels converted LTA_4 to LTC_4. These results are in accordance with earlier studies on transformation of LTA_4 and LTC_4 by cultured human and porcine endothelial cells.[18-20] In brain microvessels, however, cysteinyl-containing leukotrienes were formed only when exogenous glutathione was added together with LTA_4. This may be due to depletion of intracellular glutathione stores during isolation of the tissue or to species differences. Alternatively, the discrepancy may indicate that the brain endothelium posesses less capacity to produce LTC_4 from LTA_4 as compared to endothelium from peripheral tissue. Preliminary results indicate that the choroid plexus has very limited capacity to transform LTA_4 to LTC_4 (Karnushina et al., unpublished). On the other hand, histochemical data indicate that the γ-GTP activity is considerably higher in cerebral microvessels, as compared to microvessels from peripheral tissue.[21] Thus, brain microvessels and choroid plexuses seem to be involved mainly in leukotriene degradation, thereby protecting the central nervous system from these bioactive substances. Although the transformation of LTC_4 to LTD_4 was rapid, the subsequent conversion to LTE_4 was relatively slow. However, in the *in vivo*

TABLE 1. Accumulation of Leukotrienes in Rat Brain Microvessels and Choroid Plexuses

	Radioactivity Ratio: Buffer/Tissue					
	Choroid Plexuses			Microvessels		
Incubation	LTC_4	LTD_4	LTE_4	LTC_4	LTD_4	LTE_4
LTC_4	40	2.5	0.6	—	8.2	3.7
LTD_4	—	10	1.2	—	14	12
LTE_4	—	—	2.4	—	—	5.2

NOTE: Choroid plexuses or cerebral microvessels were incubated with indicated leukotriene (0.5 μM, 100.000 cpm) for 10 min. at 37 °C. After separation of the buffer from the tissue, each of them was analyzed by RP-HPLC, and radioactivity was determined in collected fractions (see METHODS).

situation LTD_4 formed by the microvessels on the luminal side,[22] may be further catabolized by platelets that efficiently convert LTD_4 to LTE_4.[23] The ability of the choroid plexus to accumulate LTE_4 (TABLE 1) is in agreement with the concept that this tissue might be involved in the transport of leukotrienes from the brain.[12] However, according to our findings in the rat, LTC_4 has to be metabolized into LTE_4 prior to this accumulation (TABLE 1).

The cellular origin of leukotriene formation in the brain is presently not known. Brain microvessels did not produce leukotrienes after incubation with ionophore A23187, indicating that this tissue lacks 5-lipoxygenase activity and is therefore not the origin of leukotriene formation in the brain. Regional distribution studies, using HPLC-analysis of LTB_4 and LTC_4, demonstrated the highest LTC_4 formation in the hypothalamus, while its formation in the cerebellum and brain cortex was much lower.[24] In contrast, the capacity to produce LTB_4 was much more uniformly distributed within the rat brain. This may indicate that LTC_4 and LTB_4 are produced by different cell types, and that LTB_4 is formed by more evenly distributed cells, such as glial cells. Formation of LTB_4 by oligodendrocytes has been reported.[25] Furthermore, immunohistochemical studies revealed LTC_4-positive nerve cells in the median eminence.[2] In addition, single fibers with similar immunoreactivity were observed in other regions in the brain. This may suggest LTC_4 formation by nerve cells. Further studies to elucidate the leukotriene producing capacity in nerve and glial cells are needed.

In conclusion, the present study shows that brain microvessels and choroid plexus readily metabolize leukotrienes. A potent system for degradation of leukotrienes in the central nervous system may be of importance, since these bioactive compounds probably possess both pathophysiological and physiological roles in the central nervous system.

ACKNOWLEDGMENTS

We thank Ms. Barbro Näsman-Glaser, Ms. Inger Forsberg, Ms. Gunilla Gyllner, and Ms. Monica Hendén for skillful technical assistance.

REFERENCES

1. SAMUELSSON, B., S.-E. DAHLÉN, J. Å. LINDGREN, C. A. RAUZER & C. N. SERHAN. 1987. Leukotrienes and lipoxines: Structures, biosynthesis and biological effects. Science **237:** 1171–1176.
2. LINDGREN, J. Å., T. HÖKFELT, S. E. DAHLÉN, C. PATRONO & B. SAMUELSSON. 1984. Leukotrienes in the rat central nervous system. Proc. Natl. Acad. Sci. USA **81:** 6212–6216.
3. DEMBINSKA-KIEC', A., T. SIMMET, B. A. PESKAR. 1984. Formation of leukotriene C_4-like material by rat brain tissue. Eur. J. Pharmacol. **99:** 57–62.
4. MOSKOWITZ, M. A., K. J. KIWAK, K. HEKIMIAN & L. LEVINE. 1984. Synthesis of compounds with properties of leukotrienes C_4 and D_4 in gerbil brains after ischemia and reperfusion. Science **224:** 886–889.
5. WOLFE, L. S., H. M. PAPPIUS, R. POKRUPA & A. HAKIM. 1985. Involvement of arachidonic acid metabolites in experimental brain injury. Identification of lipoxygenase products in brain. Clinical studies on prostacyclin infusion in acute cerebral ischemia. In Advances in Prostaglandin, Thromboxane and Leukotriene Research, Vol. 15. O. Hayaishi & S. Yamamoto, Eds.: 585–588. Raven Press. New York, NY.
6. MIYAMOTO, T., J. Å. LINDGREN & B. SAMUELSSON. 1987. Isolation and identification of lipoxygenase products from the rat central nervous system. Biochim. Biophys. Acta **922:** 372–378.
7. SHIMIZU, T., Y. TAKUSAGAWA, T. IZUMI, N. OHISHI & Y. SEYAMA. 1987. Enzymatic synthesis of leukotriene B_4 in guinea pig brain. J. Neurochem. **48:** 1541–1546.
8. ROSENTHAL, A. & C. R. PACE-ASCIAK. 1983. Potent vasoconstriction of the isolated perfused rat kidney by leukotrienes C_4 and D_4. Can. J. Physiol. Pharmacol. **61:** 324–328.
9. DAHLÉN, S.-E., J. BJÖRK, P. HEDQVIST, K.-E. ARFORS, S. HAMMARSTRÖM, J. Å. LINDGREN & B. SAMUELSSON. 1981. Leukotrienes promote plasma leakage and leukocyte adhesion in postcapillary venules. In vivo effects with relevance to the acute inflammatory response. Proc. Natl. Acad. Sci. USA **78:** 3887–3891.
10. ROSENBLUM, W. I. 1985. Constricting effects of leukotrienes on cerebral arterioles of mice. Stroke **16:** 262–263.
11. BLACK, K. L. & J. T. HOFF. 1985. Leukotrienes increase blood-brain barrier permeability following intraparenchymal injections in rat. Ann. Neurol. **18:** 349–351.
12. SPECTOR, R. & E. J. GOETZL. 1985. Leukotriene C_4 transport by the choroid plexus in vitro. Science **228:** 325–327.
13. SPECTOR, R. & E. J. GOETZL. 1986. Leukotriene C_4 transport and metabolism in the central nervous system. J. Neurochem. **46:** 1308–1312.
14. DIGLIO, C. A., P. GRAMMAS, F. GIACOMELLI & J. WIENER. 1982. Primary culture of rat

cerebral microvascular endothelial cells. Isolation, growth and characterization. Lab. Invest. **46:** 554–563.
15. SZASZ, G. 1969. A kinetic photometric method for serum γ-glutamyl-transpeptidase. Clin. Chem. **15:** 124–138.
16. ALBERT, Z., M. ORLOWSKI, Z. RZUCIDLO & J. ORLOWSKA. 1966. Studies on γ-glutamyl transpeptidase activity and its histochemical localization in the central nervous system of man and different animal species. Acta Histochem. **25:** 312–320.
17. SHINE, H. D. & B. HABER. 1981. Immunochemical localization of γ-glutamyl transpeptidase in the rat CNS. Brain Res. **217:** 339–349.
18. CLAESSON, H. E. & J. HAEGGSTRÖM. 1988. Human endothelial cells stimulate leukotriene synthesis and convert granulocyte released leukotriene A_4 into leukotrienes B_4, C_4, D_4 and E_4. Eur. J. Biochem. **173:** 93–100.
19. CLAESSON, H. E. & J. HAEGGSTRÖM. 1987. Metabolism of leukotriene A_4 by human endothelial cells: Evidence for leukotriene C_4 and D_4 formation by leukocyte-endothelial cell interaction. *In* Advances in Prostaglandin, Thromboxane and Leukotriene Research, Vol. 17. B. Samuelsson, R. Paoletti & P. W. Ramwell, Eds.: 115–119. Raven Press. New York, NY.
20. FEINMARK, S. J. & P. J. CANNON. 1986. Endothelial cell leukotriene C_4 synthesis results from intercellular transfer of leukotriene A_4 synthesized by polymorphonuclear leukocytes. J. Biol. Chem. **261:** 16466–16472.
21. ORLOWSKI, M., G. SESSA, J. P. GREEN. 1974. γ-glutamyl transpeptidase in brain capillaries: Possible site of a blood-brain barrier for amino acids. Science **184:** 66–68.
22. GHANDOUR, M. S., O. K. LANGLEY & V. VARGA. 1980. Immunohistological localization of γ-glutamyl transpeptidase in cerebellum at light and electron microscope levels. Neurosci. Lett. **20:** 125–129.
23. EDENIUS, CH., K. HEIDVALL & J. Å. LINDGREN. 1988. Novel transcellular interaction—conversion of granulocyte-derived leukotriene A_4 to cysteinyl-containing leukotrienes by human platelets. Eur. J. Biochem. In press.
24. MIYAMOTO, T., J. Å. LINDGREN, T. HÖKFELT & B. SAMUELSSON. 1987. Regional distribution of leukotriene and mono-hydroxyeicosatetraenoic acid production in the rat brain. FEBS Lett. **216:** 123–127.
25. SHIRAZI, Y., D. K. IMAGAWA & M. L. SHIN. 1987. Release of leukotriene B_4 from sublethally injured oligodendrocytes by terminal complement complexes. J. Neurochem. **48:** 271–278.

Biologically Active Metabolites of the 12-Lipoxygenase Pathway Are Formed by *Aplysia* Nervous Tissue

STEVEN J. FEINMARK,[a,b,c] DANIELE PIOMELLI,[d,e]
ELI SHAPIRO,[d] AND JAMES H. SCHWARTZ[d]

[a]*Departments of Pharmacology and Medicine*
and
[d]*Howard Hughes Medical Institute*
Center for Neurobiology and Behavior
Columbia University
New York, New York 10032

INTRODUCTION

Aplysia californica is a marine mollusk that has been the subject of extensive neurobiological study. Its simple nervous system, composed of large neurons, has permitted the identification and mapping of many specific cell connections. In addition to electrophysiologic observations of these cells, the biochemical definition of the neurotransmitter content of many neurons also has been accomplished.[1]

In spite of this wealth of detail, little data have been reported on the lipid biochemistry in this species. Polyunsaturated fats, an important component of membrane phospholipids, are especially prominent in marine animals. Nevertheless, as recently as 1973, Komai *et al.*[2] suggested that these lipids were absent from a related species of *Aplysia*. We have reevaluated the fatty acid composition of *Aplysia* nervous tissue and specifically investigated the metabolism of an important polyunsaturated fat, arachidonic acid. In addition to its role as a phospholipid component, this fatty acid is the presursor of a variety of biologically active metabolites.[3] One pathway, initiated by the 12-lipoxygenase enzyme, converts arachidonate into 12-hydroperoxy-eicosatetraenoic acid (12-HPETE), which is rapidly reduced to 12(S)-hydroxy-eicosatetraenoic acid (12(S)-HETE). Although these products were first discovered in 1974,[4,5] no clear biological function had yet been assigned to them. Our studies of lipid metabolism in *Aplysia* have led to the identification of a 12-lipoxygenase pathway that is activated by physiological stimuli.[6] Furthermore, the production of several biologically active metabolites will be described in this volume. The metabolism of 12-HPETE to 12-keto-eicosatetraenoic acid is discussed elsewhere[7]; the identifica-

---

[b]An Established Investigator of the American Heart Association.
[c]Address for correspondence: Dr. S. Feinmark, Department of Pharmacology, Columbia University, 630 West 168th Street, New York, New York 10032.
[e]Present address: Laboratory of Molecular and Cellular Neuroscience, The Rockefeller University, 1230 York Avenue, New York, New York 10021.

tion and activity of an epoxy alcohol, 8-hydroxy-11,12-epoxy-eicosatrienoic acid (8-HEpETE), is the subject of this report.

METHODS

Preparation of Tissue: Biochemical Analyses

Ganglia were dissected from *Aplysia* (70–200 g; Howard Hughes Medical Institute Mariculture Resource Facility, Woods Hole, MA or Marinus, Sand City, CA), and trimmed of connective tissue. In some experiments, the ganglia were exposed to [^{3}H]arachidonic acid (2.5–25 μCi for 2–20 h) in an artificial seawater.[6] The tissue was then washed and stimulated in order to study the metabolism of its endogenous lipids as described below. In other experiments, the nervous tissue was homogenized and incubated with exogenous arachidonate (50 μM) or histamine (50 μM) in the seawater.

Preparation of Tissue: Electrophysiologic Analyses

The trimmed abdominal or cerebral ganglia were pinned to silicone plastic in a superfusion chamber (0.3–0.4 ml) with flowing artificial seawater (1–5 ml/min). Identified cell bodies were impaled with glass microelectrodes (10–20 mΩ resistance filled with 2 M potassium citrate) and identified by previously defined criteria.[6,8-10] In some experiments cells were impaled with two electrodes, one for recording voltage and the other to pass current. In a series of experiments designed to examine the stimulation of arachidonic acid metabolism by synaptic stimulation, ganglia were incubated with [^{3}H]arachidonate (see above) before the identified presynaptic (L32) and postsynaptic (L14) cells were impaled. To test for biological activity, compounds were pressure-ejected from micropipettes (10–20 μm tip diameter) positioned approximately 0.5 mm above the cell body of L14. Pressure pulses lasted 1–10 s and ejected volumes of 1–10 μl of the solutions to be tested. Solutions of 12-HPETE, 12(S)-HETE, 8-HEpETE sodium salt in alcohol were dried under nitrogen and resuspended in seawater by sonication.

Lipid Extractions and Analysis

Lipids were extracted from homogenates of nervous tissue with hexane/isopropanol (3:2; v/v) as previously described.[6] Complex lipids were transesterified by treatment with 12% boron trifluoride in methanol at 70 °C for 1 hour. The recovered fatty acid methyl esters were measured by gas chromatography (HP5840 GC, SP2340 fused silica capillary, 30 m × 0.32 mm).

Unextracted bath samples were analyzed for the presence of 12-HETE by chromatography on a Novapak C_{18} column (150 × 3.9 mm) eluted with methanol/water/acetic acid (73:27:0.1; v/v) flowing at 1 ml/min.

In other experiments, the bath medium was acidified with formic acid (pH 3.6–4.0) and extracted twice either with ethyl acetate or with diethyl ether. The dried extracts were fractionated by normal-phase HPLC (Silicar LC Si, 250 × 4.6 mm) eluted with hexane/isopropanol/acetic acid (98:2:0.1; v/v) at 1 ml/min. Purified fractions were used for further analysis by GC/MS, scintillation counting, enzymatic hydrolysis, or reversed-phase HPLC.

Preparation of Standard Epoxy Alcohols: Enzymatic Hydrolysis

Synthetic 8(R,S)-hydroxy-11,12-*trans*-epoxy-5,14-*cis*-9-*trans*-eicosatrienoic acid methyl ester was prepared by the method of Corey and Wei-Guo[11] and saponified to produce the sodium salt just before use.[12] Standard epoxy alcohols were prepared from rat lung and purified as reported.[13] Rat lung epoxide hydrolase was prepared according to Pace-Asciak et al.[13]

Purified epoxy alcohols as well as the products of their enzymatic hydrolysis were chromatographed by reversed-phase HPLC (Nucleosil C_{18}; 250 × 4.6mm) eluted with methanol/water/acetic acid (75:25:0.1; v/v) at 1 ml/min.

TABLE 1. Fatty Acids of Total Lipids in *Aplysia* Nervous System[a]

Fatty Acid	Relative Abundance (Area %)
14:0	12.2 ± 6.2
16:0	10.4 ± 3.9
18:0	10.4 ± 3.9
18:1	9.8 ± 1.6
18:2	5.3 ± 3.2
20:1[b]	4.3 ± 1.2
20:2	5.5 ± 1.9
20:4	9.9 ± 1.5
20:5	2.9 ± 1.5
22:2	4.9 ± 1.3
22:4	24.3 ± 5.9
22:6	4.2 ± 3.3
Others	10.7 ± 4.1

NOTE: Neural lipids were subjected to transmethylation and the fatty acid methyl esters identified by GC/MS. Quantitative analysis was performed by GC. The area of each peak on the chromatogram was quantified by a Hewlett-Packard integrator, which also normalized these values to the total areas of all of the peaks. Fatty acid nomenclature: the first number refers to the number of carbon atoms in the chain and the second to the number of double bonds. Arachidonic acid is 20:4; others indicate unidentified derivatives. Values are expressed as means ± SEM ($n = 4$).
[a]From Piomelli et al.[6]
[b]May contain traces of 18:3.

RESULTS AND DISCUSSION

Fatty Acid Composition of Aplysia Nervous Tissue

Aplysia neural components (neuronal cell bodies and neuropil) were isolated and homogenized, and their total cellular lipids were extracted. In some experiments, the lipid extract was fractionated into phospholipid subclasses before the fatty acid content of the extract or subclass was determined. Polyunsaturated fatty acids as a group made up over 57% of the total fatty acid content of the neural lipids, and arachidonic acid alone comprised nearly 10% of the total (TABLE 1). The distribution of fatty acids within each phospholipid subclass did not differ greatly from that found in the total lipid extract. When isolated neural components were incubated with [^{3}H]arachidonic acid, the fatty acid was rapidly incorporated into membrane phospholipids, from which it could be released by a variety of stimuli.[6]

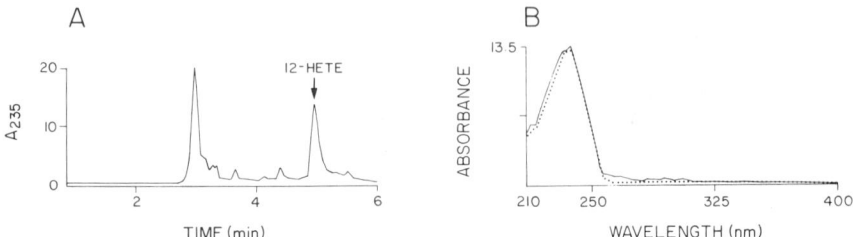

FIGURE 1. Identification of 12-HETE formed by *Aplysia* neural tissue analysis by UV spectrometry. The homogenate of central ganglia from 100 animals was incubated with arachidonic acid (50 μM) for 30 min, and the lipid extract was subjected to normal-phase HPLC purification (see METHODS). **A:** Absorbance (A, 235 nm) was monitored continuously. A major peak was observed at the retention time of the 12-HETE standard (4.8 min, indicated by the *arrow*). **B:** The full spectrum of this material (*continuous line*) was identical to that of authentic 12-HETE (*dotted line*). (From Piomelli et al.[6] Reprinted by permission from *Journal of Neuroscience*).

Identification of 12-HETE

Neural components were homogenized and incubated with exogenous arachidonate. After 30 min, lipids were extracted and fractionated by normal-phase HPLC (FIG. 1A). A major peak eluted at the retention time of authentic 12-HETE. The identity of the material was confirmed to be 12-HETE by ultraviolet spectrophotometry (FIG. 1B) and by GC/MS using negative-ion chemical ionization of the pentafluorobenzyl ester–trimethylsilyl ether (PFB-TMS) derivative and electron impact mass fragmentography of the methyl ester-TMS derivative.[6] The stereochemistry of the 12-hydroxyl is tentatively assigned to be (S) based upon the cross-reactivity of the material derived from *Aplysia* with antiserum raised against 12(S)-HETE.

Neurotransmitter-induced Synthesis of 12-HETE

Neural components were first labeled with [^{3}H]arachidonate and then exposed to histamine, a neurotransmitter in *Aplysia*.[14–16] Products isolated from the bathing

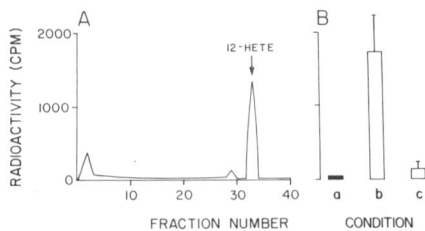

FIGURE 2. Stimulation of [^{3}H]12-HETE formation by histamine. Neural components, labeled by incubation for 2 h with [^{3}H]arachidonic acid (25 μCi/ml), were exposed for 1 min to histamine (50 μM). Samples were subjected to reversed-phase HPLC (see METHODS), and fractions were analyzed for radioactivity. **A:** Representative chromatogram typical of 4 experiments. **B:** [^{3}H]12-HETE formation under various conditions. Control, **a** ($n = 4$); histamine (50 μM), **b** ($n = 4$); histamine (50 μM) together with cimetidine (100 μM), **c** ($n = 3$). (From Piomelli et al.[6] Reprinted by permission from *Journal of Neuroscience*.)

FIGURE 3. Formation of 12-HETE produced by intracellular stimulation of L32 neurons. Labeled abdominal ganglia were stimulated as described in the legend to FIGURE 4. HPLC chromatograms of bath samples taken before (**B**) and after (**A**) stimulation. Stimulation of L32 evoked production of labeled 12-HETE. Samples were analyzed by reversed-phase HPLC for 12-HETE (see METHODS). (Modified from Piomelli et al.[6])

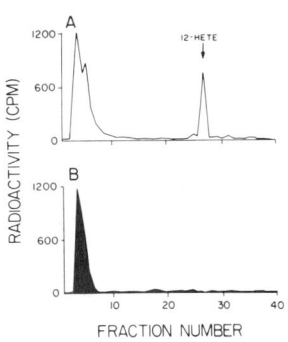

medium were fractionated by reversed-phase HPLC, and each fraction was tested for radioactivity. A single peak of labeled material was detected at a retention time identical to that of synthetic 12-HETE (FIG. 2A). Release of [^{3}H]12-HETE was significantly less during control incubations or in the presence of the histamine antagonist cimetidine (FIG. 2B).

Similar results were obtained when the putative histaminergic neuron L32 was stimulated to release its endogenous transmitter. L32 cells were identified in ganglia that had been prelabeled with [^{3}H]arachidonate. The neuron was impaled and driven electrically by three 2-s pulses, which produced 40 spikes. This protocol induced the synthesis of [^{3}H]12-HETE (450 ± 85 cpm/ganglion). No product could be detected during control periods ($n = 5$) (FIG. 3).

Production of 12-HETE after treatment with histamine or intracellular stimulation of L32 neurons suggests a potential physiologic role for metabolites of the 12-lipoxygenase pathway. When 12(S)-HETE was applied to L14 neurons, which are follower cells of L32, no effect was observed (FIG. 4). In contrast, 12-HPETE, the immediate precursor of 12-HETE, induced a response similar to that caused by histamine; both 12-HPETE and histamine cause a dual-action response of L14, similar to the response of L14 after intracellular stimulation of L32 (FIG. 4). Furthermore, L14's dual-action response to histamine could be blocked by applying bromophenacyl bromide, an inhibitor of phospholipase.[17]

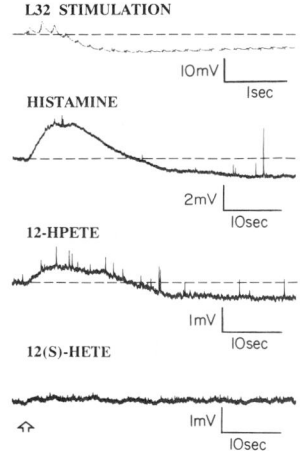

FIGURE 4. Response of L14. L14 was impaled for intracellular recording of membrane potential. **L32 stimulation:** The presynaptic cell, L32, was driven with a 5-s train of depolarizing pulses of 200 ms at 5 Hz. Each pulse produced three spikes in L32 (not shown). The resting potential of L14 was −60 mV. This response is typical but was not recorded from the same L14 used in the other recordings. **Histamine** (100 pmol over 1 s) was applied to L14 (resting potential −70 mV). **12-HPETE** (100 pmol over 3 s) was applied to L14 (resting potential −70 mV). **12(S)-HETE** (250 pmol over 5 s) was applied to L14 (resting potential −64 mV). Histamine and 12-HPETE records are from the same L14 cell. The *arrow* indicates the beginning of drug application. (From Piomelli et al.[12] Reprinted by permission from *Proceedings of the National Academy of Sciences of the United States of America*.)

Although the activity found with 12-HPETE may be inherent to this molecule, the reactive hydroperoxide is known to undergo complex metabolism (FIG. 5). In the presence of iron-containing proteins, 12-HPETE undergoes an intramolecular rearrangement to yield two diastereomeric epoxy alcohols,[13,18] 8(R,S)-hydroxy-11,12-epoxy-5,9,14-eicosatrienoic acid (8-HEpETE) and 10(R,S)-hydroxy-11,12-epoxy-5,8,14-eicosatrienoic acid (10-HEpETE). The epoxy alcohols are converted to trihydroxy acids (THETE) by an epoxide hydrolase.[18,19] In addition, 12-HPETE can be converted to carbonyl-containing molecules,[20,21] for example, the keto acid 12-keto-5,8,10,14-eicosatetraenoic acid (12-KETE). In this paper, we have studied the synthesis and physiological activity of the epoxy alcohols in *Aplysia* nervous tissue. Data on 12-KETE are reported elsewhere.[7,22]

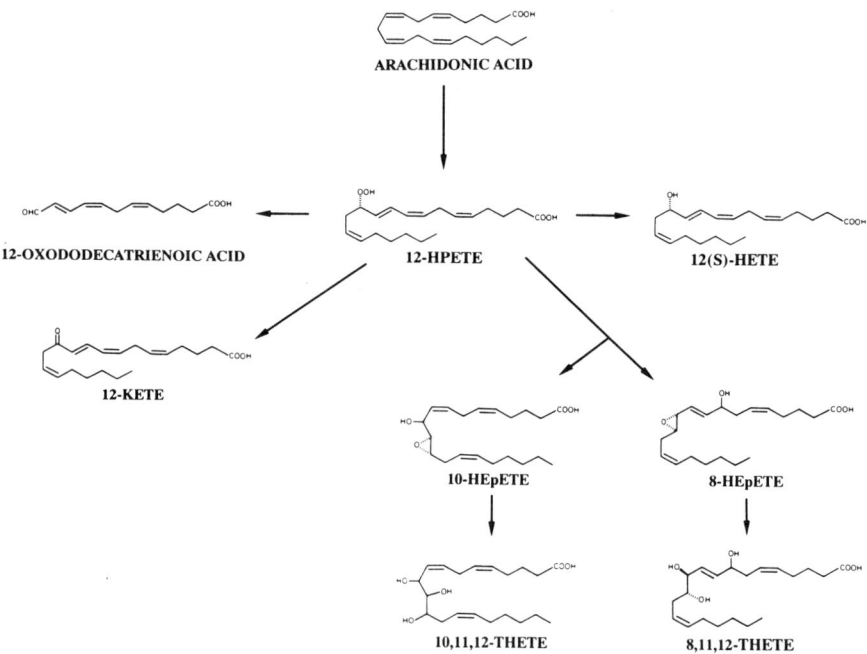

FIGURE 5. Metabolic pathways of 12-HPETE.

Homogenates of *Aplysia* nervous tissue were incubated with [³H]arachidonate and the products purified by extractive isolation followed by normal-phase HPLC. A major product was detected at the retention time reported for 8-HEpETE[13] and had the same elution characteristics as biosynthetically prepared standard 8-HEpETE. When HPLC-purified *Aplysia*-derived 8-HEpETE and standard 8-HEpETE were reanalyzed by reversed-phase HPLC, they again showed identical retention values (FIG. 6B). In addition, incubation of purified and standard 8-HEpETE with rat lung epoxide hydrolase converted both compounds to products (isomeric THETE) that were indistinguishable by HPLC analysis (FIG. 6C, D). This biochemical evidence that the *Aplysia* metabolite is 8-HEpETE was confirmed by GC/MS both in negative-ion

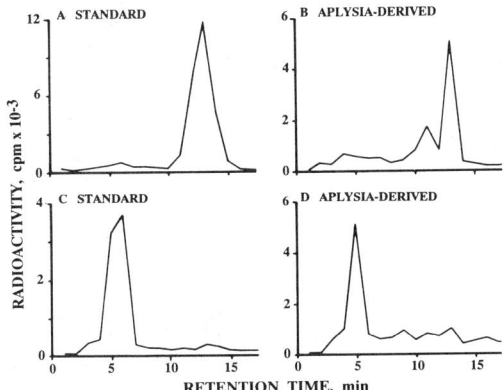

FIGURE 6. Reversed-phase HPLC analysis of purified 8-HEpETE before and after hydrolysis. **A:** [^{3}H]8-HEpETE, synthesized with rat lung 12-lipoxygenase, was applid to the HPLC. **C:** Some of this material was incubated with epoxide hydrolase before analysis. Purified *Aplysia* [^{3}H]8-HEpETE (**B**) and its enzymatic hydrolysis product (**D**) were similarly analyzed. One-min fractions of the HPLC effluent were assayed for radioactivity by liquid scintillation counting. (From Piomelli *et al.*[12] Reprinted by permission from *Proceedings of the National Academy of Sciences of the United States of America*.)

chemical ionization (pentafluorobenzyl ester, trimethylsilyl ether) and mass fragmentography (methyl ester, trimethylsilyl ether).[12]

In order to test for the physiologic production of the metabolite, L32 neurons in abdominal ganglia prelabeled with [^{3}H]arachidonic acid were driven electrically. The labeled products isolated from the bath were fractionated by normal-phase HPLC

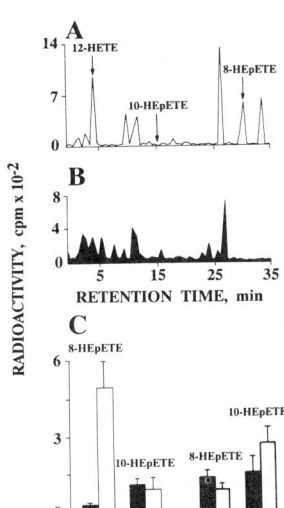

FIGURE 7. Production of metabolites from prelabeled abdominal ganglia. Ganglia were labeled with [^{3}H]arachidonate before L32 neurons were impaled and driven as described in the legend to FIGURE 4. **A:** L32 was stimulated to fire 40 spikes. The bath medium was analyzed for radioactive products by normal-phase HPLC; 1-min fractions were collected. **B:** Bath medium was collected as a control before impaling L32. **C:** [^{3}H]epoxy alcohols were quantified after L32 ($n = 4$) in the abdominal ganglion or C2 ($n = 5$) in the cerebral ganglion were stimulated intracellularly. *Solid bar:* controls; *open bar:* stimulated. Values are mean ± SEM. (From Piomelli *et al.*[12] Reprinted by permission from *Proceedings of the National Academy of Sciences of the United States of America*.)

(FIG. 7A). In addition to previously identified compounds, a major peak of material eluted at the retention time of 8-HEpETE. This material was absent in controls (FIG. 7B). Although both epoxy alcohols are produced in nearly equal amounts by the nonenzymatic rearrangement of 12-HPETE,[19] no 10-HEpETE could be detected in the experimental samples that contained significant amounts of 8-HEpETE (FIG. 7A). Interestingly, 10-HEpETE is chemically stable in contrast to its isomer, which contains an allylic epoxide and is, therefore, quite labile. Thus the appearance of

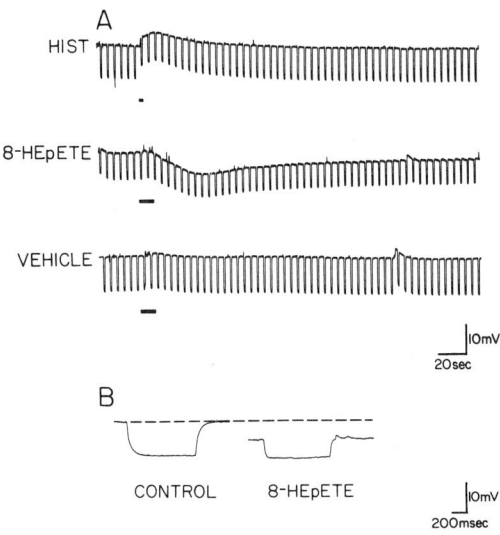

FIGURE 8. L14 response to 8-HEpETE. L14 cell was impaled with two intracellular electrodes, one to pass current and the other to record voltage. One-second hyperpolarizing current pulses were delivered at 0.2 Hz to monitor L14's input resistance. **A:** A 2-s application of histamine (1 μl; 0.1 nmol) to L14 causes a dual-action, fast depolarizing–slow hyperpolarizing response in L14 (*top trace,* HIST). Membrane potential of L14 was −60 mV. A 10-s application of 8-HEpETE (4 μl; 24 nmol) elicits a hyperpolarizing response and decreased resistance in L14 (*middle trace,* 8-HEpETE). Membrane potential of L14 was −40 mV. A 10-s application of vehicle (10 μl; prepared in parallel to the 8-HEpETE hydrolysate) to L14 causes no response and no change in input resistance (*lower trace,* VEHICLE). Membrane potential of L14 was −60 mV. **B:** In the same experiment, a second 10-s application of 8-HEpETE (3 μl; 18 nmol) again caused a hyperpolarization of L14 (*dashed line*) associated with decreased input resistance. Conductance pulses are shown at faster sweep speed to demonstrate the decrease in input resistance. L14 resting membrane potential was −60 mV.

8-HEpETE after L32 stimulation without concomitant production of 10-HEpETE suggests that this conversion is enzymatically controlled. Additional support for this idea comes from the observation that a different neural circuit (C2 and its followers in the cerebral ganglion) that is known to possess 12-lipoxygenase activity[6] does not generate epoxy alcohols (FIG. 7C). Thus, the presence of the 12-lipoxygenase alone is not sufficient to yield 8-HEpETE in an *Aplysia* neuron.

Biological Activity of 8-HEpETE

The physiologic activity of 8-HEpETE was assessed by applying the epoxy alcohol to L14 neurons. Histamine produces a dual-action response in L14 (FIGS. 4 and 8A). In contrast, 8-HEpETE induces marked hyperpolarization that appears similar to the late hyperpolarizing phase of the histamine response. No effect was detected with the vehicle control. The hyperpolarization induced by 8-HEpETE is accompanied by an increased ionic conductance (FIG. 8B). This effect has a calculated reversal potential of -77 mV (data not shown), which is similar to the conductance change and reversal potential of the slow inhibitory postsynaptic potential caused by L32 stimulation.[8] The similarities of the reversal potential and conductance changes between the hyperpolarizing effects of 8-HEpETE and synaptic activation (activation of L32) suggests a common ionic mechanism. Moreover, the differences between the response of L14 neurons to 8-HEpETE and the effect of histamine and L32 stimulation may be due to the compound nature of the dual-action synaptic response. 8-HEpETE may be responsible for the hyperpolarizing phase, while another metabolite (perhaps 12-KETE; see References 7, 22) induces the initial depolarization. Further electrophysiological and patch-clamp analysis is underway to provide direct evidence for the identity of the conductance pathways modulated by L32, histamine, and specific metabolites of arachidonic acid in L14.

We have demonstrated an active 12-lipoxygenase pathway in *Aplysia* nervous tissue. Physiologic stimulation leads to the production of several biologically active compounds, including the epoxy alcohol 8-HEpETE. Furthermore, there is some indication that the production of this epoxy alcohol is under enzymatic control. The synthesis and activity of 8-HEpETE lead us to propose that this compound may serve as a novel second messenger in the nervous system of *Aplysia*.

ACKNOWLEDGMENTS

We thank Jillayn Lindahl and Patricia Naughton for typing the manuscript and Dr. R. Zipkin of BIOMOL Research Laboratories for synthesizing 8-HEpETE and for helpful discussions.

REFERENCES

1. KANDEL, E. 1976. *Cellular Basis of Behavior*. W. H. Freeman. San Francisco, CA.
2. KOMAI, Y., S. MATSUKAWA & M. SATAKE. 1973. Lipid composition of the nervous tissue of the invertebrates *Aplysia kurodai* (gastropod) and *Cambarus clarki* (arthropod). Biochim. Biophys. Acta. **316:** 271–281.
3. NEEDLEMAN, P., J. TURK, B. A. JAKSCHIK, A. R. MORRISON & J. B. LEFKOWITH. 1986. Arachidonic acid metabolism. Annu. Rev. Biochem. **55:** 69–102.
4. HAMBERG, M. & B. SAMUELSSON. 1974. Prostaglandin endoperoxides. Novel transformations of arachidonic acid in human platelets. Proc. Natl. Acad. Sci. USA **71:** 3400–3404.
5. NUGTEREN, D. H. 1975. Arachidonate lipoxygenase in blood platelets. Biochim. Biophys. Acta. **380:** 299–307.
6. PIOMELLI, D., E. SHAPIRO, S. J. FEINMARK & J. H. SCHWARTZ. 1987. Metabolites of arachidonic acid in the nervous system of *Aplysia*: possible mediators of synaptic modulation. J. Neurosci. **7:** 3675–3686.
7. PIOMELLI, D., S. J. FEINMARK, E. SHAPIRO & J. H. SCHWARTZ. 1989. 12-keto-eicosatetraenoic acid. A biologically active eicosanoid in the nervous system of *Aplysia*. Ann. N.Y. Acad. Sci. This volume.

8. BYRNE, J. H. 1980. Neural circuit for inking behavior in *Aplysia californica*. J. Neurophysiol. **43:** 896–911.
9. BYRNE, J. H. 1980. Identification of neurons contributing to presynaptic inhibition in *Aplysia californica*. Brain Res. **199:** 235–239.
10. KRETZ, R., E. SHAPIRO & E. R. KANDEL. 1986. Presynaptic inhibition produced by an identified presynaptic inhibitory neuron. I. Physiological mechanisms. J. Neurophysiol. **55:** 113–130.
11. COREY, E. J. & S. WEI-GUO. 1984. Total synthesis of biologically active metabolites of arachidonic acid. The two 8-hydroxy-11,12(S,S)-epoxy eicosa-5, 14(Z),9(E)-trienoic acids. Tetrahedron Lett. **25:** 5119–5122.
12. PIOMELLI, D., E. SHAPIRO, R. ZIPKIN, J. H. SCHWARTZ & S. J. FEINMARK. 1989. Formation and action of 8-hydroxy-11,12-epoxy-5,9,14-eicosatrienoic acid in *Aplysia:* a possible second messenger in neurons. Proc. Natl. Acad. Sci. USA. In press.
13. PACE-ASCIAK, C. R., E. GRANSTRÖM & B. SAMUELSSON. 1983. Arachidonic acid epoxides. Isolation and structure of two hydroxy epoxide intermediates in the formation of 8,11,12- and 10,11,12-trihydroxy eicosatrienoic acids. J. Biol. Chem. **258:** 6835–6840.
14. WEINREICH, D., C. WEINER & R. McCAMAN. 1975. Endogenous levels of histamine in single neurons isolated from CNS of *Aplysia californica*. Brain Res. **84:** 341–345.
15. McCAMAN, R. E. & D. WEINREICH. 1982. On the nature of histamine mediated slow hyperpolarizing synaptic potentials in identified molluscan neurones. J. Physiol. **328:** 485–507.
16. KRETZ, R., E. SHAPIRO, C. H. BAILEY, M. CHEN & E. R. KANDEL. 1986. Presynaptic inhibition produced by an identified presynaptic inhibitory neuron. II. Presynaptic conductance changes caused by histamine. J. Neurophysiol. **55:** 131–146.
17. SHAPIRO, E., D. PIOMELLI, S. FEINMARK, S. VOGEL, G. CHIN & J. H. SCHWARTZ. 1988. The role of arachidonic acid metabolites in signal transduction in an identified neural network mediating presynaptic inhibition in *Aplysia*. Cold Spring Harbor Symp. Quant. Biol. In press.
18. PACE-ASCIAK, C. R. 1984. Arachidonic acid epoxides. Demonstration through [^{18}O]oxygen studies of an intramolecular transfer of the terminal hydroxyl group of 12(S)-hydroperoxy-eicosa-5,8,10,14-tetraenoic acid to form hydroxyepoxides. J. Biol. Chem. **259:** 8332–8337.
19. PACE-ASCIAK, C. R. 1984. Hemoglobin- and hemin-catalyzed transformation of 12L-hydroperoxy-5,8,10,14-eicosatetraenoic acid. Biochim. Biophys. Acta **793:** 485–488.
20. GLASGOW, W. C., T. M. HARRIS & A. R. BRASH. 1986. A short-chain aldehyde is a major lipoxygenase product in arachidonic acid–stimulated porcine leukocytes. J. Biol. Chem. **261:** 200–204.
21. FRUTEAU DE LACLOS, B., J. MACLOUF, P. POUBELLE & P. BORGEAT. 1987. Conversion of arachidonic acid into 12-oxo derivatives in human platelets. A pathway possibly involving the heme-catalyzed transformation of 12-hydroperoxy-eicosatetraenoic acid. Prostaglandins **33:** 315–337.
22. PIOMELLI, D., S. J. FEINMARK, E. SHAPIRO & J. H. SCHWARTZ. 1988. Formation and biological activity of 12-keto-eicosatetraenoic acid in the nervous system of *Aplysia*. J. Biol. Chem. **263:** 16591–16596.

Cerebrospinal Fluid Eicosanoids as an Index of Cerebrovascular Status[a]

RICHARD P. WHITE

Departments of Pharmacology and Neurosurgery
College of Medicine
University of Tennessee
Memphis, Tennessee 38163

It is well established that perturbation of cell membranes will cause the release of arachidonic acid (AA) and that metabolites of AA (eicosanoids) are autacoids that produce remarkably diverse cellular effects.[1] The effects become most evident in pathophysiological phenomena such as pain, edema, hemostasis (via platelet aggregation), fever, and various aspects of inflammation, including the invasion of leukocytes into traumatized tissue. Metabolites of AA are also vasoactive. It is because of these diverse effects that investigators have attempted to relate the appearance of an eicosanoid in the cerebrospinal fluid (CSF) to a particular cerebrovascular or neurological disorder. This article is a review of those attempts.

To date, the eicosanoids identified in CSF of patients include the products of cyclooxygenase: prostaglandins (PG) PGI_2 (detected as the stable metabolite 6-keto PGF_{1a} or $6KPGF_{1a}$), PGF_{2a}, PGE_2, and PGD_2, as well as thromboxane A_2 (as the stable metabolite TxB_2). The products of lipoxygenase, leukotriene C_4 (LTC_4) and 5-hydroxy-6, 8, 11, 14-eicosatetraenoic acid (5-HETE) have also been studied. In addition, a major end product of lipid peroxidation, malondialdehyde (MDA), has been identified in CSF. MDA should be a good indicator of the overall release of AA in health and disease, since the major polyunsaturated fatty acid in cell membranes is AA.[2]

ANALYSIS AND OVERVIEW OF THE DATA

Specific effects of eicosanoids on isolated human cerebral arteries has been investigated,[3-16] and the results are summarized in TABLE 1. These results suggest that most eicosanoids would reduce cerebral blood flow if sufficient quantities were produced locally in response to pathological conditions or were present in sufficient concentrations in the CSF.

The concentration of various eicosanoids in CSF has been studied in a wide variety of cerebrovascular and neurological disorders.[17-51] Some investigators obtained CSF samples sequentially over days, while others sampled only during the height of disease and at remission. Some reports present only raw data on each patient or only a range of values among patients, while other reports include complete statistical analyses. For this review, raw data of positive findings were averaged as needed and the extremes in

---

[a]This work was supported by United States Public Health Service Grant NS 21405 of the National Institutes of Health.

the range of values noted among the reports. The means obtained from the reports for a particular affliction or condition were averaged in order to obtain a composite picture of the changes in eicosanoid content that may occur in disease. However, it should be emphasized that the time course of disease varies among patients, so that grand means do not necessarily reflect the severity of the disorder. Also, CSF samples need not reveal what is occurring remotely from the tap or what had occurred at some previous time that may have caused damage. Many reports studied only specific disorders. One studied only healthy subjects.[48] Here, control values are presented separately from patients with disease.

TABLE 1. Main Responses of Isolated Human Cerebral Arteries to Eicosanoids and Some Analogues

Eicosanoid	Pial Arterioles			Basilar/Middle			References
	+	0	−	+	0	−	
AA	+			+			5, 15
PGA_1				+	0		3, 16
PGA_2				+			16
PGB_2	+						11
PGD_1		0					11
PGD_2	+			+			11, 15
PGE_1		0		+			3, 11, 12, 16
PGE_2	+			+			11, 12, 15, 16
PGF_{1a}	+			+			11, 16
PGF_{2a}	+			+			3, 5, 7, 11, 12, 15, 16
PGH_2				+			4, 12
PGI_2			−			−	5, 6, 12
$6KPGE_1$			−				5
ETYA	+						5
TxA_2				+			7, 12
TxB_2	+						11
U44069	+						11
U46619	+			+			7, 8, 11
LTC_4					0		12
LTD_4				+	0		9, 12

NOTE: Contraction indicated under (+), no response under (0), and relaxation under (−).

Some investigators reported that samples of CSF obtained from the ventricles or from the cisterns (enlarged areas of the subarachnoid space surrounding the brain) best reflect pathological conditons, whereas most CSF has been obtained by lumbar puncture, distant from the brain. The wide range of CSF values reported for any single condition may also reflect the methodology employed—radioimmunoassay (RIA), radioisotopic dilution (RD), and gas chromatography–mass spectrometry (GS/MS)—as well as the investigator's expertise. In some cases the CSF values reported here for PGE_2 and PGF_{2a} include, respectively, PGE_1 and PGF_{1a}, when the investigators were unable to distinguish between these prostaglandins.

Despite the limitations of this meta-analysis, the results clearly indicate that at some time during an acute CNS affliction, eicosanoid levels of CSF are high; whereas with chronic conditions like tumors, this elevation is less evident. Moreover, some investigators have demonstrated significant relationships between the disorder studied and CSF eicosanoids. Last, the analysis shows that the profile of eicosanoids present in human CSF is different from that reported for some laboratory animals.

SOURCE OF EICOSANOIDS IN CEREBROSPINAL FLUID

Virtually all tissue that makes contact with CSF synthesizes eicosanoids. This includes blood vessels, the choroid plexus, the leptomeninges, brain parenchyma, and, after hemorrhage, blood.[52-62] Bovine or canine cerebral arteries, for instance, reportedly synthesize PGI_2, PGE_2, PGF_{2a}, PGD_2, and TxA_2.[32,60,61] The profile of synthesis reported varies markedly among tissues. The small vessels, choroid plexus, and leptomeninges from a variety of species synthesize more PGI_2 than PGE_2, or PGF_{2a}, or TxA_2, whereas brain tissue makes mostly PGD_2, PGE_2, or PGF_{2a}, depending on the species.[32,58,59] Moreover, the profile of synthesis by specific tissues changes in animal models of hemorrhagic stroke.[32,60]

A paramount problem of identifying the role eicosanoids may play in health and disease is that the variety is so great as to tax the expertise of investigators. In the early 1970s PGE_1 and PGF_{2a} dominated the interest of investigators because these were readily available for study and produced diametrically opposite physiological effects on cerebral circulation.[63] By the 1980s leukotrienes and many other eicosanoids were being studied.[1] The clinical relevancy of relating changes in CSF concentrations of eicosanoids to disease depends both on the identification of the tissue source of the eicosanoid and the identification of the appropriate AA metabolite. The CSF is akin to the lymphatic system, being a repository for products formed by tissue interposed between the arterial and venous circulations. It is not surprising, therefore, that eicosanoid levels in CSF is elevated in response to abnormal stimuli. However, specificity may be important; for instance, PGE_2 could be a better marker for the presence of pyrogens than PGF_{2a}, and PGD_2 may be better related to cerbral vasospasm than TxA_2. Also, are leukotrienes responsible for cerebral edema?

CEREBROVASCULAR EFFECTS OF EICOSANOIDS

Experiments performed on isolated human cerebral arteries indicate that the fundamental pharmacodynamic effect of most eicosanoids is constriction (TABLE 1). This constriction may be produced with nmol concentrations.[3-16] Moreover, the contraction elicited by many eicosanoids seems to last for an indefinite period, in contrast to many other contractile agonists.[15] The maximum response achieved exceeds that of KCl, and among the prostaglandins the response to 10^{-8} M PGE_2 is comparable to the peak effect obtained with 10^{-6} M serotonin.[15] These characteristics support the concept that prostaglandins are important to the phenomenon of cerebral vasospasm.[52-57]

Because PGI_2 is a potent dilator of human cerebral arteries and will induce pain and edema, it has been considered a candidate as a mediator of migraine.[54,58] However, the stimulus for its release in migraine is unknown; and PGI_2, and even a stable analogue (Iloprost), will produce vasoconstriction at concentrations above 10^{-6} M.[8,10] Its effect on vasomotion in pathological concentrations is, therefore, open to question.

Reports indicate that leukotrienes produce either no effect on human arteries[12] or constriction that is subject to tachyphylaxis.[9] In either case, the appearance of

TABLE 2. Eicosanoid Values (pg/ml) in Cerebrospinal Fluid in Control Subjects and in Patients Suffering from Subarachnoid Hemorrhage (SAH)

Substance/Subject	6KPGF$_{1a}$	PGF$_{2a}$	PGE$_2$	PGD$_2$	TxB$_2$	LTC$_4$
Control (low)[a]						
Mean	56 (4)	48 (7)	41 (4)	84 (3)	32 (2)	108 (1)
Spread	ND–317 (7)	ND–150 (8)	ND–160 (7)	ND–220 (1)	ND–300 (4)	X
Control (high)[b]						
Mean	555 (1)	859 (2)	776 (3)		337 (2)	
Spread	ND–1590 (1)	400–4750 (2)	ND–2220 (3)		290–770 (1)	
SAH all studies[c]						
Mean	311 (3)	829 (5)	581 (1)	403 (3)	887 (3)	337 (2)
Spread	ND–1538 (6)	ND–7583 (5)	69–1804 (1)	50–1140 (2)	6–9832 (3)	X
No spasm						
Mean	221 (2)			240 (3)	263 (2)	234 (1)
Spread	ND–247 (1)			50–840 (1)	25–133 (1)	X
Spasm						
Mean	177 (2)			573 (3)	2633 (2)	440 (1)
Spread	ND–145 (1)			70–1140 (1)	1412–9832 (1)	X

NOTE: Data based on lumbar samples. Numbers in parentheses are numbers of reports cited. X = not available or appropriate. Italicized values indicate significant differences between corresponding groups of patients and/or control subjects or are based on at least one report claiming a clinical significance. ND = not detected.

[a]References include 18–20, 24, 25, 30, 32, 36, 37, 39–41, 45, 48, 49.
[b]References include 25, 26, 35, 44, 46.
[c]References include 18, 20, 21, 25–27, 29–32.

leukotrienes in the CSF would appear to be more related to cellular or vasogenic edema than to an effect on vasomotion.

A major question asked concerning the relationship between CSF eicosanoids and cerebrovascular disease has been whether their concentration is sufficient to account for the changes in cerebral blood flow observed in patients.[32] The answer appears to be negative, because the concentrations reported are in general too low to produce the effects obtained of arteries *in vitro* and because comparable concentrations of any one eicosanoid may be present in patients with and without cerebrovascular disease (TABLES 2–7). For instance, the highest average concentration reported for PGF_{2a} was 7,900 pg/ml in patients apparently free of cerebrovascular disease (TABLE 5). This is 5 times greater than any mean value reported for cerebral vasospasm (TABLE 2). It is equivalent to a 2.2×10^{-8} M solution, which *in vitro* studies indicate would be insufficient to elicit biologically significant contractions in human cerebral arteries.[3,8,15] The highest average value reported for PGE_2 is, however, sufficient (2.4×10^{-8} M); but, again, in patients who did not present evidence of cerebral

TABLE 3. Eicosanoid Concentrations (pg/ml) Reported for Patients Suffering from Stroke, Transient Ischemic Attacks (TIA), or Neoplasm

Substance/Subject	$6KPGF_{1a}$	PGF_{2a}	PGE_2	TxB_2
Stroke (ischemic)[a]				
Mean	X	789 (2)	682 (1)	X
Spread	ND–50 (1)	25–2000 (2)	150–3000 (1)	150–400 (1)
First 4 hrs				
Mean		1122 (1)		
Spread		440–2000 (1)		
12–24 hr				
Mean		576 (1)		
Spread		X		
TIA[b]				
Mean		170 (1)		
Spread		35–355 (1)		
Tumor[c]				
Mean		114 (1)		
Spread		ND–500 (2)		

NOTE: Lumbar values. Numbers in parentheses are numbers of reports cited. X = not available or appropriate. Italicized values indicate significant differences between corresponding groups of patients and/or control subjects or are based on at least one report claiming a clinical significance. ND = not detected.
[a]References include 36, 37, 39, 41.
[b]References include 37.
[c]References include 37, 42.

ischemia (TABLE 5). In any case, the concentrations reported most commonly for any of the eicosanoids fall short of directly influencing the cerebral vasculature.

However, when the source of these eicosanoids in disease becomes better understood and as more investigators study the changes in profile of synthesis with disease, the relationship between synthesis and pathology should become more apparent. None of the intracranial tissue is known to significantly degrade eicosanoids so that these lipids are removed by the circulation. One study, which dealth specifically with the disposition of eicosanoids in CSF, showed that PGF_{2a} given intrathecally had a half-life of only 8 min, yet produced vasoconstriction for several hours.[20] The results indicated that the prolonged effect was related to the eicosanoid concentration in the artery, not in the CSF. Moreover, some clinical studies performed to date implicate specific CSF eicosanoids in the pathogenesis of cerebrovascular disease.

CEREBROSPINAL FLUID EICOSANOIDS IN DISEASE

Control Values

Clinical studies can be conveniently divided into reports indicating that the CSF, on average, contained less than 100 pg/ml and those indicating that CSF exceeds 300 pg/ml. Nevertheless, in each group (TABLE 2, control (low) and (high)) appears to be present in the lowest concentration; and 6-keto PGF_{1a} (or prostacyclin) is not the major AA metabolite, as it is in unanesthetized felines.[48] The control (low) group shows good agreement between values obtained with RIA and GS/MS. The Control (high) group used RIA. Both groups contain patients with a variety of neurological complaints that

TABLE 4. Eicosanoid Concentration (pg/ml) in Cerebrospinal Fluid Reported for Patients Suffering from Central Nervous System (CNS) Infections, Elevated Intracranial Pressure, Epilepsy, Head Trauma, and Multiple Sclerosis

Substance/Subject	$6KPGF_{1a}$	PGF_{2a}	PGE_2	PGD_2
CNS infections[a]				
Mean		*648 (4)*	*1009 (1)*	
Spread		25–2196 (4)	X	
Elevated intracranial pressure[b]				
Mean	6060 (1)	800 (1)	500 (1)	425 (1)
Spread	100–15300 (1)	ND–1800 (2)	100–1100 (1)	50–800 (1)
Epilepsy[c]				
Mean		*346 (2)*		
Spread		25–2500 (2)		
Head trauma (V)[d]				
Mean	14145 (1)	529 (2)	2229 (1)	
Spread	ND–27323 (1)	ND–3349 (2)	ND–11800 (1)	
Exceptional values	167580	215843	63240	
Multiple sclerosis[e]				
Mean, all values	702 (1)	*272 (3)*	*403 (3)*	
Spread	480–900 (1)	0–1050 (3)	12–1180 (3)	
Mean, remission	673 (1)	471 (2)	436 (3)	
Spread	530–880 (1)	180–1050 (2)	12–1180 (3)	
Mean, relapse	731 (1)	335 (2)	346 (3)	
Spread	480–900 (1)	0–740	63–790 (3)	

NOTE: Lumbar values. Numbers in parentheses are numbers of reports cited. X = not available or appropriate. Italicized values indicate significant differences between corresponding groups of patients and/or control subjects or are based on at least one report claiming a clinical significance. V = ventricular tap, ND = not detected.
[a]References include 37, 42, 46, 51.
[b]References include 33, 42.
[c]References include 37, 51.
[d]References include 21, 38.
[e]References include 35, 37, 45, 49.

TABLE 5. Eicosanoid Levels (pg/ml) in Cerebrospinal Fluid Reported for Friedrich's Ataxia, Hemorrhage Infarcts, Lumbar Disk Problems, Unspecified Neurological Disorders, and Psychiatric Disorders

Substance/Subject	$6KPGF_{1a}$	PGF_{2a}	PGE_2	PGD_2	TxB_2
Friedrich's ataxia[45]					
Mean			100 (1)		
Hemorrhagic infarcts[34]					
Mean		15000 (1)	11400 (1)		
Spread		10200–18800 (1)	4300–18300 (1)		
Lumbar disk problems[34]					
Mean		8100 (1)	2200 (1)		
Spread		1300–15200 (1)	0–5500 (1)		
Other neurological disorders (OND)[33-35,45]					
Mean	667 (2)	3020 (3)	2410 (4)	0.0 (1)	
Spread	0–1590 (2)	100–10000 (3)	100–14400 (4)	X	
Psychiatric disorders[40,43-45]					
Schizophrenia					
Mean	0.0 (1)	0.0 (1)	*1030 (3)*		410 (1)
Spread	X	X	0–5740 (4)		250–690 (1)
Depression (UP)					
Mean	0.0 (1)	0.0 (1)	*840 (3)*		
Spread	X	X	0–4471 (4)		
Mania					
Mean			*148 (2)*		
Spread			50–200 (2)		

NOTE: Lumbar samples. Numbers in parentheses are numbers of reports cited. X = not available or appropriate. Italicized values indicate significant differences between corresponding groups of patients and/or control subjects or are based on at least one report claiming a clinical significance.

the investigators felt would not influence eicosanoid synthesis unduly, but some of the studies include normal subjects.

Cerebral Vasospasm and Other Diseases

One manifestation of subarachnoid hemorrhage (SAH) is vasospasm. This most commonly results from rupture of an aneurysm at the base of the brain, takes about seven days to appear, and persists for several weeks.[13,15,55] The vasoconstriction is most evident in the hemorrhaged vessel and typically involves those branches distal to the rupture in the direction of the bulk flow of CSF, although it may spread to other arteries with time.

Though this remarkable constriction appears to be essential for the development of severe neurological deficits, some patients may manifest maximum constriction, shown

TABLE 6. Ancillary Cerebrospinal Fluid Data (pg/ml) Reflecting the Role Eicosanoids May Play in Health and Disease

Substance/Subject	$6KPGF_{1a}$	PGD_2	TxB_2	LTC_4	MDA	5-HETE
Neonates[47]						
Lumbar ($n = 29$)	>50					
Lumbar and ventricular ($n = 9$)	50–100					
Lumbar ($n = 3$)	>200					
SAH[22,27,29]	Intracisternal				Lumbar	Lumbar
Control						none
No spasm[a]	306	460	5753	813	1440	none
	(93–1110)	(110–1150)	(810–1200)	(140–2600)	2740	
Spasm[b]	214	1130	4350	2582	5180	present
	(68–342)	(300–2200)	(490–900)	(700–5750)		

NOTE: Italicized values indicate significant differences between corresponding groups of patients and/or control subjects or are based on at least one report claiming a clinical significance.
[a]Number of patients without spasm for $6KPGF_{1a}$ through $LTC_4 = 24$; number without spasm for MDA = 11.
[b]Number of patients with spasm for $6KPGF_{1a}$ through $LTC_4 = 16$; number with spasm for MDA = 14.

arteriographically, without impairment of cognitive function (asymptomatic vasospasm). This indicates that other factors contribute to the loss of consciousness and death. Since a rise in intracranial pressure is commonly associated with subarachnoid hemorrhage, it is likely that cerebral edema contributes to the demise of these patients by further reducing blood flow. Recent findings indicate that LTC_4 (causing vasogenic edema?) and PGD_2 (producing vasospasm?) are the eicosanoids in CSF that best reflect the condition of the patients (TABLES 2, 7). If these are high, the patient suffers most.[18,19,23-27]

Animal studies indicate that leukotrienes are synthesized mainly by cerebral gray matter, not by arteries; but of the PGs, the rodent brain synthesizes predominantly PGD_2.[64,65] Cerebral arteries also synthesize PGD_2, but the pharmacodynamic properties of other prostaglandins suggests these, also, are important to the phenomenon of vasospasm.[10,11,15,54] The injection of blood into the CSF of animals markedly enhances the synthesis of brain leukotrienes and PGE_2 by cerebral arteries.[32,66] Moreover, cyclooxygenase inhibitors reduce the synthesis of the prostanoids by all the intracranial tissue studied[32] and prevents cerebral vasospasm in canines.[67] Despite the potency of

TABLE 7. Comparison of the Highest Concentration (pg/ml) of Eicosanoids in Cerebrospinal Fluid with That Present in the Last Cerebrospinal Fluid Tap Performed during Treatment of Hydrocephalus

Eicosanoid	Highest			Last Sample	
	Mean	%[a]	Range	Mean (pg/ml)	Range
PGD_2	1410.3	100	286–2725	102.6	0.0–308
PGE_2	867	50	630–1100	0.0	0.0
PGF_{2a}	615.5	50	222–1009	63.4	0.0–108
6-keto PGF_{1a}	668.7	100	238–1374	89.0	12–169
TxB_2	493.7	100	154–1243	178.5	135–476
LTC_4	2053.6	100	1164–3728	338.7	0.0–786

NOTE: Data from four preterm infants with intraventricular hemorrhage. Lumbar taps performed 2–4 times to relieve intracranial pressure at various intervals of time.
[a]Percent of patients with positive finding.

TxA_2, its effect is too ephemeral to account for the vasospasm, and animal[32] and clinical studies indicate that this prostanoid is not involved (TABLE 2).

Much has been speculated concerning the role prostacyclin may play in protecting the vessel from vasospasm as a natural dilator.[15,32,60,61] The synthesis of this prostanoid by arteries is significantly decreased in animal models of SAH.[32,60] However, clinical studies indicate that changes in prostacyclin production is not important to the genesis of vasospasm, and animal studies show that replacement therapy, via intra-arterial administration, has no effect on cerebral vasospasm.[27,67] Indeed, there is no convincing evidence that any vasodilator, released from the endothelium or blood-borne, will reverse an established vasospasm.[15,67]

It has been proposed that free radials generated by lipid peroxidation (mainly of AA) may be the cause of vasospasm.[54] Various hydroperoxides given intrathecally will produce vasospasm experimentally,[68] and an end product of lipid peroxidation is clearly elevated in vasospasm (TABLE 6). It has also been proposed that free radical scavengers in CSF may protect the vessel, and, when they are exhausted, vasospasm occurs.[28,68] Also, individual pharmacodynamic differences among human arteries, desensitization of arteries to many agonists, and the presence of vasodilator proteins in blood may account for the fact that cerebral vasospasm does not occur in all patients with aneurysmal rupture of cerebral arteries.[15,57] The pathogenesis of vasospasm is apparently complex, but an increased production of eicosanoids seems pivotal to its occurrence.

Experimental studies indicate that prostanoids and leukotrienes are important mediators of cerebral damage in *stroke*.[2,65,66] The cerebral hypoxia caused by thrombotic episodes evidently triggers the release of AA and generates oxygen radicals during the conversion of PGG_2 to PGH_2 as well as a number of eicosanoids, some of which cause edema and changes in cerebral blood flow.

The clinical studies performed on *stroke patients* indicate that CSF levels of PGF_{2a} and PGE_2 rise significantly (TABLE 3). In several studies the values reflected the status of the patients. TxA_2 values are generally higher than controls, but the spread of the data requires further study to establish the role this prostanoid may play in the pathogenesis of stroke. The time at which the samples of CSF are drawn appears to be critical to accurately relating eicosanoid synthesis to the encephalopathy of stroke. PGI_2 does not appear to change significantly in stroke.

The concentration of PGF_{2a} reportedly increases significantly above control values in *TIA* (transient ischemic attacks) and *tumors* (TABLE 3). The TIA patients were sampled the same day of the attack. Compared to other CNS pathologies, the rise is slight (TABLES 2–7). However, LTC_4 synthesis by tumors from patients correlates well with the cerebral edema recorded.[62]

Several reports concluded that *meningitis and other CNS infections* (TABLE 4) elevate CSF PGF_{2a}, but the only study that simultaneously evaluated PGE_2 concluded that only PGE_2 was significantly elevated with infection and that the elevation was significantly linked to fever.[46] The control values of these studies were among the highest reported for these prostaglandins (TABLE 2), but it should be noted that animal studies support the conclusion that the production of especially PGE-type prostaglandins is associated with fever.[65]

The few investigators who have studied the relationship between prostanoid levels and *intracranial pressure* (TABLE 4) concluded that there is no pattern that separates this condition from the other neurological problems studied. However, it is likely that, compared to normal subjects, many of these patients would have elevated levels. The PGI_2 concentration of 15.3 ng/ml found in one patient is certainly high (TABLE 4). In this regard, the concentration of PGF_{2a} reported was higher than that found for *epilepsy*, which was shown to be higher than controls (TABLE 4). Reports agree that PGF_{2a} is elevated in epilepsy, and one report indicates this value may rise from 559 (124–1230) to 1197 (118–2500) pg/ml after surgery.[51]

Samples of ventricular fluid from patients with *head injuries* yield some of the highest prostanoid mean values, especially for prostacyclin (TABLE 4). The concentrations found varied markedly from day to day and appeared to be significantly reduced with pentobarbital. Animal studies also indicate that head trauma increases eicosanoid synthesis more than experimental SAH and that pentobarbital anesthesia significantly reduces synthesis.[48,66] Although the leukotrienes may be the best marker for cerebral edema, it is possible that among the prostanoids PGI_2 may be a good index of inflammation, as its level appears to be most elevated in head trauma (TABLE 4). The high PGE_2 values present in head injuries might account for the cerebral vasospasm seen occasionally in these patients.[55]

The overall findings in *multiple sclerosis* suggests that PGF_{2a}, PGE_2, and PGI_2 are elevated, as compared to normal subjects; but that during remission, PGF_{2a} and PGE_2 can be higher in value than with relapse (exacerbation) of the disease (TABLE 4). The elevation during remission, if present, might reflect tissue repair, as might the elevation found in epileptics after surgery. The concentration of CSF linoleic acid rises markedly in multiple sclerosis, but this has been attributed to impairment of the blood-brain barrier and a concomitant rise in CSF albumin.[50]

Reports indicate that patients presenting a wide variety of neurological complaints (e.g., headache, vertigo, neuropathies), grouped as *other neurological disorders* by investigators, do not have detectable levels of PGD_2 and have lower CSF concentrations of other prostanoids than patients suffering from *lumbar disk problems* (TABLE 5). In turn, patients suffering *hemorrhage infarcts* manifest higher values than those with disk problems (TABLE 5). The PGE_2 evident in the CSF of patients with *Friederich's ataxia* appears within normal range (TABLE 5).

The few studies performed on psychiatric patients suggest that CSF values for PGE_2 are lowest for mania and highest for schizophrenia, with values for depression between these. Investigators concluded that TxA_2 was within normal limits and that prostacyclin and PGF_{2a} were absent (TABLE 5). This review does not distinguish between PGE_1 and PGE_2; but Kaiya[69] summarizes the arguments that PGE_1 is deficient in schizophrenia, while PGE_2 levels should rise, and reports on the limited success of treating these patients intravenously with PGE_1.

SPECIAL STUDIES ON NEONATES AND SUBARACHNOID HEMORRHAGE

An earlier report[33] that PGI_2 was the major CSF prostaglandin found in 8 of 12 adult patients with varying complaints prompted Rennie *et al.*[47] to determine if that eicosanoid might be prominent in neonates, especially premature infants with suspected sepsis. They concluded that PGI_2 (as 6-keto PGF_{1a}) is not a major prostaglandin in the CSF of human infants (TABLE 6).

The analysis of bloody CSF removed at the time of aneurysmal surgery shows that the levels of PGD_2 and LTC_4 are significantly elevated in adults who suffer from vasospasm over those who do not (TABLE 6). The concentration of malondialdehyde is also more evident in patients with vasospasm (TABLE 6), indicating that lipid peroxidation is more prominent. The lipid peroxide 5-HETE has been identified in the CSF of SAH patients (TABLE 6).

Preliminary observations ($n = 4$) indicate that LTC_4 is the most conspicuous eicosanoid in the CSF of premature infants with *hemorrhagic hydrocephalus* (C. W. Leffler and R. P. White, unpublished data). Moreover, the concentration of LTC_4 and other identified eicosanoids drops dramatically with successful treatment (TABLE 7). The stimulus for the increased synthesis is apparently blood, because blood administered into the lateral ventricles of rabbits also enhances LTC_4 synthesis.[66] LTC_4 may be a marker for neurological damage from blood, as it is high in these premature infants and high in the adults most severely affected by SAH. In contrast, our previous observations indicated that prostanoids are not always present in the CSF of infants after intraventricular hemorrhage, as shown by the following percentages: PGD_2 73%, PGF_2 34%, PGE_{2a} 55%, 6-keto PGF_{1a} 82%, and TxB_2 64%. In any case, the concentration of six eicosanoids decreases significantly as the signs of hemorrhagic hydrocephalus disappear (TABLE 7).

EPILOGUE

It is evident from this review that no single eicosanoid is pathognomonic of the disorders studied and that the recorded CSF concentrations vary greatly among patients suffering from specific disorders. Nevertheless, eicosanoid levels are on average significantly elevated in a variety of neurological afflictions, indicating enhanced synthesis during the course of disease. Synthesis is likely to be highest in patients with severe acute injury, to be intermediate when the condition is not life-threating, to wane as clinical status improves, and to be lowest in normal individuals. The earlier low values occasionally reported in single CSF samples of severely ill patients[20,21,51] may reflect posttraumatic events, because close monitoring of SAH patients shows that high CSF levels of certain eicosanoids is predictive of cerebral vasospasm.[18,19,23–27,70] In addition, the more inclusive studies indicate that changes in the profile of synthesis best reflect the disease investigated.

The most extraordinary single values reported for $6KPGF_{1a}$ (4.5×10^{-7} M), PGF_{2a} (6.1×10^{-7} M), and PGE_2 (1.8×10^{-7} M) were obtained from patients with head injury (TABLE 4). The highest single concentrations reported for PGD_2 (6.2×10^{-9} M), TxB_2 (2.7×10^{-7} M), and LTC_4 (0.2×10^{-9} M) were seen in SAH (TABLES 2 and 6). Although some eicosanoids are vasoactive at these concentrations *in vitro*, the CSF levels found in most patients appear to be insufficient per se to influence vasomotor tone. Moreover, high concentrations may be present in patients without cerebrovascular disease. Nevertheless, the clinical data become more pertinent when the vasculature is considered as the source of the CSF eicosanoid studied. In this regard, the data obtained during the past twenty years from laboratory experiments and clinical observations have provided a more realistic assessment of the tissue sources and significance of eicosanoids in health and disease.

ACKNOWLEDGMENTS

The author thanks Mrs. Marion Johnson for her expert assistance.

REFERENCES

1. MONCADA, S., R. J. FLOWER & J. R. VANE. 1985. Prostaglandins, prostacyclin, thromboxane A, and leukotrienes. *In* The Pharmacological Basis of Therapeutics. 7th edit. A. G. Gilman, L. S. Goodman, T. W. Rall. & F. Murad, Eds.: 660–673. Macmillan. New York, NY.
2. BAKAY, R. A. E., K. M. SWEENEY & J. H. WOOD. 1986. Pathophysiology of cerebrospinal fluid in head injury. Neurosurgery **18**: 234–243.
3. ALLEN, G. S., C. J. GROSS, L. A. FRENCH & S. N. CHOU. 1976. Cerebral arterial spasm. Part 5: *In vitro* contractile activity of vasoactive agents including human CSF on human basilar and anterior cerebral arteries. J. Neurosurg. **44**: 594–600.
4. BOULLIN, D. J., S. BUNTING, W. P. BLASO, T. M. HUNT & S. MONCADA. 1979. Responses of human and baboon arteries to prostaglandin endoperoxides and biologically generated and synthetic prostacyclin: Their relevance to cerebral arterial spasm in man. Br. J. Clin. Pharmacol. **7**: 139–147.
5. BRANDT, L., B. LJUNGGREN, K.-E. ANDERSSON, B. HINDFELT & T. USKI. 1981. Effects of indomethacin and prostacyclin on isolated human pial arteries contracted by CSF from patients with aneurysmal SAH. J. Neurosurg. **55**: 877–883.
6. HARDEBO, J. E., J. HANKO & CH. OWMAN. 1983. Species variation in the cerebrovascular response to neurotransmitters and related vasoactive agents. Gen. Pharmacol. **14**: 135–136.
7. PAUL, K. S., E. T. WHALLEY, C. FORSTER, R. LYE & J. DUTTON. 1982. Prostacyclin and cerebral vessel relaxation. J. Neurosurg. **57**: 334–340.
8. SCHRÖR, K. & R. VERHEGGEN. 1988. Use of human post-mortem cerebral blood vessels to study vasospasm. Trends Pharmacol. Sci. **9**: 71–74.

9. TAGARI, P., G. H. DU BOULAY, V. AITKEN & D. J. BOULLIN. 1983. Leukotriene D_4 and the cerebral vasculature *in vivo* and *in vitro*. Prostagland. Leuk. Med. **11:** 281–297.
10. USKI, T., K.-E. ANDERSSON, L. BRANDT, L. EDVINSSON & B. LJUNGGREN. 1983. Responses of isolated feline and human cerebral arteries to prostacyclin and some of its metabolites. J. Cereb. Blood Flow Metab. **3:** 238–245.
11. USKI, T. K., K.-E. ANDERSSON, L. BRANDT & B. LJUNGGREN. 1984. Characterization of the prostanoid receptors and of the contractile effects of prostaglandin F_{2a} in human pial arteries. Acta Physiol. Scand. **121:** 369–378.
12. VON HOLST, H., E. GRANSTROM, S. HAMMARSTROM, B. SAMUELSSON & L. STEINER. 1982. Effect of Leucotrienes C_4, D_4, prostacyclin and thromboxane A_2 on isolated human cerebral arteries. Acta Neurochir. **62:** 177–185.
13. WHITE, R. P. 1987. Comparison of the inhibitory effects of antithrombin III, a_2-macroglobulin, and thrombin in human basilar arteries: Relevance to cerebral vasospasm. J. Cereb. Blood Flow Metab. **7:** 68–73.
14. WHITE, R. P. 1987. Responses of human basilar arteries to vasoactive intestinal polypeptide. Life Sci. **41:** 1155–1163.
15. WHITE, R. P. & J. T. ROBERTSON. 1987. Pharmacodynamic evaluation of human cerebral arteries in the genesis of vasospasm. Neurosurgery **21:** 523–531.
16. YASHON, D., R. J. BROWN & W. E. HUNT. 1977. Vasoactive properties of prostaglandin compounds on the in vitro human basilar artery. Surg. Neurol. **8:** 111–115.
17. BOULLIN, D. J., L. BRANDT, B. LJUNGGREN & P. TAGARI. 1981. Vasoconstrictor activity in cerebrospinal fluid from patients subjected to early surgery for ruptured intracranial aneurysms. J. Neurosurg. **55:** 237–245.
18. GAETANI, P., R. RODRIGUEZ Y BAENA, V. SILVANI, F. RAINOLDI & P. PAOLETTI. 1986. Prostacyclin and vasospasm in subarachnoid hemorrhage from ruptured intracranial aneurysm. Acta Neurol. Scand. **73:** 33–38.
19. GAETAMO, P., V. SILVANI, M. T. CRIVELLARI, T. VIGANO, R. RODRIQUEZ Y BAENA & P. PAOLETTI. 1986. Prostaglandin D_2 monitoring in human CSF after subarachnoid hemorrhage: The possible role of prostaglandin D_2 in the genesis of cerebral vasospasm. Ital. J. Neurol. Sci. **7:** 81–88.
20. HAGEN, A. A., J. N. GERBER, C. C. SWEELEY, R. P. WHITE & J. T. ROBERTSON. 1977. Levels and disappearance of prostaglandin F_{2a} in cerebral spinal fluid: A clinical and experimental study. Stroke **8:** 672–675.
21. LA TORRE, E., C. PATRONO, A. FORTUNA & D. GROSSI-BELLONI. 1974. Role of prostaglandin F_2 in human cerebral vasospasm. J. Neurosurg. **41:** 293–299.
22. NAKAMURA, T., N. SUZUKI, I. HISHINUMA, Y. ISHIKAWA, T. SASAKI & T. ASANO. 1984. Appearance of 5-hydroxy eicosatetraenoic acid in cerebrospinal fluid after subarachnoid haemorrhage. Med. Biol. **62:** 125–128.
23. RODIGUEZ Y BAENA, R., P. GAETANI, G. FOLCO, U. BRANZOLI & P. PAOLETTI. 1985. Cisternal and lumbar CSF concentration of arachidonate metabolites in vasospasm following subarachnoid hemorrhage from ruptured aneurysm: Biochemical and clinical considerations. Surg. Neurol. **24:** 428–432.
24. RODRIGUEZ Y BAENA, R., P. GAETANI, G. FOLCO, T. VIGANO & P. PAOLETTI. 1986. Arachidonate metabolites and vasospasm after subarachnoid haemorrhage. Neurol. Res. **8:** 25–32.
25. RODRIGUEZ Y BAENA, R., P. GAETANI, G. GRIGNANI, L. PACCHIARINI, T. VIGANO, D. R. SCALABRINI, V. SILVANI, G. FOLCO & P. PAOLETTI. 1987. Role of arachidonate metabolites in the genesis of cerebral vasospasm. *In* Advances in Prostaglandin, Thromboxane, and Leukotriene Research, Vol. 17. B. Samuelsson, R. Paoletti & P. W. Ramwell, Eds.: 938–942. Raven Press. New York, NY.
26. RODRIGUEZ Y BAENA, R., P. GAETNI & P. PAOLETTI. 1988. A study on cisternal CSF levels of arachidonic acid metabolites after aneurysmal subarachnoid hemorrhage. J. Neurol. Sci. In press.
27. RODRIGUEZ Y BAENA, R., P. GAETANI, V. SILVANI, T. VIGANO, M. T. CRIVELLARI & P. PAOLETTI. 1987. Cisternal and lumbar CSF levels of arachidonate metabolites after subarachnoid haemorrhage: An assessment of the biochemical hypothesis of vasospasm. Acta Neurochir. **84:** 129–135.

28. SAKAKI, S., H. KUWABARA & S. OHTA. 1986. Biological defence mechanism in the pathogenesis of prolonged cerebral vasospasm in the patients with ruptured intracranial aneurysms. Stroke **17:** 196–202.
29. SASAKI, T., T. TANISHIMA, T. ASANO, Y. MAYANAGI & K. SANO. 1979. Significance of lipid peroxidation in the genesis of chronic vasospasm following rupture of an intracranial aneurysm. Acta Neurochir. Suppl. **28:** 536–540.
30. SEIFERT, V., D. STOLKE, V. KAEVER & H. DIETZ. 1987. Arachidonic acid metabolism following aneurysm rupture. Surg. Neurol. **27:** 243–252.
31. SUZUKI, N., T. NAKAMURA, S. IMABAYASHI, Y. ISHIKAWA, T. SASAKI & T. ASANO. 1983. Identification of 5-hydroxy eicosatetraenoic acid in cerebrospinal fluid after subarachnoid hemorrhage. J. Neurochem. **41:** 1186–1189.
32. WALKER, V., J. D. PICKARD, P. SMYTHE, S. EASTWOOD & S. PERRY. 1983. Effects of subarachnoid haemorrhage on intracranial prostaglandins. J. Neruol. Neurosurg. Psychiatry **46:** 119–125.
33. ABDEL-HALIM, M. S., J. EKSTEDT & E. ÄNGÅRD. 1979. Determination of prostaglandin F_{2a}, E_2, D_2 and 6-keto-F_{1a} in human cerebrospinal fluid. Prostaglandins **17:** 405–409.
34. AIZAWA, Y. & K. YAMADA. 1976. Determination of prostaglandin F_{2a} and E_2 contents in human cerebrospinal fluid by the radioisotope dilution method. Prostaglandins **11:** 43–50.
35. BOLTON, C., A. M. TURNER & J. L. TURK. 1984. Prostaglandin levels in cerebrospinal fluid from multiple sclerosis patients in remission and relapse. J. Neuroimmunol. **6:** 151–159.
36. CARASSO, R. L., J. VARDI, J. M. RABAY, U. ZOR & M. STREIFLER. 1977. Measurement of prostaglandin E2 in cerebrospinal fluid in patients suffering from stroke. J. Neurol. Neurosurg. Psychiatry **40:** 967–969.
37. EGG, D., M. HERALD, E. RUMPL & R. GUNTHER. 1980. Prostaglandin F_{2a} levels in human cerebrospinal fluid in normal and pathological conditions. J. Neurol. **222:** 239–248.
38. ELLIS, C. K., R. K. NARAYAN & E. F. ELLIS. 1981. GC/MS analysis of prostaglandins in ventricular cerebrospinal fluid from head injured humans. Prostaglandins Med. **7:** 157–161.
39. FAGAN, S. C., D. CASTELLANI & F. M. GENGO. 1986. Prostanoid concentrations in human CSF following acute ischaemic brain infarction. Clin. Exp. Pharmacol. Physiol. **13:** 629–632.
40. GERNER, R. H. & J. E. MERRILL. 1983. Cerebrospinal fluid prostaglandin E in depression, mania, and schizophrenia compared to normals. Biol. Psychiatry **18:** 565–569.
41. KOSTIC, V. S., B. M. DJURICIC & B. B. MRSULJA. 1984. Cerebrospinal fluid prostaglandin F_{2a} in stroke patients: No relationship to the degree of neurological deficit. Eur. Neurol. **23:** 291–295.
42. LANDAW, I. S. & C. W. YOUNG. 1977. Measurement of prostaglandin F_{2a} levels in cerebrospinal fluid of febrile and afebrile patients with advanced cancer. Prostaglandins **14:** 343–353.
43. LINNOILA, M., A. R. WHORTON, D. R. RUBINOW, R. W. COWDRY, P. T. NINAN & R. N. WATERS. 1983. CSF prostaglandin levels in depressed and schizophrenic patients. Arch. Gen. Psychiatry **40:** 405–406.
44. MATHÉ, A. A., G. SEDVALL, F. A. WIESEL & H. NYBACK. 1980. Increased content of immunoreactive prostaglandin E in cerebrospinal fluid of patients with schizophrenia. Lancet **1:** 16–17.
45. MERRILL, J. E., R. H. GERNER, L. W. MYERS & G. W. ELLISON. 1983. Regulation of natural killer cell cytotoxicity by prostaglandin E in the peripheral blood and cerebrospinal fluid of patients with multiple sclerosis and other neurological diseases. J. Neuroimmunol. **4:** 223–237.
46. PHILLIPP-DORMSTON, W. K. & R. SIEGERT. 1975. Prostaglandins in cerebrospinal fluid of patients during various infectious diseases. Klin. Wachenschr. **53:** 1167–1168.
47. RENNIE, J. M., J. DOYLE & R. W. I. COOKE. 1986. Levels of 6-ketoprostaglandin F_{Ia} in neonatal cerebrospinal fluid. Early Human Dev. **13:** 295–297.
48. ROMERO, S. D., D. CHYATTE, D. E. BYER, J. C. ROMERO & T. L. YAKSH. 1984. Measurement of prostaglandins in the cerebrospinal fluid in cat, dog, and man. J. Neurochem. **43:** 1642–1649.
49. ROSNOWSKA, M., W. CENDROWSKI, Z. SOBOCINSKA & A. WIECZORKIEWICZ. 1981.

Prostaglandins E_2 and F_{2a} in the cerebrospinal fluid in patients with multiple sclerosis. Acta Med. Pol. **22:** 97–103.
50. SEIDEL, D., R. HEIPERTZ & B. WEISNER. 1980. Cerebrospinal fluid lipids in demyelinating disease. J. Neurol. **222:** 177–182.
51. WOLFE, L. S. & O. A. MAMER. 1975. Measurement of prostaglandin F_{2a} levels in human cerebrospinal fluid in normal and pathological conditions. Prostaglandins **9:** 183–192.
52. WHITE, R. P. 1979. Multiple origins of cerebral vasospasm. *In* Cerebrovascular Diseases. T. R. Price & E. Nelson, Eds.: 307–319. Raven Press. New York, NY.
53. WHITE, R. P. 1980. Overview of the pharmacology of vasospasm. *In* Cerebral Arterial Spasm. R. H. Wilkins, Ed.: 229–236. Williams & Wilkins. Baltimore, MD.
54. WHITE, R. P. & A. A. HAGEN. 1982. Cerebrovascular actions of prostaglandins. Pharm. Ther. **18:** 313–331.
55. WHITE, R. P. 1983. Vasospasm—Experimental findings. *In* Intracranial Aneurysms, Vol. 1. J. L. Fox, Ed.: 218–249. Springer-Verlag. New York, NY.
56. WHITE, R. P., A. A. HAGEN & J. T. ROBERTSON. 1983. Prostaglandins in cerebrospinal fluid. *In* Neurobiology of Cerebrospinal Fluid, Vol. 2. J. H. Wood, Ed.: 579–590, Plenum. New York, NY.
57. WHITE, R. P. 1988. Pharmacodynamic features of delayed cerebral vasospasm. *In* Cerebral Vasospasm. R. H. Wilkins, Ed.:373–382. Raven Press, New York, NY.
58. GAUDET, R. & L. LEVINE. 1980. Transient cerebral ischemia and brain cyclooxygenase products: Relevance to migraine. Prostaglandin Ther. **6:** 1–2.
59. ABDEL-HALIM, M. S., H. VON HOLST, B. MEYERSON, C. SACHS & E. ÄNGGARD. 1980. Prostaglandin profiles in tissue and blood vessels from human brain. J. Neurochem. **34:** 1331–1333.
60. MAEDA, Y., E. TANI & T. MIYAMOTO. 1981. Prostaglandin metabolism in experimental cerebral vasospasm. J. Neurosurg. **55:** 779–785.
61. HAGEN, A. A., R. P. WHITE & J. T. ROBERTSON. 1979. Synthesis of prostaglandins and thromboxane B_2 by cerbral arteries. Stroke **10:** 306–309.
62. BLACK, K. L., J. T. HOFF, J. E. MCGILLICUDDY & S. S. GEBARSKI. 1986. Increased leukotriene C_4 and vasogenic edema surrounding brain tumors in humans. Ann. Neurol. **19:** 592–595.
63. DENTON, I. C., R. P. WHITE & J. T. ROBERTSON. 1972. The effects of prostaglandins E_1, A_1 and F_{2a} on the cerebral circulation of dogs and monkeys. J. Neurosurg. **36:** 34–42.
64. MOSKOWITZ, M. A., K. J. KIWAK, K. HEKIMIAN & L. LEVINE. 1984. Synthesis of compounds with properties of leukotrienes C_4 and D_4 in gerbil brains after ischemia and reperfusion. Science **224:** 886–889.
65. WOLFE, L. S. 1982. Eicosanoids: Prostaglandins, thromboxanes, leukotrienes, and other derivatives of carbon-20 unsaturated fatty acids. J. Neurochem. **38:** 1–14.
66. KIWAK, K. J., M. A. MOSKOWITZ & L. LEVINE. 1985. Leukotriene production in gerbil brain after ischemic insult, subarachnoid hemorrhage, and concussive injury. J. Neurosurg. **62:** 865–869.
67. WHITE, R. P. & J. T. ROBERTSON. 1983. Comparison of piroxicam, meclofenamate, ibuprofen, aspirin, and prostacyclin in a chronic model of cerebral vasospasm. Neurosurgery **12:** 40–46.
68. ASANO, T., T. SASAKI, T. KOIDE, K. TAKAKURA & K. SANO. 1984. Experimental evaluation of the beneficial effect of an antioxidant on cerebral vasospasm. Neurol. Surg. **6:** 49–53.
69. KAIYA, H. 1984. Prostaglandin E_1 treatment of schizophrenia. Biol. Psychiatry **19:** 457–463.
70. CHEHRAZI, B., S. GIRI & M. R. JOY. 1988. Role of prostaglandins and vasoactive amines in cerebral vasospasm (abstract). Stroke **19:** 132.

Eicosanoids and the Blood-Brain Barrier

REYNOLD SPECTOR

*Merck Sharp & Dohme Research Laboratories
Rahway, New Jersey 07065*

Eicosanoids play important roles in the central nervous system (CNS).[1,2] However, much is unknown about the pharmacokinetics of the eicosanoids and their precursors in the CNS. One of several unanswered questions is: How do essential fatty acids enter the brain from the blood? It is clear that the eicosanoids are synthesized in the brain from essential fatty acids.[3] Since essential fatty acids cannot be synthesized *in situ*, they must enter the brain from the blood, by mechanisms that are unclear (see below).[3,4] Second, the eicosanoids, including the prostaglandins and leukotrienes, do not readily enter the brain from the blood when they are injected into the blood.[5] An excellent example is the disposition of intravenously injected leukotriene C in the CNS; this eicosanoid does not enter the brain or cerebrospinal fluid (CSF) to any degree after intravenous injection.[5,6] Finally, there is substantial evidence that eicosanoids, including the peptidoleukotrienes and prostaglandins, are transported between the CNS—especially the extracellular space of the brain and the CSF—and blood by specific, carrier-mediated transport systems within the CNS.[2,5,6,7,8]

The purposes of this communication are to review: (1) how fatty acids, the precursors of eicosanoids, enter the brain from the blood; and (2) how the peptidoleukotrienes and prostaglandins traverse the blood-brain and blood-CSF barriers. Both of these eicosanoids are transported from the extracellular space of the brain and CSF into the blood by carrier-mediated active transport systems within the choroid plexus and possibly the brain capillaries.[2,6,7,9]

Before beginning, the anatomical and physiological basis of the blood-brain and blood-CSF barriers is worth briefly reviewing.[1,10] The brain is protected from fluctuations in its internal milieu better than any other organ in the body.[1,10] This is accomplished, at least in part, by the blood-brain and blood-CSF barriers.[1,10] It is worth noting that there is no barrier to the diffusion of substances between the extracellular space of the brain and the CSF. The anatomical systems that isolate the brain from the blood include the cerebral capillaries, which are joined by tight endothelial junctions and are termed collectively the blood-brain barrier, and the choroid plexus, of which the epithelial cells are also joined by tight junctions.[1,10] Moreover, the CSF compartment is surrounded by the arachnoid membrane, which is similarly joined by tight junctions.[1,10]

Thus, both the brain and CSF are isolated from the blood by anatomical barriers. These barriers are effective in retarding the entry into the brain of large and small (e.g., mannitol and salts) water-soluble molecules by simple diffusion.[1,10] In contrast, there is no specific anatomic barrier to the transport of lipid-soluble substances between blood and brain.[1,10] It is worth noting that the eicosanoids and their long-chain fatty acid precursors are almost completely ionized at pH 7.4 and would not be expected to be transported through the blood-brain or blood-CSF barriers in their ionized forms.[3] Moreover, these long-chain fatty acids are extensively bound to plasma proteins, a phenomenon that should further retard their exit from plasma.[3]

The anatomical blood-brain and blood-CSF barriers, if unmodified, would preclude the proper function of the brain because they would exclude the water-soluble nutrients required for the maintenance of the viability and functions of nerve cells.[1,10]

In fact, specialized transport systems at the blood-brain and blood-CSF barriers enable the brain to be nourished adequately; these transport systems include the carrier-mediated transport system for fatty acids to be discussed below. The specialized systems in the cerebral capillaries and choroid plexus are able to transfer not only fatty acids but also glucose, amino acids, nucleosides, and vitamins.[1,10]

The nourishing systems described above do not adequately protect the brain from water-soluble substances that exhibit neurotoxicity or alter neuronal function adversely.[1] An example is penicillin, which causes seizures when injected directly into the CSF or cerebral ventricles.[1] However, intravenous injection of penicillin does not lead to seizures, except after massive injections, because the concentration of penicillin in the CSF and extracellular space of the brain is maintained at approximately 1% of that in plasma.[1] In short, the brain is protected by several mechanisms. First, as described above, water-soluble substances (e.g., penicillin) do not penetrate the blood-brain or blood-CSF barrier well.[1] Second, the choroid plexus and possibly, in some cases, the cerebral capillary endothelial cells have an important "cleansing" role. The choroid plexus epithelial cells can eliminate certain toxic or useless substances from the extracellular space of the brain and CSF by pumping them from the CSF back into the blood.[1,11] These systems for pumping certain water-soluble substances (e.g., penicillin) from the CSF into the blood are crucial to understanding the pharmacokinetics of the eicosanoids in the central nervous system to be discussed below.[1,11] A teleological explanation for these functions of the choroid plexus is that they prevent the buildup in the CNS of potentially deleterious substances.[1] The eicosanoids, which are vasoactive and have other properties, might damage the CNS. Hence, rapid transfer of these substances from the CSF into the blood would remove them from the CNS for detoxification by either the liver or kidneys.

FATTY ACID TRANSPORT INTO THE BRAIN

Fatty acids, including essential fatty acids, are continually required by developing and adult mammals.[3,4] Essential and significant amounts of nonessential fatty acids enter the brain from the blood.[3,4] Since, as components of triglycerides and phospholipids, fatty acids are not transported from the blood into the brain via the blood-brain barrier, we postulated that there must be specific transport systems for essential and long-chain fatty acids at the blood-brain barrier. Otherwise, they would not be expected to pass from the blood into the brain because: (1) they bind tightly to plasma proteins (> 99% bound), (2) they are almost completely ionized at pH 7.4 (> 99%), and (3) fatty acids do not readily flip from one side of the plasma membrane to the other.[3] However, Morand et al.[12] showed that palmitic and lignoceric acids entered the brain from the blood more readily than stearic acid did, and Pardridge and Mietus[13] documented that palmitic acid (C_{16}) did, in fact, cross the blood-brain barrier from plasma in small amounts, notwithstanding the fact that more than 99% of the palmitic acid was bound to plasma proteins. These investigators also hypothesized that there may be an exchange mechanism for fatty acids at the blood-brain barrier.[13] Oldendorf and Pardridge had previously demonstrated that short-chain fatty acids readily enter the brain by a saturable, probenecid-sensitive transport system at the blood-brain barrier.[14]

With this background, we instituted a series of studies to measure the transport of medium-chain, long-chain, and essential fatty acids through the blood-brain barrier.[3] We employed an *in situ* rat brain perfusion technique that allowed calculation of the permeability–surface area (PS) products of various labeled compounds.[3] No protein

TABLE 1. Effects of Various Inhibitors on [^{14}C]Octanoic Acid Permeability–Surface Area (PS) Products

Inhibitor; Concentration	PS Product[a] $s^{-1} \times 10^{-2}$	Percent Control
Control; 0.5 μM [^{14}C]octanoic acid	1.52 ± 0.13 (12)	—
Sodium octanoate; 0.25 mM	1.22 ± 0.21 (10)	80
Sodium octanoate; 1.0 mM	0.77 ± 0.13 (8)	51[b]
Sodium octanoate; 2.5 mM	0.78 ± 0.10 (4)	51[b]
Sodium octanoate; 10.0 mM	0.68 ± 0.10 (6)	45[b]
Sodium butyrate; 10.0 mM	0.97 ± 0.12 (6)	64[b]
Probenecid; 1.0 mM	0.85 ± 0.16 (9)	56[b]
D-Pantothenic acid; 1.0 mM	1.58 ± 0.14 (8)	104
L-Leucine; 1.0 mM	1.31 ± 0.17 (4)	86

[a] All values are means ± SEM, with the number of determinations in parentheses. The PS products for [^{14}C]octanoate were determined in the forebrain using 7-s perfusions with various concentrations of unlabeled sodium octanoate or, in some cases, other potential inhibitors and [^{3}H]inulin in the perfusate.[3]
[b] $p < 0.05$ when compared with control; Dunnett's test.

was placed in the perfusate, which consisted of a well-oxygenated balanced salt solution at 37 °C with a pH = 7.4.[3]

In the first series of studies, shown in TABLE 1, we measured the ability of various concentrations of octanoate, probenecid, D-pantothenic acid, and leucine in the cerebral perfusate to inhibit the transfer of (^{14}C) octanoic acid across the blood-brain barrier.[3] In these studies, 0.5 μM (^{14}C) octanoic acid was extracted approximately 30% as well from the perfusate as (^{14}C) diazepam, which is completely extracted as it passes through the cerebral circulation.[3] As shown in TABLE 1, our results clearly showed that a portion of the (^{14}C) octanoate transfer from the perfusate into the substance of the brain was inhibited by octanoate and probenecid, but not by D-pantothenic acid and, leucine. These results suggest that octanoic acid, like short-chain fatty acids, enters the brain at least in part by a saturable transport system at the blood-brain barrier.

The effects of various inhibitors on (^{14}C) myristic acid PS products at the blood-brain barrier of rats is shown in TABLE 2.[3] In studies with (^{14}C) myristic acid and

TABLE 2. Effects of Various Inhibitors on [^{14}C]Myristic Acid Permeability–Surface Area (PS) Products

Inhibitor; Concentration	PS Product[a] $s^{-1} \times 10^{-2}$	Percent Control
Control; 0.5 μM [^{14}C]myristic acid[b]	4.77 ± 0.32 (12)	—
Probenecid; 1.0 mM	2.17 ± 0.21 (10)	45[c]
Sodium octanoate; 10 mM	1.08 ± 0.07 (4)	23[c]
Sodium butyrate; 10 mM	2.25 ± 0.24 (8)	47[c]
L-Leucine; 1.0 mM	4.44 ± 0.19 (4)	93

[a] All values are means ± SEM, with the number of determinations in parentheses. The PS products in the forebrain for [^{14}C]myristic acid were determined using 7-s perfusions and calcium-free buffers, as in TABLE 1.[3]
[b] Self-inhibition of [^{14}C]myristic acid transport by unlabeled myristic acid could not be measured because of the limited solubility of myristic acid in the buffer solution.
[c] $p < 0.05$ compared to control; Dunnett's test.

(^{14}C) linoleic acid (see below), the $CaCl_2$ was omitted from the perfusate to prevent the formation of calcium salts and erratic scintillation spectroscopic assays.[3] Myristic acid, a 14-carbon saturated fatty acid, was completely cleared in one pass through the cerebral circulation by the brain. However, probenecid, sodium octanoate, and sodium butyrate—but not leucine—decreased the entry of (^{14}C) myristic acid from the perfusate into the brain. These data suggest that approximately three-quarters of the (^{14}C) myristic acid entered the brain from the perfusate by a saturable transport system. The system is specific in that leucine had no effect on myristic acid PS products.

The PS products of the essential fatty linoleic acid at the blood-brain barrier are shown in Table 3.[3] Here the PS product is much lower than that of the shorter myristic acid and is comparable to that of octanoic acid. Approximately 25% of the (^{14}C) linoleic acid was cleared from the perfusate into the brain. However, the entry of (^{14}C) linoleic acid was not inhibited by probenecid (1 mM) or sodium octanoate (10 mM).

Thus, medium-chain and, to a greater extent, long-chain saturated fatty acids enter the brain in large part by a probenecid-sensitive mechanism at the blood-brain barrier. However, the essential linoleic acid entered the brain as readily as octanoic acid from the perfusate, but the entry of linoleic acid was not inhibited by probenecid or a high concentration of sodium octanoate.

TABLE 3. Effects of Various Inhibitors on [^{14}C]Linoleic Acid Permeability–Surface Area (PS) Products

Inhibitor; Concentration	PS Product[a] $s^{-1} \times 10^{-2}$	Percent Control
Control; 0.5 μM	1.22 ± 0.12 (12)	—
Linoleic acid; 10 μM	1.44 ± 0.18 (8)	118
Probenecid; 1.0 mM	1.24 ± 0.11 (12)	102
Sodium octanoate; 10 mM	0.99 ± 0.12 (7)	82

[a]All values are means ± SEM, with the number of determinations in parentheses. The PS products for [^{14}C]linoleic acid were determined in the forebrain using 7-s perfusions and calcium-free buffers, as in TABLE 1.[3]

These results are consistent with previous data about the transport of saturated fatty acids at the blood-brain barrier.[12–14] Also, fatty acid transport systems have been described in other cells.[3] In adult mammals, since there is no or minimal net transfer of fatty acids in a single pass through the brain, fatty acids must also be transported in the reverse direction from the brain into plasma.[3,12–14] The exact mechanism of the probenecid-sensitive transport system for saturated fatty acids at the blood-brain barrier remains to be determined. Once within the brain, fatty acids can be oxidized to CO_2, elongated, or converted into amino acids or complex lipids, including eicosanoids and other substances, especially by cerebral capillaries.[3] We were unable to inhibit the transport of the essential fatty acid linoleic acid through the blood-brain barrier with probenecid or octanoate (TABLE 3) as we were the transport of the saturated medium-chain and long-chain fatty acids (TABLES 1 and 2). The explanation for these differences is not clear but might be related to the two double bonds in linoleic acid that alter the shape and solubility of this compound compared to the very flexible saturated fatty acids.[3] The transfer of arachidonic acid and other long-chain unsaturated essential fatty acids between blood and brain remains to be established.

EICOSANOID TRANSPORT FROM THE CEREBROSPINAL FLUID AND EXTRACELLULAR SPACE OF THE BRAIN

In a series of elegant papers, Bito and his colleagues showed that various prostaglandins and certain prostaglandin analogues were rapidly transported from the CSF into the blood by a mechanism postulated to be within the choroid plexus.[2,7,8] These investigators showed that *in vitro* the isolated rabbit choroid plexus was able to concentrate several prostaglandins, including $PGF_{2\alpha}$ and PGE_1, by an energy-dependent, probenecid-sensitive process.[7] In *in vivo* ventriculocisternal perfusion experiments with rabbits, these investigators were also able to show that prostaglandin $PGF_{2\alpha}$ was rapidly cleared from the CSF.[2] Moreover, the clearance was inhibited by $PGF_{2\alpha}$ itself, probenecid, and bromocresol green, but not iodide, which is transported by a separate transport system. The authors concluded that the removal of prostaglandins from the extracellular fluid of the brain and CSF is mediated by a saturable, facilitated transport process across both the choroid plexus and possibly the cerebral capillaries.[1,2,7] The authors speculated that removal of prostaglandins from the extracellular space of the brain and CSF was the primary mechanism for the termination of action of these potent, endogenously produced autocoids.

More recently, we studied the transfer of leukotrienes from the CNS into blood both *in vitro* and *in vivo*.[6,9] We showed that in the isolated rabbit choroid plexus *in vitro*, LTC_4 was concentrated by a specific energy-dependent transport system (TABLE 4).[9] *In vivo*, the clearance of LTC_4 from the CNS was rapid. Moreover, after the intraventricular injection of LTC_4, LTC_4 was transported from the CNS by a probenecid-sensitive mechanism much more rapidly than mannitol (TABLE 5).[6] This was not due to significant metabolism of the LTC_4.[6] Finally, the system was specific in

TABLE 4. *In Vitro* Uptake of [^{3}H]LTC_4 by Rabbit Choroid Plexus

Experimental Condition	Uptake of [^{3}H]LTC_4 (T/M Ratio)[a]	% Control
Control; 3.0 nM	68.4 ± 5.1 (35)	
4°	5.2 ± 0.5 (6)	8[b]
Dinitrophenol and iodoacetate, both 2 mM	6.0 ± 0.6 (6)	9[b]
N-Ethylmaleimide, 2 mM	15.2 ± 5.4 (10)	22[b]
Probenecid, 1 mM	14.5 ± 2.1 (11)	21[b]
LTC_4, 1.6 μM	55.4 ± 7.3 (7)	81
LTD_4, 1.0 μM	80.6 ± 4.2 (10)	117
Tolazoline, 2 mM	52.5 ± 7.0 (10)	76
Cysteine, 2 mM	65.5 ± 7.1 (10)	96
Glutathione, 2 mM	64.8 ± 5.0 (5)	95
Sodium iodide, 2 mM	65.6 ± 3.1 (5)	96
2.5-min incubation	10.1 ± 0.8 (5)	15
5.0-min incubation	19.8 ± 3.4 (10)	29
10.0-min incubation	43.6 ± 3.7 (26)	64
Forebrain slices	2.2 ± 0.2 (6)	3[b]
Red blood cells	0.2 ± 0.1 (6)	0[b]

NOTE: Choroid plexuses and control tissues and cells were incubated at 37 °C in medium containing [^{3}H]LTC_4 and other compounds for 15 min, unless otherwise specified.[9]

[a] The tissue-to-medium (T/M) ratios are mean ± standard error of the results of the number of experiments indicated in parentheses.[9]

[b] All 15-min percentage values so designated differed significantly ($p < 0.01$) from the control value at 15 min by Dunnett's test of multiple comparisons with a control.

TABLE 5. Ratio of $[^3H]/[^{14}C]$ in Tissue Divided by Ratio of $[^3H]/[^{14}C]$ in Injectate

	Control ($n = 5$)	Probenecid ($n = 4$)	Cysteine ($n = 4$)	Unlabeled LTC$_4$ (Carrier) ($n = 4$)
CSF	0.31 ± 0.01	0.67 ± 0.02^a	0.25 ± 0.02	0.40 ± 0.2^{a,b}
Choroid plexus	1.5 ± 0.2	1.3 ± 0.1	0.5 ± 0.1^a	3.0 ± 0.06
Left brain	0.35 ± 0.04	0.50 ± 0.03^a	0.16 ± 0.01^a	0.36 ± 0.02
Right brain	0.34 ± 0.07	0.48 ± 0.03	0.17 ± 0.01	0.32 ± 0.02
Total^c	0.33 ± 0.02	0.60 ± 0.02^a	0.20 ± 0.01^a	0.39 ± 0.02

NOTE: Rabbits were injected intraventricularly with 2.5 μCi $[^3H]LTC_4$, 0.3 μCi $[^{14}C]$mannitol and, in some cases, 0.9 mg prebenecid, 1.8 mg cysteine, or 1.4 μg unlabeled LTC$_4$.[15] After 2 hr, the $[^3H]$ and $[^{14}C]$ content of the tissue was determined, and the ratio of $[^3H]/[^{14}C]$ in the tissue was divided by the ratio of $[^3H]/[^{14}C]$ in the injectate. Each value is the mean ± SEM of the results of studies of the number of rabbits shown in parentheses. Ratios that are less than 1.0 signify that $[^3H]LTC_4$ was cleared more rapidly than the $[^{14}C]$mannitol marker of passive diffusion in the central nervous system.
$^a p < 0.05$ (two-tailed Dunnett's test).
^{b}The concentration of unlabeled LTC$_4$ in the CSF withdrawn after 2 hr was 0.14 μM.
^{c}Total equals total $[^{14}C]$ and $[^3H]$ radioactivity in the CSF, choroid plexus, and brain.

that it was not inhibited by the weak-base tolazoline that blocks the transport of weak bases from CSF.[6]

The choroid plexus transports both prostaglandins and peptidoleukotrienes from the extracellular space of the brain and CSF into the blood.[1,2,6,7,9] The prostaglandins and peptidoleukotrienes are, thus, two examples of many substances that not only do not penetrate the blood-brain barrier well, but if they do, are transported from the CSF and the brain.[1,5,15] This would presumably be of advantage to mammals, since these eicosanoids have important physiological functions in the CNS. Moreover, maintaining low concentrations of these substances within the CNS would preserve the capacity of any receptors in the CNS for these eicosanoids to sense small changes in local concentrations.[2,15]

In conclusion, the mechanisms by which fatty acids enter the CNS are not clear. However, in the case of linoleic acid, simple diffusion appears to explain the extant data best, unlike the saturated long-chain fatty acids, which enter the brain at least in part by a saturable transport system at the blood-brain barrier. However, it is very clear that both the prostaglandins and peptidoleukotrienes are actively removed from the extracellular space of the brain and CSF by transport systems that exist in large part within the choroid plexus and possibly cerebral capillaries. Since eicosanoids are not readily degraded or accumulated by neuronal or glial cells, it appears that the active transport of eicosanoids from the CSF and extracellular space of the brain is the body's method for bringing physiological actions on nervous and other cells in the CNS to an end.[2,7,15]

REFERENCES

1. BRADBURY, M. 1979. The Concept of a Blood-Brain Barrier. John Wiley. Chichester, England.
2. BITO, L. Z., H. DAVSON & J. R. HOLLINGSWORTH. 1976. Facilitated transport of prostaglandins across the blood-cerebrospinal fluid and blood-brain barriers. J. Physiol. **256:** 273-285.

3. SPECTOR, R. 1988. Fatty acid transport through the blood-brain barrier. J. Neurochem. **50:** 639–643.
4. DHOPESHWARKAR, G. A. 1973. Uptake and transport of fatty acids into the brain and the role of the blood-brain barrier system. Adv. Lipid Res. **11:** 109–142.
5. APPELGREN, L. E. & S. HAMMARSTROM. 1982. Distribution and metabolism of ^{3}H-labeled leukotriene C_3 in the mouse. J. Biol. Chem. **257:** 531–535.
6. SPECTOR, R. & E. J. GOETZL. 1986. Leukotriene C_4 transport and metabolism in the central nervous system. J. Neurochem. **46:** 1308–1312.
7. BITO, L. Z., H. DAVSON & E. V. SALVADOR. 1976. Inhibition of in vitro concentrative prostaglandin accumulation by prostaglandins, prostaglandin analogues and by some inhibitors of organic anion transport. J. Physiol. **256:** 257–271.
8. BITO, L. Z. & M. C. WALLENSTEIN. 1977. Transport of prostaglandins across the blood-brain and blood-aqueous barriers and the physiological significance of these absorptive transport processes. Exp. Eye Res. Suppl.: 229–243.
9. SPECTOR, R. & E. J. GOETZL. 1985. Leukotriene C_4 transport by the choroid plexus in vitro. Science **228:** 325–327.
10. SPECTOR, R. 1986. Nucleoside and vitamin homeostatis in the mammalian central nervous system. Ann. N. Y. Acad. Sci. **481:** 221–230.
11. SPECTOR, R. & A. V. LORENZO. 1974. Inhibition of penicillin transport from the cerebrospinal fluid after intracisternal innoculation of bacteria. J. Clin. Invest. **54:** 316–325.
12. MORAND, O., M. MASSON, N. BAUMANN & J. M. BOURRE. 1981. Exogenous [1-^{14}C]lignoceric acid uptake by neurons, astrocytes and myelin, as compared to incorporation of [1-^{14}C]palmitic and stearic acids. Neurochem. Int. **3:** 329–334.
13. PARDRIDGE, W. M. & L. J. MIETUS. 1980. Palmitate and cholesterol transport through the blood-brain barrier. J. Neurochem. **34:** 463–466.
14. PARDRIDGE, W. M., J. D. CONNOR & I. L. CRAWFORD. 1975. Permeability changes in the blood-brain barrier: Causes and consequences. CRC Crit. Rev. Toxicol. **3:** 159–199.
15. SPECTOR, R. & E. J. GOETZL. 1986. Commentary—Role of concentrative leukotriene transport systems in the central nervous system. Biochem. Pharmacol. **35:** 2849–2853.

PART III. ARACHIDONIC ACID AND ITS METABOLITES IN SIGNAL TRANSDUCTION

The Relationship between Phospholipases A_2 and C in Signal Transduction

EDUARDO G. LAPETINA AND MICHAEL F. CROUCH

*Molecular Biology Department
Burroughs Wellcome Co.
Research Triangle Park, North Carolina 27709*

Arachidonic acid can be released from membrane phospholipids of platelets in response to a number of receptor-mediated signals. The enzymes most responsible for this activation are phospholipase A_2[1] and, to a lesser degree, 1,2-diacylglycerol lipase.[2] In this paper, we will describe some of the studies on phospholipase A_2 activation that we have carried out and also some other published work that has helped us understand some of the physiological control mechanisms of this enzyme.

The importance of phospholipase A_2 in receptor-mediated platelet activation varies with both the type and the strength of agonist used. As examples, collagen and epinephrine are absolutely dependent on the release of arachidonic acid for stimulation of platelet secretion and aggregation, whereas thrombin depends on arachidonic acid release only when used at low concentration; at higher doses the ability of thrombin to activate platelets is independent of arachidonic acid metabolites. The most relevant arachidonic acid metabolites for platelet stimulation are endoperoxides and thromboxane A_2.

THE ROLE OF PHOSPHOLIPASE C IN ACTIVATION OF PHOSPHOLIPASE A_2

Calcium and Inositol Trisphosphate

It is now thought that upon stimulation of platelets with an agonist, the initial phospholipid response of the cell is inositol phospholipid hydrolysis by a phospholipase C.[1] This is followed by the activation of phospholipase A_2.[1] The sequential nature of these responses has often led to the conclusion that some products of phosphoinositide hydrolysis are responsible for phospholipase A_2 activation.[1]

The phosphodiesteratic cleavage of phosphatidylinositol-4,5-bisphosphate yields the two second messenger molecules, inositol trisphosphate (IP3) and 1,2-diacylglycerol (DAG).[3] IP3 has been shown in many cell types, including the platelet, to release intracellular Ca^{2+} less stores.[3,4] Since it has been clearly established that activation of platelets with the Ca^{2+} ionophore A23187 was able to raise the intracellular Ca^{2+} concentration and also activate phospholipase A_2, a possible link between the two receptor-activated enzymes has been established: receptor activation of phospholipase C induced the formation of IP3, which then raised the intracellular Ca^{2+} concentration. This Ca^{2+} signal then directly induced phospholipase A_2 stimulation and release of arachidonic acid.

Support for this concept came from experiments that showed that IP3 would induce thromboxane A_2 formation in permeabilized platelets and that platelet aggregation and secretion induced by IP3 were sensitive to inhibitors of arachidonic acid metabolism.[5,6] Thus, these studies implied that the mobilization of Ca^{2+} by IP3 was sufficient to induce phospholipase A_2 activation.

Despite these results, there are indications that phospholipase A_2 is not primarily under the control of the prevailing Ca^{2+} level in the intact cell. Pollock et al.[7] have shown that the activation of phospholipase A_2 by collagen could be accomplished at cytosolic Ca^{2+} levels of around 115 nM, whereas the Ca^{2+} ionophore ionomycin induced a significant release of arachidonic acid only when this compound had elevated the cytosolic Ca^{2+} level to about 1 μM. These results strongly suggested that collagen activated phospholipase A_2 independently of changes in the cellular Ca^{2+} concentration.[7]

Work from our laboratory has also suggested that the same may be true for other agonists.[8,9] Alpha-thrombin is a potent agonist for all platelet responses,[10,11] including that of phospholipase A_2. Gamma-thrombin is produced by proteolysis of alpha-thrombin, and is a less potent agonist. We have compared the abilities of alpha- and gamma-thrombins, and platelet activating factor (PAF) to stimulate phospholipase A_2 and mobilized cellular Ca^{2+} stores.[9] We found that alpha-thrombin elevated the cytosolic Ca^{2+} concentration to about 1 μM and increased arachidonic acid release by 6-fold.[9] Both gamma-thrombin and PAF induced the release of Ca^{2+} stores also, but only to maxima of 350 nM each.[9] The peak responses to these two agonists were the same, although gamma-thrombin produced a more sustained response. In contrast, only gamma-thrombin could induce a detectable release of arachidonic acid in our system.[9] Thus, there appeared to be a dissociation of the ability of an agonist to induce Ca^{2+} mobilization and the activation of phospholipase A_2. In addition, epinephrine, which alone did not activate phospholipase A_2, was able to potentiate the alpha-thrombin-induced release of arachidonic acid.[9] However, we could not detect any potentiation of the peak release of Ca^{2+} when these two agents were added together.[9]

The reasons for the disparity between the data using IP3 on permeabilized cells to activate phospholipase A_2 and that of agonists on whole cells are not clear. However, it is possible that the high concentrations of IP3 required to activate phospholipase A_2 in permeabilized platelets may represent nonphysiological levels or that the permeabilized cell is not a realistic model for studying phospholipase A_2 activation.

Diacylglycerol and Protein Kinase C

The other immediate product of phospholipase C activation is 1,2-diacylglycerol,[1,3] which is a known activator of protein kinase C.[12] This enzyme, which can also be activated by the tumor-promoting phorbol esters, phosphorylates a major 40-kDa protein substrate in platelets.[1,2] A recent report by Touqui et al.[13] implicated the 40-kDa protein in phospholipase A_2 activity. These proteins are known collectively as *lipocortins*. Touqui et al. suggested that the 40-kDa protein was a lipocortin, based on the ability of a monoclonal antibody to inhibit its anti–phospholipase A_2 activity against renocortin. This antibody immunoprecipitated a 40-kDa protein phosphorylated in platelets pretreated with thrombin or phorbol ester.[13] Based on this data and a previous report that had shown that phorbol esters were able to elicit arachidonic acid release in the presence of Ca^{2+} ionophores, they suggested that the 40-kDa protein was a lipocortin with intrinsic anti–phospholipase A_2 activity. When cells were stimulated, protein kinase C phosphorylated this protein, thus reducing its anti–phospholipase A_2 activity and allowing arachidonic acid liberation.

We have challenged this proposal by comparing 40-kDa protein phosphorylation in response to alpha-thrombin with that of gamma-thrombin and examining the resulting phospholipase A_2 activation. We found that gamma-thrombin, particularly in the presence of epinephrine, was capable of stimulating 40-kDa protein phosphorylation to the same degree as that of alpha-thrombin, but was 6–7 times less potent at activating phospholipase A_2. That is, we could find no correlation between 40-kDa protein phosphorylation and stimulation of phospholipase A_2. Pollock et al.[7] have further presented evidence that phorbol esters are without effect on phospholipase A_2 in the presence of Ca^{2+} ionophore—a result that contests that of Mobley and Tai.[14] Similarly, we could not detect any release of arachidonic acid in response to concentrations of phorbol ester that maximally phosphorylated the 40-kDa protein (unpublished).

THE ROLE OF GTP-BINDING PROTEINS IN PHOSPHOLIPASE A_2 ACTIVATION

Thus far, we are left without any convincing evidence for a relationship between the receptor stimulation of phospholipase C and phospholipase A_2. One may, therefore, postulate that the receptor may activate these two enzymes by mechanisms that diverge at the receptor level: there may be separate transducing elements from the receptor to each of these enzymes.

There has been a recent flurry of interest in the possibility that receptors control the activity of phospholipase C by first altering the state of a "GTP-binding protein." This class of proteins (or G proteins), first described for their involvement in the adenylate cyclase system, are heterotrimeric. They are composed of alpha, beta, and gamma subunits. The beta and gamma subunits are highly homologous, whereas the alpha subunits show a great heterogeneity and appear to convey specificity. Receptors that stimulate cyclase are linked to Gs (the adenylate cyclase stimulatory G protein), whereas those that inhibit adenylate cyclase appear in general to be linked to Gi (inhibitory G protein). The alpha subunit is the GTP-binding component and is thought to be separated from the beta/gamma complex after receptor stimulation. When this occurs, the alpha subunit appears to activate certain processes, such as the stimulation of adenylate cyclase (alpha-s).

It has recently been shown that phospholipase A_2 of mast cells is sensitive to GTP analogs[15] and that inactivation of Gi with pertussis toxin inhibits phospholipase A_2 activation of thryoid cells. In addition, Jelsema and Axelrod[18] have shown that the beta/gamma dimer of G proteins is capable of activating phospholipase A_2 in retinal rod outer segments. In total, these results lend support to the proposal that there may be a direct link between the receptor and phospholipase A_2 via a GTP-binding protein in some cells.

Although the possible contribution for such a G protein involvement in the platelet has not been well examined, we have found evidence that does not support this view, at least for the inhibitory GTP-binding protein Gi. As mentioned above, pertussis toxin is able to inactivate Gi, and this occurs by the toxin-catalyzed ADP-ribosylation of the alpha subunit of Gi.[1,10,16] This acts to inhibit the receptor–GTP-binding protein interaction. When the toxin is introduced to the cell in the presence of radioactively labeled NAD, one can label the ADP-ribosylated Gi, and so obtain a measure of the amount of undissociated Gi that is present in a cell.[1,10,16] If one stimulates platelets with an agonist and dissociates the Gi, it is then no longer a substrate for pertussis toxin–induced ADP-ribosylation, and there is reduced labeling of Gi.[10,16] By this method, one can ascertain if a receptor type is or is not coupled to Gi.

When we did this experiment with alpha-thrombin, we found a potent decrease in the ADP-ribosylation of Gi, indicating dissociation of most of the alpha subunits from the beta/gamma dimers of Gi.[10] The same pattern was found for gamma-thrombin, with a decrease in labeling of Gi in the presence of pertussis toxin.[10] However, gamma-thrombin is a very weak agonist for phospholipase A_2.[9] These experiments suggest, therefore, that the ability of an agonist to dissociate Gi does not convey an ability to activate phospholipase A_2.

Of course, we have addressed only the question of Gi and know nothing about what these agonists may do to other GTP-binding proteins of the platelet. However, we can conclude with some confidence that the beta/gamma subunits do not contribute significantly to the stimulation of phospholipase A_2 in the activated platelet, since dissociation of Gi would act to supply these within the plasma membrane.

CONCLUSION

The mechanism by which agonists stimulate phospholipase A_2 of platelets is still much of a mystery. We have presented a discussion that suggests that neither Ca^{2+}, protein kinase C, or dissociation of the inhibitory GTP-binding protein Gi is solely responsible for activating this enzyme. We cannot exclude the possibility that there may be some contribution of each pathway for some agonists, and that the contribution may change with agonist concentration or potency. These possibilities await further clarification.

REFERENCES

1. LAPETINA, E. G. 1986. Inositide-dependent and independent mechanisms. *In* Phosphoinositides and Receptor Mechanisms. J. Putney, Ed.: 271–286. Alan R. Liss. New York, NY.
2. MAHADEVAPPA, V. G. & B. J. HOLUB. 1986. Diacylglycerol lipase pathway is a minor source of released arachidonic acid in thrombin-induced human platelets. Biochem. Biophys. Res. Commun. **134:** 1327–1333.
3. BERRIDGE, M. J. & R. F. IRVINE. 1984. Inositol triphosphate, a novel second messenger in cellular signal transduction. Nature **312:** 315–321.
4. O'ROURKE, F. A., S. P. HALENDA, G. B. ZAVOICO & M. B. FEINSTEIN. 1985. Inositol 1,4,5-triphosphate releases Ca^{2+} from Ca^{2+}-transporting membrane vesicle fraction derived from human platelets. J. Biol. Chem. **260:** 956–962.
5. WATSON, S. P., M. RUGGIERO, S. L. ABRAHAMS & E. G. LAPETINA. 1986. Inositol 1,4,5-triphosphate induces aggregation and release of 5-hydroxytryptamine from saponin-permeabilized human platelets. J. Biol. Chem. **261:** 5368–5372.
6. AUTHI, K. S., B. J. EVENDEN & N. CRAWFORD. 1986. Metabolic and functional consequences of introducing inositol 1,4,5-triphosphate into saponin-permeabilized human platelets. Biochem. J. **233:** 707–718.
7. POLLOCK, W. K., T. S. RINK & R. F. IRVINE. 1986. Liberation of [^{3}H]arachidonic acid and changes in cytoxolic free calcium in fura-2-loaded human platelets stimulated by ionomycin and collagen. Biochem. J. **235:** 869–877.
8. CROUCH, M. F. & E. G. LAPETINA. 1986. Phosphorylation of the 47 kDa protein in gamma-thrombin-stimulated human platelets does not activate phospholipase A2: Evidence against lipocortin. Biochem. Biophys. Res. Commun. **141:** 459–465.
9. CROUCH, M. F. & E. G. LAPETINA. 1988. No direct correlation between Ca^{2+} mobilization and dissociation of G_i during platelet phospholipase A_2 activation. Biochem. Biophys. Res. Commun. **153:** 21–30.
10. CROUCH, M. F. & E. G. LAPETINA. 1988. A role for G_i in control of thrombin receptor-phospholipase-C coupling in human platelets. J. Biol. Chem. **263:** 3363–3371.
11. CROUCH, M. F. & E. G. LAPETINA. 1988. The NA^+/H^+ antiporter is not involved in potentiation of thrombin-induced responses by epinephrine. Biochem. Biophys. Res. Commun. **151:** 178–186.

12. NISHIZUKA, Y. 1984. The role of protein kinase C in cell surface signal transduction and tumour promotion. Nature **308:** 693–697.
13. TOUQUI, L., B. ROTHHUT, A. M. SHAW, A. FRADIN, B. B. VERGAFTIG & I. RUSSO-MARIE. 1986. Platelet activation–a role for a 40K antiphospholipase A2 protein indistinguishable from lipocortin. Nature **321:** 177–180.
14. MOBLEY, A. & H. H. TAI. 1985. Synergistic stimulation of thromboxane biosynthesis by calcium ionophore and phorbol ester or thrombin in human platelets. Biochem. Biophys. Res. Commun. **130:** 717–723.
15. OKANO, Y., K. YAMADA, K. YANO & Y. NOZAWA. 1987. Guanosine 5'-(gamma-thio)triphosphate stimulates arachidonic acid liberation in permeabilized rat peritoneal mast cells. Biochem. Biophys. Res. Commun. **145:** 1267–1275.
16. JELSEMA, C. L. & J. AXELROD. 1987. Stimulation of phospholipase A2 in bovine rod outer segment by the beta gamma subunits of transducin and its inhibition by the alpha subunit. Proc. Natl. Acad. Sci. USA **84:** 3623–3627.
17. LAPETINA, E. G., B. REEP & K. J. CHANG. 1986. Treatment of human platelets with trypsin, thrombin, or collagen inhibits the pertussis toxin-induced ADP-ribosylation of a 41-kDa protein. Proc. Natl. Acad. Sci. USA **83:** 5880–5883.

# Regulation of Phospholipase A_2 and Phospholipase C in Rod Outer Segments of Bovine Retina Involves a Common GTP-binding Protein but Different Mechanisms of Action

CAROLE L. JELSEMA

Laboratory of Cell Biology
National Institute of Mental Health
Bethesda, Maryland 20892

INTRODUCTION

Activation of receptors on the cell surface by neurotransmitters, hormones, and other ligands is coupled to changes in effector systems within the cell by action of membrane-bound, signal-transducing GTP-binding proteins (G proteins). These G proteins are heterotrimers that, upon binding of activated receptors and exchange of GTP for the GDP bound to the α subunit, dissociate into their component α and $\beta\gamma$ subunits (FIG. 1).[1,2] The dissociated G protein subunits then interact with and modulate the activity of intracellular regulatory proteins, such as adenylate cyclase. The GTP-bound α subunit of the G protein G_s and the $\beta\gamma$ subunits of the G protein G_i are, for example, responsible for the stimulation and inhibition, respectively, of adenylate cyclase.[3] Other effector systems coupled by signal-transducing G proteins include cAMP and cGMP phosphodiesterases;[4,5] the Ca^{++}, K^+, and Na^+ ion channels;[6-10] phospholipase C,[11-13] and phospholipase A_2.[14-20]

While activation of phospholipase A_2 has been shown to be modulated by G proteins in a variety of systems,[14-21] a direct link between stimulation of phospholipase A_2 and the activation of a specific G protein has been demonstrated only in the rod outer segments (ROS) or photoreceptor membranes of bovine retina.[14,15] In this system, the G protein transducin has been shown to couple the light activation of rhodopsin to stimulation of both cGMP phosphodiesterase[5] and phospholipase A_2[14,15] (FIG. 1). Since the end products of phospholipase C activation can lead to stimulation of phospholipase A_2 and vice versa,[22,23] and phospholipase C has been demonstrated to be under G protein regulation in a variety of systems,[11-13] the question has arisen as to whether the G protein–mediated regulation of phospholipase A_2 occurs independent of the G protein–dependent regulation of phospholipase C. In both platelets and thyroid cells, the two phospholipase activities have been shown to be independent of one another, as indicated by the ability of neomycin to block phospholipase C activity without affecting phospholipase A_2 activity.[20,21] However, the inhibitory effect of neomycin occurs at the level of the phospholipase C substrate,[24] not at the level of the G protein, and therefore does not directly address the uniqueness of the G protein regulation of the two phospholipases. Similarly, the observation that the two phospholipases have different pertussis toxin sensitivities[20,21] does not eliminate the possibility that a common G protein may be involved in the regulation of both phospholipases while employing different mechanisms of action.

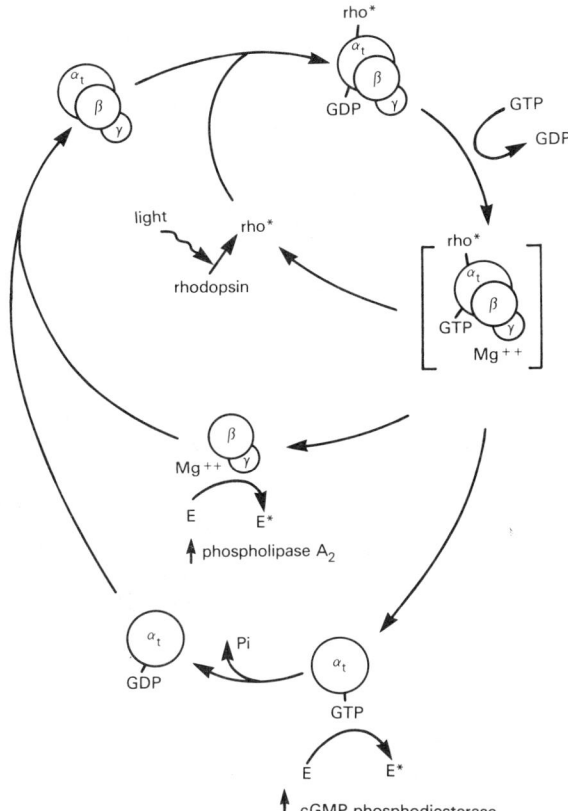

FIGURE 1. The role of the GTP-binding protein transducin in the light activation of cGMP phosphodiesterase and phospholipase A_2. In the bovine retina, transducin couples the light activation of rhodopsin to increases in both cGMP phosphodiesterase and phospholipase A_2 activity.[5,14] Initiation of the signal begins with light activation of rhodopsin and binding of photolysed rhodopsin (rho*) to the α subunit of the GTP-binding protein, transducin ($\alpha_t\beta\gamma$). Upon binding of rho*, there is an exchange of GTP for GDP at the guanine nucleotide binding site on the α_t subunit, followed by dissociation of the α and $\beta\gamma$ subunits. At the same time, rho* is released to interact with and activate another molecule of transducin, leading to amplification of the signal. Transduction of the signal occurs upon interaction of the GTP-bound α_t with the cGMP phosphodiesterase inhibitor,[48] leading to activation of the enzyme. At the same time, the dissociated $\beta\gamma$ subunits cause the stimulation of phospholipase A_2 by an as-yet-undetermined mechanism. Termination of the signal occurs upon the hydrolysis of GTP by action of a GTPase intrinsic to the α_t subunit, leading to reassociation of the inactive heterotrimer.

Light also stimulates phospholipase C activity in bovine ROS[25,26] by a G protein–dependent mechanism.[25] This factor, in combination with the reported role of the G protein transducin in the light activation of phospholipase A_2,[14,15] makes this system ideal for determining the mechanism for the G protein–mediated regulation of phospholipase A_2. Specifically, the questions to be addressed include the extent to which the G protein–mediated light activation of phospholipase A_2 and phospholipase

C occur by action of the same G protein(s) and the specific role of the G protein transducin in the stimulation of phospholipase A_2, whether it occurs by direct activation of enzyme activity or by inactivation of an inhibitor.

EXPERIMENTAL PROCEDURES

Preparation of Rod Outer Segments and Isolation of Transducin

Dark-adapted rod outer segments of bovine retina were isolated and purified as previously described[14] using retina that were dissected under dim red light. Transducin-depleted ROS were prepared from purified, dark-adapted ROS by extensive washing (six times each) first with isotonic, then with hypotonic buffers.[14,27] This procedure routinely extracts 75 to 80% of the membrane transducin from dark-adapted ROS, based on the loss of GTPγS-binding from the membranes.[14] In contrast, similar washing of purified ROS prepared from light-activated ROS does not remove transducin unless GTP is added to the membranes.[27] Transducin was, therefore, isolated from purified, light-activated ROS membranes that had been extensively washed as described above, then extracted with GTP to remove the transducin.[28] Excess GTP was separated from the transducin by chromatography.[29] Transducin accounted for 95% of the protein extracted by GTP, as determined by using 12% polyacrylamide gels that had been silver stained. Based on the absence of cross-reactivity with available antibodies to other G proteins, it was determined that the GTP-binding protein extracted from purified, light-activated ROS by GTP was primarily, if not exclusively, transducin (data not shown).

Isolation of Transducin Subunits

Transducin subunits were separated chromatographically using heptylsepharose[30] (prepared by reaction of heptylamine with CL-4B Sepharose; Pharmacia). For subunit separation, transducin was activated by the procedure of Sternweis,[30] diluted to a final concentration of 0.25 mg protein per ml in 0.2% cholate/1.5 M NaCl/0.25 M Tris-HCl, pH 8.0/0.05 M $MgCl_2$/0.01 M EGTA (TME buffer), then added to the heptylsepharose column (20 ml of packed heptyl Sepharose per 6 mg of transducin). The α and the βγ subunits were eluted using a 200-ml linear cholate/NaCl gradient (0.6% cholate/1.25 M NaCl to 1.4% cholate/0.5 M NaCl) in TME buffer after an initial 50-ml linear gradient of 0.2% cholate/1.5 M NaCl to 0.6% cholate/1.25 M NaCl. Fractions containing the isolated α and βγ subunits were identified by gel electrophoresis of aliquots of the fractions on SDS polyacrylamide gels[31] using a 5% stacking gel and a 12% running gel. Samples were prepared by the method of Neer et al.,[32] and loaded onto the gels; the proteins were separated by electrophoresis,[31] then visualized by silver stain (Bio-Rad).[33] The fractions containing either the α or the βγ subunits were pooled, concentrated by filtration (Amicon YM10), then dialyzed overnight with several changes of TME to remove the cholate and/or NaCl as well as residual GTP, Al^{+3}, and F^- ions, all of which interfere with either the phospholipase A_2 assay per se or with experiments designed to determine the effect of subunit reassociation. The transducin subunits were stored at 4 °C and used within 3 days of the initial extraction of the transducin.

Isolation of Calpactin

Calpactin was isolated from human placenta by the procedure of Soric and Gordon,[34] involving the calcium-dependent adsorption of calpactin to a DEAE-Sephacel column and its elution with EGTA.

Phospholipase A_2 Assay

In vitro phospholipase A_2 assays were performed on isolated, dark-adapted ROS using 1-palmitoyl-2-[^{14}C-arachidonyl]phosphatidylcholine as the substrate. Radiolabeled substrate (10^7 dpm/ml) was prepared by evaporation of the solvent under N_2 and addition of 0.12 M Tris-HCl, pH 8.8. The lipids were dispersed by a 5-min sonication using a Branson sonicating water bath, then made into a micellar suspension by a 15-sec sonication with a Kontes microprobe tip immediately prior to the assay. For the in vitro assays using soluble porcine pancreatic phospholipase A_2 (500 ng), unlabeled diarachidonylphosphatidylcholine (0.08 mg/ml) was added to the radiolabeled substrate to provide for a lipid environment in lieu of membrane. Reactions were initiated by addition of 20 μl of the sonicated, radiolabeled substrate to dark-adapted ROS membranes (20 μg, unless otherwise specified) or to soluble porcine pancreatic phospholipase A_2 (500 ng) in a reaction mixture containing a final concentration of 4 mM glutathione, 0.6 mM NaCl, 40 mM $MgCl_2$, 5 mM $CaCl_2$, 30 mM Tris-HCl, pH 8.8, in a total volume of 80 μl. Incubations were at 37 °C either under dim red light or white light (300 watts). Reactions were stopped at zero time (to determine the amount of nonenzymatic hydrolysis) and at specified times thereafter by addition of 100 μl 1 N formic acid. Despite saturating substrate concentrations, the reaction proved to be linear for only 15 min.[14] The assay was, therefore, routinely stopped at 10 min to ensure that measurements were taken in the linear phase. Samples were extracted by addition of 400 μl N-heptane. After vortexing, samples were centrifuged (3 min, Eppendorf microfuge) to separate the phases and aliquots (100 μl) of the upper phase analyzed for the release of [^{14}C]-dpm following addition of 10 mls Biofluor (New England Nuclear). The radioactivity of the samples was measured using an LKB scintillation counter programmed to correct for quenching, counting efficiency, and the spill of [^{14}C]-dpm into the [^{3}H] channel. To ensure that the [^{14}C]-dpm measured was representative of [^{14}C]-arachidonic acid released, reaction products were separated by thin layer chromatography using chloroform/methanol/water (63:27:4) on Whatman LK6D plates. To correct for the loss of the released [^{14}C]-arachidonic acid during lipid extraction, [^{3}H]-arachidonic acid (2000 dpm/50 μl) was added to each sample prior to the final extraction step, and the percent [^{3}H]-dpm recovered was employed to correct for the loss of [^{14}C]-dpm. Following subtraction of the nonspecific hydrolysis observed in the zero-time control, phospholipase A_2 activity was expressed as nmol [^{14}C]-arachidonic acid released/min/mg protein.

Phospholipase C Assay

In vitro assays of phospholipase C were performed on isolated, dark-adapted ROS using L-3-phosphatidylinositol [2-^{3}H-inositol] as the substrate. Unlabeled phosphoinositides and phosphatidylserine (0.08 mg/ml) in a 2:1 ratio were added to the radiolabeled substrate (10^7 dpm/ml), and the solvent was evaporated under N_2. After addition of 0.12 M Tris-HCl, pH 7.5, the lipids were dispersed as described above and micelles prepared by a 15-sec sonication with a Kontes microtip probe immediately prior to the assay. Reactions were initiated by addition of 20 μl of the sonicated, radiolabeled substrate to dark-adapted ROS membranes (20 μg, unless otherwise specified) in a reaction mixture containing a final concentration of 4 mM glutathione, 0.6 mM NaCl, 40 mM $MgCl_2$, 200 μM $CaCl_2$, 30 mM Tris-HCl, pH 7.5, in a final volume of 80 μl. Incubations were at 37 °C either under dim red light or white light (300 watts). Reactions were stopped at zero time (to determine the amount of nonenzymatic hydrolysis) and at specified times thereafter by addition of 1.5 ml methanol:chloroform (2:1, v/v). Despite saturating substrate concentrations, the reaction proved to be linear for less than 20 min.[25] The assay was, therefore, routinely stopped at 10 min to ensure that measurements were taken in the linear phase. Samples were extracted by a modified Bligh and Dyer extraction involving further addition of 0.5 ml chloroform and 0.8 ml 0.12 M HCl. Samples were then vortexed and centrifuged (1000 × g, 10 min) to separate the phases and aliquots (1 ml) of the water-soluble upper phase analyzed for the release of [^{3}H]-dpm following evaporation of the methanol to minimize quenching. After addition of 10 mls Biofluor (New England Nuclear), the radioactivity of the samples was measured as described above using an LKB scintillation counter. The reaction products were analyzed by Dowex chromatography[35] to ensure that [^{3}H]-dpm measured was representative of the released [^{3}H]-inositol phosphate. To correct for the loss of the released [^{3}H]-inositol phosphate during lipid extraction, [^{14}C]-myo-inositol-1-phosphate (2000 dpm/50 μl) was added to each sample prior to the final extraction step, and the percent [^{14}C]-dpm recovered was used to correct for the loss of [^{3}H]-dpm. Following subtraction of the nonspecific hydrolysis observed in the zero-time control, phospholipase C activity was expressed as pmol [^{3}H]-inositol phosphate released/min/mg protein.

Toxin Treatment

Dark-adapted ROS membranes were treated with activated pertussis toxin (10 ng/ml) or cholera toxin (50 ng/ml) in the absence of light for 2 h at 30 °C in an incubation mixture containing 50 mM potassium phosphate, pH 7.5, 20 mM thymidine, 1 mM ATP, 5 mM $MgCl_2$ and 1 mM nicotinamide adenine dinucleotide (NAD).[14] Toxins were activated by incubation with 20 mM dithiothreitol in 50 mM glycine, pH 8.0, for 10 min at 30 °C.[14] To avoid loss of transducin from the toxin-treated membranes, the membranes were not washed free of the toxins prior to the assay. Consequently, both toxins and NAD were present during the subsequent 10-min enzyme assays. This is particularly important since cholera toxin–induced ADP-ribosylation of transducin, assessed by radiolabeling of the α subunit of transducin by [^{32}P]-NAD, was observed only in membranes that were subsequently exposed to light during the 10-min time interval required for enzyme assays (data not presented). This is consistent with the report that cholera toxin–induced ADP-ribosylation occurs only in light-activated ROS.[36]

GTPγS Binding

The G protein content of ROS membranes was assessed both before and after extraction of transducin by measuring the [^{35}S]-GTPγS-binding capacity of the membranes using nitrocellulose filters (Type HA, Millipore).[30]

Materials

L-3-phosphatidyl [2-^{3}H]inositol and 1-palmitoyl-2-[^{14}C]-arachidonylphosphatidylcholine were from New England Nuclear. Cholera toxin and pertussis toxin were from List Biological Laboratories (Campbell, CA) and GDPβS and GTPγS from Boehringer Mannheim. Actin was purchased from Sigma. The G_s, G_i, and G_o subunits and the G protein arf were kindly provided by Dr. R. Kahn, the G protein antibodies by Dr. S. Mumby.

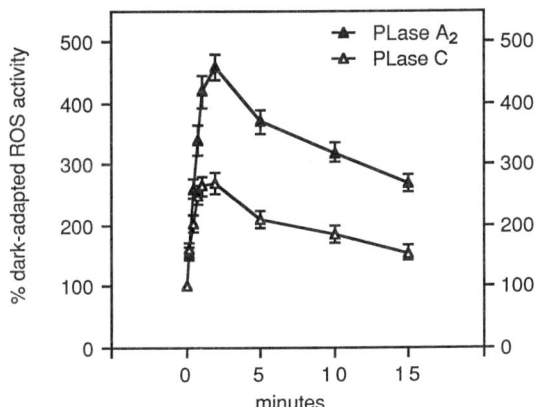

FIGURE 2. Time course for the light activation of phospholipase A_2 and phospholipase C in dark-adapted bovine rod outer segments (ROS). Phospholipase A_2 and phospholipase C activities were measured as nmol [^{14}C]-arachidonic acid or pmol [^{3}H]-inositol phosphate released from either [^{14}C]-arachidonylphosphatidylcholine or phosphatidyl-[^{3}H]-inositol, respectively, upon incubation of dark-adapted bovine ROS membranes under either dim red light or 300-watt white light. Preparation of dark-adapted ROS membranes and the phospholipase assay conditions were as described under EXPERIMENTAL PROCEDURES. Data on the light activation of the phospholipase (PLase) A_2 (▲) and phospholipase C (△) are presented as % dark-adapted (basal) activity. To minimize fluctuations in activity due to varying amounts of transducin in different ROS preparations, values were normalized to a transducin content of 3.6 pmol/mg protein based on the binding of [^{35}S]-GTPγS. The results are mean ± SE ($n = 4$).

RESULTS

Light Stimulates both Phospholipases A_2 and C

In dark-adapted photoreceptor membranes of bovine retina, both phospholipase A_2 and phospholipase C are stimulated several-fold upon exposure to light when assayed *in vitro* using exogenous [^{14}C]-arachidonylphosphatidylcholine and phosphatidyl-[^{3}H]-inositol, respectively, as the substrates (FIG. 2). Plotting the increases in phospholipase activities as a percentage of the dark-adapted ROS activities, the rapid light-induced rise in both enzyme activities can easily be observed. Although maximal differences between the dark-adapted and light-activated enzymes were reached after two minutes' exposure to light, this was due to a slower rise in basal activities in response to the dim red light[14,25] and not to transient increases in the phospholipase activities. To eliminate the potential variability in the percent increase, assays were performed for 10 minutes, during the linear phases of both enzyme activities.[14,25]

Both basal and light-activated phospholipase A_2 activities were significantly higher than the phospholipase C activities present in bovine ROS. In dark-adapted ROS, the phospholipase A_2 activity was orders of magnitude higher (29.4 nmol [^{14}C]-arachidonate released/min/mg protein) than the phospholipase C activity (0.7 pmol [^{3}H]-inositol phosphate released/min/mg protein) (see TABLE 1). The light-stimulated increase in phospholipase A_2 activity was 4- to 5-fold higher than the basal (i.e., dark-adapted) activity, while the light-induced increase in phospholipase C activity reached a maximum of 2- to 3-fold higher than the basal activity.

GTPγS, GDPβS, and Neomycin Effects on Phospholipase A_2 and C Activities Indicate Fundamental Differences in the G Protein Regulation of These Two Light-Activated Enzymes

To determine whether GTP-binding proteins function in the regulation of phospholipases in these membranes, the effects of GTPγS and GDPβS on the phospholipase activities of dark-adapted and light-activated ROS were examined. GTPγS, which induces dissociation of G proteins and stabilizes G proteins in their active, dissociated state,[2] would be expected to stimulate both the basal and light-activated phospholipases. GDPβS, in contrast, stabilizes the inactive, associated state of the G proteins and would be expected to inhibit the stimulation of the phospholipases without affecting basal activities.[36] Addition of 100 μM GTPγS to dark-adapted ROS led to a marked increase in both phospholipase A_2 and phospholipase C activities, mimicking the effect of light (FIGS. 3A, 3B).[14,25] Addition of GTPγS to light-activated ROS, however, did not further enhance the light activation of these phospholipases, but rather inhibited the light effects of both enzymes (FIGS. 3A, 3B).[14,25] The inhibitory effect of GTPγS on light-activated ROS suggests the existence of another G protein (or proteins), which, upon activation, is capable of inhibiting the light-stimulated but

TABLE 1. Phospholipase A_2 and Phospholipase C Activities of Transducin-rich and Transducin-poor Rod Outer Segments (ROS) in the Presence or Absence of Light and/or GTPγS or the Phospholipase Activators Melittin and Deoxycholate

	Phospholipase A_2 Activity (Nmol ^{14}C-Arachidonate Released/Min/Mg Protein) ± Melittin		Phospholipase C Activity (Pmol ^{3}H-Inositol Phosphate Released/Min/Mg Protein) ± Deoxycholate	
	−	+	−	+
Transducin-rich ROS				
Dark-adapted ROS	29.4 ± 2.6	275.2 ± 22.1	0.78 ± 0.03	5.23 ± 0.65
+ GTPγS	110.5 ± 12.7	n.d.[a]	2.69 ± 0.07	n.d.
+ Light	133.6 ± 24.2	280.4 ± 18.1	3.13 ± 0.12	5.65 ± 0.82
+ Light + GTPγS	40.1 ± 1.9	n.d.	2.07 ± 0.08	n.d.
Transducin-poor ROS				
Dark-adapted ROS	46.1 ± 2.7	237.5 ± 24.7	0.43 ± 0.07	1.58 ± 0.11
+ GTPγS	18.9 ± 0.8	n.d.	0.49 ± 0.06	n.d.
+ Light	63.8 ± 3.5	262.7 ± 14.8	0.47 ± 0.05	1.62 ± 0.14
+ Light + GTPγS	62.1 ± 5.1	n.d.	0.43 ± 0.09	n.d.

[a] n.d. = not determined.

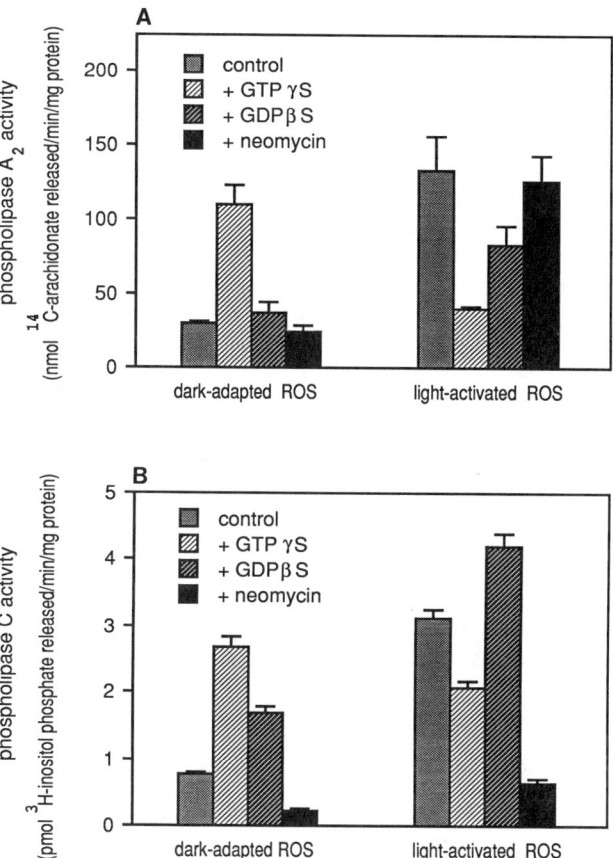

FIGURE 3. GTPγS, GDPβS, and neomycin effects on phospholipase A_2 and phospholipase C indicate the two enzyme activities are independent of each other. Phospholipase A_2 and phospholipase C activities were assayed in the presence of dim red light or 300-watt white light using 20 μg of dark-adapted rod outer segments (ROS). ROS membrane preparations and phospholipase assay conditions were as described under EXPERIMENTAL PROCEDURES. Incubations were for 10 min in the presence or absence of 100 μM GTPγS, GDPβS, or neomycin. Values from separate experiments were normalized as indicated in the legend to FIG. 2. Results are mean ± SE (n = 3). (A) Phospholipase A_2 activity, nmol [^{14}C]-arachidonate released/min/mg protein; (B) Phospholipase C activity, pmol [^{3}H]-inositol phosphate released/min/mg protein.

not the basal phospholipase A_2 and phospholipase C activities. This dual regulation of enzyme activity by both a stimulatory and an inhibitory G protein is reminiscent of the G protein regulation of adenylate cyclase, where activation of G_i leads to inhibition of G_s-stimulated adenylate cyclase without affecting basal activity.[3]

Both phospholipase A_2 and C were similarly affected by exposure to light and/or addition of GTPγS, indicating a degree of similarity in the G protein regulation of these light-activated enzymes. Addition of GDPβS, however, had markedly different effects on the two phospholipases. GDPβS inhibited the light-activated but not the basal phospholipase A_2 activity (FIG. 3A), which is consistent with a role for a stimulatory G protein in the light activation of phospholipase A_2. In contrast, GDPβS stimulated both basal and light-activated phospholipase C (FIG. 3B), suggesting that this enzyme may be under tonic inhibition by an inhibitory G protein, with stimulation of the enzyme occurring by removal of this inhibitory control. Furthermore, these results indicate that, despite the fact that the two phospholipases are both regulated by G proteins and activated by light, there are fundamental differences in the G protein regulation of these two enzymes.

Although the difference in the GDPβS effects on the two phospholipases suggested that the two enzyme activities were independent of one another, to further demonstrate this, the effect of the phospholipase C inhibitor, neomycin, was assessed. Neomycin, which inhibited both basal and light-activated phospholipase C (FIG. 3B), had no effect on phospholipase A_2 activity (FIG. 3A), indicating that, in this tissue, phospholipase A_2 activity did not require prior action of phospholipase C or vice versa. This did not, however, address the similarity or dissimilarity of the G protein–mediated regulation of the two phospholipases.

Pertussis and Cholera Toxin Effects on the Two Phospholipases Suggest the Independence of the G Protein Regulation of the Two Enzyme Activities

Transducin, the major G protein of the retina, binds photolysed rhodopsin,[2] suggesting that this G protein may function in the light activation of phospholipases A_2 and C. Transducin serves as a substrate for both pertussis and cholera toxin, with the pertussis toxin–induced ADP-ribosylation of transducin observed to stabilize this G protein in its associated, inactive state.[37,38] To assess the potential role of transducin in the activation of these phospholipases, both enzymes were assayed following treatment of dark-adapted ROS with either pertussis or cholera toxin. Pertussis toxin treatment of dark-adapted ROS inhibited both basal (i.e., dark-adapted) and light-induced phospholipase A_2 activities (FIG. 4A),[14] which is consistent with a role for transducin as the G protein mediating the light-induced stimulation of this phospholipase. In contrast, pertussis toxin stimulated both basal and light-activated phospholipase C,[25] an effect similar to that of GDPβS (compare FIGS. 3B and 4B). This lends support to the concept that phospholipase C is under tonic inhibitory control by a G protein and suggests that this inhibitory G protein is a pertussis toxin–sensitive G protein. Transducin may, however, still function in the stimulation of phospholipase C by interacting with and inactivating the inhibitory G protein.

Both phospholipases were inhibited by cholera toxin but differed in whether the toxin affected the basal or the light activated enzyme. With phospholipase A_2 activity, only the light-stimulated activity was inhibited (FIG. 4A), whereas with phospholipase C, only basal activity was inhibited (FIG. 4B). Although transducin is a substrate for cholera toxin, it has not been established whether the toxin acts to stabilize the active, dissociated or the inactive, associated state of this G protein. The ability of cholera toxin to inhibit the GTPase activity of transducin[38,39] does not address the mechanism of action, since both cholera toxin, when acting on G_s,[40] and pertussis toxin, when acting on either G_i,[41] or transducin,[39] inhibit the GTPase activities of their G protein substrate. However, the observation that transducin appears to be ADP-ribosylated by cholera toxin only in the light or upon addition of Gpp(NHp)[38] suggests that the toxin acts on the dissociated, that is, the activated, state of transducin. Assuming the toxin is acting either to activate or to stabilize the activated state of its G protein substrate(s), similarly to its effect on G_s,[40] the inhibition of light-activated but not basal phospholipase A_2 is inconsistent with a cholera-toxin effect on transducin. Were cholera toxin

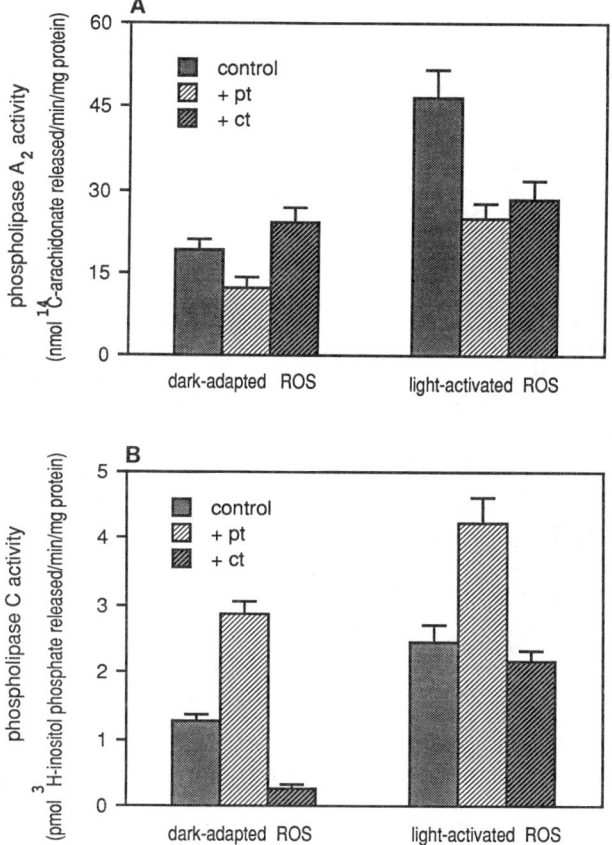

FIGURE 4. Pertussis toxin and cholera toxin differentially affect phospholipase A_2 and phospholipase C activity. Phospholipase A_2 and C activities were assayed in the presence of dim red light or 300-watt white light using 20 μg of dark-adapted rod outer segments (ROS) previously treated with pertussis (pt; 10 ng/ml) and/or cholera toxin (ct; 50 ng/ml). Membrane preparation, phospholipase assays, and toxin treatments were as described under EXPERIMENTAL PROCEDURES. Values from separate experiments were normalized as indicated in the legend to FIG. 2. Results are mean ± SE ($n = 4$). (**A**) Phospholipase A_2 activity, nmol [^{14}C]-arachidonate released/min/mg protein; (**B**) Phospholipase C activity, pmol [^{3}H]-inositol phosphate released/min/mg protein.

acting on transducin to stabilize the inactive heterotrimer, similarly to the action of pertussis toxin on transducin,[37] one would expect the effects of cholera toxin to mimic the effects of pertussis toxin and inhibit both the basal and the stimulated enzyme, rather than having selective effects on either basal or light-induced activity. These results appear to preclude action of the toxin on transducin and suggest that activation of another cholera toxin–sensitive G protein, possibly G_s, is responsible for the GTPγS-mediated inhibition of the light-activated phospholipase A_2 (FIG. 3A).

Cholera toxin inhibited basal phospholipase C, but had no effect on light-stimulated phospholipase C activity (FIG. 4B). The absence of a stimulatory or inhibitory effect of the toxin on the light activation of phospholipase C again suggests that the cholera-toxin effect is not on transducin, but rather on another cholera toxin–sensitive, light-insensitive G protein whose activation causes further inhibition of phospholipase C. This would be consistent with an activating effect of the toxin on a G protein that tonically inhibits phospholipase C.

Removal of Transducin from Dark-Adapted Rod Outer Segments Correlates with the Loss of Light- and GTPγS-Stimulated Phospholipase Activities

The fact that both phospholipases were activated by light strongly suggests a role for the rhodopsin-binding G protein transducin in the stimulation of these enzymes. While the pertussis toxin–induced inhibition of phospholipase A_2 supports a role for transducin in the light activation of phospholipase A_2, the ability of pertussis toxin to stimulate rather than inhibit phospholipase C indicates that this enzyme is under tonic inhibitory control by another pertussis toxin–sensitive G protein. This does not preclude the possibility that transducin may yet function in the light stimulation of phospholipase C by blocking the action of this inhibitory G protein.

To address more directly the potential role of transducin in the light activation of both phospholipases, transducin was removed from the dark-adapted ROS with repeated washings and the transducin-depleted ROS analyzed for phospholipase activities in the presence or absence of light. Using [^{35}S]-GTPγS-binding as a measure of the transducin content of the ROS membranes,[14] removal of 75% of the transducin from the membranes was paralleled by a loss of both the light- and GTPγS-induced activation of the two phospholipases (TABLE 1). This loss of phospholipase A_2 activation upon removal of transducin was not accompanied by a loss of phospholipase A_2 per se, since stimulation of the membrane with melittin, a phospholipase A_2 activator,[42] led to comparable activity in both transducin-rich and transducin-poor ROS (TABLE 1). Removal of transducin, therefore, correlated with the loss of light- and GTPγS-induced phospholipase A_2 activity, supporting a role for transducin in the light activation of this enzyme. Removal of transducin also unmasked the G protein observed to inhibit the light-activated enzyme (FIG. 3A) such that addition of GTPγS to transducin-poor ROS now resulted in inhibition of phospholipase A_2, not activation (TABLE 1).

Upon removal of transducin, phospholipase C activity also lost its sensitivity to light and GTPγS (TABLE 1). However, further examination revealed that phospholipase C activity itself also appeared to be lost upon repeated washing of the dark-adapted membranes (TABLE 1). This was assessed by stimulating the membranes with deoxycholate, a phospholipase C enhancer.[43] While melittin-stimulated phospholipase A_2 activity was the same in both transducin-rich and transducin-poor ROS, there was a significant loss of detergent-stimulated phospholipase C activity in the transducin-poor ROS (TABLE 1). The loss of light- and GTPγS-induced phospholipase C activity, therefore, cannot be directly attributed to the removal of transducin, although it may be a factor.

Exogenous Transducin Added to Transducin-poor Red Outer Segments Restores the Light Activation of Both Phospholipases, but Activation of Phospholipase C Requires an Additional Factor

To further determine whether there is a role for transducin in the light activation of the phospholipases, exogenous transducin was added back to the transducin-poor ROS in the presence or absence of light. Addition of exogenous transducin was able to restore the light activation of phospholipase A_2 in dark-adapted, transducin-poor ROS (FIG. 5A),[14,15] but was unable to restore the light activation of phospholipase C (FIG. 5B).[25] To restore the light activation of phospholipase C required both exogenous transducin as well as a soluble factor, although the factor alone had no effect on

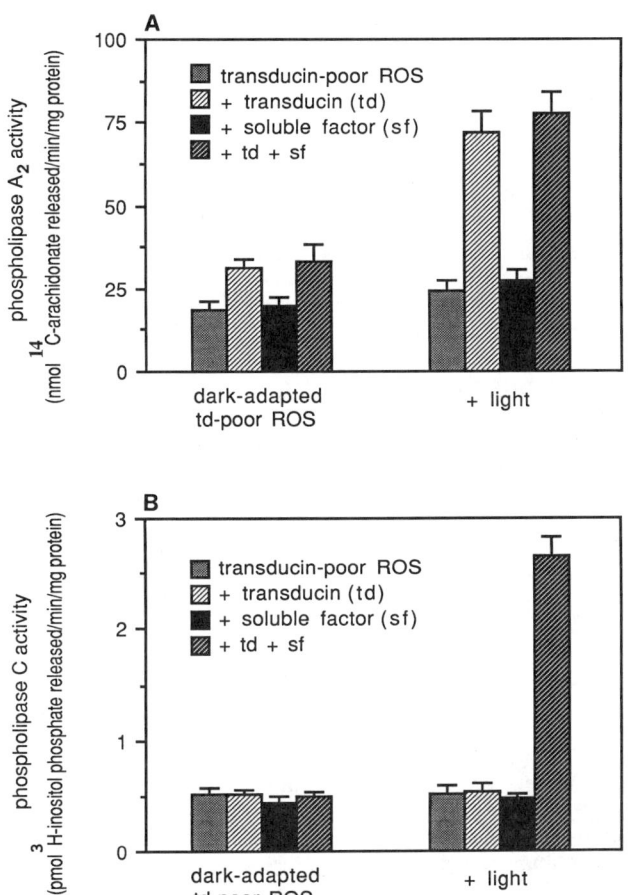

FIGURE 5. Exogenous transducin alone restores the light activation of phospholipase A_2 in dark-adapted, transducin-poor rod outer segments (ROS), while light activation of phospholipase C requires the presence of an added factor. Phospholipase A_2 and C activities were assayed in the presence or absence of exogenous transducin (td; 500 ng) and/or a concentrated supernatant fraction (sf or soluble factor; 500 ng) using dark-adapted, transducin-poor ROS (td-poor ROS; 20 μg) incubated 10 min under either dim red light or 300-watt white light. Preparation of td-poor ROS, isolation and purification of transducin, preparation of the supernatant fraction, and the phospholipase assays were as described under EXPERIMENTAL PROCEDURES. Values were normalized to a transducin content of 0.8 pmol GTPγS bound/mg protein. Results are mean ± SE ($n = 3$). (**A**) Phospholipase A_2 activity, nmol [^{14}C]-arachidonate released/min/mg protein; (**B**) Phospholipase C activity, pmol [^{3}H]-inositol phosphate released/min/mg protein.

phospholipase C activity (FIG. 5B). Addition of transducin that had been previously ADP-ribosylated was unable to restore the activation of either phospholipase (data not presented), indicating that it was the dissociated state of the transducin that was important in the light activation of the two enzymes.

Transducin α and βγ Subunits Have Contrasting Roles in the Modulation of Phospholipase A_2 and Phospholipase C Activity

The isolated, purified subunits of transducin were added to transducin-poor ROS membranes in the presence or absence of light to determine the role of the individual subunits in the activation of the two phospholipases. As previously reported[14] and illustrated here (FIG. 6A), the βγ subunits were found to stimulate phospholipase A_2. The α subunit, while slightly stimulatory when added alone, was able to inhibit the βγ-induced increase in phospholipase A_2 when added under nondissociating conditions (FIG. 6A). These results suggest that the inhibitory effect of the α subunit on the βγ-induced increase in phospholipase A_2 activity occurs as a result of facilitating subunit reassociation (see FIG. 10).

In contrast, phospholipase C activity was stimulated by addition of the α subunit of transducin, while the βγ subunits inhibited phospholipase C activity when added in the absence of light (FIG. 6B). In the presence of light, however, the βγ subunits stimulated the enzyme; and, when added together with the α subunit, the stimulatory effects of the α and βγ subunits were additive (FIG. 6B). These results suggest that the βγ subunits have an effect on phospholipase C activity independent of the action of the α subunit. In view of the pertussis toxin- and GDPβS-induced stimulation of basal and activated phospholipase C (FIGS. 3A, 4A) and the GTPγS-mediated inhibition of the light-activated enzyme (FIG. 3A), there appears to be not only tonic inhibition of phospholipase C by a G protein, but inhibition of the light-activated enzyme upon activation of a G protein. It is unclear, however, whether inhibition is mediated by the α or βγ subunits of this inhibitory G protein. The ability of the βγ subunits of transducin both to inhibit phospholipase C activity and to prevent the α-induced increase in phospholipase C activity in the absence of light (FIG. 6B), together with the tonic inhibition of the enzyme, suggest that inhibition of phospholipase C may be a function of the βγ subunits that are present in membranes in excess of the G protein α subunits.[2,3] The stimulatory effect of the α subunit of transducin would then occur by combining with and inactivating the βγ subunits of this inhibitory G protein (see FIG. 10). The inhibitory effects of the βγ subunits of transducin on phospholipase C activity in the absence of light is consistent with this concept, but their ability to actively stimulate phospholipase C activity in the presence of light is, at present, difficult to explain mechanistically.

In Vitro Experiments Suggest That the βγ Subunits Stimulate Phospholipase A_2 Activity by Removal of an Inhibitor

The transducin subunits had no direct effect on soluble pancreatic phospholipase A_2 activity (FIG. 7), while addition of calpactin, a phospholipase A_2 inhibitor thought to act by binding phospholipid substrate,[44] decreased phospholipase A_2 activity nearly 40% (FIG. 7). In the presence of calpactin, addition of the α subunit of transducin led to

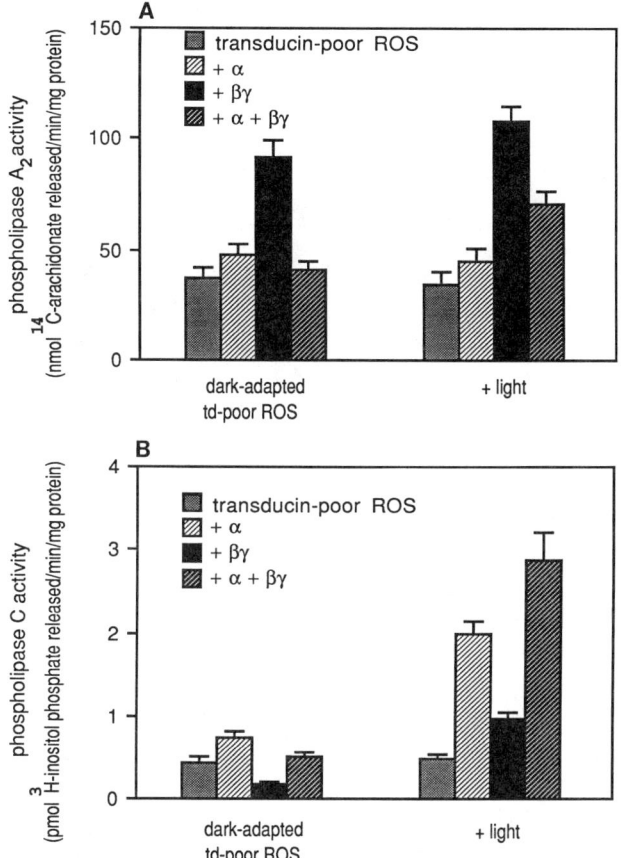

FIGURE 6. The $\beta\gamma$ subunits of transducin stimulate phospholipase A_2 activity in transducin-depleted rod outer segments (ROS) in the presence or absence of light, while phospholipase C activity was inhibited in the absence of light and stimulated in the presence of light. Dark-adapted, transducin-poor ROS (td-poor ROS) were incubated with α and/or $\beta\gamma$ subunits of transducin (5 ng to 5 μg/100 μl assay volume; data presented is for 50 ng) under either dim red light or 300-watt white light. The isolation of transducin, the separation and concentration of the α and $\beta\gamma$ subunits, the preparation of dark-adapted, transducin-depleted ROS, and the phospholipase assays were as described under EXPERIMENTAL PROCEDURES. Values were normalized to a transducin content of 0.8 pmol GTPγS bound/mg protein. Results are mean ± SE ($n = 3$). (A) Phospholipase A_2 activity, nmol [^{14}C]-arachidonate released/min/mg protein; (B) Phospholipase C activity, pmol [^{3}H]-inositol phosphate released/min/mg protein.

further inhibition of phospholipase A_2 activity, whereas addition of the $\beta\gamma$ subunits prevented the calpactin-induced inhibition of phospholipase A_2 (FIG. 6). These preliminary studies indicate that the $\beta\gamma$ subunits of transducin do not directly stimulate the enzyme but, rather, may act to block the action of an inhibitor.

Similar results were obtained upon addition of other G protein subunits. The α

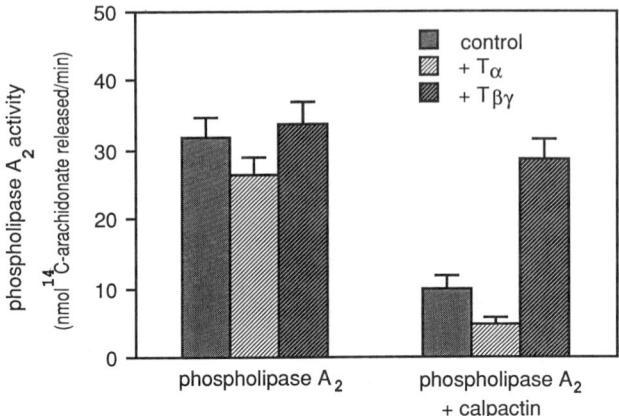

FIGURE 7. The isolated transducin subunits, in the absence of a direct effect on pancreatic phospholipase A_2, modulate the calpactin-induced inhibition of phospholipase A_2. The effect of isolated α (T_α) and $\beta\gamma$ ($T_{\beta\gamma}$) subunits of transducin (50 ng) on soluble porcine pancreatic phospholipase A_2 (500 ng) was examined *in vitro* in the presence or absence of calpactin (50 ng), an inhibitor of phospholipase A_2.[44] The phospholipase A_2 assay procedure, the preparation of dark-adapted transducin-poor rod outer segments (ROS), and isolation of both the transducin subunits and calpactin were as described under EXPERIMENTAL PROCEDURES. Results are expressed as nmol ^{14}C-arachidonate released/min/mg protein $\pm$ SE ($n = 3$).

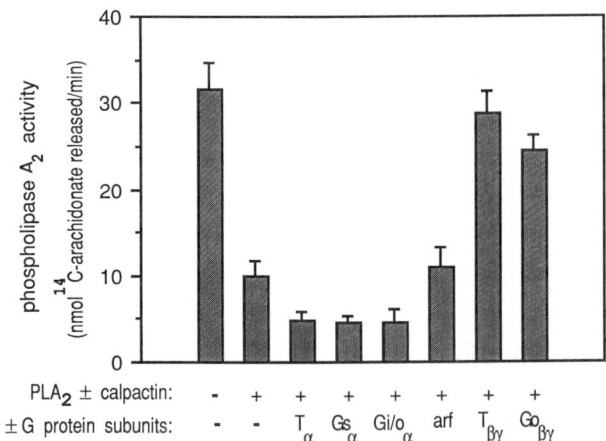

FIGURE 8. The $\beta\gamma$ subunits of G proteins prevent the calpactin-induced inhibition of phospholipase A_2, while G protein α subunits further inhibit the enzyme. The isolated α subunits of transducin, G_s and a mixture of G_i and G_o (G_i/G_o), were analyzed along with the $\beta\gamma$ subunits of transducin or G_o and the GTP-binding ADP-ribosylating factor (arf)[45] for an effect on soluble pancreatic phospholipase A_2 (500 ng) *in vitro* in the presence or absence of calpactin (50 ng), an inhibitor of phospholipase A_2.[44] The phospholipase A_2 assay procedure and the preparation of the α and $\beta\gamma$ subunits and calpactin were as described under EXPERIMENTAL PROCEDURES. Results are mean $\pm$ SE ($n = 3$).

subunits of G_s and a mixture of G_i and G_o (G_i/G_o) enhanced the inhibitory effect of calpactin, while the $\beta\gamma$ subunits of G_o prevented the calpactin-induced inhibition (FIG. 8). The 21-kDa GTP-binding ADP-ribosylation factor (arf)[45] had no effect in this system. Actin, which binds to calpactin,[46] also prevented the calpactin-mediated inhibition of phospholipase A_2 and acted synergistically with the $\beta\gamma$ subunits to stimulate phospholipase A_2 in this *in vitro* system (FIG. 9). These results suggest that the $\beta\gamma$ subunits may stimulate phospholipase A_2 by removing an inhibitor. It is not clear whether calpactin is itself present in the ROS membranes, although there has been a report of a protein present in bovine ROS that exhibits immunoreactivity to the calpactin antibody.[47]

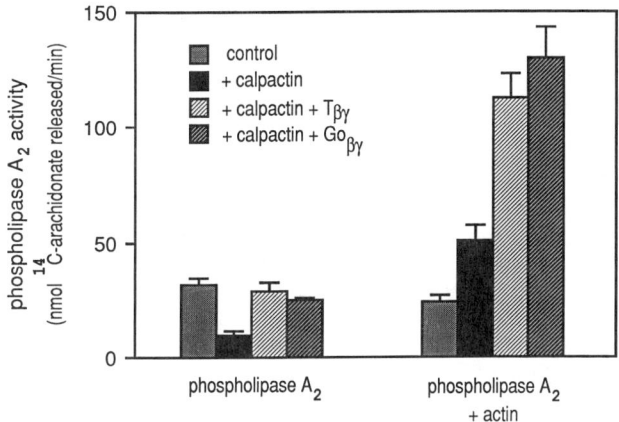

FIGURE 9. The $\beta\gamma$ subunits act synergistically with actin to stimulate phospholipase A_2 by preventing the calpactin-mediated inhibition of phospholipase A_2. The effect of the $\beta\gamma$ subunits of transducin (50 ng) on soluble porcine pancreatic phospholipase A_2 (500 ng) was examined in the presence or absence of calpactin (50 ng), a phospholipase A_2 inhibitor,[44] and/or actin (50 ng), a cytoskeletal protein that interacts with calpactin.[45] The phospholipase A_2 assay procedure and the preparation of the $\beta\gamma$ subunits and calpactin were as described under EXPERIMENTAL PROCEDURES. Results are mean $\pm$ SE ($n = 3$).

DISCUSSION

In bovine ROS, both phospholipase A_2 and phospholipase C appear to be under dual regulation by stimulatory and inhibitory G proteins, with transducin functioning as the stimulatory G protein in the light activation of both phospholipases. Despite these similarities, the activation of the two phospholipases occurs independently, and the G protein regulation of the two enzymes is fundamentally different. Phospholipase C is under tonic inhibitory control by a pertussis toxin–sensitive, inhibitory G protein, with transducin functioning in the light activation of phospholipase C by preventing the action of this inhibitory G protein. Phospholipase A_2 activity, in contrast, is not under tonic inhibition by a G protein, and transducin plays a more direct role in the light activation of this phospholipase. Activation of phospholipase A_2 by transducin, however, does not appear to involve direct stimulation of the enzyme, but rather, is suggested to act by blocking the action of a phospholipase A_2 inhibitor such as calpactin.[44,47] This is analogous to the role of the GTP-bound α subunit of transducin in the light activation of cGMP phosphodiesterase, where activation occurs by inactivation of an inhibitor.[48] While phospholipase A_2 activity is not under tonic inhibition by a G protein, the activated enzyme is susceptible to regulation by an inhibitory G protein. The G protein responsible for the inhibition of phospholipase A_2 activity is sensitive to cholera toxin and inhibits the activated, but not the basal, enzyme activity.

The results supporting a role for transducin in the light activation of phospholipase A_2 in bovine retinal rod outer segments include: (1) the ability of GTPγS to mimic and GDPβS to prevent the light activation of phospholipase A_2 (FIG. 3A);[14] (2) the ability of pertussis toxin, which ADP-ribosylates the α subunit of transducin and stabilizes this G protein in its inactive, associated state,[37] to inhibit the light activation of transducin (FIG. 4A);[14] (3) the loss of light- and GTPγS-induced phospholipase A_2 activity upon removal of transducin from dark-adapted ROS without loss of phospholipase A_2 per se (TABLE 1);[14] and (4) the ability of exogenous transducin to restore the light- and GTPγS-induced increase in phospholipase A_2 in dark-adapted, transducin-depleted ROS (FIG. 5A).[14,15] In the modulation of phospholipase A_2 by transducin, the $\beta\gamma$ subunits function in the activation of the enzyme, while the α subunits block the $\beta\gamma$-induced increase in phospholipase A_2 (FIG. 6A).[15] The inhibitory effect of the α subunit appears to occur by facilitating reassociation of the inactive heterotrimer, based on the observation that the α subunit inhibits the $\beta\gamma$-induced increase in phospholipase A_2 activity only under nondissociating conditions (FIG. 6A).[15]

Inhibition of light-activated phospholipase A_2 (FIG. 3A) appears to occur by action of another cholera toxin–sensitive G protein, as indicated by the ability of either GTPγS or cholera toxin to inhibit the light-stimulated but not the basal enzyme activity (FIGS. 3A, 4A). Moreover, addition of GTPγS to transducin-depleted ROS resulted in inhibition rather than stimulation of phospholipase A_2, even in dark-adapted ROS (TABLE 1). Removal of transducin, therefore, appeared to unmask the presence of an inhibitory G protein that normally was in evidence only upon activation of the phospholipase. The mechanism for this G protein–mediated inhibition of phospholipase A_2, it is suggested, occurs by interaction of the dissociated α subunit of this cholera toxin–sensitive, "inhibitory" G protein (possibly G_s) with the $\beta\gamma$ subunits of transducin, resulting in inhibition of the $\beta\gamma$-activated phospholipase A_2 (FIG. 10). The GTPγS-induced inhibition of basal phospholipase A_2 observed in transducin-depleted ROS may relate to the observation that these membranes, while depleted of transducin, are actually enriched in the $\beta\gamma$ subunits relative to the α subunit. This results in an actual increase in basal activity (TABLE 1),[14] an increase that can be blocked by the dissociated α subunits of the cholera toxin–sensitive, inhibitory G protein upon activation of transducin-poor ROS with GTPγS.

Phospholipase A_2 activity in bovine ROS is independent of phospholipase C activity, although both enzymes are light-activated and are under dual regulation by G proteins. The independence of the two phospholipases and the fundamental difference in the G protein regulation of these enzymes is indicated by: (1) the absence of an inhibitory effect of neomycin on basal or light-activated phospholipase A_2 activity while inhibiting phospholipase C activity (FIG. 3); (2) the ability of both GDPβS and pertussis toxin to stimulate basal and light-induced phospholipase C activity while inhibiting the light activation of phospholipase A_2 (FIGS. 3, 4), suggesting that phospholipase C, but not phospholipase A_2, is under tonic inhibitory control by a pertussis toxin–sensitive G protein; (3) the observation that exogenous transducin alone restores the light activation of phospholipase A_2 in transducin-poor ROS, whereas restoration of the light-induced phospholipase C activity requires the presence of both transducin and a soluble factor (FIG. 5); and (4) the contrasting role of the

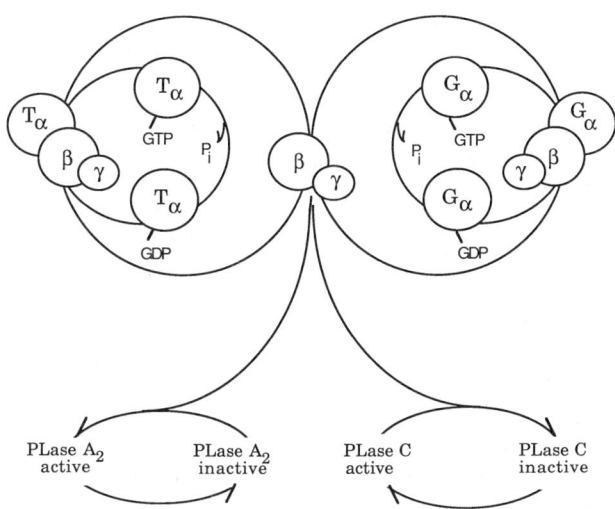

FIGURE 10. Regulation of phospholipase A_2 and phospholipase C activity in bovine retina involves a common stimulatory G protein, transducin, but different inhibitory G proteins. Transducin (T), which dissociates into the T_α and $T_{\beta\gamma}$ subunits upon binding of photolysed rhodopsin and exchange of GTP for GDP, couples the light activation of both phospholipase (PLase) A_2 and phospholipase C.[14,15,25] The mechanism proposed for the transducin-mediated light activation of phospholipase C involves tonic inhibition of the enzyme by the $\beta\gamma$ subunits that are common to all G proteins and are present in membranes in excess of G protein α subunits.[3] The transducin-mediated stimulation of phospholipase C activity occurs by action of the T_α subunit, which blocks the $\beta\gamma$-induced inhibition of the phospholipase by facilitating the reassociation of an inactive $T_{\alpha\beta\gamma}$ heterotrimer. Addition of $T_{\beta\gamma}$ inhibited phospholipase C activity when added to dark-adapted rod outer segments and, under nondissociating conditions, blocked the T_α-induced stimulation of the enzyme. Inhibition of light-activated phospholipase C occurs by GTPγS-induced dissociation of a pertussis toxin–sensitive inhibitory G protein (illustrated here as $G_{\alpha\beta\gamma}$), resulting in release of inhibitory $G_{\beta\gamma}$ subunits. In contrast, in the modulation of phospholipase A_2 activity, the $T_{\beta\gamma}$ subunits stimulated phospholipase A_2 activity, while addition of T_α, under nondissociating conditions, prevented the $\beta\gamma$-induced increase in phospholipase A_2 activity. Phospholipase A_2 activity is also susceptible to inhibitory control, but by a cholera toxin–sensitive G protein (presumed to be G_s but illustrated here as $G_{\alpha\beta\gamma}$) that blocks light-induced phospholipase A_2 activity by interaction of G_α with the stimulatory $\beta\gamma$ subunits. The light activation of the two phospholipases thus occurs by action of a common stimulatory G protein, transducin, but by action of different subunits. Inhibition of light-activated phospholipase A_2, however, occurs by action of a cholera toxin–sensitive G protein, while phospholipase C activity is inhibited by a pertussis toxin–sensitive G protein. In addition, phospholipase C, but not phospholipase A_2, is under tonic inhibitory control by G proteins in this system.

transducin α and $\beta\gamma$ subunits in the modulation of phospholipase A_2 and phospholipase C activity, with the $\beta\gamma$ subunits of transducin stimulating phospholipase A_2 activity while inhibiting phospholipase C activity in the absence of light, and the α subunit inhibiting the $\beta\gamma$-induced increase in phospholipase A_2 while stimulating phospholipase C activity (FIG. 6).[15]

The stimulatory effect of the $\beta\gamma$ subunits on phospholipase A_2 (FIG. 6A), it is suggested, results from inhibition of an inhibitor, rather than by direct activation of the enzyme, as indicated by: (1) the absence of a direct stimulatory effect of the $\beta\gamma$ subunits on enzyme activity in an *in vitro* model system using soluble porcine pancreatic phospholipase A_2 (FIG. 7); (2) the ability of the $\beta\gamma$ subunits of both transducin and G_o to prevent the inhibition of phospholipase A_2 by calpactin, a phospholipase A_2 inhibitor,[44,47] while the α subunits of various G proteins enhanced the inhibition (FIG. 8); (3) the ability of actin, which binds calpactin,[46] to also prevent the calpactin-induced inhibition of phospholipase A_2 (FIG. 9); and (4) the synergistic effect of actin and the $\beta\gamma$ subunits in blocking the calpactin-mediated inhibition of phospholipase A_2 activity (FIG. 9). The physiological relevance of the calpactin-induced inhibition of phospholipase A_2 has been challenged on the basis of its interaction with the phospholipid substrate rather than the enzyme.[44] In addition, studying the effects of the G protein subunits on a soluble rather than a membrane-bound phospholipase A_2 may markedly affect the results. Nevertheless, the absence of a direct stimulatory effect of the $\beta\gamma$ subunits on phospholipase A_2 activity, in combination with their ability to block the calpactin-induced inhibition of the enzyme—particularly in the presence of actin—makes this an attractive model for the $\beta\gamma$-induced increase in phospholipase A_2 activity, although calpactin may not be the physiologically relevant phospholipase A_2 inhibitor in the bovine ROS.

The mechanism proposed for the transducin-mediated, light-induced increase in phospholipase A_2 activity involves interaction of the $\beta\gamma$ subunits of transducin with an inhibitor of phospholipase A_2 (FIG. 10), resulting in activation of the enzyme. Inhibition of light-activated, but not basal, phospholipase A_2 activity occurs by action of a cholera toxin–sensitive G protein, presumably by the release of an α subunit capable of binding and thereby preventing the $\beta\gamma$-induced stimulation of phospholipase A_2. Phospholipase C activity, in contrast, is under tonic inhibitory control by an inhibitory G protein, and the transducin-mediated, light-induced increase in phospholipase C activity occurs by preventing the action of this inhibitory G protein (FIG. 10), resulting in disinhibition of the enzyme activity. In the activation of phospholipase C, however, it appears to be the α subunit of transducin that relieves the inhibition, while the $\beta\gamma$ subunits function to inhibit the stimulatory effect of the α subunit in the absence of light. The light activation of the two phospholipases in bovine ROS thus occurs by action of the same G protein, transducin, but involves fundamentally different mechanisms of action.

REFERENCES

1. STRYER, L., J. B. HURLEY & B. K.-K. FUNG. 1981. Curr. Top. Membr. Transp. **15:** 93–108.
2. BOURNE, H. & L. STRYER. 1986. Annu. Rev. Cell. Biol. **2:** 397–420.
3. GILMAN, A. G. 1987. Annu. Rev. Biochem. **56:** 615–649.
4. ELKS, M. L., P. A. WATKINS, V. C. MANGANIELLO, J. MOSS, E. HEWLETT & M. VAUGHAN. 1983. Biochem. Biophys. Res. Commun. **116:** 593–598.
5. FUNG, B. K.-K., J. B. HURLEY & L. STRYER. 1981. Proc. Natl. Acad. Sci. USA **78:** 152–156.
6. DUNLAP, K., G. G. HOLZ & S. G. RANE. 1987. Trends Neurosci. **10:** 241–244.
7. COHEN-ARMON, M. & M. SOKOLOVSKY. 1986. J. Biol. Chem. **261:** 12498–12505.
8. YATANI, A., J. CODINA, A. M. BROWN & L. BIRNBAUMER. 1987. Science **235:** 207–211.
9. LOGOTHETIS, D. E., Y. KURACHI, J. GALPER, E. NEER & D. E. CLAPHAM. 1987. Nature **325:** 321–326.
10. LEWIS, D. L., F. F. WEIGHT & A. LUINI. 1986. Proc. Natl. Acad. Sci. USA **83:** 9035–9039.
11. COCKCROFT, S. & B. D. GOMPERTS. 1985. Nature **314:** 534–536.
12. UHING, R. J., V. PRPIC, H. JIANG & J. H. EXTON. 1984. J. Biol. Chem. **261:** 2140–2146.
13. UI, M. 1984. Trends Pharmacol. Sci. **5:** 277–279.
14. JELSEMA, C. L. 1987. J. Biol. Chem. **262:** 163–168.

15. JELSEMA, C. L. & J. AXELROD. 1987. Proc. Natl. Acad. Sci. USA **84**: 3623–3627.
16. AXELROD, J., R. M. BURCH & C. L. JELSEMA. 1988. Trends Neurosci. **11**: 117–123.
17. BOKOCH, G. M., T. KATADA, J. K. NORTHUP, M. UI & A. G. GILMAN. 1984. J. Biol. Chem. **259**: 3560–3567.
18. BURCH, R. M., C. L. JELSEMA & J. AXELROD. 1988. J. Pharmacol. Exp. Ther. **244**: 765–773.
19. NAKASHIMA, S., T. TOHMATSU, H. HALTON, A. SUGANAMA & Y. NOZAWA. 1987. J. Biol. Chem. **101**: 1055–1058.
20. FUSE, I. & H.-H. TAI. 1987. Biochem. Biophys. Res. Commun. **146**: 659–665.
21. BURCH, R. M., A. LUINI & J. AXELROD. 1986. Proc. Natl. Acad. Sci. USA **83**: 7201–7205.
22. IRVINE, R. F., A. J. LETCHER & R. M. C. DAWSON. 1979. Biochem. J. **179**: 497–500.
23. MOBLEY, A. & H.-H. TAI. 1985. Biochem. Biophys. Res. Commun. **130**: 717–723.
24. SCHACHT, J. 1976. J. Neurochem. **27**: 1119–1124.
25. JELSEMA, C. L. & J. AXELROD. 1987. *In* Sensory Transduction (Discussions in Neurosciences), Vol. 4. A. J. Hudspeth, P. R. MacLeish, F. L. Margolis & T. N. Wiesel, Eds.: 79–84. Foundations for the Study of the Nervous System. Geneva.
26. GHALAYINI, A. & R. E. ANDERSON. 1984. Biochem. Biophys. Res. Commun. **124**: 503–506.
27. KUHN, H. 1980. Nature **283**: 587–589.
28. STERNWEIS, P. C. & A. G. GILMAN. 1982. Proc. Natl. Acad. Sci. USA **79**: 4888–4891.
29. BAEHR, W., M. J. DEVLIN & M. L. APPLEBURY. 1979. J. Biol. Chem. **254**: 11669–11677.
30. STERNWEIS, P. C. & J. D. ROBISHAW. 1984. J. Biol. Chem. **259**: 13806–13813.
31. LAEMMLI, U. K. 1970. Nature (London) **227**: 680–685.
32. NEER, E. J., J. M. LOK & L. WOLF. 1984. J. Biol. Chem. **259**: 14222–14229.
33. WRAY, W., T. BOULIKAS, V. P. WRAY & R. HANCOCK. 1981. Anal. Biochem. **118**: 197–203.
34. SORIC, J. & J. A. GORDON. 1986. J. Biol. Chem. **261**: 14490–14495.
35. BERRIDGE, M. J. 1983. Biochem. J. **212**: 849–858.
36. ECKSTEIN, F., D. CASSEL, H. LEVKOVITZ, M. LOWE & Z. SELINGER. 1979. J. Biol. Chem. **254**: 9829–9834.
37. VAN DOP, C., G. YAMANAKA, F. STEINBERG, R. D. SEKURA, C. R. MANCLARK, L. STRYER & H. R. BOURNE. 1984. J. Biol. Chem. **259**: 23–26.
38. ABOOD, M. E., J. B. HURLEY, M.-C. PAPPONE, H. R. BOURNE & L. STRYER. 1982. J. Biol. Chem. **257**: 10540–10543.
39. WATKINS, P. A., J. MOSS, D. L. BURNS, E. L. HEWLETT & M. VAUGHAN. 1984. J. Biol. Chem. **259**: 1378–1381.
40. CASSEL, D. & Z. SELINGER. 1977. Proc. Natl. Acad. Sci. USA **74**: 4185–4189.
41. BURNS, D. L., E. L. HEWLETT, J. MOSS & M. VAUGHAN. 1983. J. Biol. Chem. **258**: 1435–1438.
42. HABERMAN, E. 1972. Science **117**: 413–414.
43. BILLAH, M. M., E. G. LAPETINA & P. CUATRECASAS. 1980. J. Biol. Chem. **255**: 10227–10231.
44. DAVIDSON, F. F., E. A. DENNIS, M. POWELL & J. R. GLENNEY. 1987. J. Biol. Chem. **262**: 1698–1705.
45. GLENNEY, J. 1986. J. Biol. Chem. **261**: 7247–7252.
46. KAHN, R. A. & A. G. GILMAN. 1986. J. Biol. Chem. **261**: 7906–7911.
47. HUANG, K. S., B. P. WALLNER, R. J. MATTALIANO, R. TIZARD, C. BURNE, L. FREY, K. L. RAMACHANDRAN, J. TANG, J. E. SMART & R. B. PEPINSKY. 1986. Cell **46**: 191–199.
48. HURLEY, J. B. & L. STRYER. 1982. J. Biol. Chem. **257**: 11094–11099.

Mechanisms Involved in the Action of Prostaglandins as Modulators of Neurotransmission[a]

LARS E. GUSTAFSSON[b]

*Institute of Environmental Medicine and
Department of Physiology
Karolinska Institute
Stockholm, Sweden*

INTRODUCTION

Prostaglandins have a broad spectrum of actions on autonomic neuroeffector transmission. They may alter transmitter release as well as effector responsiveness, and often both effects are present, as originally observed[1] and extensively reviewed.[2-7] The end response is the sum of all the pre- and postjunctional effects. To cover all the possibilities of action one would have to organize the problem into a "Roman square" (FIG. 1). Failure to consider all possibilities for arachidonate action and lack of measurement of transmitter release may well explain some of the earlier controversies concerning whether prostaglandins modulate cholinergic transmitter release, for example, and whether this modulation is stimulatory or inhibitory.[5] Furthermore, species *and* organ differences are likely involved. Most important, prostaglandins of the E type have a strong stimulatory effect on certain smooth muscles, leading to postjunctional enhancement of contractile repsonses. An example will be given below, where it can also be demonstrated that endogenous arachidonate turnover alters effector responsiveness. Transmitter concentration profiles at nerve terminals might be difficult to imitate by the application of exogenous transmitter, and exogenously applied transmitter might act via receptors with characteristics or transducer mechanisms different from those of innervated receptors. Therefore, quantitative analysis of effector response can merely allow *speculations* on whether a simultaneous prejunctional effect is at hand, but *conclusive* evidence requires measurement of transmitter release, often a difficult task. An illustration of how careful analysis must be applied is the situation in the dog trachealis muscle, where interaction between a number of arachidonates with the cholinergic neurotransmission and comparison with interaction with exogenous acetylcholine might suggest a prejunctional effect, whereas analysis of excitatory junction potentials indicates a lack of prejunctional effect.[8] Over the last decade, in different reports the whole spectrum of influence has been suggested (inhibition, no effect, or stimulation) for prostaglandin effects on transmitter release or action,[8-22] although conclusive evidence is often lacking. As measured by transmitter overflow, prostaglandins E_2 and I_2 may inhibit endogenous noradrenaline release in the

---

[a]This work was supported by the Swedish MRC (Projects 7919 and 4342), the Swedish Society of Medicine, the Torsten Foundation, the Ragnar Söderberg Foundation, the Institute of Environmental Medicine, and the Karolinska Institute.

[b]Address for correspondence: Dr. Lars Gustafsson, Department of Physiology, Karolinska Institute, P.O. Box 60 400, S-104 01 Stockholm, Sweden.

rabbit heart,[19] although PGE_2 is a preferential presynaptic and PGI_2 a postsynaptic modulator in the kidney.[23] PGI_2 may increase noradrenaline release in canine isolated veins.[9] Prostaglandins may also inhibit the release of bombesin and somatostatin in the rat stomach,[24] as indicated by the effect of indomethacin on mediator release. Inhibition of cyclooxygenase failed to alter endogenous noradrenaline release in canine skeletal muscle *in vivo*.[25] A thromboxane/endoperoxide mimetic has been shown to increase the overflow of noradrenaline in the isolated vas deferens.[26] The lipoxygenase product 12-HETE (12-hydroxyeicosatetraenoic acid) has been implicated in the modulation of neuron activity by the synaptic action of histamine in *Aplysia*.[27,28] Other neuromodulatory agents may act indirectly via stimulation of cyclooxygenase activity.[29-31]

The mechanism by which transmitter release is altered by prostaglandins is not known. In the cerebral cortex inhibition of spontaneous neuronal activity by vasoactive intestinal peptide (VIP) and noradrenaline might involve an arachidonate-induced increase in cAMP;[30] and in neuroblastoma-glioma cells prostaglandins of the D, E, and F types may increase intracellular cGMP, perhaps secondary to a calcium increase independent of voltage-sensitive calcium channels.[32] Alterations in nerve membrane

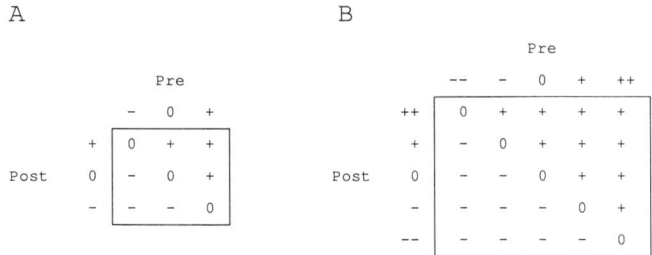

FIGURE 1. Panel A: Theoretical end effect of a neuromodulatory agent with pre- and/or postjunctional action (denoted by Pre and Post, respectively), as organized with a Roman square. + indicates stimulation, − indicates inhibition, 0 indicates no action. End effect (within *square*) can clearly be different from pre- or postjunctional action. Panel B: If the inhibitory and stimulatory pre- or postjunctional actions are graded by introducing just two levels of quantity (thus, + + and − − added), it can easily be realized that the quality of the end effect may even be opposite that of the pre- or postjunctional action.

resting and action potential have been considered as a mechanism for prostaglandin neuromodulation,[2,4] although direct interference with calcium turnover seems a stronger candidate.[2] In peripheral autonomic nerves, the adrenergic agonist clonidine may inhibit transmitter release by modifying the nerve terminal action potential.[33] In the same model system, prostaglandins also inhibit transmitter release, but fail to alter the nerve terminal action potential.[34]

When cyclooxygenase inhibitors are used to block formation of endogenous arachidonate metabolites, confounding effects may be obtained, leading to difficulties in interpretation regarding the role of endogenous prostaglandins in transmitter release. In isolated tissues inhibition of cyclic nucleotide phosphodiesterases is one such action,[35] which could lead to inhibition of contractile responses via smooth muscle relaxation. Other possible effects are calcium antagonism[36,37] or interference with protein phosphorylation.[38,39] In whole organs, inhibition of cyclooxygenase might lead to a decrease in the formation of vasodilator prostaglandins, leading in turn to decreased oxygenation. Hypoxia is a potent stimulus for release not only of prostaglandins but also of purines such as adenosine,[40–42] which usually are vasodilatory, although in the kidney they may induce vasoconstriction.[43–45] Furthermore, adenosine and other purines are effective modulators of adrenergic, cholinergic, and other neurotransmitter release.[5,45,46] The release of purines thus may obscure the effect of cyclooxygenase blockade on neurotransmitter release as well as on effector responses.[47] Whether cyclooxygenase inhibitors may release purines in isolated smooth muscle is presently unclear.

One way of addressing the interaction between arachidonate metabolism and purine release would be to use adenosine receptor antagonists. Alkylxanthines such as

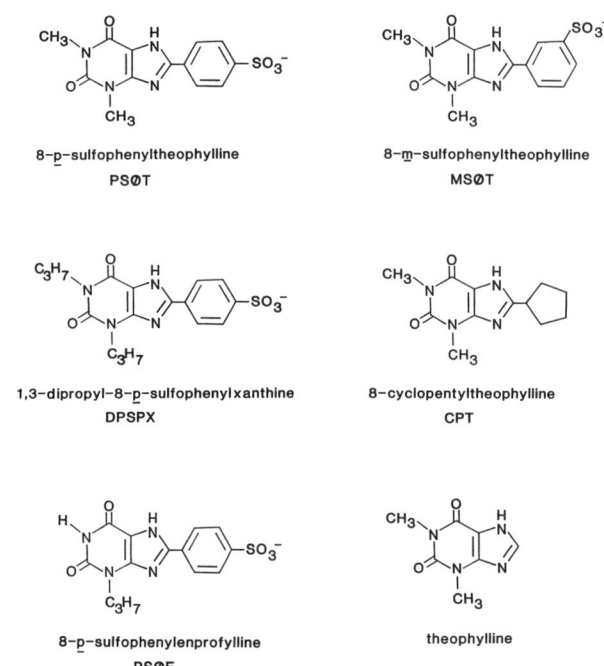

FIGURE 2. Structures and abbreviations for xanthines used in this study.

theophylline are competitive adenosine antagonists, but they are complicated to use due to their phosphodiesterase inhibitory actions.[48] Sulfo derivatives of xanthines may offer an interesting alternative, since they are permanently charged at physiological pH.[48–50] The aim of the present study was to investigate possible pre- and postjunctional effects of PGs and PG synthesis inhibitors, and the effects of these agents on purine overflow; and to try to synthesize some novel sulfo derivatives of alkylxanthines that may be used in studies of the relative role of purine and PG mechanisms in the regulation of neuroeffector transmission. The structures of 8-substituted alkylxanthines used in the present study are given in FIGURE 2. A brief account of the synthesis and partial use of 8-*m*-sulfophenyltheophylline has been presented elsewhere.[51]

METHODS

Smooth Muscle Preparations

Bovine iris sphincter preparations and plexus-containing longitudinal muscle preparations of guinea pig ileum were prepared and stimulated in Tyrode's solution in 5-ml organ baths as previously described.[5,52] Guinea pig urinary bladder smooth muscle was prepared by mounting urinary bladders on a glass rod and removing spiral muscle strips from underlying mucosa. Contractile responses to transmural nerve stimulation (3-Hz, 0.2-ms pulses in groups of 15 at 1-min intervals) were monitored isotonically or isometrically. Stimulation of postganglionic autonomic nerves was verified by application of tetrodotoxin, hexamethonium, or atropine. Release of acetylcholine from ileum preparations was measured before and during stimulation by groups of 840 3-Hz, 1-ms pulses at 20-min intervals in the presence of eserine (3×10^{-6} M).

Quantitation of Acetylcholine

Tissue perifusates were put on ice, immediately adjusted to pH 6 with HCl, and frozen. The content of acetylcholine was assayed on the dorsal muscle of the leech (*Hirudo medicinalis,* kept at 4 °C until ½ h before the experiment). Two muscle strips were obtained from each animal and were mounted at approximately 1 g of tension with an auxotonic lever. The leech muscles were continuously superfused with eserinized Tyrode's solution, 1 ml/min at 25°C, and standards and unknowns were injected into the superfusate immediately before the prewarming coil (delay to contact and contact time approximately 10 s each).

Rabbit Kidney Perfused in Situ

Rabbits (2.5–3.5 kg, either sex) were anesthetized with sodium pentobarbital iv and ventilated via a tracheal cannula. The left kidney was perfused with blood from the carotid artery via a catheter inserted into the renal artery. The catheter was equipped with side branches for drug infusions and monitoring of perfusion pressure. At 10–30 min before the experiments the catheter was connected to a Sigmamotor perfusion pump for perfusion at constant but pulsatile flow, which was set to initially match kidney perfusion pressure against systemic blood pressure, and which was usually obtained at about 10 ml/min. The renal nerve was crushed proximally and placed on electrodes for stimulation distally (pulses of 5–10 Hz, 0.2–1 ms, 2–7 V delivered in 15–60-s series—i.e., 75–600 pulses—at 5–20-min intervals).

Rabbit Kidney Perfused in Vitro

Animals were anesthetized as above and the kidney similarly cannulated. In addition, catheters were placed in the ureter and the renal vein. The kidney was then flushed with saline, moved to an organ chamber at 37°C, and perfused with Tyrode's solution at a constant flow (10 ml/min). Purine release was monitored as release of ^{14}C after preinfusion with 10 μCi ^{14}C-adenine. Nerve stimulation was performed as in the preceding section.

Synthesis of Alkylxanthines

The general procedure for synthesis of alkylxanthines was according to a method for synthesis of 8-*p*-sulfophenyltheophylline,[50] with modifications. An approach with direct sulfonylation was also tried.

I. 8-p-*Sulfophenyltheophylline*

Method 1a. An equimolar (0.005 or 0.01 mol each) solution of 5,6-diamino-1,3-dimethyluracil (Aldrich) and *p*-sulfobenzoic acid (Kodak) was prepared in 20 or 40 ml water and adjusted to pH 6–7. EDAC [1-ethyl-3-(3-dimethylaminopropyl)-carbodiimide, Sigma] was added in 50% excess, and pH was brought to 4–5 by HCl, with further additions of acid until pH was stable. The intermediate formed was either isolated in ice-cold methanol or (the more efficient procedure) cyclized directly by 5 min boiling after addition of 10 M NaOH to a concentration of 2.5 M. Hereafter, the final product (white crystals) was obtained by several reprecipitations in methanol from solutions obtained in dilute NaOH and neutralized by concentrated HCl. The typical yield was 50–70%.

Method 1b. 8-Phenyltheophylline (25 mg, Calbiochem) was directly sulfonylated by heating (approx. 200°C) in concentrated sulfuric acid (0.3 ml), until its color changed to moderate brown. A precipitate was obtained with diethyl ether ion by slowly introducing the chilled sulfuric acid solution into ice-cold diethyl ether (2 ml). Sham-reacted solutions failed to give a precipitate. The precipitate was washed with ether and cold ethanol, dissolved in water, made slightly alkaline by slow introduction into a 6% (w/v) solution of $NaHCO_3$, dried, and redissolved in water. By chromatography (for method, see below) the precipitate was found to contain three major UV-absorbing peaks, one of which co-chromatographed with 8-*p*-sulfophenyltheophylline. The yield was poor, especially with prolonged reaction times.

II. 8-m-*Sulfophenyltheophylline*

8-*m*-Sulfophenyltheophylline was prepared according to Method 1a from 5,6-diamino-1,3-dimethyluracil and *m*-sulfobenzoic acid (Na^+ salt, Kodak). White crystals soluble in water were formed, with a yield of 70%.

III. 8-p-*Sulfophenylenprofylline [3-propyl-8-(p-sulfophenyl)xanthine]*

8-*p*-Sulfophenylenprofylline [3-propyl-8-(*p*-sulfophenyl)xanthine] was prepared from 5,6-diamino-1-propyluracil (courtesy of Dr. G. Kjellin, Draco) and *p*-sulfobenzoic acid (K^+ salt, Kodak) by a modification of Method 1a. Thus, in water or pure methanol a solution of diamine and sulfonic acid could not be simultaneously obtained at the required pH, and carbodiimide coupling was inefficient. In a 55/45 (v/v) water/methanol mixture a good suspension and partial solution of the diamine as well as the sulfonic acid could be prepared. During addition of EDAC, HCl to pH 4–5, with heating (60–70°C), a complete solution was obtained, as the reaction proceeded and methanol evaporated. Cyclization was performed directly by addition of NaOH and boiling. Isolation was accomplished by 2 reprecipitations in methanol at −20°C. White crystals soluble in water, slightly soluble in ethanol or methanol at room temperature, were formed, with a yield of 25%.

Identity of Xanthines

The xanthines (synthesized according to Method 1a with modifications) gave expected proton NMR spectra (courtesy of Dr. Ulla Jacobsson, Royal Technical Institute, Stockholm). 8-p-Sulfophenyltheophylline synthesized according to Method 1a co-chromatographed with and had a UV absorbance spectrum (below) identical to a commercial sample (Research Biochemicals, Natick, MA).

Chromatography and Ultraviolet Spectra

A Nucleosil (Macherey-Nagel) 5-μm C_{18} bonded silica column (4.6 × 200 mm) was eluted at 0.7 ml/min with 30% methanol in 0.01 M ammonium phosphate in water, pH 6. Samples (10–6000 pmol) were dissolved in 0.01 M ammonium phosphate and injected in 10–100 μl. Peaks were detected by monitoring at 254 nm (LDC UV III monitor) followed by an LKB 2140 Rapid Spectral diode array detector allowing repeated (at 2-s intervals) UV spectra from 190 to 350 nm, obtained via sampling on an IBM PC (LKB Wavescan software).

RESULTS AND DISCUSSION

Isolated Smooth Muscle Preparations

Administration of PGE_2 (1–25 × 10^{-9} M) to either guinea pig ileum longitudinal muscle or bovine iris sphincter markedly enhanced contractile responses to postganglionic cholinergic nerve stimulation. The effects were reversible and reproducible (FIG. 3). At higher concentrations (20–50 × 10^{-9} M), an increase in basal tone was obtained. When indomethacin (1–10 x 10^{-6} M) was applied, a decrease in muscle tone was obtained in preparations having a moderate to high basal tone. Moreover, a decrease in contractile responses to nerve stimulation was observed in the iris and ileum preparations. The effects of indomethacin were mimicked by application of eicosatetraynoic acid. Application of PGE_2 enhanced contractile responses to the cholinergic transmitter acetylcholine, whereas eicosatetraynoic acid inhibited these responses (FIG. 3), suggesting a postjunctional stimulatory action of both exogenous and endogenous prostaglandins on the cholinergic neurotransmission. In order to elucidate a prejunctional action, measurement of acetylcholine overflow was made. In six ileum longitudinal muscle preparations, PGE_2 failed to modify the overflow of acetylcholine from eserinized preparations, as quantified on the dorsal muscle of the leech. This outcome is a statistically significant lack of effect at the 5% level of probability. A representative experiment is shown in FIGURE 4. PGE_2 did not modify the sensitivity of the assay muscle to acetylcholine, whereas indomethacin strongly decreased the sensitivity, precluding measurement of acetylcholine overflow in the presence of this compound. Thus a prejunctional effect could not be verified by this method, and the other data suggest that the dominating effect is a postjunctional stimulatory effect of endogenous cyclooxygenase products.

It is of interest that the inhibitory effect of indomethacin on contractile responses to nerve stimulation could not be reversed fully by the application of PGE_2 (FIG. 3). This

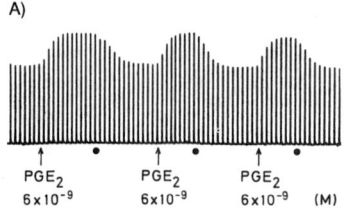
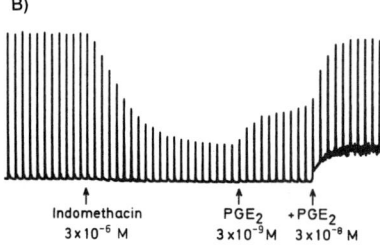
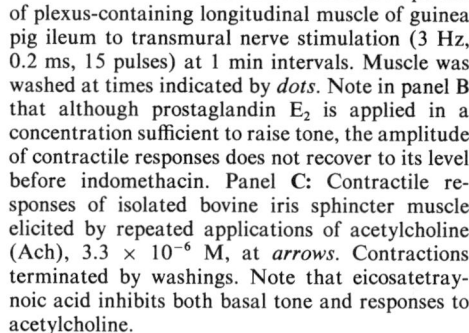
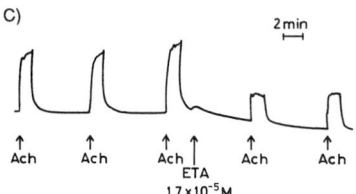

FIGURE 3. Panels **A** and **B**: Contractile responses of plexus-containing longitudinal muscle of guinea pig ileum to transmural nerve stimulation (3 Hz, 0.2 ms, 15 pulses) at 1 min intervals. Muscle was washed at times indicated by *dots*. Note in panel B that although prostaglandin E_2 is applied in a concentration sufficient to raise tone, the amplitude of contractile responses does not recover to its level before indomethacin. Panel **C**: Contractile responses of isolated bovine iris sphincter muscle elicited by repeated applications of acetylcholine (Ach), 3.3×10^{-6} M, at *arrows*. Contractions terminated by washings. Note that eicosatetraynoic acid inhibits both basal tone and responses to acetylcholine.

suggests that there are other actions of indomethacin. In a previous study, we observed that indomethacin could decrease acetylcholine overflow, an effect which was not fully reversed by PGE_2.[53] Thus, either other cyclooxygenase products modulate the neurotransmission by facilitating transmitter release or indomethacin has other inhibitory effects—for example, interference with purine mechanisms, leading to increased purine levels. Preliminary experiments that attempted to monitor purine overflow from ileum preparations after incubation with ^{14}C-adenine failed because of a high basal release of purines, which was perhaps due to interfering effects such as tissue hypoxia

FIGURE 4. Overflow of acetylcholine in the guinea pig ileum longitudinal muscle, as quantified on the dorsal muscle of the leech (*Hirudo medicinalis*). Note the lack of effect of prostaglandin on both basal (*short columns*) and stimulation-evoked (*tall columns*) transmitter overflow.

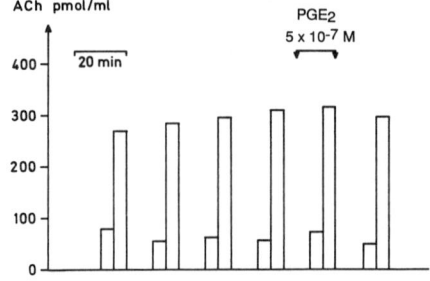

(data not shown). Therefore, a perfused organ—the isolated kidney—was investigated.

Isolated Rabbit Kidney

Upon preinfusion with ^{14}C-adenine, the kidney exhibited a reproducible outflow of radioactivity after an initial 20-min rinsing period (FIG. 5). The tissue labeling is mainly in adenine nucleotides, and the outflow of purines consists mainly of inosine, hypoxanthine, and adenosine.[54] Increments in purine overflow were obtained during renal nerve stimulation. During infusion of indomethacin ($1-10 \times 10^{-6}$ M) (FIG. 5) or aspirin (data not shown), marked augmentation of basal purine overflow was obtained. Usually, both vasoconstrictor responses[47] as well as purine outflow (FIG. 5), elicited by renal nerve stimulation, were increased during infusion of cyclooxygenase inhibitor. The vasoconstrictor effect of indomethacin as well as the enhancement of responses to renal nerve stimulation by indomethacin were augmented by infusion of the adenosine uptake inhibitors dipyridamole or dilazep ($1-100 \times 10^{-6}$ M).

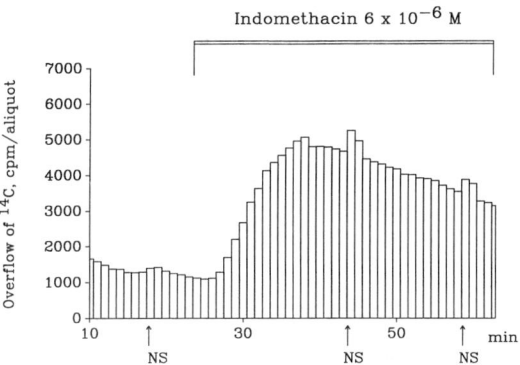

FIGURE 5. Overflow of ^{14}C in isolated perfused (Tyrode's solution) rabbit kidney after preinfusion of 10 μCi ^{14}C-adenine. Renal nerve stimulation (5-Hz, 1-ms pulses delivered in 60-s series—i.e., 300 pulses—at 10-20-min intervals) is indicated by NS. There was increased outflow of radiolabel during infusion of indomethacin.

Rabbit Kidney in Vivo

In order to verify that the effect of indomethacin was present also *in vivo*, experiments were performed in anesthetized rabbits. Intravenous infusion of indomethacin caused effects similar to those of the adenosine uptake inhibitor dilazep, leading to increased perfusion pressure and increased responses to renal nerve stimulation in the *in situ* blood-perfused kidney. Furthermore, combination of intravenous indomethacin and dilazep gave more than additive effects in inducing vasoconstriction and especially in enhancing responses to renal nerve stimulation (FIG. 6).

Intravenous administration of equimolar amounts of the adenosine antagonists theophylline or 8-*p*-sulfophenyltheophylline antagonized the effects of both indomethacin and dilazep. However, theophylline also had the capacity to decrease both systemic blood pressure and renal perfusion pressure, even in the presence of adenosine receptor blockade by 8-*p*-sulfophenyltheophylline (FIG. 6). One explanation for this might be that there is an intracellular effect such as the accumulation of cAMP due to the capacity of theophylline to inhibit the phosphodiesterase, since the nonpenetrating xanthine 8-*p*-sulfophenyltheophylline[48–50] had much less vasodilator effect and often instead increased systemic blood pressure (FIG. 6).

Sulfophenyl Alkylxanthines

In order to obtain a set of sulfophenylxanthines with, it was hoped, different capacities as adenosine antagonists, two novel alkylxanthines were synthesized; 8-*m*-sulfophenyltheophylline and 8-*p*-sulfophenylenprofylline. These compounds should share with 8-*p*-sulfophenyltheophylline the characteristic of remaining mainly

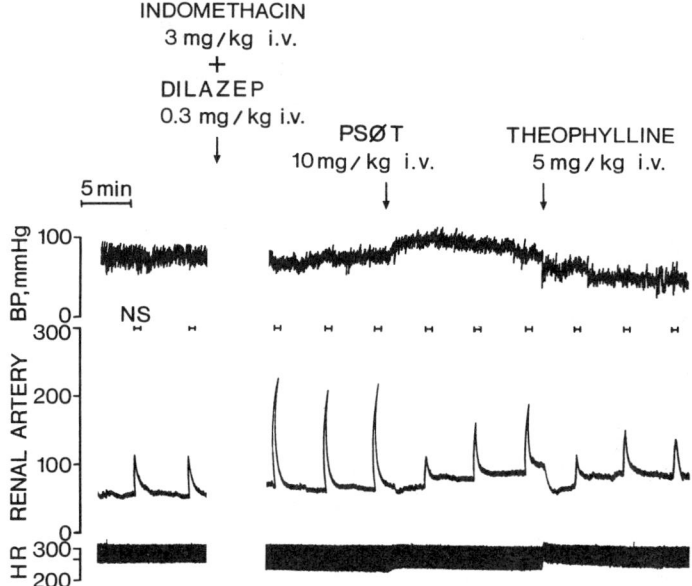

FIGURE 6. Systemic (femoral) arterial pressure (BP, *top panel*), renal perfusion pressure (Renal Artery, *middle panel*) and heart rate (HR, *bottom panel*) of the anesthetized rabbit. Renal nerve stimulation (NS; 3-Hz, 1-ms pulses delivered in 30-s series—i.e., 90 pulses—at 5-min intervals) is indicated by *horizontal bars*. Note the augmenting effect of dilazep and indomethacin iv, and the antagonism of this effect by 8-*p*-sulfophenyltheophylline (PSØT) and theophylline.

extracellular, due to the presence of the sulfo group. Thus they should have negligible effect on phosphodiesterases and in consequence be devoid of the ability to directly affect smooth muscle relaxation. They should thereby offer tools that would allow correlations between their capacity as adenosine antagonists and their capacity to alter biological responses, thus permitting firmer conclusions regarding the involvement of purine effects at adenosine receptors in such responses. The enprofylline analog was chosen for synthesis because enprofylline has been shown to be a weak adenosine antagonist with some selectivity for certain types of adenosine effects.[55] The 8-*m*-sulfophenyltheophylline compound was chosen for synthesis because *meta* substituents on the 8-phenyl ring might reduce receptor affinity.[56] Low affinity was an

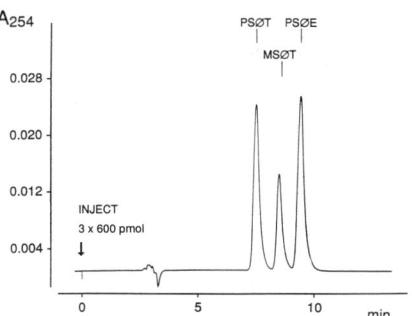

FIGURE 7. Separation of 8-sulfophenyl xanthines on a Nucleosil 5-μm C_{18} column (4.9 × 200 mm, mobile phase: 30% methanol in 0.01 M ammonium phosphate (v/v), pH 6, 0.7 ml/min). At *arrow* 600 pmol of each of the xanthines was injected. Abbreviations as in FIGURE 2.

explicit objective because a compound with relatively high affinity was already at hand (1,3-dipropyl-8-*p*-sulfophenylxanthine, DPSPX);[50] to obtain a set of sulfo compounds with a great range of affinities, a low-affinity compound would have to be found. A simple method, which included direct cyclization, was first established by trying alterations in an existing method for the synthesis of 8-*p*-sulfophenyltheophylline.[50] The result was verified by an alternate method of synthesis, direct sulfonylation. When chromatographed alone, the xanthines synthesized according to Method 1a gave single chromatographic peaks and could be resolved upon simultaneous injection into the chromatograph (FIG. 7). 8-*p*-sulfophenyltheophylline and 8-*p*-sulfophenylenprofylline had nearly identical UV absorbance spectra (FIG. 8). The capacity of the xanthines to

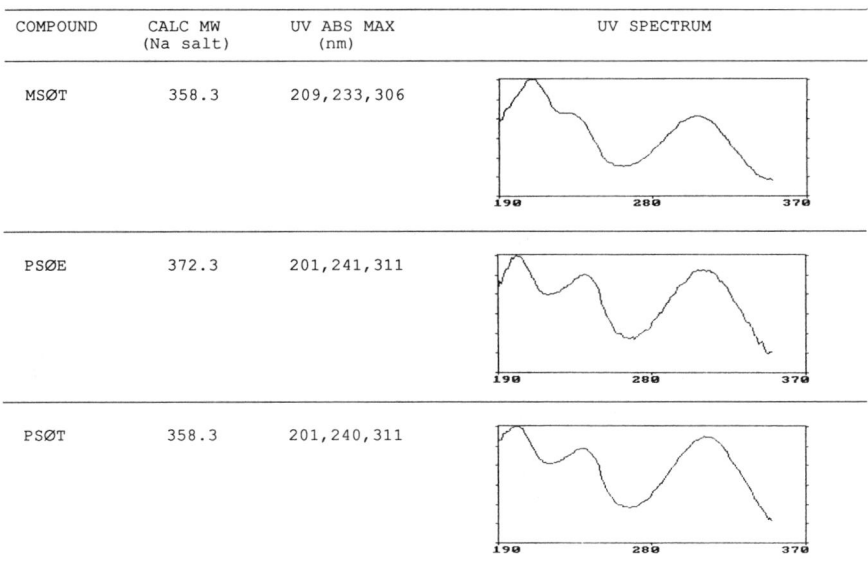

FIGURE 8. Calculated molecular weights, ultraviolet absorbance maxima, and absorbance spectra for the xanthines as obtained online in HPLC solvent, pH 6. Abbreviations as in FIGURE 2.

antagonize adenosine effects were characterized in guinea pig ileum and urinary bladder models, which are representative of prejunctional and postjunctional effects of adenosine, respectively.[57] Comparison was made with two other known alkylxanthine adenosine antagonists,[50,58] 8-cyclopentyltheophylline and 1,3-dipropyl-8-p-sulfophenylxanthine (FIG. 2).

All the 8-substituted xanthines investigated showed competitive adenosine receptor antagonism, as analyzed by Schild plot analysis. As can be seen from TABLE 1, 1,3-dipropyl-8-p-sulfophenylxanthine, 8-p-sulfophenyltheophylline, and 8-p-sulfophenylenprofylline were nonselective between the two different models for adenosine action. 8-cyclopentyltheophylline was quite selective for the prejunctional effect of adenosine in the guinea pig ileum (A_1 receptor), whereas 8-m-sulfophenyltheophylline was moderately selective for the postjunctional smooth muscle relaxing effect of adenosine in the guinea pig urinary bladder (A_2 receptor). None of the sulfonic derivatives showed smooth muscle relaxing action per se, whereas 8-cyclopentyltheophylline exhibited some inhibitory action at 10^{-6} M and above. Since the potencies of the sulfo derivatives exhibited a range between 10^{-7} M to 10^{-4} M, this series of compounds offers blockers with the required range of potencies necessary for analysis of the biological role of purines in physiological situations. They should be of utility also in situations with pharmacological manipulation—for example, with cyclooxygenase inhibitors having putative indirect actions via interference with purine mechanisms. The usefulness of the sulfo derivatives has been verified by the demonstration of

TABLE 1. Adenosine Antagonism by 8-Substituted Alkylxanthines as Quantified by Schild Analysis

	Guinea Pig		
Antagonist	Ileum (A_1 Receptor)	Bladder (A_2 Receptor)	Ratio A_2/A_1
PSØT	5.8	5.9	1.26
MSØT	4.5	5.3	6.3
PSØE	4.3	4.4	1.26
DPSPX	6.8	7.0	1.6
CPT	7.3	6.1	0.063

NOTE: Data are pA_2 values for the antagonism by the xanthines of inhibitory effects of 2-chloroadenosine (ileum) or 5'-N-ethylcarboxamide-adenosine (bladder) on contractile responses to nerve stimulation. Abbreviations as in FIGURE 2.

a regulatory role of adenosine on skeletal muscle microvessels *in vivo*, studied by intravital microscopy.[59] By means of these compounds, further analysis of the relative role of purines and prostaglandins in the regulation of neurotransmission is presently under way.

CONCLUSIONS

Prostaglandins exert powerful postjunctional effects leading to the enhancement of cholinergic neurotransmission in some systems. A prejunctional effect is not demonstrable, either because it is nonexistent or because of inherent methodological problems. In adrenergic neurotransmission both PGE_2 and PGI_2 may inhibit neurotransmitter release. Other cyclooxygenase products, such as thromboxane/endoperoxides, might be prejunctional stimulators. In several systems studies of effector responses indicate both stimulatory, inhibitory, or no effects of various arachidonates on neuroeffector transmission. The role of endogenous arachidonate metabolites as studied by cyclooxygenase inhibitors might be difficult to evaluate because of interference, by the inhibitors, with purine mechanisms in turn modulating neurotransmission pre- or postjunctionally. A series of 8-substituted alkylxanthines—including two novel sulfonic derivatives—that are adenosine receptor antagonists is suggested for use in these situations.

ACKNOWLEDGMENTS

Dr. Ulla Jacobsson kindly performed NMR analysis. The skillful technical assistance of Ms. Ulla Palmertz and Ms. Lena Stelius is gratefully acknowledged.

REFERENCES

1. HEDQVIST, P. & J. BRUNDIN. 1969. Inhibition by prostaglandin E_1 of noradrenaline release and of effector response to nerve stimulation in the cat spleen. Life Sci. **8:** 389–395.
2. HEDQVIST, P. 1977. Basic mechanisms of prostaglandin action on autonomic neurotransmission. Annu. Rev. Pharmacol. Toxicol. **17:** 259–279.
3. STARKE, K. 1977. Regulation of noradrenaline release by presynaptic receptor systems. Rev. Physiol. Biochem. Pharmacol. **77:** 1–124.
4. WESTFALL, T. C. 1977. Local regulation of adrenergic neurotransmission. Physiol. Rev. **57:** 659–728.
5. GUSTAFSSON, L. 1980. Studies on modulation of transmitter release and effector responsiveness in autonomic cholinergic neurotransmission. Acta Physiol. Scand. **110** (Suppl. 489): 1–28.
6. GÜLLNER, H.-G. 1983. The interactions of prostaglandins with the sympathetic nervous system—A review. J. Auton. Nerv. Syst. **8:** 1–12.
7. WENNMALM, M. 1987. Purines and prostaglandins as modulators of adrenergic neurotransmission in the isolated rabbit heart. Thesis, Karolinska Institutet, Stockholm.
8. SERIO, R. & E. E. DANIEL. 1988. Thromboxane effects on canine trachealis neuromuscular function. J. Appl. Physiol. **64:** 1979–1988.
9. HERMAN, A. G., T. J. VERBEUREN, S. MONCADA & P. M. VANHOUTTE. 1978. Effect of prostacyclin on myogenic activity and adrenergic neuroeffector interaction in canine isolated veins. Prostaglandins **16:** 911–921.
10. HEMKER, D. P. & J. W. AIKEN. 1980. Modulation of autonomic neurotransmission by PGD_2: Comparison with effects of other prostaglandins in anesthetized cats. Prostaglandins. **20:** 321–332.
11. BEDWANI, J. R. & S. E. HILL. 1980. Facilitation of sympathetic neurotransmission in the rat anococcygeus muscle by prostaglandins D_2 and F_2. Br. J. Pharmacol. **69:** 609–614.
12. NAKAHATA, N., H. NAKANISHI & T. SUZUKI. 1980. A possible negative feedback control of excitatory transmission via prostaglandins in canine small intestine. Br. J. Pharmacol. **68:** 393–398.
13. NAKAHATA, N., H. NAKANISHI & T. SUZUKI. 1980. Difference between the inhibitory actions of prostaglandins E_1 and verapamil in canine small intestine. Eur. J. Pharmacol. **63:** 335–340.
14. TRACHTE, G. J. 1985. The influence of prostaglandins on neurotransmission in the rabbit isolated vas deferens. Prostaglandins **29:** 47–59.
15. FULLER, R. W., C. M. DIXON, C. T. DOLLERY & P. J. BARNES. 1986. Prostaglandin D_2 potentiates airway responsiveness to histamine and methacholine. Am. Rev. Respir. Dis. **133:** 252–254.

16. DANIEL, E. E., C. DAVIS & V. SHARMA. 1987. Effects of endogenous and exogenous prostaglandin in neurotransmission in canine trachea. Can. J. Physiol. Pharmacol. **65:** 1433–1441.
17. TAMAOKI, J., K. SEKIZAWA, P. D. GRAF & J. A. NADEL. 1987. Cholinergic neuromodulation by prostaglandin D_2 in canine airway smooth muscle. J. Appl. Physiol. **63:** 1396–1400.
18. TAMAOKI, J., K. SEKIZAWA, M. L. OSBORNE, I. F. UEKI, P. D. GRAF & J. A. NADEL. 1987. Platelet aggregation increases cholinergic neurotransmission in canine airway. J. Appl. Physiol. **62:** 2246–2251.
19. WENNMALM, M., G. A. FITZGERALD, A. WENNMALM. 1987. Prostacyclin as a neuromodulator in the sympathetically stimulated rabbit heart. Prostaglandins **33:** 675–692.
20. YOSHITOMI, T. & Y. ITO. 1988. Effects of indomethacin and prostaglandins on the dog iris sphincter and dilator muscles. Invest. Ophthalmol. Vis. Sci. **29:** 127–132.
21. AGRAWAL, D. K., S. BHIMJI & J. H. MCNEILL. 1987. Effect of chronic experimental diabetes on vascular smooth muscle function in rabbit carotid artery. J. Cardiovasc. Pharmacol. **9:** 584–593.
22. GUSTAFSSON, B. I. & D. S. DELBRO. 1988. Effects of indomethacin on non-adrenergic, non-cholinergic motility of stomach and small intestine. Eur. J. Pharmacol. **147:** 67–72.
23. HEDQVIST, P. 1979. Actions of prostacyclin (PGI_2) on adrenergic neuroeffector transmission in the rabbit kidney. Prostaglandins **17:** 249–258.
24. BENDER, H., A. PFEFFER & V. SCHUSDZIARRA. 1987. Effect of indomethacin on bombesin-like immunoreactivity, somatostatin and gastrin secretion from rat stomach. Clin. Physiol. Biochem. **5:** 268–275.
25. KAHAN, T. 1987. Prejunctional adrenergic receptors and sympathetic neurotransmission: Studies in canine skeletal muscle vasculature *in situ*. Acta Physiol. Scand. **560:** 1–38.
26. TRACHTE, G. J. 1986. Thromboxane agonist (U46619) potentiates norepinephrine efflux from adrenergic nerves. J. Pharmacol. Exp. Ther. **237:** 473–477.
27. PIOMELLI, D., A. VOLTERRA, N. DALE, S. A. SIEGELBAUM, E. R. KANDEL, J. H. SCHWARTZ & F. BELARDETTI. 1987. Lipoxygenase metabolites of arachidonic acid as second messengers for presynaptic inhibition of Aplysia sensory cells. Nature **328:** 38–43.
28. PIOMELLI, D., E. SHAPIRO, S. J. FEINMARK & J. H. SCHWARTZ. 1987. Metabolites of arachidonic acid in the nervous system of Aplysia: Possible mediators of synaptic modulation. J. Neurosci. **7:** 3675–3686.
29. SAYE, J., S. B. BINDER, G. J. TRACHTE & M. J. PEACH. 1986. Angiotensin peptides and prostaglandin E_2 synthesis: Modulation of neurogenic responses in the rabbit vas deferens. Endocrinology **119:** 1895–1903.
30. SCHAAD, N. C., M. SCHORDERET & P. J. MAGISTRETTI. 1987. Prostaglandins and the synergism between VIP and noradrenaline in the cerebral cortex. Nature **328:** 637–640.
31. WIKLUND, N. P. & L. E. GUSTAFSSON. 1988. Agonist and antagonist characterization of the P_2-purinoceptors in the guinea pig ileum. Acta Physiol. Scand. **132:** 15–21.
32. MIWA, N., H. SUGINO, R. UENO & O. HAYAISHI. 1988. Prostaglandin induces Ca^{2+} influx and cyclic GMP formation in mouse neuroblastoma X rat glioma hybrid NG108-15 cells in culture. J. Neurochem. **50:** 1418–1424.
33. BROCK, J. A. & T. C. CUNNANE. 1987. Characteristic features of transmitter release from sympathetic nerve terminals. Blood Vessels **24:** 253–260.
34. BROCK, J. A. & T. C. CUNNANE. 1987. Investigation of the mechanism of inhibition by prostaglandin E_1 of electrically evoked transmitter release from sympathetic nerves of the guinea-pig vas deferens *in vitro* J. Physiol.(London) **394:** 11P.
35. GRYGLEWSKI, R. J. 1979. Screening and assessment of the potency of anti-inflammatory drugs *in vitro*. Handb. Exp. Pharmacol. **50, II:** 3–43.
36. NORTHOVER, B. J. 1971. Mechanism of the inhibitory action of indomethacin on smooth muscle. Br. J. Pharmacol. **41:** 540–564.
37. NORTHOVER, B. J. 1977. Indomethacin—a calcium antagonist. Gen. Pharmacol. **8:** 293–296.
38. KANTOR, H. S. & M. HAMPTON. 1978. Indomethacin in submicromolar concentrations inhibits cyclic AMP-dependent protein kinase. Nature **276:** 841–842.
39. CATALÁN, R. E., M. D. ARAGONES, A. M. MARTINEZ, M. ARMIJO & M. PINA. 1980. Effect of indomethacin on the cyclic AMP-dependent protein kinase. Eur. J. Pharmacol. **63:** 187–190.

40. FREDHOLM, B. B., P. HEDQVIST, K. LINDSTRÖM & M. WENNMALM. 1982. Release of nucleosides from the rabbit heart by sympathetic nerve stimulation. Acta Physiol. Scand. **116:** 285–295.
41. EDLUND, A., B. B. FREDHOLM, P. PATRIGNANI, C. PATRONO, Å. WENNMALM & M. WENNMALM. 1983. Release of two vasodilators, adenosine and prostacyclin, from isolated rabbit hearts during controlled hypoxia. J. Physiol. **340:** 487–501.
42. BERNE, R. M., J. M. GIDDAY, H. E. HILL, R. R. CURNISH & R. RUBIO. 1987. Adenosine in the local regulation of blood flow: Some controversies. *In* Topics and Perspectives in Adenosine Research. E. Gerlach & B. F. Becker, Eds: 395–405. Springer-Verlag. Berlin.
43. OSSWALD, H. 1975. Renal effects of adenosine and their inhibition by theophylline in dogs. Naunyn-Schmiedeberg's Arch. Pharmacol. **288:** 79–86.
44. HEDQVIST, P. & B. B. FREDHOLM. 1976. Effects of adenosine on adrenergic neurotransmission; Prejunctional inhibition and postjunctional enhancement. Naunyn-Schmiedeberg's Arch. Pharmacol. **293:** 217–223.
45. FREDHOLM, B. B. & P. HEDQVIST. 1980. Modulation of neurotransmission by purine nucleotides and nucleosides. Biochem. Pharmacol. **29:** 1635–1643.
46. FREDHOLM, B. B., M. DUNER-ENGSTRÖM, J. FASTBOM, B. JONZON, E. LINDGREN, C. NORDSTEDT, F. PEDATA & I. VAN DER PLOEG. 1987. Interactions between the neuromodulator adenosine and the classic transmitters. *In* Topics and Perspectives in Adenosine Research. E. Gerlach & B. F. Becker. Eds.: 505–520. Springer-Verlag. Berlin.
47. GUSTAFSSON, L. E. 1985. Interaction between prostaglandin and purine systems on neurotransmission in the kidney. *In* Advances in Prostaglandin, Thromboxane, and Leukotriene Research, Vol. 15. O. Hayaishi & S. Yamamoto, Eds.: 565–567. Raven Press. New York, NY.
48. GUSTAFSSON, L. E. 1984. Adenosine antagonism and related effects of theophylline derivatives in guinea pig ileum longitudinal muscle. Acta Physiol. Scand. **122:** 191–198.
49. DALY, J. W. 1982. Adenosine receptors: Targets for future drugs. J. Med. Chem. **25:** 197–207.
50. DALY, J. W., W. PADGETT, M. T. SHAMIM, P. BUTTS-LAMB & J. WATERS. 1985. 1,3-Dialkyl-8-(p-sulfophenyl)xanthines: Potent water-soluble antagonists for A_1 and A_2-adenosine receptors. J. Med. Chem. **28:** 487–492.
51. GUSTAFSSON, L. E., A. ÖHLEN, M. PERSSON & P. HEDQVIST. 1987. Evidence for physiological role of purines in regulation of mammalian skeletal muscle vascular tone. *In* Microcirculation—An Update, Vol. 2. M. Tsuchiya, M. Asano, Y. Mishima & M. Oda, Eds.: 525–526. Elsevier. Amsterdam.
52. GUSTAFSSON, L. E., N. P. WIKLUND, J. LUNDIN & P. HEDQVIST. 1985. Characterization of pre- and postjunctional adenosine receptors in guinea-pig ileum. Acta Physiol. Scand. **123:** 195–203.
53. GUSTAFSSON, L., P. HEDQVIST & G. LUNDGREN. 1980. Pre- and postjunctional effects of prostaglandin E_2, prostaglandin synthetase inhibitors and atropine on cholinergic neurotransmission in guinea pig ileum and bovine iris. Acta Physiol. Scand. **110:** 401–411.
54. FREDHOLM, B. B. & P. HEDQVIST. 1978. Release of ^{3}H-purines from [^{3}H]-adenine labelled rabbit kidney following sympathetic nerve stimulation, and its inhibition by α-adrenoceptor blockade. Br. J. Pharmacol. **64:** 239–245.
55. FREDHOLM, B. B. & C. G. PERSSON. 1982. Xanthine derivatives as adenosine receptor antagonists. Eur. J. Pharmacol. **81:** 673–676.
56. BRUNS, R. F., J. W. DALY & S. H. SNYDER. 1983. Adenosine receptor binding: Structure-activity analysis generates extremely potent xanthine antagonists. Proc. Natl. Acad. Sci. USA **80:** 2077–2080.
57. GUSTAFSSON, L. E. 1987. The guinea pig urinary bladder as a model for adenosine A_2 receptors. Abstracts, Tenth International Congress of Pharmacology, Sydney, August 23–28, 1987: 0230.
58. BRUNS, R. F., G. H. LU & T. A. PUGSLEY. 1987. Adenosine receptor subtypes: Binding studies. *In* Topics and Perspectives in Adenosine Research. E. Gerlach & B. F. Becker, Eds.: 59–73. Springer. Berlin.
59. GUSTAFSSON, L. E., M. G. PERSSON, A. ÖHLEN, P. HEDQVIST & L. LINDBOM. 1989. Adenosine modulation of vascular tone in skeletal muscle of the rabbit. Naunyn-Schmiedeberg's Arch. Pharmacol. Physiol. In press.

The Role of Arachidonic Acid and Its Metabolites in the Release of Neuropeptides[a]

SERGIO R. OJEDA,[b] HENRYK F. URBANSKI,[b]
MARIE-PIERRE JUNIER,[c] AND JORGE CAPDEVILA[d]

[b]Division of Neuroscience
Oregon Regional Primate Research Center
Beaverton, Oregon 97006

[c]Unité de Radioimmunologic Analytique
Institute Pasteur
75724 Paris, France

[d]Department of Medicine and Biochemistry
Vanderbilt Medical School
Nashville, Tennessee 37232

THE METABOLISM OF ARACHIDONIC ACID

Arachidonic acid is derived from the essential fatty acid linoleic acid. It is transformed into a variety of biologically active metabolites via three main enzymatic pathways, which are initiated by either cyclooxygenase, lipoxygenase, or epoxygenase activities. While activation of the cyclooxygenase pathway leads to the biosynthesis of prostaglandins (PGs) and thromboxanes,[1] lipoxygenation of arachidonic acid via either 5-, 12- or 15-lipoxygenase enzymes results in the formation of leukotrienes and several hydroxy acids (HETEs) (for references and review, see References 1 and 2).

More recently, a NADPH-dependent, cytochrome P-450-mediated monooxygenation of arachidonic acid that results in the formation of a series of regioisomeric epoxyeicosatrienoic acids has been described.[3] The enzymatic activity that initiates the metabolism of arachidonic acid through this pathway has been termed epoxygenase.[4]

THE PRESENCE OF ARACHIDONIC ACID METABOLITES IN THE BRAIN

The presence of PGs in the brain was recognized more than 20 years ago,[5] an initial finding that was rapidly confirmed and extended by other investigators (for references see Reference 6). Several years later, evidence was provided that the brain can also metabolize arachidonic acid to thromboxane B_2, and that this compound is, in fact, a major cyclooxygenase product in the cerebral cortex.[7] Very recently, the leukotrienes LTC_4, LTD_4, and LTE_4 have been isolated from incubates of rat brain, and regional differences in LTC_4 synthesis have been reported.[8] Another product of lipoxygenase

---

[a]This work was supported by National Institutes of Health Grants RR-00163 and HD-09988 (Project IV). Publication No. 1617 from the Oregon Regional Primate Research Center, Beaverton, Oregon.

activity produced in the brain is 12-HETE, which has been isolated from the cerebral cortex[9] and found to be a predominant lipoxygenase product in the rat hypothalamus.[10] The capacity of brain tissue to metabolize arachidonic acid through the epoxygenase pathway has also been demonstrated in the rat hypothalamus.[4,11] Incubation of hypothalamic microsomes with exogenous ^{14}C-labeled arachidonic acid has been shown to result in the NADPH-dependent formation of several metabolites, among which 5, 6-epoxyeicosatrienoic acid (5, 6-EET) and its hydration product 5, 6-dihydroeicosatrienoic acid (5, 6-DHET), have been identified by mass spectrometric analysis.[4] The other regioisomeric epoxy acids 8, 9–11, 12-, and 14, 15-EET have recently been found to be endogenous constituents of the hypothalamus.[11] Thus, it is clear that the central nervous system (CNS) has the capability of producing an entire spectrum of arachidonic acid metabolites. The function of these substances, however, is still incompletely understood.

ARACHIDONIC ACID METABOLITES AND NEUROPEPTIDE RELEASE

Recent reports have begun to explore the functional relationship between neuropeptides and arachidonic acid metabolites in peripheral systems[12,13] and the cerebral vasculature.[14] For instance, evidence has been presented that vasoactive intestinal peptide (VIP) and calcitonin gene-related peptide (CGRP) inhibit LTC_4 release from lung tissue,[12] and that substance P increases arachidonic acid release and prostaglandin E_2 (PGE_2) synthesis in iris sphincter muscle.[13] Both substance P and VIP have been shown to dilate cerebral blood vessels, possibly by stimulating PG-induced cyclic AMP formation.[14] In a series of elegant experiments, and taking advantage of the simple nervous system of the mollusc aplysia, Piomelli and colleagues have provided unambiguous evidence that lipoxygenase metabolites mediate the inhibitory synaptic actions that the neuropeptide FMRF amide exerts on sensory neurons.[15,16] The inhibitory effect of FMRF amide was reproduced by arachidonate, suppressed by an inhibitor of phospholipase activity, and mimicked by 12-hydroperoxyeicosatetraenoic acid (12-HPETE). Moreover, FMRF amide stimulated the formation of the stable hydroxy acids 5-hydroxyeicosatetraenoic acid (5-HETE) and 12-HETE from clusters of sensory neurons dissected from pleural ganglia.

Most of what is known about the involvement of arachidonic acid metabolites in neuropeptide release in mammals, however, has been derived from studies concerning a family of neuropeptides that control the secretion of anterior pituitary hormones. These peptides are produced in several brain areas, but they are preferentially synthesized in the hypothalamus. Two of them, luteinizing hormone-releasing hormone (LHRH) and somatostatin (SRIF), will be discussed in more detail in this article. The former controls the secretion of pituitary gonadotropins and also appears to exert modulatory effects within the CNS. The latter exerts a tonic inhibitory influence on the release of growth hormone from the adenohypophysis and modulates CNS synaptic transmission.

LUTEINIZING HORMONE–RELEASING HORMONE

The first indication that PGs were involved in the process of LHRH release was provided independently by two laboratories that showed that PGE_1 or PGE_2 injected into the third ventricle of the rat brain induced release of luteinizing hormone (LH) into the blood stream.[17,18] A similar injection into the anterior pituitary gland was ineffective[17] and thus strongly implicated the CNS as the site of action for the PGs to stimulate LH release. Direct confirmation of this inference was provided by the finding that intraventricular injection of PGE_2 increased LHRH in both hypophyseal portal plasma and the venous effluent from the brain.[19,20] Further confirmation came from the finding that PGE_2-induced LH release could be prevented by administration of antibodies to LHRH.[21]

PGE_2 appears to act at two main anatomical sites to bring about LHRH release: the medial basal hypothalamus–median eminence region and the preoptic–anterior hypothalamic area.[22] That PGE_2 acts directly within the LHRH-secreting neurons has been suggested by *in vivo* pharmacological studies that demonstrated that neither monoaminergic, cholinergic, nor serotoninergic receptor blockers were able to prevent the release of LH induced by intracerebral injection of PGE_2.[23]

Experiments involving *in vivo* suppression of PG synthesis have further supported a physiological role for PGs in the mechanism of LHRH release. In ewes, the administration of indomethacin, an inhibitor of cyclooxygenase, has been shown to suppress the increase in LH secretion induced by estradiol in the face of an increased pituitary responsiveness to LHRH.[24] In the rat, indomethacin depresses the high LH levels seen in ovariectomized animals, inhibits pulsatile LH release, prevents the postcastration rise in LH that follows gonadectomy, and inhibits the LH discharge induced by ovarian steroids, also in spite of uninhibited pituitary responsiveness to LHRH.[25] 5, 8, 11, 14-eicosatetraynoic acid, an inhibitor of enzymatic arachidonic acid metabolism, also depresses plasma LH levels when injected intraventricularly into ovariectomized rats.[25] Other investigators have demonstrated that microinjection of aspirin, a nonsteroidal inhibitor of cyclooxygenase activity, into the anterior hypothalamus suppresses progesterone-induced ovulation.[26] Furthermore, the microinjection of N-0164, a PGE and thromboxane antagonist, into the medial basal hypothalamic–median eminence region of proestrous rats has been shown to suppress the preovulatory LH surge,[27] as judged by the inhibition of ovulation. In female rabbits, the release of LH induced by cervical stimulation is preceded by an increase in PGE_2 levels in the cerebrospinal fluid;[28] administration of melatonin abolishes not only the increase in PGE_2 formation but also the LH surge, thus suggesting that PGE_2 is a component in the sequence of events by which cervical-vaginal stimulation induces reflex LH secretion in this species.

The development of *in vitro* systems either to perifuse hypothalamic fragments[29] or to statically incubate median eminence (ME) nerve terminals[30] has permitted the assessment of the formation of PGE_2 in hypothalamic tissue in response to neurotransmitters and the establishment of the relationship of this formation of PGE_2 to LHRH release.

The first *in vitro* evidence that PGE_2 is an effective stimulator of LHRH release was obtained in a perifusion system of hypothalamic fragments that included the preoptic area and the medial basal hypothalamus.[29] In other experiments, exposure of ME fragments to norepinephrine (NE), a neurotransmitter known to be stimulatory to gonadotropin release, was found to induce a dose-related increase in PGE_2 accumulation in the incubation medium and a concomitant increase in LHRH release.[31] Dopamine, which either stimulates or inhibits LH release *in vivo,* was found consistently to stimulate LHRH release *in vitro* but to have little effect on PGE_2 formation. That the stimulatory effect of NE on LHRH release is PGE_2-mediated is evidenced by the finding that indomethacin prevents the LHRH response to NE without altering the effect of PGE_2 on LHRH release (FIG. 1). To define the receptor type involved in mediating the stimulatory effect of NE on LHRH secretion, we conducted experiments to examine the effect of α- and β-adrenergic receptor blockers on the NE-induced LHRH and PGE_2 release.[32] The results demonstrate that the effect of NE is mediated by α-adrenoreceptors because phentolamine, an α-adrenergic receptor blocker, inhibited in a dose-related manner the increase in PGE_2 and LHRH induced by NE. Blockade of β-adrenoreceptors with propranolol was ineffective. Other researchers have further demonstrated, by using specific agonists and antagonists to α-adrenoreceptor subtypes, that the effect of NE is mediated by $α_1$ receptors.[33] Indeed, an increase in PGE_2 synthesis appears to be essential for NE, acting through α-adrenergic receptors, to exert its stimulatory effect on cyclic AMP (cAMP) formation within the CNS.[34]

Little is known regarding the effects of PGE_2 on the release of other hypothalamic

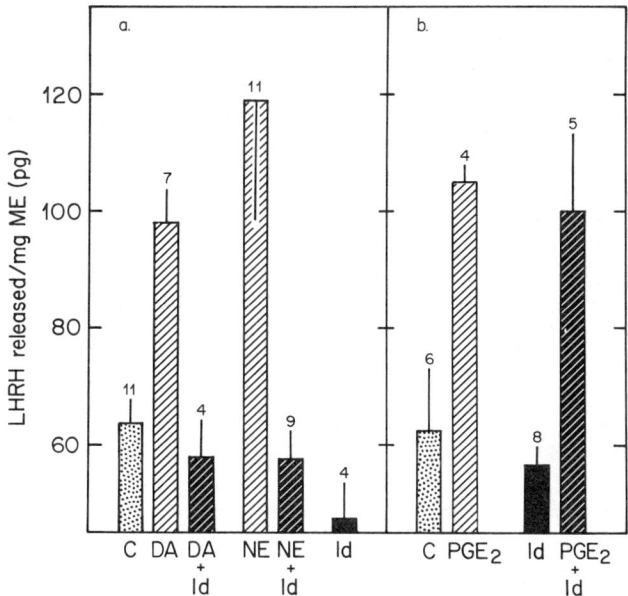

FIGURE 1. Effect of *in vitro* inhibition of prostaglandin (PG) synthesis with indomethacin (Id; 100 μM) on catecholamine-induced (**a**) or PGE_2-induced (**b**) LHRH release. Tissues were preincubated for 15 min in the presence of Id. The medium was then replaced by fresh medium containing the catecholamine or PGE_2 in the presence of the same concentration of Id. DA (dopamine) and NE (norepinephrine) were used at a concentration of 60 μM. PGE_2 was used at a concentration of 2.8 μM. C = control. (From Ojeda *et al.*[31] Reprinted by permission from *Endocrinology*.)

neuropeptides. Earlier *in vivo* experiments failed to show an effect of PGEs on the release of hypothalamic thyrotropin-releasing hormone but suggested a stimulatory action on the release of corticotropin-releasing hormone and prolactin-releasing factors (for reviews, see References 35 and 36). More recent *in vitro* experiments have shown that PGE_2 is ineffective in releasing either SRIF[37] or neuropeptide Y (NPY)[38] from ME nerve terminals.

In contrast to these observations, a now sizable body of evidence derived from *in vitro* experiments strongly implicates PGE_2 as a physiological component of the LHRH-secreting system. For instance, PGE_2 can induce release of LHRH long before puberty.[39] As puberty approaches, the increasing output of estradiol from the developing ovaries induces a preovulatory surge of gonadotropins, which results from both a discharge of LHRH and an increased pituitary response to the decapeptide. Examination of the capacity of the medial basal hypothalamus to metabolize arachidonic acid through the cyclooxygenase pathway has revealed a pubertal increase in the formation of PGE_2, particularly during the first proestrus.[40] (This phase of puberty corresponds to the day of the first preovulatory surge of gonadotropins.) Intriguingly, the increase in PGE_2 synthesis was not associated with changes in the formation of $PGF_{2\alpha}$, PGI_2, PGD_2, or thromboxane B_2 from exogenous arachidonic acid, suggesting that a specific increase in PGE_2 formation is an event directly associated with the peripubertal activation of the reproductive hypothalamus. The estrogen dependence of this event has been demonstrated by the finding that treatment of juvenile animals with estradiol (using a dose capable of inducing a preovulatory surge of gonadotropins) increases the capacity of the hypothalamus to synthesize PGE_2 (FIG. 2).

More recent *in vitro* experiments with ME nerve terminals[39] have demonstrated that *in vivo* pretreatment of the animals with estradiol, using a dose and mode of administration that induce a preovulatory surge of LH, enhances the formation of PGE_2 in response to NE and increases the release of LHRH in response to both NE (FIG. 3) and PGE_2. These observations, however, do not identify the biochemical site(s) where estradiol acts to modify the intracellular pathway that transduces the noradrenergic stimulatory signal into LHRH release. One of these sites may be the cyclooxygenase enzyme complex itself[41] because of the facilitatory effect of estradiol on the synthesis of PGE_2 from exogenous arachidonic acid. An increase in cyclooxygenase activity does not, however, explain the selective increase in PGE_2 formation without significant alteration in thromboxane B_2 or the other PGs examined. Hence, an effect of estradiol on PGH_2 isomerase activity appears to be a more plausible explanation.

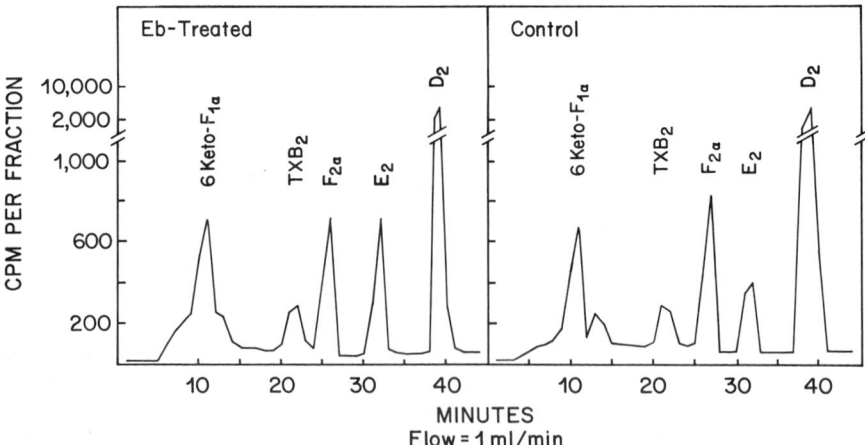

FIGURE 2. Representative HPLC elution profiles of cyclooxygenase products resulting from the metabolism of arachidonic acid by hypothalamic homogenates of juvenile rats treated with estradiol benzoate (Eb). Female rats 29 days old were injected sc with Eb (10 μg) 27 h before being killed. Control animals received an oil injection. For each group one of three profiles is represented. (From Ojeda & Campbell.[40] Reprinted by permission from *Endocrinology*.)

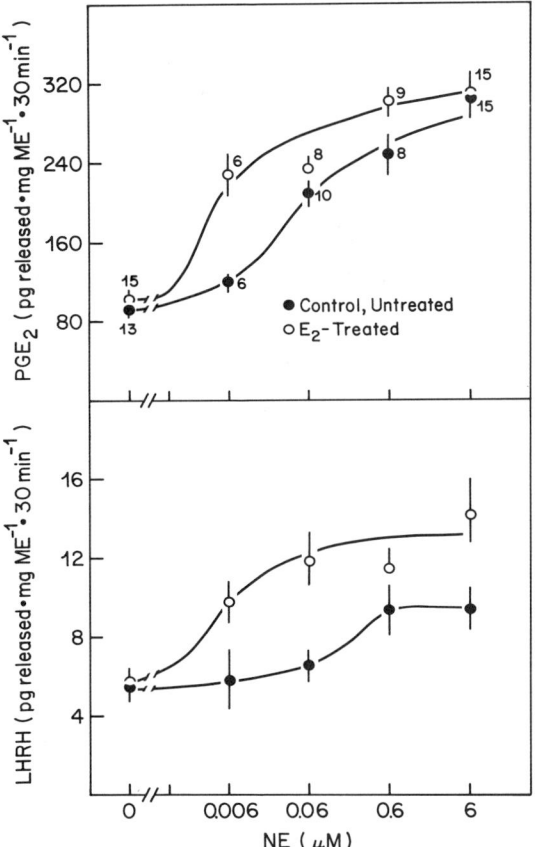

FIGURE 3. Effect of *in vivo* simulation of preovulatory serum estradiol levels on the *in vitro* release of PGE_2 (*top*) and LHRH (*bottom*) from the median eminence (ME) of juvenile 28-day-old female rats in response to norepinephrine (NE). Estradiol was provided in sc Silastic capsules at a concentration (400 μg/ml corn oil) that reproduces serum estradiol levels on the day of first proestrus. The estradiol-containing capsules were implanted 48 h before the experiment. (From Ojeda *et al.*[39] Reprinted by permission from *Neuroendocrinology*.)

The finding that ovariectomy at the beginning of the juvenile period results in almost complete loss of the LHRH response to PGE_2 two weeks later[39] suggests that the development of the capacity of LHRH neurons to respond to PGE_2 is regulated by the secretory activity of the immature ovary. During the adult estrous cycle, the release of LHRH at proestrus appears to depend upon a sequential increase in the PGE_2 response to NE and in the LHRH response to PGE_2.[42] The former event is associated with the beginning of the preovulatory LH surge, the latter coincides with the peak of the LH discharge. That progesterone is involved in enhancing the LHRH response to PGE_2 is suggested by the observation that administration of the steroid in the morning of proestrus significantly advances the time of enhanced LHRH response to PGE_2.[42]

Like LHRH, the release of PGE_2 from ME nerve terminals in response to depolarizing agents is dependent upon the extracellular concentration of calcium (Ca^{2+}). Removal of extracellular Ca^{2+} or incubation of the nerve terminals with verapamil, a blocker of voltage-sensitive Ca^{2+} channels, almost completely prevents the increase in PGE_2 and LHRH release induced by a depolarizing concentration of potassium (K^+).[43,44] In contrast, the stimulatory effect of PGE_2 on LHRH is only partially dependent on extracellular Ca^{2+}.[45,46] PGE_2 can elicit LHRH release in the absence of extracellular Ca^{2+}, even if a submillimolar concentration of verapamil is added to the incubation medium.[46] When MEs were loaded with ^{45}Ca and the release of the isotope from the tissue was examined in a perifusion system, it was found that PGE_2 increased Ca^{2+} efflux regardless of the absence of extracellular Ca^{2+} (FIG. 4). Thus, it appears that the mechanism of PGE_2 action on LHRH release involves

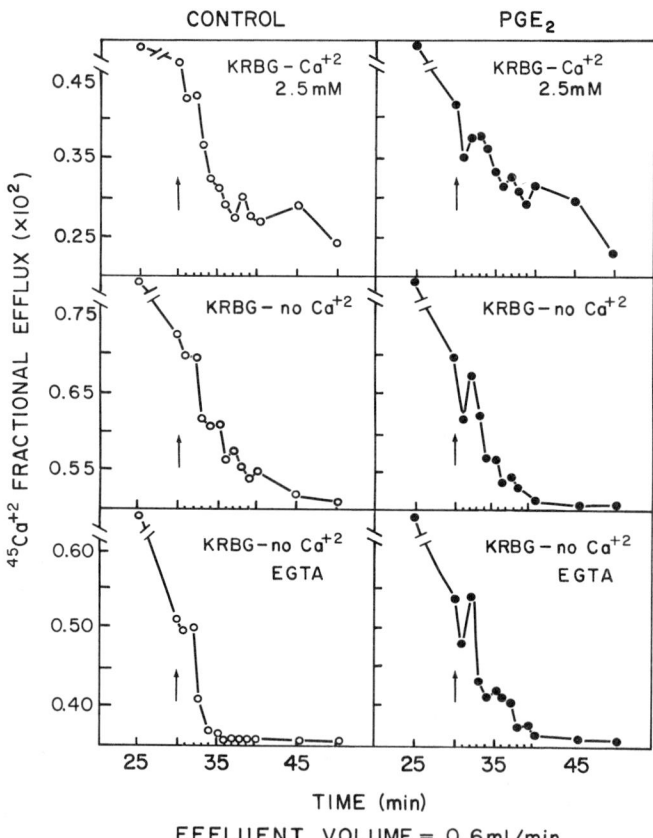

FIGURE 4. Effect of PGE_2 on $^{45}Ca^{2+}$ efflux from median eminence nerve terminals perifused with Krebs Ringer bicarbonate-glucose buffer (KRBG)-2.5 mM Ca^{2+} (*upper panels*), KRBG-no Ca^{2+} (*middle panels*), and KRBG-no Ca^{2+} with 10^{-4} M EGTA (*lower panels*). The MEs were preincubated in Ca^{2+} free medium for 1 h with frequent medium changes (see Ref. 46 for details) and then loaded with $^{45}Ca^{2+}$ (12 μCi/ml KRBG) for 2 h at 37°C in Ca^{2+}-free medium. Note the almost instantaneous increase in Ca^{2+} efflux (1 min) elicited by the PG (*arrows*). (From Ojeda & Negro-Vilar.[46] Reprinted by permission from *Endocrinology*.)

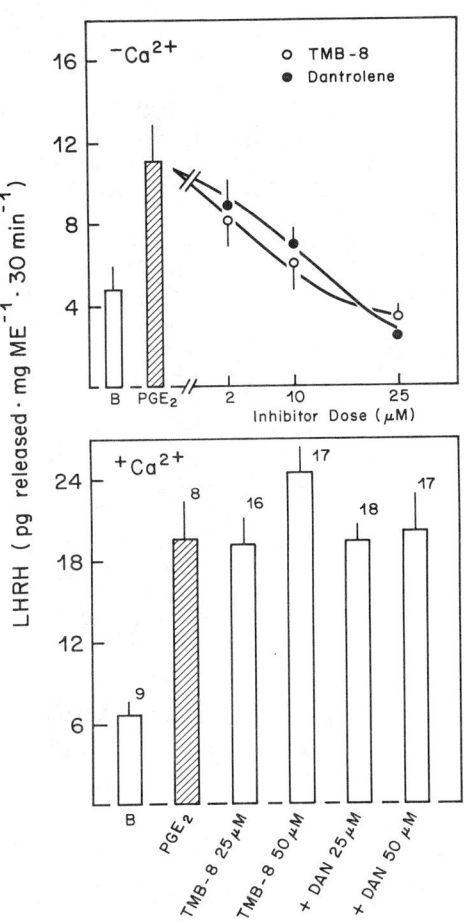

FIGURE 5. Effect of blockers of intracellular Ca^{2+} mobilization on PGE_2 (2.8 μM)-induced LHRH release from median eminence (ME) of juvenile female rats *in vitro* in the absence (*upper panel*) or presence (*lower panel*) of Ca^{2+}. In the upper panel each bar or point represents the mean of 6–12 MEs. In the lower panel numbers on top of the bars indicate the number of MEs per group. B = basal release; DAN = dantrolene. (From Ojeda et al.[47] Reprinted by permission of *Brain Research*.)

translocation of Ca^{2+} from intracellular stores. Very recently, we found[47] that exposure of ME terminals to 8-(diethylamino)-octyl-3,4,5-trimethoxybenzoate (TMB-8) or dantrolene, two blockers of intracellular Ca^{2+} mobilization, abolishes the LHRH response to PGE_2 (FIG. 5). As expected, this inhibitory effect can be counteracted by raising extracellular Ca^{2+} to physiological levels. Interestingly, the effect of PGE_2 on LHRH release has been found to be independent of calmodulin. Exposure of ME nerve terminals to either of five different inhibitors of calmodulin activity, or to an inhibitor of calmodulin-dependent kinase activity, does not affect the LHRH response to PGE_2. A similar independent response occurs when A-23187, a Ca^{2+} ionophore, is used instead of PGE_2. In contrast, A-23187–induced PGE_2 formation is inhibited by blockers of calmodulin activity, indicating that synthesis of PGE_2 in ME nerve terminals depends on both Ca^{2+} influx into the nerve terminal and binding of Ca^{2+} to calmodulin. The Ca^{2+}-calmodulin interaction likely results in activation of phospholipase A_2, which releases arachidonic acid membrane phospholipids and makes it available to the cyclooxygenase.

A series of experiments performed independently by two laboratories have provided *in vitro* evidence for an involvement of cAMP in LHRH release.[48-50] Stimulation of adenylate cyclase activity with either forskolin, cholera toxin, or pertussis toxin was shown to enhance the release of LHRH without affecting PGE_2 formation[49] (FIG. 6). Since NE induces both cAMP and PGE_2 formation,[31,34] and PGE stimulates cAMP synthesis,[47,48,50] the sequence of steps mediating NE-induced LHRH release is likely to begin with the activation of PGE_2 synthesis, followed by activation of cAMP formation.[50,51]

In recent experiments,[47] we have obtained evidence that activation of cAMP synthesis is not an obligatory component in the mechanism by which PGE_2 induces LHRH release. Omission of Ca^{2+} from the incubation medium prevented the effect of forskolin on LHRH release, but not the stimulation of cAMP accumulation. This is in marked contrast to the effect of PGE_2 on LHRH, which is not prevented by reducing extracellular Ca^{2+} levels. Interestingly, inhibition of calmodulin activity or of intracellular Ca^{2+} mobilization in the presence of normal extracellular Ca^{2+} levels prevented the effect of PGE_2 on cAMP accumulation, but failed to affect the release of LHRH induced by the PG. Thus, it appears that PGE_2 can evoke LHRH release in a cyclic AMP–independent manner. In addition, these results suggest that the effect of PGE_2

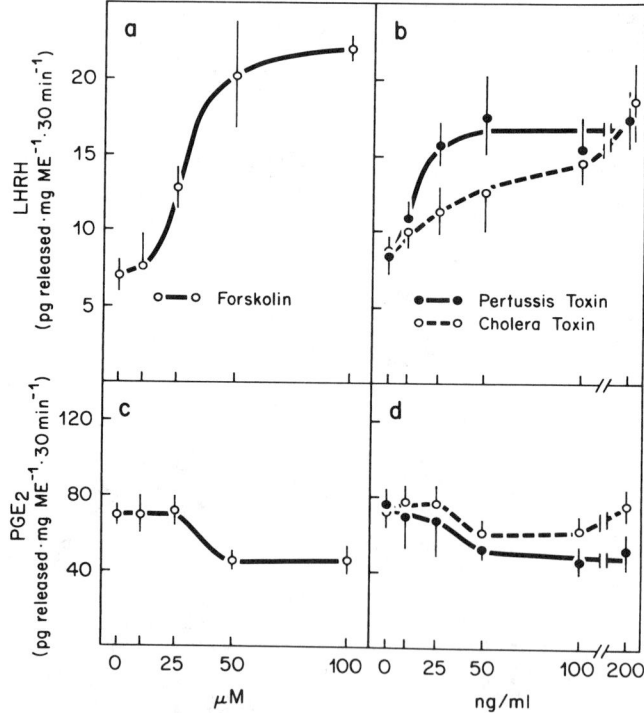

FIGURE 6. Divergent effects of forskolin, cholera toxin, and pertussis toxin on the *in vitro* release of LHRH (**a** and **b**) and PGE_2 (**c** and **d**) from median eminence (ME) nerve terminals of juvenile 28-day-old female rats. Notice that all three probes enhance LHRH release but fail to increase PGE_2 release. Each point represents the mean of 4–10 individual determinations. (From Ojeda *et al.*[49] Reprinted by permission from *Endocrinology*.)

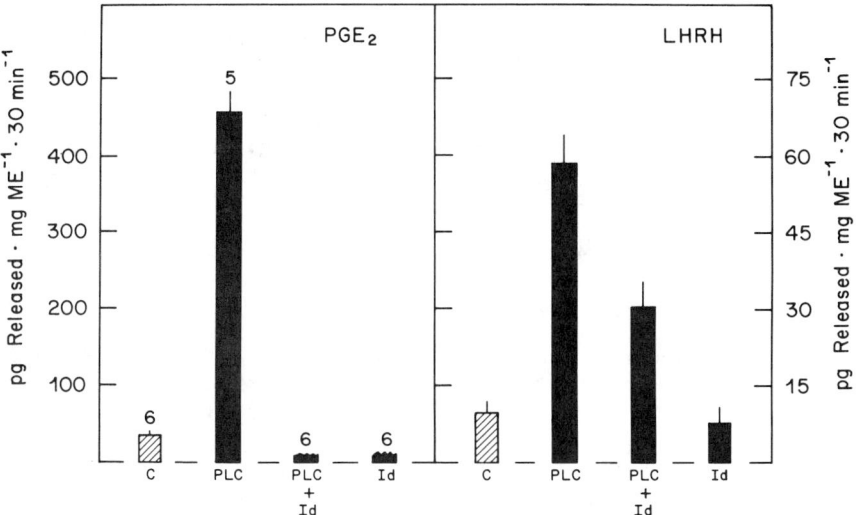

FIGURE 7. Inhibitory effect of *in vitro* blockade of cyclooxygenase activity with indomethacin (Id, 50 μM) on phospholipase C (PLC) (0.25 unit/ml)–induced PGE_2 and LHRH release from median eminences (MEs) of juvenile female rats. Numbers above bars indicate the number of individual MEs per group. C = control, basal release. *Incomplete bars* indicate undetectable PGE_2 levels. (From Ojeda *et al.*[52] Reprinted by permission from *Proceedings of the National Academy of Sciences of the United States of America*.)

on cAMP formation involves calmodulin activation and mobilization of Ca^{2+} from intracellular stores possibly located in the cell membrane.

Taken altogether, the above observations permit the conclusion that PGE_2 induces LHRH release from ME nerve terminals through a mechanism that involves both translocation of Ca^{2+}, from possibly more than one intracellular storage site, and stimulation of cAMP formation. This latter event, however, is not essential for PGE_2 to exert its stimulatory effect. Calmodulin is also involved, but its participation is limited to well-defined steps in the cascade (i.e., formation of PGE_2 from membrane phospholipids and PGE_2-induced activation of adenylate cyclase).

Recent evidence,[52,53] supports the involvement of protein kinase C (PKC), a Ca^{2+}-activated, phospholipid-dependent kinase,[54] in the process of LHRH release. In experiments performed on ME nerve terminals of juvenile female rats, it was found that two known stimulators of PKC activity, dioctanolylglycerol (DiC8) and the phorbol ester 4β-phorbol 12β-myristate 13α-acetate (PMA), elicited LHRH release.[52] Exposure of the MEs to PMA failed to enhance PGE_2 releases, indicating that the effect of this agent on LHRH release was independent of PGE_2. Interestingly, using MEs from adult male rats, other authors found that activation of PKC activity by the diacylglycerol analog didecanoylglycerol induced PGE_2 formation through a phospholipase A_2–mediated mechanism but failed to evoke LHRH release unless lipoxygenation of arachidonic acid was prevented.[53] While this observation suggests an inhibitory involvement of lipoxygenase metabolites in PKC-induced LHRH release, it is clear from the results of both laboratories that the PKC pathway can induce LHRH release independently of PGE_2. Exposure of the MEs to phospholipase C (PLC) markedly increases LHRH and PGE_2 release; however, if cyclooxygenase activity is blocked by indomethacin only, the effect of PLC on PGE_2 is abolished (FIG. 7).[52,53] The release of LHRH is reduced by about 50%, suggesting that this fraction may represent the contribution of PGE_2, whereas the rest can be attributed to an independent PKC-mediated process. The complementarity of these two pathways is further suggested by the observation that concomitant exposure of the MEs to PGE_2 plus DiC8 or PMA, or forskolin plus DiC8 or PMA, results in an additive effect on LHRH release.[52] In contrast, the simultaneous exposure of MEs to PGE_2 and forskolin results in an increase in LHRH release that is greater than that elicited by either PGE_2 or forskolin alone.[51,52]

The nature of the neurotransmitter that activates PKC in LHRH nerve terminals is unknown. Although there is evidence that NE, acting through α_1 receptors, increases PLC activity,[55] in our experiments NE and DiC8 had an additive effect suggesting that a neurotransmitter other than NE may be the primary signal for PKC activation in the ME. It is possible, however, that the activation of PKC activity by NE is submaximal or compartmentalized[56] and preferentially routed through the arachidonate cascade.[57] The elevation in intracellular Ca^{2+} levels induced first by the interaction of NE with α_1-adrenoreceptors[55] and subsequently by PGE_2 may then, by increasing the binding of PKC to the plasma membrane,[58] prime the LHRH terminal to the direct effect of DiC8 or PMA. Thus, activation of PKC by these agents would readily enhance the LHRH response to NE. Alternatively, NE and DiC8 may be activating different PKC species,[59] which may have a different intraneuronal subdistribution.

Evidence has recently been presented[10,60] that the lipoxygenase products 12-HETE, 5-HETE, and LTC_4 can stimulate LHRH release *in vitro*. In particular, LTC_4 has been shown to be maximally effective at a concentration as low as 10^{-16} M.[60] These arachidonic acid metabolites may not be involved in NE-induced LHRH release because of the effectiveness of indomethacin, a cyclooxygenase inhibitor, in suppressing the NE effect. LHRH neurons are, however, subjected to a variety of excitatory and inhibitory inputs, and thus the stimulatory effect of neurotransmitters other than NE may well be mediated by lipoxygenase products. In regard to the epoxygenase pathway, results from our laboratory have shown that LHRH release is not affected by two of the epoxyacids (11, 12 and 14, 15-EET) and is only slightly increased by 5, 6-EET, at micromolar concentrations.[4] We do not know whether the epoxyacid 8, 9-EET, recently shown to be the predominant EET produced in the hypothalamus[11] and to be extremely effective in releasing somatostatin (*vide infra*), may also induce LHRH release. If such a stimulatory effect indeed exists, it would raise the intriguing possibility that 8, 9-EET mediates the action of a neurotransmitter other than NE on LHRH release.

SOMATOSTATIN

The release of SRIF from the hypothalamus is not affected by the cyclooxygenase products PGE_2 or $PGF_{2\alpha}$.[37] On the contrary, if cyclooxygenase activity is blocked with indomethacin, an elevation of basal SRIF secretion from ME nerve terminals and an inhibitory effect of PGE_2 on this basal release become apparent.[37] The lipoxygenase product 12-HETE, which stimulates LHRH release at submicromolar levels, is ineffective in altering SRIF release.[10]

In contrast to the inability of these arachidonic acid metabolites to affect SRIF release, the secretion of SRIF is markedly increased by the epoxygenase products 5, 6-EET[4] (FIG. 8), 11, 12-EET, and, in particular, 8, 9-EET.[11] The hydration product of 5, 6-EET, 5, 6-DHET, is also effective,[4] but at a much higher concentration. The differences in potency between these compounds are remarkable. While the maximal effect of 8, 9-EET is observed at 10^{-12} M, 5, 6-EET and 5, 6-DHET are maximally effective at 10^{-8} and 10^{-6} M, respectively.

That these epoxygenase products are physiological constituents of the hypothalamus was first suggested by the finding that incubation of hypothalamic microsomes with exogenous ^{14}C-arachidonic acid resulted in the NADH-dependent, cytochrome P-450–mediated formation of both 5, 6-EET and its hydration product 5, 6-DHET.[4] More recently, we have taken advantage of the development of improved gas chromatography/mass spectral methods for the separation and isolation of EETs[61] and have demonstrated that 5, 6-EET, 11, 12-EET, and 8, 9-EET are endogenous products of arachidonic acid metabolism in the hypothalamus. We have further demonstrated,

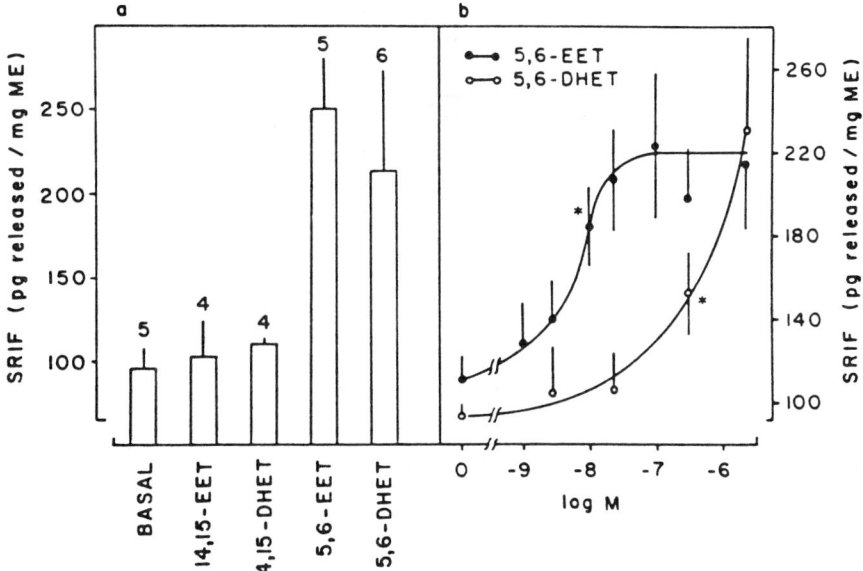

FIGURE 8. (a) Effect of epoxygenase products (2.5 μM) on the *in vitro* release of somatostatin (SRIF) from median eminence (ME) nerve terminals. 5, 6-DHET: $p < 0.05$; and 5, 6-EET: $p < 0.01$ vs. basal control. (b) Effect of different concentrations of 5, 6-EET and 5, 6-DHET on SRIF release from the ME *in vitro*. Each point is the mean of 9–20 determinations (5, 6-EET) or 4–9 determinations (5, 6-DHET). * = first significant ($p < 0.05$) increase over control flasks. (From Capdevila *et al.*[4] Reprinted by permission from *Endocrinology*.)

by comparing gas chromatography retention times and mass spectral fragmentation patterns, that 8, 9-EET is a major endogenous product of epoxygenase in the hypothalamus.[11]

The role that these epoxyacids may play in the regulation of neuropeptide release is not yet well established. Nevertheless, the marked effectiveness of 5, 6- and 8, 9-EET is stimulating SRIF release from the ME strongly suggests their involvement in this process. The recent demonstration that the imidazole derivatives clotrimazole and ketoconazole inhibit the release of somatostatin induced by the neurotransmitter dopamine[11] further suggest that epoxygenase products are components of the signal transduction mechanism that mediates the effect of certain neurotransmitters. Clotrimazole and ketoconazole are potent general inhibitors of microsomal cytochrome P-450 function, and of the arachidonic acid epoxygenase in particular.[62]

CONCLUSIONS

It now appears clear that different arachidonic acid metabolites may subserve different functions within the central nervous system. The concept that emerges from the information so far obtained is that products of each one of the pathways of arachidonic acid metabolism may play a role in mediating the effect of neurotransmitters on neuropeptide release, and that particular neurotransmitters may utilize different arachidonic acid metabolites to exert their effects on neuropeptide-secreting neurons. The observations presented in this article provide an initial example of this concept by furnishing evidence that the effect of NE on LHRH release is mediated by PGE_2, a cyclooxygenase product, and that the effect of dopamine on SRIF release may be mediated by 8, 9- and 5, 6-EET, two products of epoxygenase activity. The neurotransmitter(s) that utilizes the lipoxygenase products 12-HETE, LTC_4, and 5-HETE as mediators of their stimulatory effect on LHRH release remain to be determined.

ACKNOWLEDGMENT

We thank Ms. Janie Gliessman for typing the manuscript.

REFERENCES

1. NEEDLEMAN, P., J. TURK, B. A. JAKSCHIK, A. B. MORRISON & J. B. LEFKOWITH. 1986. Arachidonic acid metabolism. Annu. Rev. Biochem. **55:** 69–102.
2. SAMUELSSON, B. 1982. The leukotrienes: An introduction. In Leukotrienes and Other Lipoxygenase Products. B. Samuelsson & R. Paoletti, Eds.: 1–17. Raven Press. New York, NY.
3. CHACOS, N., J. R. FALCK, C. WIXTROM & J. CAPDEVILA. 1982. Novel epoxides formed during the liver cytochrome P-450 oxidation of arachidonic acid. Biochem. Biophys. Res. Commun. **104:** 916–922.
4. CAPDEVILA, J., N. CHACOS, J. R. FALCK, S. MANNA, A. NEGRO-VILAR & S. R. OJEDA. 1983. Novel hypothalamic arachidonate products stimulate somatostatin release. Endocrinology **113:** 421–423.
5. SAMUELSSON, B. 1964. Identification of a smooth muscle-stimulating factor in bovine brain. Biochim. Biophys. Acta **84:** 218–219.
6. WOLFE, L. S. 1975. Possible roles of prostaglandins in the nervous system. In Advances in Neurochemistry, Vol. 1. B. W. Agranoff & M. H. Aprison, Eds.: 1–49. Plenum. New York, NY.
7. WOLFE, L. S., K. ROSTWOROWSKI & J. MARION. 1976. Endogenous formation of the prostaglandin endoperoxide metabolite, thromboxane B_2, by brain tissue. Biochem. Biophys. Res. Commun. **70(3):** 907–913.
8. LINDGREN, J. A., T. HOKFELT, S.-E. DAHLEN, C. PATRONO & B. SAMUELSSON. 1984. Leukotrienes in the rat central nervous system. Proc. Natl. Acad. Sci. USA **81:** 6212–6216.
9. SANTEBIN, L., C. SPAGNUOLO, C. GALLI & G. GALLI. 1978. A mass fragmentographic procedure for the simultaneous determination of HETE and $PGF_{2\alpha}$ in the central nervous system. Prostaglandins **16(6):** 985–988.
10. GEROZISSIS, K., B. VULLIEZ, J. M. SAAVEDRA, R. C. MURPHY & F. DRAY. 1985.

Lipoxygenase products of arachidonic acid stimulate LHRH release from rat median eminence. Neuroendocrinology **40:** 272–276.

11. JUNIER, M.-P., F. DRAY, I. BLAIR, J. CAPDEVILA, E. DISHMAN, J. R. FLACK & S. R. OJEDA. Hypothalamic epoxyeicosatrienoic acids mediate dopamine-induced somatostatin release. Submitted for publication.
12. TIPPINS, J. R., V. DIMARZO & H. R. MORRIS. 1987. Effect of vasoactive intestinal peptide and calcitonin gene-related peptide on leukotriene release from guinea pig and rat lung. *In* Advances in Prostaglandin, Thromboxane and Leukotriene Research, Vol. 17B. B. Samuelsson, R. Paoletti & P. W. Ramwell, Eds.: 1028–1032. Raven Press. New York, NY.
13. YOUSUFZAI, S. Y., R. A. AKHTAR & A. A. ABDEL-LATIF. 1986. Effects of substance P on inositol triphosphate accumulation, on contractile responses and on arachidonic acid release and (prostaglandin) biosynthesis in rabbit iris sphincter muscle. Exp. Eye Res. **43(2):** 215–226.
14. PALMER, G. C. 1986. Neurochemical coupled actions of transmitters in the microvasculature of the brain. Neurosci. Biobehav. Rev. **10(2):** 79–101.
15. PIOMELLI, D., A. VOLTERRA, N. DALE, S. A. SIEGELBAUM, E. R. KANDEL, J. H. SCHWARTZ & F. BELARDETTI. 1987. Lipoxygenase metabolites of arachidonic acid as second messengers for presynaptic inhibition of Aplysia sensory cells. Nature **328:** 38–43.
16. PIOMELLI, D., E. SHAPIRO, S. J. FEINMARK & J. H. SCHWARTZ. 1987. Metabolites of arachidonic acid in the nervous system of Aplysia: Possible mediators of synaptic modulation. J. Neurosci. **7(11):** 3675–3686.
17. HARMS, P. G., S. R. OJEDA & S. M. MCCANN. 1973. Prostaglandin involvement in the hypothalamic control of gonadotropin and prolactin release. Science **181:** 760–761.
18. SPIES, H. G. & R. L. NORMAN. 1973. Luteinizing hormone release and ovulation induced by the intraventricular infusion of prostaglandin E_1 into pentobarbital blocked rats. Prostaglandins **4:** 131–141.
19. WARBERG, J., R. L. ESKAY & J. C. PORTER. 1976. Prostaglandin E_2-induced release of LHRH into hypophysial portal blood. Endocrinology **97:** 816–824.
20. OJEDA, S. R., J. E. WHEATON & S. M. MCCANN. 1975. Prostaglandin E_2-induced release of luteinizing hormone-releasing factor (LRF). Neuroendocrinology **17:** 283–287.
21. CHOBSIENG, P., Z. NAOR, Y. KOCH, U. ZOR & H. R. LINDNER. 1975. Stimulatory effect of prostaglandin E_2 on LH release in the rat. Evidence for hypothalamic site of action. Neuroendocrinology **17:** 12–17.
22. OJEDA, S. R., H. E. JAMESON & S. M. MCCANN. 1977. Hypothalamic areas involved in prostaglandin (PG) induced gonadotropin release. I. Effect of PGE_2 and $PGF_{2\alpha}$ implants on luteinizing hormone release. Endocrinology **100:** 1585–1594.
23. HARMS, P. G., S. R. OJEDA & S. M. MCCANN. 1976. Failure of monoaminergic and serotoninergic receptor blockers to prevent prostaglandin E_2-induced LH release. Endocrinology **98:** 318–323.
24. CARLSON, J. C., B. BARCIKOWSKI, V. CARGILL & J. A. MCCRACKEN. 1974. The blockade of LH release by indomethacin. J. Clin. Endocrinol. Metab. **39:** 399–402.
25. OJEDA, S. R., P. G. HARMS & S. M. MCCANN. 1975. Effect of inhibition of prostaglandin synthesis on gonadotropin release in the rat. Endocrinology **97:** 843–854.
26. LABBSETWAR, A. P. & A. ZOLVICK. 1973. Evidence for the hypothalamic interaction between prostaglandins and catecholamines in promoting gonadotropin secretion for ovulation. Nature **249:** 55–56.
27. BOTTING, J. H., E. A. LINTON & S. A. WHITEHEAD. 1977. Blockade of ovulation in the rat by a prostaglandin antagonist (N-0164). J. Endocrinol. **75:** 335–336.
28. LEACH, C. M., J. A. REYNOLDSON & G. D. THORBURN. 1982. Release of E prostaglandins into the cerebrospinal fluid and its inhibition by melatonin after cervical stimulation in the rabbit. Endocrinology **110:** 1320–1324.
29. GALLARDO, E. & V. D. RAMIREZ. 1977. A method for the superfusion of rat hypothalami: Secretion of luteinizing hormone-releasing hormone. Proc. Soc. Exp. Biol. Med. **155:** 79–84.
30. NEGRO-VILAR, A., S. R. OJEDA & S. M. MCCANN. 1979. Catecholaminergic modulation of LHRH release by median eminence terminals in vitro. Endocrinology **104:** 1749–1751.
31. OJEDA, S. R., A. NEGRO-VILAR & S. M. MCCANN. 1979. Release of prostaglandin E

(PGEs) by hypothalamic tissue: Evidence for their involvement in catecholamine-induced LHRH release. Endocrinology **104:** 617–624.
32. OJEDA, S. R., A. NEGRO-VILAR & S. M. MCCANN. 1982. Evidence for involvement of α-adrenergic receptors in norepinephrine-induced PGE_2 and LHRH release from the median eminence. Endocrinology **110:** 409–412.
33. HEAULME, M. & F. DRAY. 1984. Noradrenaline and prostaglandin E_2 stimulate LHRH release from rat median eminence through distinct 1-alpha-adrenergic and PGE_2 receptors. Neuroendocrinology **39:** 403–407.
34. PARTINGTON, C. R., M. W. EDWARDS & J. W. DALY. 1980. Regulation of cyclic AMP formation in brain tissue by α-adrenergic receptors: Requisite intermediary of prostaglandins of the E series. Proc. Natl. Acad. Sci. USA **77:** 3024–3028.
35. HEDGE, G. A. 1977. Roles for the prostaglandins in the regulation of anterior pituitary secretion. Life Sci. **20:** 17–34.
36. OJEDA, S. R., Z. NAOR & A. NEGRO-VILAR. 1979. The role of prostaglandins in the control of gonadotropin and prolactin secretion. Prostaglandins Med. **5:** 249–275.
37. OJEDA, S. R., A. NEGRO-VILAR, A. ARIMURA & S. M. MCCANN. 1980. On the hypothalamic mechanism by which prostaglandin E_2 stimulates growth hormone release. Neuroendocrinology **31:** 1–7.
38. SAHU, A., S. P. KALRA, W. R. CROWLEY, T. L. O'DONOHUE & P. S. KALRA. 1987. Neuropeptide Y levels in microdissected regions of the hypothalamus and in vitro release in response to KCl and prostaglandin E_2: Effects of castration. Endocrinology **120:** 1831–1836.
39. OJEDA, S. R., H. F. URBANSKI, K. H. KATZ & M. E. COSTA. 1986. The activation of estradiol positive feedback at puberty: Estradiol sensitizes the LHRH releasing system at two different biochemical steps. Neuroendocrinology **43:** 259–266.
40. OJEDA, S. R. & W. B. CAMPBELL. 1982. An increase in hypothalamic capacity to synthesize PGE_2 precedes the first preovulatory surge of gonadotropins. Endocrinology **111:** 1031–1037.
41. CHANG, W. C., J. NAKAO, H. ORIMO & S. I. MUROTA. 1980. Stimulation of prostaglandin cyclooxygenase and prostacyclin synthetase activities by estradiol in rat aortic smooth muscle cells. Biochim. Biophys. Acta **620:** 472–482.
42. DEPAOLO, L., S. R. OJEDA, A. NEGRO-VILAR & S. M. MCCANN. 1982. Alterations in the responsiveness of median eminence luteinizing-hormone-releasing hormone nerve terminals to norepinephrine and prostaglandin E_2 in vitro during the rat estrous cycle. Endocrinology **110:** 1999–2005.
43. DROUVA, S. V., J. EPELBAUM, M. HERY, L. TAPIA-ARANCIBIA, E. LAPLANTE & C. KORDON. 1981. Ionic channels involved in the LHRH and SRIF release from rat mediobasal hypothlamus. Neuroendocrinology **32:** 155–162.
44. OJEDA, S. R. & A. NEGRO-VILAR. 1984. Release of prostaglandin E_2 from the hypothalamus depends on extracellular Ca^{2+} availability: Relation to LHRH release. Neuroendocrinology **39:** 442–447.
45. RAMIREZ, V. D., E. GALLARDO & D. HARTTER. 1980. Factors altering the secretion of LHRH from superfused fragments of rat hypothalamus. J. Endocrinol. Invest. **3:** 29–36.
46. OJEDA, S. R. & A. NEGRO-VILAR. 1985. Prostaglandin E_2-induced LHRH release involves mobilization of intracellular Ca^{2+}. Endocrinology **116:** 1763–1770.
47. OJEDA, S. R., H. F. URBANSKI, K. H. KATZ & M. E. COSTA. 1988. Prostaglandin E_2 releases luteinizing hormone-releasing hormone from the female juvenile hypothalamus through a Ca^{2+}-dependent, calmodulin-independent mechanism. Brain Res. **441:** 339–351.
48. RAMIREZ, V. D., K. KIM & D. DLUZEN. 1985. Progesterone action on the LHRH and nigrostriatal dopamine neural systems: In vitro and in vivo studies. Recent Prog. Horm. Res. **41:** 421–472.
49. OJEDA, S. R., H. F. URBANSKI, K. H. KATZ & M. E. COSTA. 1985. Stimulation of cyclic AMP production enhances luteinizing hormone-releasing hormone release without increasing prostaglandin E_2 synthesis. Studies in prepubertal female rats. Endocrinology **117:** 1175–1178.
50. KIM, K. & V. D. RAMIREZ. 1986. Effects of prostaglandin E_2, forskolin and cholera toxin on

cAMP production and in vitro LHRH release from the rat hypothalamus. Brain Res. **386:** 258–265.
51. BARNEA, A. & G. CHO. 1987. Copper amplification of prostaglandin E_2 stimulation of the release of luteinizing hormone-releasing hormone is a post-receptor event. Proc. Natl. Acad. Sci USA **84:** 580–584.
52. OJEDA, S. R., H. F. URBANSKI, K. H. KATZ, M. E. COSTA & P. M. CONN. 1986. Activation of two different but complementary biochemical pathways induces release of hypothalamic luteinizing hormone-releasing hormone. Proc. Natl. Acad. Sci. USA **83:** 4932–4936.
53. NEGRO-VILAR, A., D. CONTE & M. VALENCA. 1986. Transmembrane signals mediating neural peptide secretion: Role of protein kinase C activators and arachidonic acid metabolites in luteinizing hormone-releasing hormone secretion. Endocrinology **119:** 2796–2802.
54. KIKKAWA, U., Y. TAKAI, R. MINAGUSHI, S. INOHARA & Y. NISHIZUKA. 1982. Calcium-activated, phospholipid-dependent protein kinase from rat brain. J. Biol. Chem. **257:** 13341–13348.
55. ZATZ, M. 1985. Denervation supersensitivity of the rat pineal to norepinephrine-stimulated [^{3}H] inositide turnover revealed by lithium and a convenient procedure. J. Neurochem. **45:** 95–100.
56. WOLF, M., H. LEVINE III, W. W. MAY, JR., P. CUATRECASAS & N. SAHYOUN. 1985. A model for intracellular translocation of protein kinase C involving synergism between Ca^{2+} and phorbol esters. Nature **317:** 546–549.
57. HO, A. K. & D. C. KLEIN. 1987. Activation of α_1-adreno receptors, protein kinase C, or treatment with intracellular free Ca^{2+} elevating agents increases pineal phospholipase A_2 activity. J. Biol. Chem. **262:** 11764–11770.
58. MAY, W. S., JR., N. SAHYOUN, M. WOLF & P. CUATRECASAS. 1985. Role of intracellular calcium mobilization in the regulation of protein kinase C-mediated membrane processes. Nature **317:** 549–551.
59. ONO, Y., U. KIKKAWA, K. OGITA, T. FUJII, T. KUROKAWA, Y. ASAOKA, K. SEKIGUCHI, K. ASE, K. IGARASHI & Y. NISHISUKA. 1987. Expression and properties of two types of protein kinase C: Alternative splicing from a single gene. Science **236:** 1116–1120.
60. GEROZISSIS, K., C. ROUGEOT & F. DRAY. 1986. Leukotriene C_4 is a potent stimulator of LHRH secretion. Eur. J. Pharmacol. **121:** 159–160.
61. TOTO, R., A. SIDDHANTA, S. MANNA, B. PRAMANIK, J. R. FALCK & J. CAPDEVILA. 1987. Arachidonic acid epoxygenase: Detection of epoxyeicosatrienoic acids in human urine. Biochim. Biophys. Acta **919:** 132–139.
62. CAPDEVILA, J., L. GIL, M. ORELLANA, L. J. MARNET, I. MASON, P. YADAGIRI & J. R. FALCK. 1988. Inhibitors of cytochrome P-450 dependent arachidonic acid metabolism. Arch. Biochem. Biophys. **261:** 257–263.

12-Keto-Eicosatetraenoic Acid

A Biologically Active Eicosanoid in the Nervous System of *Aplysia*

DANIELE PIOMELLI,[a,b,c] STEVEN J. FEINMARK[d]
ELI SHAPIRO,[a] AND JAMES H. SCHWARTZ[a]

[a]*Howard Hughes Medical Institute*
Center for Neurobiology and Behavior
and
[d]*Departments of Pharmacology and Medicine*
Columbia University
New York, New York 10032

INTRODUCTION

In the neural tissue of *Aplysia*, the neurotransmitter histamine and the peptide FMRFamide evoke release of 12-hydroxyeicosatetraenoic acid (12-HETE), a stable end product of the 12-lipoxygenase pathway.[1,3] The short-lived precursor of 12-HETE, 12-HPETE, simulates electrophysiological responses induced by FMRFamide in sensory cells[3,4] and by histamine in L14 cells,[2] suggesting that this hydroperoxide or one of its metabolites serves as intracellular signal to mediate the synaptic actions of FMRFamide and histamine. Several novel metabolites derived from 12-HPETE have recently been identified in mammalian tissues.[5–8] Therefore, it is possible that 12-HPETE produces its effects in *Aplysia* neurons only after conversion to an active metabolite.

Here, we report that a metabolite of 12-HPETE, 12-KETE, is released when *Aplysia* nervous tissue is stimulated by applying histamine. We also show that application of 12-KETE, like 12-HPETE, produces electrophysiological responses similar to those evoked by histamine in two identified *Aplysia* neurons, L10 and L14.

EXPERIMENTAL PROCEDURES

Aplysia weighing 70–200 g (Howard Hughes Medical Institute Mariculture Research Facility, Woods Hole Oceanographic Institution, Woods Hole, MA; and Marinus, Sand City, CA) were kept in aquaria at 15 °C. Homogenates of nervous tissue and isolated neural components (cell bodies and neuropil) were prepared as described previously.[1]

---

[b]Fellow of the Louis and Rose Klosk Fund.
[c]Address for correspondence: Dr. Daniele Piomelli, Laboratory of Molecular and Cellular Neuroscience, The Rockefeller University, 1230 York Avenue, New York, New York 10021.

Extraction of Lipids

Acetone (0–4 °C) was added to homogenates (1:1, v/v) and the precipitate removed by low-speed centrifugation. Metabolites were extracted twice with ethyl acetate (2 vol) after acidifying the supernatant to pH 3.5. The organic layers were combined, dried over sodium sulfate, and evaporated under vacuum. Samples from experiments with prelabeled nervous tissue were extracted with ethyl acetate without prior addition of acetone.

High-Performance Liquid Chromatography

Analytical normal-phase HPLC was performed using a silica column (250 × 4.6 mm, 5 μm; Supelco, Bellefonte, PA) eluted isocratically with hexane:isopropanol:acetic acid (98:2:0.1, v/v/v) at a flow rate of 1 ml/min. Absorbance was monitored continuously at 270 nm, and full UV spectra were obtained with a diode-array spectrophotometer (Hewlett-Packard 1090M, Palo Alto, CA); 30-sec fractions were collected and radioactivity counted by liquid scintillation. For purifications on a preparative scale, we used a Polygosil silica column (500 × 10 mm, 10 μm; Alltech, Deerfield, IL) eluted with the same solvent system at a flow rate of 3 ml/min. Reversed-phase HPLC was performed with a Nucleosil C18 column (250 × 4.6 mm, 5 μm, Alltech) eluted isocratically with methanol:water:acetic acid (65:35:0.1) at a flow rate of 1 ml/min; absorbance was monitored at 280 nm. In some experiments, carbonyl groups were reduced to alcohols by adding 1–2 mg of sodium borohydride to samples dissolved in ethanol (0.1 ml) and incubating for 15 min at 0–4 °C. Samples were then filtered through glass wool and dried under nitrogen. The resulting products were separated by normal-phase HPLC as described above with the UV detector set at 235 nm.

Gas Chromatography/Mass Spectrometry

Metabolites were purified by preparative normal-phase HPLC (see above), and converted to the methyl ester by treating the purified material with an excess of ethereal diazomethane for 2 min. To prepare the pentafluorobenzyl (PFB) esters, we incubated samples with pentafluorobenzyl bromide (35% in 10 μl acetonitrile) and diisopropylethylamine (10 μl) diluted with acetonitrile (30 μl) for 10 min at room temperature. To prepare methoxime derivatives, the esterified samples were exposed to methoxylamine hydrochloride (1% in pyridine, 20 μl) for 1 h at 60 °C.

Analyses were performed on a Hewlett-Packard 5987A GC/MS fitted with an HP-1 capillary column (12 m, Hewlett-Packard, Palo Alto, CA) using helium as the carrier gas. For electron impact analyses the column temperature was programmed from 150 to 250 °C at a rate of 30 °C/min. We kept the injector at 250 °C and the source at 200 °C. Carrier flow was regulated at a constant head pressure of 52 kPa and the voltage kept at 25 eV. Negative ion chemical ionization analyses were done using methane as the ionizing gas (source pressure approximately 0.8 torr). We kept the injector at 250 °C and the source at 150 °C. Oven temperature was kept at 60 °C for 1 min and then raised to 320 °C at a rate of 30 °C/min.

Preparation of Standards

12-KETE and 12-oxo-5,8,10-dodecatrienoic acid (12-ODTE) were prepared from 12-HPETE as described by Fruteau de Laclos et al.[7] 12-KETE was also prepared by oxidation of 12-HETE with activated manganese dioxide.[7]

Intracellular recordings

Abdominal ganglia were pinned ventral side up to Sylgard, a silicone plastic (Dow Chemical, Midland, MI), in a chamber continuously superfused with supplemented artificial seawater at room temperature. The connective tissue sheath was removed by dissection; L14 neurons, identified as previously described,[9,10] were impaled with one or two glass recording microelectrodes filled with potassium citrate (1–5 MΩ resistance). Compounds to be tested were ejected with pressure from a glass micropipette placed approximately 0.5 mm from the cell body. Samples from stock solutions of 12-HPETE, 12-KETE, and 12(S)-HETE (kept in hexane or ethanol at -20 °C) were dried under nitrogen, reconstituted in the seawater, and sonicated for 15 sec.

RESULTS AND DISCUSSION

Several biologically active molecules can be formed from 12-HPETE. Among the metabolites that have been identified thus far are 12-KETE,[7] 12-ODTE,[6,7] and several isomeric epoxy alcohols.[5,11,12] The possibility that 12-HPETE must be metabolized to produce its action in *Aplysia* neurons is suggested by an observation of Belardetti et al.:[4] the increased opening of K_S^+ channels evoked by 12-HPETE occurs only in cell-attached (but not in cell-free) patches of sensory neuron membranes. This suggests that a cytosolic component, possibly an enzyme, is required to metabolize the hydroperoxy acid further.

We describe here a novel bioactive metabolite formed in nervous tissue of *Aplysia*, the keto-acid 12-KETE. Identification was carried out by HPLC, UV spectrometry, and GC/MS in lipid extracts of the nervous tissue incubated with exogenous arachidonic acid or 12-HPETE. Homogenates of *Aplysia* nervous tissue were incubated with arachidonic acid (50 μM, 30 min), and the metabolites formed were analyzed by normal-phase HPLC (FIG. 1A). Several unidentified components with absorption maxima at 270 nm were observed (compounds a_1, a_2, and b).

The UV spectra of compounds a_1 and a_2 (FIG. 1A, inset) indicated the presence of a dienone or dienal chromophore, with maximal absorbance at 273 nm for a_1, and 271 nm for a_2. After they were purified by normal-phase HPLC, we also analyzed compounds a_1 and a_2 by reversed-phase HPLC, where they eluted as a single component (FIG. 1B). UV spectral analysis (FIG. 1B, inset) showed a pronounced bathochromic shift in absorbance (λ max = 280 nm). A spectral shift caused by the increased polarity of the solvent is characteristic of conjugated dienones and dienals.[6,7]

The presence of a conjugated carbonyl group was confirmed by reducing the methyl esters of the two compounds with sodium borohydride. Analysis of the reduced methyl esters of a_1 and a_2 by normal-phase HPLC revealed two components with UV absorbance near 235 nm (FIG. 1C): the first (a_1) eluted with the retention time of 12-HETE methyl ester and had an absorption maximum at 235 nm (FIG. 1C, inset), typical of cis-trans conjugated dienes. The second component (a_2) had a maximal absorbance near 231 nm, compatible with a trans-trans diene. This suggests that the

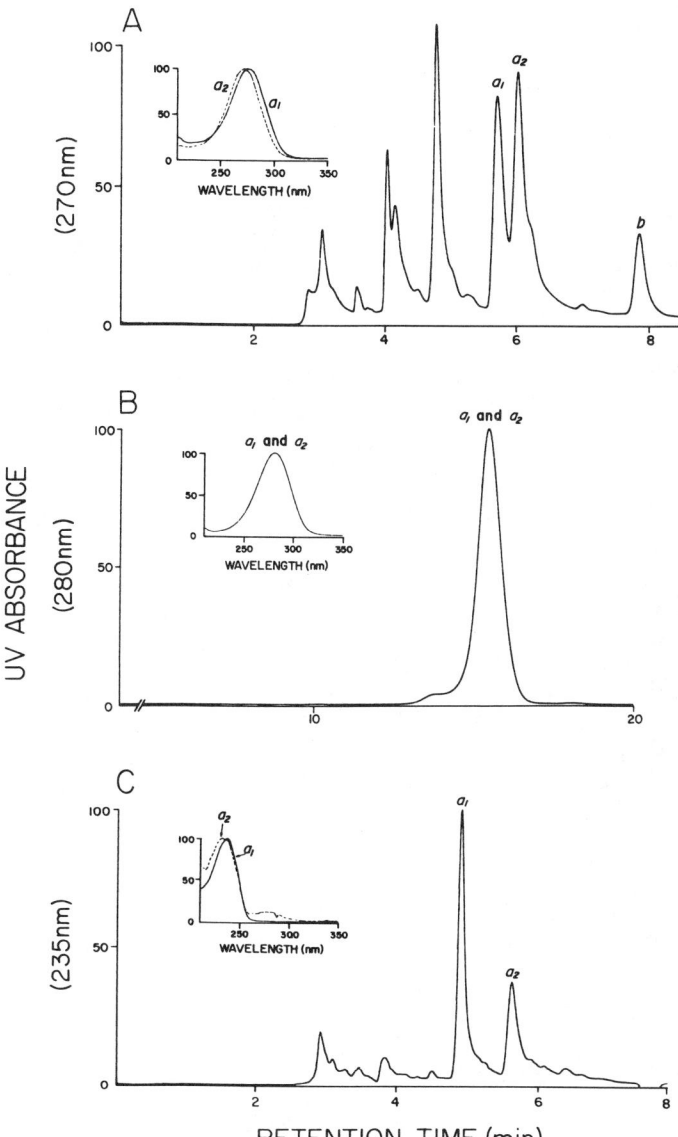

FIGURE 1. Isolation and characterization of 12-keto-5,8,10,14-eicosatetraenoic acid (12-KETE) from incubations of *Aplysia* nervous tissue with arachidonic acid (100 μM). **A:** normal-phase HPLC. Extracted lipids were fractionated on a silica column eluted with hexane:isopropanol:acetic acid (98:2:0.1, v/v/v) at 1 ml/min. UV absorbance was monitored at 270 nm. **B:** reversed-phase HPLC analysis of compounds a_1 and a_2 after they had been purified by normal-phase HPLC. Fractions containing 12-KETE, reduced to dryness and redissolved in the mobile phase, were applied to a Nucleosil C18 column eluted with methanol:water:acetic acid (65:35:0.1, v/v/v) at 1 ml/min. UV absorbance was monitored at 280 nm. **C:** normal-phase HPLC of the alcohols resulting from reduction of a_1 and a_2 with sodium borohydride. These alcohols were fractionated on a silica column as described above. UV absorbance was monitored at 235 nm. *Insets* show spectra obtained with a flow-through diode-array spectrophotometer of the compounds in the HPLC mobile phase (see EXPERIMENTAL PROCEDURES). (From Piomelli *et al.*[15] Reprinted by permission from the *Journal of Biological Chemistry*.)

reduction of the compounds with sodium borohydride yields two alcohols, 12-hydroxy-5,8,10,14($ZZEZ$)-eicosatetraenoic acid methyl ester (12-HETE methyl ester) and its geometric isomer, 12-hydroxy-5,8,10,14($ZEEZ$)-eicosatetraenoic acid.

As shown by radiolabeling experiments, compounds a_1 and a_2 are derived from arachidonic acid. Normal-phase HPLC analysis resolved two major radioactive components (FIG. 2): the first contained [^{3}H]arachidonate added as substrate as well as [^{3}H]12-HETE, and the second corresponded to compounds a_1 and a_2. Formation of these products was inhibited (>95%, $n = 2$) by incubation of the homogenates with the lipoxygenase inhibitor nordihydroguaiaretic acid (NDGA) (30 μM), but not by aspirin, a cyclooxygenase blocker (0.5 mM). This suggests that a 12-lipoxygenase enzyme catalyzes the biosynthesis of this metabolite from arachidonic acid.

In accord with this idea, we found that compounds a_1 and a_2 could also be formed when nervous tissue was incubated with 12-HPETE (50 μM, 10 min, data not shown). Boiling the tissue did not affect the conversion of exogenous 12-HPETE to these compounds, however, confirming previous reports that exogenous 12-HPETE can be converted nonenzymatically: conversion of fatty acid hydroperoxides to keto-acids and aldehydes can be catalyzed by hematin or by heme-containing proteins.[7,13,14]

Compounds a_1 and a_2 have the HPLC retention values and UV spectra of authentic 12-KETE prepared by incubating 12-HPETE with hemoglobin or by oxidation of 12-HETE with manganese dioxide. This identification was confirmed by GC/MS. Negative-ion chemical ionization analysis of pentafluorobenzyl (PFB) esters of metabolites a_1 and a_2 showed that these compounds eluted together and produced a mass spectrum identical to that of authentic 12-KETE, with only one prominent ion at m/z 317 (M $-$ 181, loss of PFB) (FIG. 3A).

Additional structural analysis was carried out by electron impact GC/MS. The methyl esters of compounds a_1 and a_2 were eluted from the GC with a carbon chain value of 21.8 (FIG. 3B), as previously reported for 12-KETE methyl ester.[7] Ions of high intensity were observed at m/z 332 (M$^+$), 314 (M$^+$ $-$ 18, loss of H$_2$O), 301

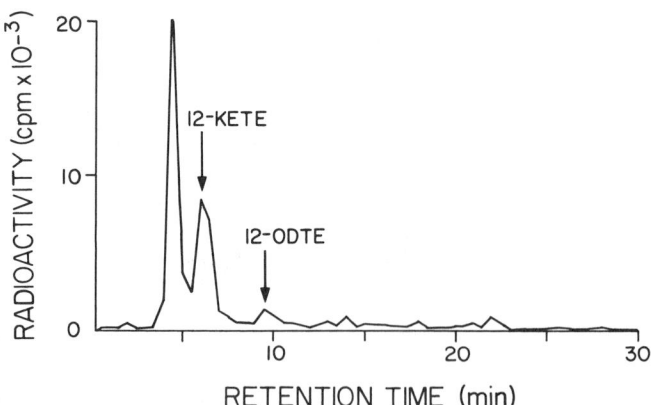

FIGURE 2. HPLC purification of radioactive compounds a_1 and a_2. Nervous tissue was incubated for 30 min with [^{3}H]arachidonic acid (12.5 μCi). The radioactive products were extracted and fractionated by normal-phase HPLC as described in the legend to FIG. 1. Radioactivity in fractions (0.5 min) was counted by liquid scintillation. 12-KETE = 12-keto-5,8,10,14-eicosatetraenoic acid; 12-ODTE = 12-oxo-5,8,10-deodecatrienoic acid. (From Piomelli et al.[15] Reprinted by permission from the *Journal of Biological Chemistry*.)

FIGURE 3. GC/MS analyses of compounds a_1 and a_2. **A:** Negative-ion chemical ionization mass spectrum of the pentafluorobenzyl (PFB) esters of a_1 and a_2. The MS source was held at 150 °C, and methane (0.8 torr) was the ionizing gas. The base peak in the spectrum represents the loss of the PFB-ester group leaving the carboxylate anion. **B:** mass spectrum of the methyl esters of a_1 and a_2. The MS source was held at 200 °C, and the ionizing voltage was set to 25 eV. (From Piomelli et al.[15] Reprinted by permission from the *Journal of Biological Chemistry*.)

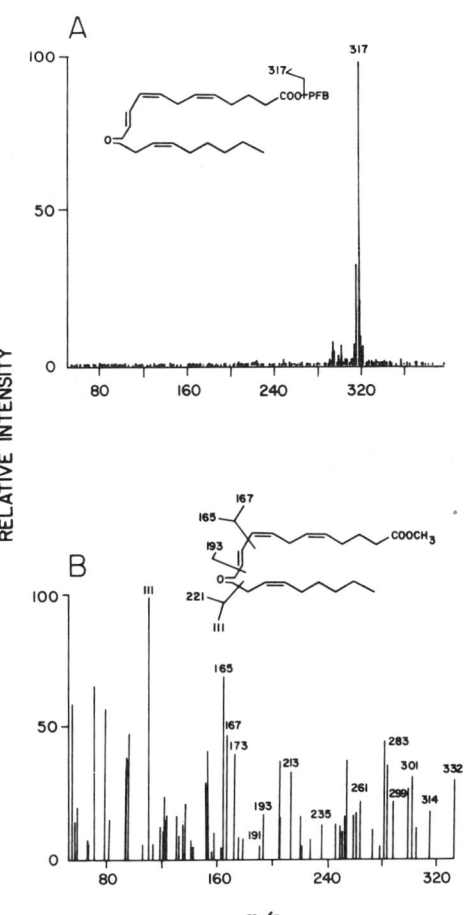

($M^+ - 31$, loss of CH_3O), 299 ($M^+ - [18 + 15]$), 283 ($M^+ - [31 + 18]$), 261 (loss of $CH_2 - (CH_2)_3CH_3$), 235 (beta-cleavage, with loss of C14 to C20), 221 (loss of CH_2—CH = CH—$(CH_2)_4$—CH_3), 193 (loss of C12–C20), 167 and 165 and 111 (base peak).

Stimulation of [³H]12-KETE Production by Neurotransmitter

Histamine stimulates the generation of [³H]12-HETE in *Aplysia* nervous tissue prelabeled with [³H]arachidonic acid.[1] Using a similar experimental protocol, we found that application of histamine caused nearly a 10-fold increase in radioactivity associated with 12-KETE compared to controls ($p < 0.05$, Student's t-test) (FIG. 4).

In addition to 12-KETE, other products of 12-HPETE are formed in *Aplysia* nervous tissue, including the short-chain aldehyde 12-oxododecatrienoic acid (12-ODTE) and two epoxy alcohols, 8-hydroxy-11,12-epoxyeicosatrienoic and 10-

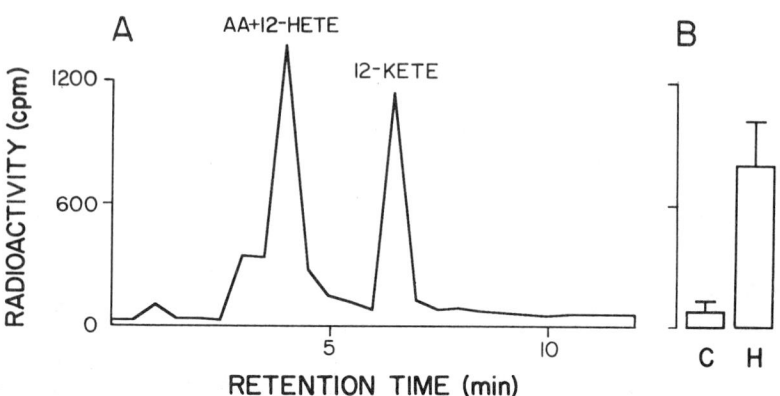

FIGURE 4. Stimulation of [^{3}H]12-KETE formation by histamine. Nervous tissue, labeled in artificial seawater for 2 h with [^{3}H]arachidonic acid (25 μCi/ml), was exposed for 1 min to histamine (100 μl, final concentration 50 μM). Products were then extracted from 50-μl samples of the incubation medium and subjected to normal-phase HPLC as described in the legend to FIG. 1. Radioactivity in fractions (0.5 min) was counted by liquid scintillation. A: representative chromatogram typical of four experiments. Analysis of material in the peak eluting before 12-keto-5,8,10,14-eicosatetraenoic acid (12-KETE) by reversed-phase HPLC reveals that it contains arachidonic acid (AA) (88%) and 12-hydroxyecosatetraenoic acid (12-HETE) (12%). B: Amounts of [^{3}H]12-KETE formed during exposure to histamine (H) or artificial seawater (control, C). Error bars represent the SEM, n = 4. (From Piomelli et al.[15] Reprinted by permission from the *Journal of Biological Chemistry*.)

hydroxy-11,12,epoxy-eicosatrienoic acids.[2,15,16] Application of histamine selectively releases [^{3}H]12-HETE and [^{3}H]12-KETE, however, On the other hand, after intracellular stimulation of the identified neuron L32, prelabeled abdominal ganglia release [^{3}H]12-HETE[1] and [^{3}H]8-hydroxy-11,12-epoxy-eicosatrienoic acid.[2] The reason for the difference in metabolites released by the two physiological treatments still remains to be determined. One possibility is that activation of specific receptors may result in the release of specific metabolites because the receptors activated by histamine might be a different subset of histaminergic receptors from those activated by the transmitter released endogenously by L32. Alternatively, while all the known actions of L32 cells are simulated by histamine and L32 PSPs are sensitive to cimetidine, a histamine antagonist in *Aplysia*,[17,18] it is still uncertain whether L 32 cells are definitively histaminergic.[19]

In preliminary experiments, we found that intracellular stimulation of C2, an identified histaminergic neuron in the cerebral ganglion of *Aplysia*,[19,20] results in release of [^{3}H]12-KETE. Stimulating C2 did not evoke the formation of [^{3}H]12-ODTE or of the epoxy alcohols, however. These results further support the idea that activation of specific histamine receptors at some synapses leads to the formation of 12-KETE.

Physiological Activity of 12-KETE on Identified Aplysia *Neurons*

Pharmacological experiments with L14 and L10, neurons of the abdominal ganglion, suggest that 12-KETE participates in the intracellular transduction of some of the actions of histamine. Each identified cell shows different and characteristic electrophysiological responses to histamine. In L14, histamine rapidly depolarizes the membrane, which is typically followed by a longer-lasting hyperpolarization.[18]

In the majority of neurons tested, applications of 12-HPETE or 12-KETE (1–2 nmol) from an extracellular puff micropipette produced a response similar to that evoked by histamine (FIG. 5, TABLE 1). Similar puffs of 12(S)-HETE were ineffective.

L10, a mixed-action neuron regulating heart and kidney function,[21] responds to histamine with a slow hyperpolarization, caused by increased K^+ conductance and decreased Ca^{2+} conductance.[18] A similar inhibitory response in L10 cells was produced by 12-KETE (TABLE 1). In only 30% of the cells tested was 12-HPETE effective, however; and 12(S)-HETE was again ineffective (TABLE 1). A possible explanation is that, as applied by the puffing micropipette, the metabolites are not completely accessible to critical sites in L10 at the concentrations used. Further experiments, using L10 neurons in culture, would be useful to test this idea.

The biological actions of 12-KETE that we have observed are in agreement with the hypothesis that conversion of 12-HPETE to the keto-acid is necessary for some of the effects of the hydroperoxy acid. Voltage-clamp and patch-clamp studies would show whether these 12-lipoxygenase products affect the same ion channels modulated by the endogenous transmitter.

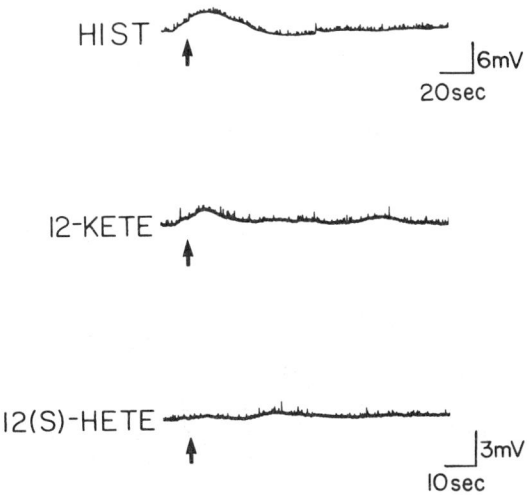

FIGURE 5. Effect of histamine and 12-lipoxygenase products on the membrane potential of L14. 1–2 nmoles of a test substance were ejected by pressure (5 sec, 6 psi) from a glass micropipette situated about 0.5 mm from the cell body of a L14 impaled with a voltage-sensitive microelectrode. Histamine (HIST) and 12-keto-5,8,10,14-eicosatetraenoic acid (12-KETE) elicited early depolarizing responses followed by a small slow hyperpolarization. 12(S)-hydroxy-5,8,10,14-eicosatetraenoic acid [12(S)-HETE] was ineffective in changing the membrane potential. The histamine response measured in this particular specimen was larger and longer-lasting than the response to 12-KETE (note difference in calibration of the electrophysiological traces). (From Piomelli *et al.*[15] Reprinted by permission from the *Journal of Biological Chemistry*.)

TABLE 1. Responses of Identified *Aplysia* Neurons to Histamine and Metabolites of Arachidonic Acid[a]

Treatment[b]	Experiments	Observations[c]	Responses[d]	Percent of Responses of Each Type		
				Depolarizing	Hyperpolarizing	Dual-Action[e]
Cell L14						
Histamine	28	58	54	11	2	87
12-KETE	6	18	16	12	25	62
12(S)-HETE	7	20	4	—[f]	—[f]	—[f]
12-HPETE	15	34	28	—[g]	—[g]	—[g]
Cell L10						
Histamine	15	35	33	0	100	0
12-KETE	3	11	8	0	100	0
12(S)-HETE	5	12	1	—[f]	—[f]	—[f]
12-HPETE	9	18	6	—[g]	—[g]	—[g]

NOTE: Compounds were applied to cells L14 and L10 as described in the legend to FIG. 5 and EXPERIMENTAL PROCEDURES.
[a] From Piomelli *et al.*[15]
[b] 12-KETE = 12-keto-5,8,10,14-eicosatetraenoic acid; 12(S)-HETE = 12(S)-hydroxy-5,8,10,14-eicosatetraenoic acid; 12-HPETE = 12-hydroperoxy-5,8,10,14-eicosatetraenoic acid.
[c] Within an experiment, each cell was tested as many as four times. The number of observations refers to the total number of times each of the compounds was applied.
[d] Total responses of all three types.
[e] Depolarizing/hyperpolarizing.
[f] Ineffective.
[g] Not determined.

SUMMARY

The lipoxygenase product 12-hydroperoxy-5,8,10,14-eicosatetraenoic acid (12-HPETE), simulates the synaptic responses produced by the modulatory transmitter histamine and the neuroactive peptide Phe-Met-Arg-Phe-amide (FMRFamide) in identified neurons of the marine mollusk *Aplysia californica*.[1,2] The 12-lipoxygenase pathway has not yet been fully characterized, but 12-HPETE is known to be metabolized further. Therefore, we began to search for other metabolites in order to investigate whether the actions of 12-HPETE might require its conversion to other active products. We have identified 12-keto-5,8,10,14-eicosatetraenoic acid (12-KETE) as a metabolite of 12-HPETE formed by *Aplysia* nervous tissue. 12-KETE was identified in incubations of the tissue with arachidonic acid using HPLC, UV spectrometry, and gas-chromatography/mass spectrometry. [^{3}H]12-KETE is formed from endogenous lipid stores in nervous tissue, labeled with [^{3}H]arachidonic acid upon stimulation by application of histamine. In L14 and L10 cells, identified neurons in the abdominal ganglion, applications of 12-KETE elicit changes in membrane potential similar to those evoked by histamine. Another metabolite of 12-HPETE, 12(s)-hydroxy-5,8,10,14-eicosatetraenoic acid [12(S)-HETE], is inactive. These results support the hypothesis that 12-HPETE and its metabolite, 12-KETE, participate in transduction of histamine responses in *Aplysia* neurons.

ACKNOWLEDGMENTS

We are grateful to Wayne Glasgow and Alan R. Brash, Vanderbilt University, for providing 12-ODTE and 12-KETE and for helpful suggestions; and to Jillayn Lindahl for her expert and cheerful assistance in typing the manuscript.

REFERENCES

1. PIOMELLI, D., E. SHAPIRO, S. J. FEINMARK & J. H. SCHWARTZ. 1987. Metabolites of arachidonic acid in the nervous system of *Aplysia*: Possible mediators of synaptic modulation. J. Neurosci. **7**: 3675–3686.
2. SHAPIRO, E., D. PIOMELLI, S. FEINMARK, S. VOGEL, G. CHIN & J. H. SCHWARTZ. 1988. The role of arachidonic acid metabolites in signal transduction in an identified neural network mediating presynaptic inhibition in *Aplysia*. Cold Spring Harbor Symp. Quant. Biol. **53**. In press.
3. PIOMELLI, D., A. VOLTERRA, N. DALE, S. A. SIEGELBAUM, E. R. KANDEL, J. H. SCHWARTZ & F. BELARDETTI. 1987. Lipoxygenase metabolites of arachidonic acid as second messengers for presynaptic inhibition of *Aplysia* sensory cells. Nature **328**: 38–43.
4. BELARDETTI, F., M. ROSOLOWSKY & W. CAMPBELL. 1987. Action of 12-hydroperoxyeicosatetraenoic acid (12-HPETE) on the S-K$^+$ channel in cell-free patches from *Aplysia* sensory neurons. Biophys. J. **53**: 144a.
5. PACE-ASCIAK, C. R., E. GRANSTROM & B. SAMUELSSON. 1983. Arachidonic acid epoxides. Isolation and structure of two hydroxy epoxide intermediates in the formation of 8,11,12 and 10,11,12-trihydroxy eicosatrienoic acids. J. Biol. Chem. **258**: 6835–6840.
6. GLASGOW, W. C., T. M. HARRIS & A. R. BRASH. 1986. A short-chain aldehyde is a major lipoxygenase product in arachidonic acid–stimulated leukocytes. J. Biol. Chem. **261**: 200–204.
7. FRUTEAU DE LACLOS, B., J. MACLOUF, P. POUBELLE & P. BORGEAT. 1987. Conversion of arachidonic acid into 12-oxo derivatives in human platelets, a pathway possibly involving the heme-catalyzed transformation of 12-hydroperoxyeicosatetraenoic acid. Prostaglandins **33**: 315–317.

8. PACE-ASCIAK, C. R., 1988. Formation and metabolism of hepoxilin A_3 in the rat brain. Biochem. Biophys. Res. Comm. **151:** 493–498.
9. CAREW, T. & E. R. KANDEL. 1977. Inking in *Aplysia californica*. I. Neural circuit of an all-or-none behavioral response. J. Neurophysiol. **40:** 692–707.
10. BYRNE, J. H., E. SHAPIRO, N. DIERINGER & J. KOESTER. 1979. Biophysical mechanisms contributing to inking behavior in *Aplysia*. J. Neurophysiol. **42:** 1233–1250.
11. WALKER, I. C., R. L. JONES & N. H. WILSON. 1979. The identification of an epoxy-hydroxy acid as a product from the incubation of arachidonic acid with washed blood platelets. Prostaglandins **18:** 173–178.
12. BRYANT, R. W. & J. M. BAILEY. 1979. Isolation of a new lipoxygenase metabolite of arachidonic acid, 8,11,12-trihydroxy-5,9,14-eicosatrienoic acid from human platelets. Prostaglandins **17:** 9–18.
13. FRUTEAU DE LACLOS, B. & P. BORGEAT. 1988. Conditions for the formation of the oxo derivatives of arachidonic acid from platelet 12-lipoxygenase and soybean 15-lipoxygenase. Biochim. Biophys. Acta **958:** 424–433.
14. DIX, T. A. & L. J. MARNETT. 1985. Conversion of linoleic acid hydroperoxide to hydroxy, keto, epoxyhydroxy and trihydroxy fatty acids by hematin. J. Biol. Chem. **260:** 5351–5357.
15. PIOMELLI, D., S. J. FEINMARK, E. SHAPIRO & J. H. SCHWARTZ. 1988. Formation and biological activity of 12-keto-eicosatetraenoic acid in the nervous system of *Aplysia*. J. Biol. Chem. **263:** 16591–16596.
16. FEINMARK, S. J., D. PIOMELLI, E. SHAPIRO & J. H. SCHWARTZ. 1989. Biologically active metabolites of the 12-lipoxygenase pathway are formed by *Aplysia* nervous tissue. Ann. N.Y. Acad. Sci. This volume.
17. KRETZ, R., E. SHAPIRO & E. R. KANDEL. 1986. Presynaptic inhibition produced by an identified presynaptic neuron. I. Physiological mechanisms. J. Neurophysiol. **55:** 113–130.
18. KRETZ, R., E. SHAPIRO, C. H. BAILEY, M. CHEN & E. R. KANDEL. 1986. Presynaptic inhibition produced by an identified presynaptic inhibitory neuron. II. Presynaptic conductance changes caused by histamine. J. Neurophysiol. **55:** 131–146.
19. SCHWARTZ, J. H., A. ELSTE, E. SHAPIRO & H. GOTOH. 1986. Biochemical and morphological correlates of transmitter type in C2: An identified histaminergic neuron in *Aplysia*. J. Comp. Neurol. **245:** 401–421.
20. WEINREICH, D., D. WEINER & R. E. MCCAMAN. 1975. Endogenous levels of histamine in single neurons isolated from CNS of *Aplysia californica*. Brain Res. **84:** 341–345.
21. KOESTER, J. & U. T. KOCH. 1987. Neural control of the circulatory system of *Aplysia*. Experientia **43:** 972–980.

Antagonistic Modulation of S-K$^+$ Channel Activity by Cyclic AMP and Arachidonic Acid Metabolites

Role for Two G Proteins[a]

ANDREA VOLTERRA[b] AND STEVEN A. SIEGELBAUM

Department of Pharmacology
Center for Neurobiology and Behavior
Howard Hughes Medical Institute
Columbia University
New York, New York 10032

INTRODUCTION: SYNAPTIC MODULATION AND LEARNING

The excitatory synaptic connection between mechanoreceptor sensory neurons and motorneurons in the marine snail *Aplysia californica* provides a useful model for studying the molecular mechanisms underlying synaptic modulation and their relevancy in learning. Thus, the sensory-motor synapse represents a very simple neural circuit mediating a defensive reflex in *Aplysia*, the gill and siphon withdrawal reflex. Environmental stimuli can modify the strength of this synaptic connection and thereby modulate the animal's behavioral response. Different kinds of electrical stimuli to the tail have been shown to cause either sensitization or inhibition of the withdrawal reflex.[1] This dual modulation of the reflex is due to activation by tail shock of, respectively, facilitatory and inhibitory interneurons that synapse onto the presynaptic terminals of the sensory neurons.

Sensitization is caused by the activation of a modulatory circuit causing presynaptic facilitation at the sensory-motor synapse, with an increase of transmitter release from the presynaptic terminals. In contrast, behavioral inhibition involves activation of a presynaptic inhibitory input at the same synapse and results in a decrease of transmitter release from the sensory neuron's terminals. Although all the elements of the facilitatory and inhibitory circuits have not yet been identified, it is known that a group of facilitatory neurons utilizes serotonin (5-HT) as a transmitter, whereas other neurons utilize the two related small cardioactive peptides (SCPa and SCPb). Presynaptic inhibition is thought to be, at least in part, mediated by cells containing the tetrapeptide Phe-Met-Arg-Phe-NH2 (FMRFamide), a molluscan neuropeptide displaying sequence homology with the enkephalins. Moreover, application of exogenous 5-HT and FMRFamide on sensory neurons mimics, respectively, presynaptic facilitation and inhibition induced by behavioral sensitization and inhibition (FIG. 1).

CELLULAR AND IONIC BASIS OF PRESYNAPTIC MODULATION

What is the cellular and ionic mechanism underlying presynaptic facilitation and inhibition in *Aplysia* sensory neurons? Direct application of 5-HT to the sensory

---

[a]This work was supported in part by National Institutes of Health Grant NS-19569.
[b]Present address: Center of Neuropharmacology and Institute of Pharmacological Sciences, University of Milan, Via Balzaretti, 9, 20133 Milan, Italy.

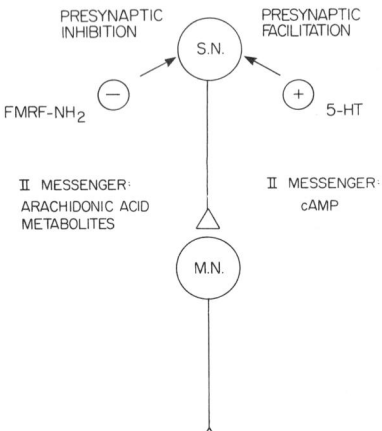

FIGURE 1. Schematic diagram for two types of presynaptic modulation of the sensory-motor synapse that mediates the gill and siphon withdrawal reflex in *Aplysia*. **Left:** the tetrapeptide FMRFamide produces presynaptic inhibition mediated by lipoxygenase metabolites of arachidonic acid. **Right:** Serotonin (5-HT) produces presynaptic facilitation through a cyclic AMP cascade. S.N. = sensory neurons; M.N. = motor neurons.

neurons leads to a slow depolarization associated with a decrease in membrane conductance, an increase in action potential duration, and an increase in transmitter release from the sensory neuron terminals (FIG. 2A). These effects are, at least in part, due to a modulatory decrease in a specific K^+ current by 5-HT, named the S current because of its sensitivity to serotonin.[2] Prolongation of the action potential duration by reduction of this outward K^+ current is thought to indirectly increase Ca^{++} influx into the sensory neuron terminals, therefore enhancing transmitter release. However, other contributory mechanisms to presynaptic facilitation independent of K^+ channel modulation have recently been identified.[3,4,5]

Application of FMRFamide to the sensory neurons leads to a series of inhibitory effects that are the opposite of those seen during facilitation. Thus, FMRFamide induces a slow hyperpolarization of the sensory neuron membrane, accompanied by an increase in membrane conductance, a decrease in action potential duration, and a decrease in transmitter release from the sensory neuron terminals (FIG. 2B). In molluscan neurons FMRFamide has been shown to have several actions on ionic currents, including an increase in an inward Na^+ current,[6,7] an increase[6] and decrease[8-11] in separate outward K^+ currents, and a decrease in a voltage-dependent inward Ca^{++} current.[9-12] Combined activation of a K^+ current and decrease of a Ca^{++} current by FMRFamide was observed in the sensory neurons as well as in other *Aplysia* neurons[11-14] and is thought to account for the presynaptic inhibitory action of the peptide.

We were particularly interested in the initial study by Erxleben *et al.*,[8] which suggested that the FMRFamide-sensitive K^+ current had properties similar to the S current. This finding raised the question as to whether the S channel could be modulated in opposing directions by distinct neurotransmitters.

UP- AND DOWN-MODULATION OF A SINGLE CLASS OF K^+ CHANNELS BY FACILITATORY AND INHIBITORY TRANSMITTERS

With the introduction of the patch-clamp technique, it became possible to study neurotransmitter actions at the molecular level of single channel function. One important goal of our initial single channel studies was to identify the K^+ channel modulated by 5-HT and to characterize the mode of action of 5-HT on single channel function. Since the mean current carried by a population of channels is given by $I = N_f \times p_o \times i$, where N_f is the number of functional channels, p_o is the probability that a given channel is open, and i is the single channel amplitude, a modulatory transmitter could alter the net ionic current carried by a population of channels by altering any one of these three parameters.

Using single channel recording, we identified a background K^+ channel in the sensory neurons that is active at the resting potential and whose gating (opening and closing reaction) is relatively independent of voltage and insensitive to internal Ca^{++} concentration.[15] However, application of 5-HT to the bathing solution appeared to decrease N_f, the number of functional channels in a cell-attached patch (FIG. 3A). No change in single channel current amplitude or in the open probability of the remaining

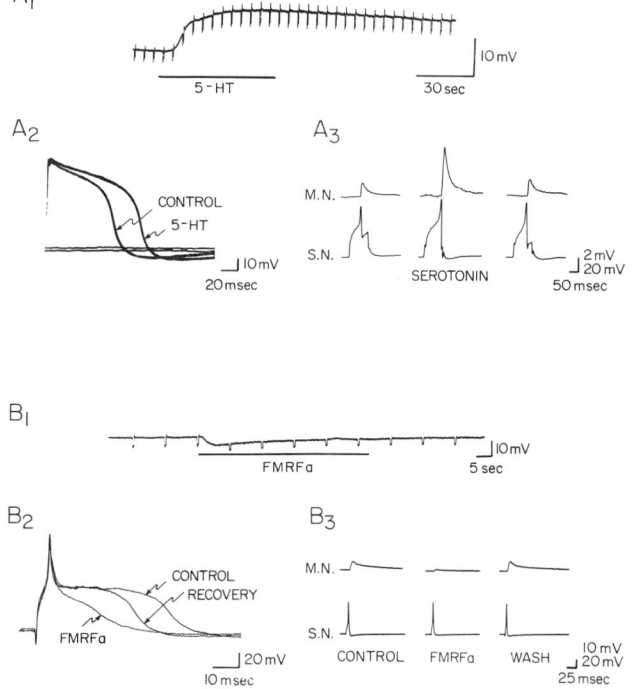

FIGURE 2. Effects of serotonin (A) and FMRFamide (B) on resting and action potentials in the sensory cell and on synaptic transmission between sensory and motor neurons. **A:** Serotonin (10 μM) causes a slow depolarization of the membrane resting potential with a decrease in conductance (seen as an increase in the voltage response to constant negative current pulses, A_1), an increase in the action potential duration (A_2), and an enhancement in sensory-motor transmission (A_3). A_3: *top trace* shows fast excitatory postsynaptic potentials (EPSPs) in the motor neuron in response to action potential stimulation in the sensory neuron (*bottom trace*). **B:** FMRFamide (10 μM) produces a slow hyperpolarization of the sensory neuron resting potential, accompanied by an increase in membrane conductance (B_1), a reversible decrease in action potential duration (B_2), and a reduction in the fast EPSP in follower motor neuron (B_3: *upper traces*) in response to firing an action potential in sensory neuron (B_3: *lower traces*).

active channels was detected. Therefore, 5-HT closes a fraction of the active S channels in the patch. This effect is all-or-nothing in that channels that still open in the presence of 5-HT appear to open and close normally, whereas channels once closed by 5-HT remain closed for prolonged times.

By contrast, application of the inhibitory peptide FMRFamide to the bath caused a consistent increase in S channel activity in the cell-attached patch (FIG. 3B). In the presence of FMRFamide, the mean S current through the patch (I) is increased several-fold over a broad range of membrane potentials. Is FMRFamide increasing I by increasing N_f (i.e., the mirror image of 5-HT modulation), p_o, or i? Direct inspection of the single channel current records shows that FMRFamide (like 5-HT)

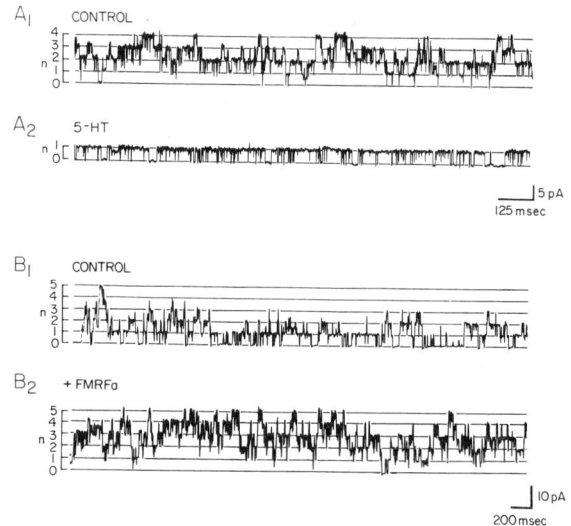

FIGURE 3. Action of serotonin (A) and FMRFamide (B) on single S channel current. (A_1) Channel activity (control) in absence of serotonin due to random openings and closings of four active S-K^+ channels present in the patch (*left-hand ordinate* gives the number of channels simultaneously open). (A_2) After application of serotonin (10 μM), three of the four channels close, whereas the remaining one continues to open and close normally. (B_1) Control trace from another patch containing five active S channels. After application of 2 μM FMRFamide (B_2) there is a significant increase in channel activity, with more channels overlapping in the open state. However, the maximal number of open channels does not change.

has no significant effect on i, the single channel current amplitude. Thus FMRFamide must act either on N_f or p_o. Three lines of evidence suggest that FMRFamide does not increase the number of functional channels in the patch, but rather increases the probability that a functional channel is in the open state. The first way to estimate the number of functional channels in a patch is simply to count the maximum number of overlapping channel openings during a long recording. Despite a four-fold increase in mean channel current, as seen in FIGURE 3B, the maximum number of overlapping events does not change. Next, we can obtain a more quantitative estimate for N_f and p_o from a binomial analysis of the observed probabilities that a given number of channels is open simultaneously. The binomial analysis confirms that there is no change in N_f

with FMRFamide and that the increase in mean channel current is due to an increase in p_o. Finally, in an experiment with a patch that contained only a single active S channel, FMRFamide produced a large increase in channel open probability without recruiting any silent channels. Therefore, we conclude that FMRFamide acts on the S channel by increasing p_o, the probability of finding the channel in the open state.

These experiments show that a single class of K^+ channels is, indeed, the target of distinct and functionally antagonistic modulatory mechanisms, resulting in the down-modulation of channel activity by 5-HT and the up-modulation of channel activity by FMRFamide. However, although FMRFamide and 5-HT modulate the same S channel in opposing directions, the actions of the two transmitters are not precisely mirror images of one another and appear to involve different modes of action on single channel function.

TWO DISTINCT SECOND-MESSENGER SYSTEMS MEDIATE THE ANTAGONISTIC MODULATION OF S CHANNEL FUNCTION BY FACILITATORY AND INHIBITORY TRANSMITTERS

The single channel experiments described above provide another important piece of information: both 5-HT and FMRFamide must act on the S channels through a second messenger. Thus, the patch pipette in the cell-attached mode forms a very stable, high resistance seal with the cell membrane that is thought to prevent diffusion of transmitters or other ligands from outside to inside the pipette. As a result, in the case of the nicotinic acetylcholine receptor of skeletal muscle (which is directly opened by transmitter binding to a single receptor-channel macromolecular complex), acetylcholine has to be introduced in the patch pipette to open channels under the pipette. By contrast, both 5-HT and FMRFamide modulate the S channels present in the patch when applied to the bathing solution outside the pipette. This observation implies that internal second messengers must exist that diffuse within the cell to couple the 5-HT and FMRFamide receptors to the K^+ channels under the pipette.

cAMP-Dependent Protein Phosphorylation Mediates the Action of Facilitatory Transmitters

One feature common to the strong tail stimuli that produce sensitization and to the application of either 5-HT or SCP to the sensory neurons is an increase in the intracellular levels of cAMP.[16] Moreover, injection of cAMP or the cAMP-dependent protein kinase into the sensory neurons simulates presynaptic facilitation.[17] These observations suggest that cAMP is the second messenger mediating the effects of 5-HT on the sensory cell, including the modulation of the S channels. To test this hypothesis directly, cAMP was intracellularly injected in sensory neurons while monitoring S channel activity under a patch pipette. cAMP was able to close single S channels in the patch in an all-or-nothing manner identical to that seen with 5-HT (FIG. 4A).[15] Moreover, direct application of the catalytic subunit of purified cAMP-dependent protein kinase to S channels in cell-free inside-out patches (where the internal surface of the membrane is exposed to the bathing solution) was also tested and resulted in prolonged all-or-none S channel closure (FIG. 4B).[18]

Thus, cAMP-dependent protein phosphorylation appears to be the molecular mechanism through which 5-HT, as well as the other facilitatory transmitters, act to decrease S channel activity. The substrate phosphoprotein involved in channel

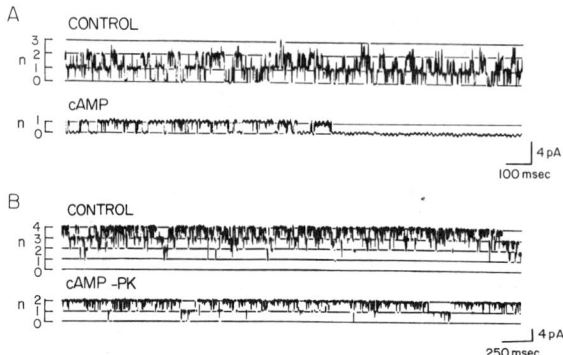

FIGURE 4. Action of cAMP (A) and the catalytic subunit of cAMP-dependent protein kinase (cAMP-PK, B) on single S channel current. (A) Control, current in absence of cAMP: three channels open and close randomly in this patch. cAMP: following iontophoretic injection into the sensory neuron of cAMP, only one channel remains open, and after a while this last channel closes. (B) Control, record from a cell-free inside-out patch (where the internal surface of the membrane is exposed to the bathing solution) containing four active channels. cAMP-PK: after addition of cAMP-PK plus Mg-ATP, two channels close and the current level fluctuates from zero to two channels open.

modulation is either the channel itself or an intermediate regulatory protein present in the small cell-free patch of membrane.

Lipoxygenase Metabolites of Arachidonic Acid Mediate the Action of the Inhibitory Transmitters

What is the identity of the second messenger recruited by FMRFamide? As 5-HT closes the S channels through the cAMP pathway, an obvious possibility is that FMRFamide decreases the resting cAMP concentration and thus leads to channel opening. However, no changes in cAMP levels in the sensory neurons are seen in response to FMRFamide.[10] Our single channel results also do not support a decrease in cAMP as the mode of FMRFamide action, because this would be expected to lead to an increase in the number of functional channels (N_f) in the patch (i.e., the converse of the action of 5-HT) rather than the increase in open probability observed.

A number of lines of evidence also argue against a role for the phosphatidylinositol metabolites produced through phospholipase C—that is, IP3 and diacylglycerol—as mediators of FMRFamide action. Thus, IP3 injections do not mimic the S current activation or Ca^{++} current depression induced by FMRFamide in *Aplysia* neurons.[12] Phorbol esters, when applied to sensory neurons, lead to presynaptic facilitation of transmitter release, an effect opposite to the presynaptic inhibition seen with FMRFamide.[4] Also, cGMP and sodium nitroprusside (an agent able to increase cGMP levels in some tissues) proved ineffective in simulating the action of FMRFamide.[12]

The first clue as to the nature of the second messenger utilized by FMRFamide action came from a biochemical study of arachidonic acid metabolism in *Aplysia*.[19] This study showed that arachidonic acid is a prominent component of *Aplysia* membranes and is metabolized by two major kinds of enzymatic pathways, a cyclooxygenase pathway and at least two (5- and 12-) lipoxygenase pathways. Moreover, release of arachidonic acid from neural membranes is a receptor-mediated process, induced by the modulatory transmitter histamine and blocked by the histamine receptor antagonist cimetidine.

To determine whether the inhibitory actions of FMRFamide might involve arachidonic acid metabolism, we began a combined biophysical and biochemical study (in collaboration with D. Piomelli, N. Dale, E. R. Kandel, J. H. Schwartz, and F. Belardetti).[20]

One key finding in this study was that FMRFamide causes release of certain lipoxygenase metabolites of arachidonic acid from isolated sensory neuron clusters preincubated with ^{3}H-arachidonic acid. Following 1-min exposure to FMRFamide, a large increase in radioactivity was found associated with HPLC fractions correspond-

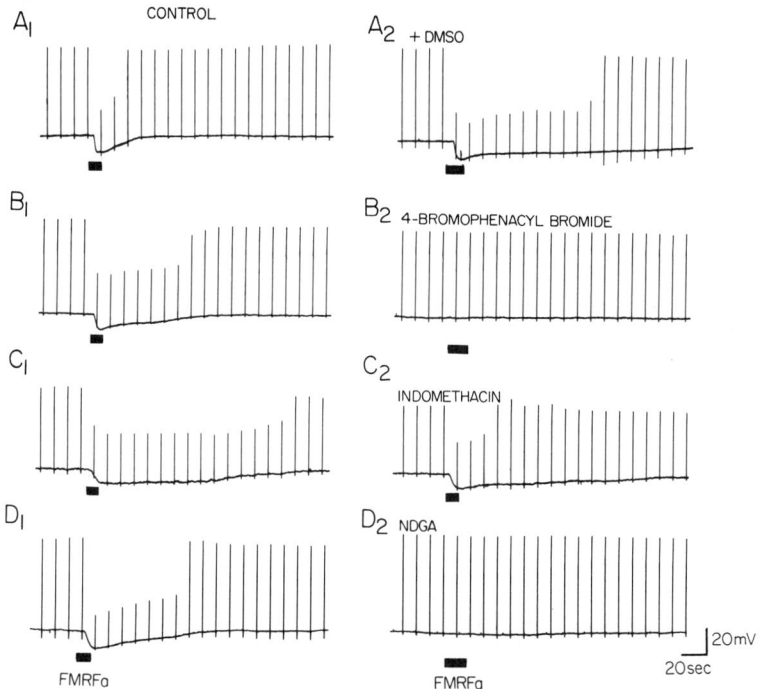

FIGURE 5. Action of inhibitors of arachidonic acid metabolism on the response to FMRFamide, as shown by chart records of membrane potential under current clamp from sensory cells in culture. Larger brief upward deflections are action potentials elicited by depolarizing current pulses. Smaller upward deflections are the passive depolarizations following action potential blockade. The *bars* mark the time of application of 2 μM FMRFamide. A–D: representative tracings from four different experiments. *Left* (A_1–D_1): control responses to the peptide. *Right* (A_2–B_2): responses to a second application of FMRFamide to the same cells after superfusion of a test compound. A_2: after superfusion with dimethylsulfoxide in artificial sea water (DMSO 1/10000). B_2, C_2, D_2: after superfusion of a sea water-DMSO mixture, containing in addition: (B_2) the phospholipase inhibitor 4-bromophenacylbromide (10 μM); (C_2) the cyclooxygenase blocker indomethacyn (5 μM); (D_2) the lipoxygenase inhibitor nordihydroguaiaretic acid (NDGA, 5 μM).

ing to 5- and 12-HETE. The effect of FMRFamide was relatively specific, since 5-HT did not lead to the release of these metabolites.

Is this effect of the peptide related to its action in channel modulation? Experiments utilizing inhibitors of arachidonic acid metabolism support this view. Thus, bromophenacylbromide (FIG. 5B), as well as mepacrine—two phospholipase inhibitors that block release of arachidonic acid from membranes—were able to block the hyperpolarizing response of the sensory neurons to FMRFamide. To dissect out which of the subsequent enzymatic reactions is involved in the action of FMRFamide, we used two other inhibitors—nordihydroguaiaretic acid (NDGA), which preferentially blocks lipoxygenases; and indomethacin, a cyclooxygenase blocker. While indomethacin had no effect (FIG. 5C), NDGA largely blocked the response to FMRFamide (FIG. 5D).

These results confirm the idea that the effects of FMRFamide are mediated by arachidonic acid metabolites and suggest that lipoxygenase, rather than cyclooxygenase, metabolites are involved in the response. One prediction from these observations is that either arachidonic acid or its active lipoxygenase products should mimic the effects of FMRFamide on sensory cell ionic conductances. Our results confirm that arachidonic acid application leads to a hyperpolarization of the sensory neuron, an increase in resting conductance, a decrease in action potential duration, and a decrease in transmitter release. FIGURE 6 illustrates and compares some of these effects with the action of FMRFamide. Using the voltage-clamp technique, we also showed that arachidonic acid increases an outward K^+ current identical to the S current activated

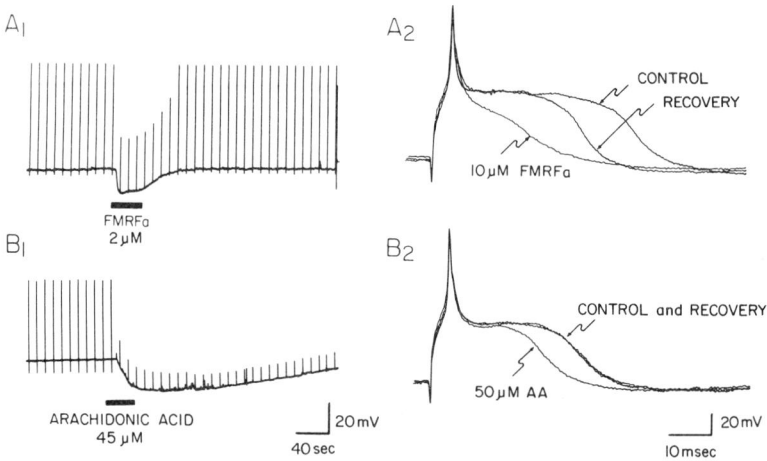

FIGURE 6. Arachidonic acid (B) simulates the action of FMRFamide (A) on whole cell potential responses. A_1 and B_1: changes in membrane potential and spike firing in response to FMRFamide (2 µM, A_1) or arachidonic acid (45 µM, B_1). The *solid bars* indicate periods of application. Upward spikes are action potentials elicited once every 10 sec by brief depolarizing constant current stimuli. The smaller spikes reflect action potential inhibition and are the passive depolarizing responses to the current steps. The slower time course of the arachidonate-induced hyperpolarization most likely reflects the time required for diffusion (or transport) across the plasma membrane and metabolism. A_2 and B_2: FMRFamide (A_2) and arachidonic acid (B_2) cause a reversible decrease in action potential duration. Action potentials recorded from sensory neuron in an intact abdominal ganglion in presence of 50 mM TEA (tetraethylammonium).

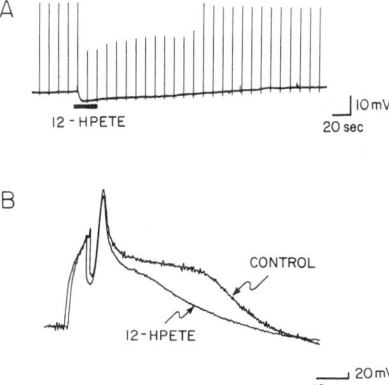

FIGURE 7. Effect of 12-HPETE on membrane and action potentials. **A:** effect of 1.5 μM 12-HPETE on resting potential and stimulated action potentials (brief upward spikes) in sensory neuron in culture. 12-HPETE inhibited spike firing for about 2 min (during this period the smaller spikes were subthreshold). **B:** effect of 60 μM 12-HPETE on action potential duration recorded from sensory neuron in intact abdominal ganglion in presence of 50 mM TEA (tetraethylammonium).

by FMRFamide. Finally, single channel studies confirm that exogenous application of arachidonate increases S channel opening.

Which lipoxygenase pathway is involved in the action of FMRFamide? We first tested the ability of 5- and 12-HETE, the two metabolites detected in response to FMRFamide application, to simulate the peptide's effects on resting and action potential. Neither of these metabolites was effective. However, the short-lived hydroperoxy intermediate 12-HPETE simulated both the FMRFamide-induced hyperpolarization and shortening of the action potential (FIG. 7). The corresponding 5-lipoxygenase product, 5-HPETE, displayed a weaker effect on action potential duration and had little effect on resting potential.

Therefore, 12-HPETE is a good candidate for the active second messenger in FMRFamide's action. However, 12-HPETE has been shown in other systems to be further metabolized to a family of compounds, including two epoxy-hydroxyderivatives (named epoxilins) and their hydrolytic products, the trioxilins.[21] Thus, the possibility exists that 12-HPETE could be further processed in *Aplysia* sensory neurons so that the metabolite ultimately responsible for S channel modulation by FMRFamide is not 12-HPETE but a metabolite of this intermediate compound, as suggested by Piomelli et al.[22]

INTERACTION OF FMRFamide AND 5-HT PATHWAYS

Although FMRFamide and 5-HT activate separate second messenger pathways, the two cascades do interact (FIG. 8). FIGURE 8A shows that application of FMRFamide during continuous exposure to 5-HT antagonizes the depolarizing action of 5-HT and hyperpolarizes the membrane to around the same level initially reached in response to FMRFamide alone. One possible mechanism by which FMRFamide could antagonize the 5-HT response is through an inhibitory GTP binding protein (G_i) that inhibits adenylate cyclase.[23] However, biochemical studies show that FMRFamide does not inhibit either basal or 5-HT–stimulated adenylate cyclase activity in *Aplysia*.[10,24]

Another compelling line of evidence that argues against the possibility that the interaction between the two cascades takes place at the level of adenylate cyclase

228 ANNALS NEW YORK ACADEMY OF SCIENCES

activity is the ability of FMRFamide to antagonize the effects of exogenously applied cAMP, as well as 5-HT, on the S channel. FIGURE 8B shows the interaction between FMRFamide and cAMP at the single channel level. In this experiment, there were initially four active S channels in the patch. The cell was then exposed to a membrane-permeant analog of cAMP, whereupon two of the four active channels closed. As seen from a binomial analysis (FIG. 8C), the open probability of the two remaining active channels was unchanged, confirming the all-or-none action of 5-HT and cAMP. Upon application of FMRFamide to the bathing solution in the continued presence of cAMP the two silent channels reopened, and there was a general increase

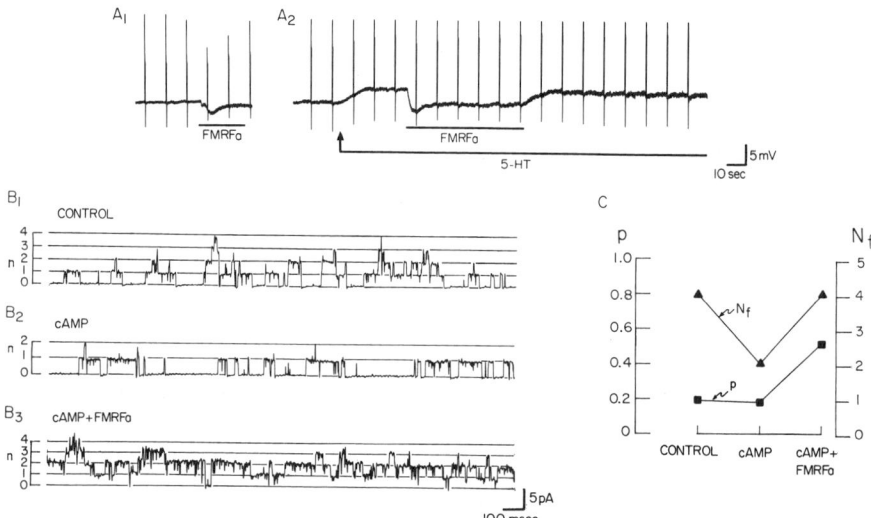

FIGURE 8. FMRFamide antagonizes S channel closure produced by serotonin and cAMP. **A:** membrane potential recordings showing a slow hyperpolarizing response to 2 μM FMRFamide alone (A_1) and on top of the depolarizing response to continuous 5-HT (1 μM) application (A_2). **B:** single channel recording from cell-attached patch under control conditions (B_1), after application of 0.1 mM dibutyryl-cAMP to the bath (B_2), and in presence of dibutyryl-cAMP plus 20 μM FMRFamide (B_3). **C:** binomial analysis of experiment shown in B. In control conditions there were four active channels with an open probability of 0.2. cAMP closes two of the active channels with no change in the open probability (p) of the remaining active channels. Subsequent addition of FMRFamide reopens the two closed channels and increases the open probability (of all four active channels) to 0.5. N_f = number of functional channels.

in open probability of all four channels. Thus, while FMRFamide does not recruit new channels under resting conditions (in the absence of 5-HT or cAMP), the peptide can reopen channels previously closed by 5-HT or cAMP.

One attractive possibility is that, in addition to a modulatory action on the S channel to increase its open probability, FMRFamide also activates a phosphoprotein phosphatase that dephosphorylates channels closed by cAMP and thus leads to their reopening. Preliminary results of a collaborative study with D. Sweatt and E. R. Kandel indicate that FMRFamide is, indeed, able to decrease the basal and cAMP-stimulated level of phosphorylation in a well-defined small group of sensory cell proteins. We are currently investigating whether such a mechanism also occurs at the S channel level and is mediated by the arachidonic acid cascade.

MECHANISMS FOR THE RECEPTOR-MEDIATED RELEASE OF ARACHIDONIC ACID IN *APLYSIA* SENSORY NEURONS

How is the binding of FMRFamide to its membrane receptor coupled to the release of arachidonic acid? How do the lipoxygenase metabolites lead to an increase in S channel opening?

Several mechanisms have been described in vertebrate cells for receptor-induced release of arachidonic acid from membrane phospholipids, including indirect activation of phospholipase A2 following an increase in intracellular Ca^{++},[25] intracellular alkalinization due to Na^+/H^+ exchange,[26] or direct phospholipase activation via G proteins.[27]

In a study in collaboration with H. Blumenfeld, B. Bug, N. Buttner, and D. Sweatt[28] we investigated whether FMRFamide altered resting levels of internal Ca^{++} or pH. The intracellular Ca^{++} levels were measured using the fluorescent Ca^{++} indicator dye Fura-2. No changes in resting intracellular Ca^{++} levels were detected in response to FMRFamide concentrations that induced marked effects on the sensory cell S current. The role of Na^+/H^+ exchange was studied first by replacing external Na^+ with the cell-impermeant cation N-methyl-d-glucamine. Na^+ removal significantly reduced the S current response to FMRFamide, leaving the response to arachidonic acid unaltered. Thus, there is a Na^+ sensitivity at a stage leading to arachidonic acid release. However, when the sensory cell internal pH was measured with the pH-sensitive dye BCEF, no changes were seen in response to FMRFamide application. FMRFamide also did not speed the recovery from acidification following exposure to NH3, arguing against a marked stimulation of the Na^+/H^+ exchange. The inhibition of the FMRFamide response in Na^+-free medium could be related to an observed decrease in internal pH of 0.3 pH units seen upon Na^+ removal.

These results indicate that the FMRFamide-induced release of arachidonic acid in *Aplysia* sensory neurons does not require an increase in internal Ca^{++} or pH. By contrast, we have recently demonstrated a role for a G protein at a stage before arachidonic acid release, and this mechanism may directly couple the FMRFamide receptor to phospholipase activation.[29,30]

ROLE OF A PERTUSSIS TOXIN–SENSITIVE G PROTEIN IN THE MODULATION OF THE S CHANNEL BY LIPOXYGENASE METABOLITES

As a first step towards analyzing the role of G proteins in the response to FMRFamide, we studied the effects of iontophoretic intracellular injection of GTP-gamma-S, an irreversible activator of G proteins,[31] on sensory cell membrane potential and ionic current. FIGURE 9A shows that GTP-gamma-S produces a slow, irreversible hyperpolarization associated with an increase in input conductance. Voltage-clamp experiments show that this hyperpolarization is due to activation of an outward conductance with the characteristics of the S current. Moreover, GTP-gamma-S alters the kinetics of the normally transient hyperpolarization in response to FMRFamide (see FIG. 2) into a partly or completely irreversible response (FIG. 9B). The persistent activation of S current with FMRFamide under these conditions suggests that the peptide does indeed activate a G protein, leading to an increased turnover of guanine nucleotides and enhanced rate of incorporation of GTP-gamma-S.

Independent evidence for an obligatory role for G proteins in the action of FMRFamide comes from experiments where the effects of two G-protein inhibitors were tested. Pressure injection into the sensory neuron of pertussis toxin, a bacterial toxin that blocks the activation of several distinct G proteins through ADP-rybosilation,[32] almost completely abolished the FMRFamide-induced hyperpolarization in a long-lasting manner (FIG. 10), but had no significant effect on the depolarization induced by 5-HT (FIG. 11). Iontophoretic injection of GDP-beta-S, another G-protein inhibitor,[33] also reduced the response to FMRFamide, although very high concentrations of this nucleotide are required (FIG. 12A).

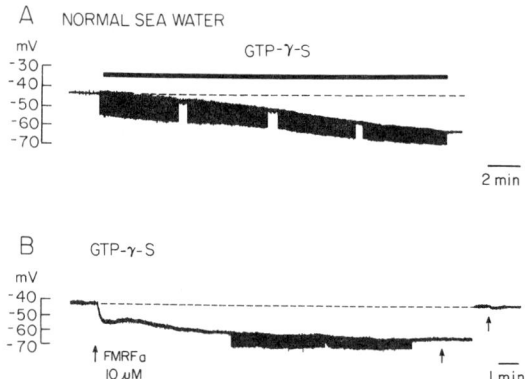

FIGURE 9. Effect of GTP-gamma-S on sensory neuron membrane potential (A), and on the FMRFamide-induced hyperpolarization (B). **A:** Membrane potential response to iontophoretic injection of GTP-gamma-S into sensory neurons. Microelectrode contained 25 mM GTP-gamma-S in 0.5 M KCL. Nucleotide injection into the cell using four 5-min periods of -0.2 nA current pulses (500 ms long at a frequency of 1 Hz). Input resistance given by amplitude of hyperpolarizing response to current pulses (regions with thickened trace). **B:** Response to FMRFamide (10 µM) under current clamp soon after impalement of sensory neuron with GTP-gamma-S (25 mM)–containing electrode. Note that before first application of FMRFamide (*first arrow*), membrane potential is stable. FMRFamide induces rapid hyperpolarization, from which there is only a small initial recovery. A second, slower phase of hyperpolarization is then seen (even though FMRFamide has been completely washed out at this time). GTP-gamma-S is then actively injected (thickened region of trace); and 10 min after injection, a maximal degree of hyperpolarization is reached, and responses to subsequent applications of FMRFamide are blocked at final hyperpolarized potential (*second arrow*) or when membrane is depolarized to original resting potential by outward current injection (*third arrow*).

At this point, our experiments clearly indicate a role for G proteins in the action of FMRFamide. Where in the arachidonic acid cascade does this G protein act? Is it involved at an early stage, perhaps coupling the receptor to arachidonate release, or is it involved at a late stage, for instance coupling the lipoxygenase metabolites to K^+ channel activation? To investigate these questions, we first studied the effects of pertussis toxin injection on the response to exogenously applied arachidonic acid. While pertussis toxin consistently inhibits the response to FMRFamide, it has little effect on the hyperpolarizing response to arachidonic acid (FIG. 11). This suggests that a pertussis toxin–sensitive G protein is involved in the cascade at an early stage, before arachidonic acid release. If this is the case, we should expect that blockers of arachidonic acid metabolism should also block the FMRFamide-like action of

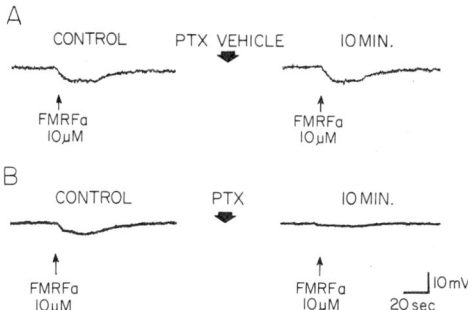

FIGURE 10. Effect of pertussis toxin (PTX) injection on FMRFamide-induced hyperpolarization. *Left:* FMRFamide responses before injections (control). *Right:* FMRFamide responses after injections. **A:** Pressure injection (through a 20–200-ms pulse of about 65 psi, controlled by an electrovalve) of PTX vehicle (50 mM NaCl, 0.5 M KCl, 10 mM dithiothreitol, 10 mM NAD^+, buffered with 10 mM sodium phosphate at pH 7.6) has little effect on response to FMRFamide (10 μM). **B:** Pressure injection of PTX (0.1 μg/μl in the above-described vehicle) largely inhibits response to FMRFamide. Right traces obtained 40 min after pressure injections. PTX produced no significant changes in input resistance or membrane potential.

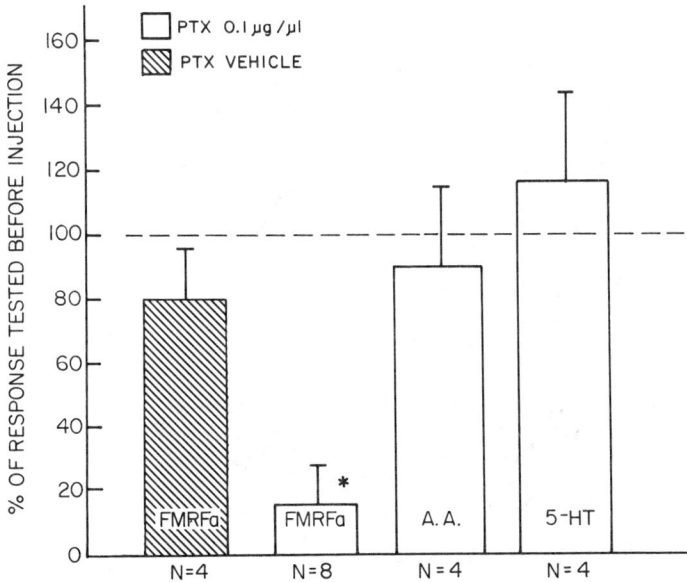

FIGURE 11. Mean effects of injection of either PTX vehicle (*cross-hatched histogram*) or active toxin (*open histograms*) on membrane potential response to different agents. 100% value represents the preinjection control response. From the left: Injection of PTX vehicle reduces only slightly the FMRFamide-induced hyperpolarization (average of 4 experiments: *error bars* show standard deviation). By contrast, PTX significantly reduces the FMRFamide response (average of 8 experiments), but leaves the arachidonic acid–induced hyperpolarization virtually unchanged (A.A., average of 4 experiments). Finally, PTX does not block the depolarization induced by 5-HT, instead causing a slight increase in the magnitude of the slow depolarization with this transmitter (average of 4 experiments). *$p < 0.001$ vs. preinjection test (Student *t* test).

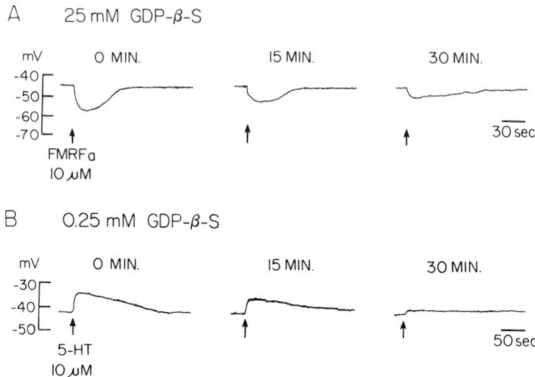

FIGURE 12. GDP-beta-S blocks responses to FMRFamide (A) and 5-HT (B). **A:** The hyperpolarizing response to FMRFamide (10 μM) is reduced by 50% 30 min after iontophoretic injection from microelectrode containing 25 mM GDP-beta-S in 0.5 M KCl. The injection protocol is identical to the one described in the legend to FIG. 9 for GTP-gamma-S injection. **B:** The depolarizing response to 5-HT (10 μM) is reduced by more than 80% 30 min after injection of 0.25 mM GDP-beta-S. At 2.5 mM, this nucleotide completely blocks the 5-HT response (not shown).

GTP-gamma-S to increase the S current and hyperpolarize the neuron. Indeed, we find that after preincubation of the sensory neurons with either the phospholipase inhibitor 4-bromophenacylbromide or the lipoxygenase inhibitor NDGA, the hyperpolarizing responses to both FMRFamide and GTP-gamma-S were blocked (data not shown).

Interestingly, under these conditions, where the FMRFamide response was completely abolished, GTP-gamma-S injection now resulted in a slow, irreversible depolarization accompanied by a decrease in input conductance. This effect resembles the normal, decreased conductance depolarization seen with 5-HT or cAMP (see FIG. 2). A likely explanation for this result is that GTP-gamma-S injection normally activates a stimulatory G protein (G_s), which leads to production of cAMP and closure of the S channels. In the absence of arachidonic acid blockers, apparently the FMRFamide pathway activated by GTP-gamma-S overrides the 5-HT pathway, just as we have previously seen (FIG. 8).

Supportive evidence for a G_s-like protein in the sensory neurons comes from a prior study that showed that a G protein couples the 5-HT receptor to stimulation of adenylate cyclase.[34] We confirmed the presence of this G protein by showing that the 5-HT–induced depolarization is blocked by GDP-beta-S (FIG. 12B). The response to 5-HT proved more sensitive to blockade with GDP-beta-S than the response to FMRFamide by at least 2 orders of magnitude (see FIG. 12). This lends support to the view that structurally distinct G proteins underlie the responses to 5-HT and FMRFamide. As further evidence that GTP-gamma-S leads to activation of the G_s-like G protein, we find the GTP-gamma-S in the presence of the lipoxygenase blocker NDGA transforms the kinetics of the normally reversible response to 5-HT into an irreversible, or only partially reversible, response (FIG. 13C). In the absence of arachidonate blockers it is impossible to detect this effect of GTP-gamma-S, because its hyperpolarizing action overwhelms the response to 5-HT (FIG. 13B).

Thus the dual modulation of the S channel by 5-HT and FMRFamide appears to involve distinct G proteins that activate distinct second-messenger cascades. While the G protein involved in the 5-HT cascade appears related to G_s (based on its ability to stimulate adenylate cyclase and PTX insensitivity), the FMRFamide-activated G protein, although PTX sensitive, does not appear related to G_i. Thus, as mentioned above, FMRFamide does not decrease resting cAMP levels or inhibit activation of adenylate cyclase with 5-HT.[10,24] Further evidence against a prominent G_i-like effect with FMRFamide comes from our finding that GTP-gamma-S in the presence of blockers of arachidonate metabolism leads to an excitatory response that appears to reflect activation of the cAMP cascade. If FMRFamide inhibited cAMP production through G_i, this inhibition should prevail in the presence of the arachidonate blockers, where GTP-gamma-S should still activate G_i.[35]

POSSIBLE ROLES FOR THE EICOSANOIDS IN NEURONAL SIGNALING

In this review we have seen that lipoxygenase metabolites of arachidonic acid mediate the presynaptic inhibitory action of the tetrapeptide FMRFamide in *Aplysia* sensory neurons. Presynaptic inhibition at sensory-motor synapses has been proven to be an important component of behavioral inhibition in *Aplysia*. Aversive stimuli can produce inhibition as well as sensitization of the gill and siphon withdrawal reflex.[1] Recently Mackey and co-workers have shown that inhibition following an electrical shock to the tail of the animal can be pharmacologically blocked by NDGA, whereas the facilitatory component of tail shock is preserved.[36]

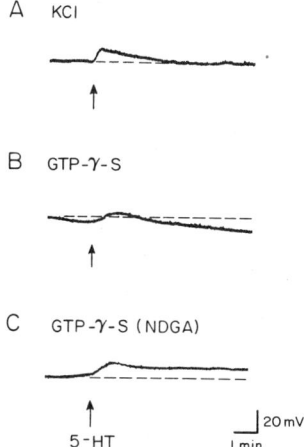

FIGURE 13. The GTP-gamma-S effect on 5-HT–induced depolarization is unmasked in the presence of arachidonate blockers. A: Normal, transient depolarization following application of 5-HT (10 μM) to a cell impaled with a 0.5-M KCl electrode. Note that the resting potential recovers to the initial level after washout of the transmitter. B: When a cell is impaled with an electrode containing 25 mM GTP-gamma-S in 0.5 M KCl, a continuous, slow, hyperpolarizing process is seen (compare with FIG. 9A). Application of 10 μM 5-HT results in a depolarizing response that is rapidly overwhelmed by the hyperpolarizing process. C: If the cell has previously been superfused with the lipoxygenase blocker NDGA (50 μM, 0.5% DMSO for 2 h) to block the FMRFamide pathway and then impaled with the 25-mM GTP-gamma-S + 0.5-M KCl electrode as in B, no hyperpolarizing process is now seen. Moreover, the transient depolarization following application of 10 μM 5-HT becomes irreversible, even after washout of the transmitter. Thus, the selective blockade of the intracellular FMRFamide cascade reveals the GTP-gamma-S activation of the 5-HT cascade.

This function for the arachidonic acid cascade is probably not unique to FMRFamide or to *Aplysia* sensory cells. Dopamine also produces presynaptic inhibition at the sensory-motor connection.[37] Recently Y. Yaari at Columbia has shown that dopamine, acting through a D2-like receptor, is able to induce an increase in the sensory neuron S current and that this effect is inhibited by NDGA (but not by indomethacin).

Morever, Piomelli et al.[19] have shown that both intracellular stimulation of the putative histaminergic neurons of the L32 cluster in the *Aplysia* abdominal ganglion and direct histamine application are able to induce the production of eicosanoids and, in particular, 12-HETE. An interesting functional parallel to the mode of action of FMRFamide on the sensory cells is that both L32 stimulation and histamine application cause presynaptic inhibition of the interneuron L10. The ionic mechanism of this effect seems to involve both an increase in a K^+ conductance and a decrease in a voltage-dependent Ca^{++} conductance.[14,38]

Many transmitters have been shown to produce presynaptic inhibition in vertebrates with similar ionic mechanisms. In the dorsal root ganglion sensory cells that mediate response to painful stimuli, such transmitters include enkephalins, acting through mu and delta opioid receptors, dynorphin, acting on kappa opioid receptors;[39] norepinephrine, through alpha-2 receptors; and GABA (γ-aminobutyric acid), through GABA-B receptors.[40] Therefore, it will be of interest to investigate whether there is a role for arachidonic acid metabolism in the inhibitory action of these transmitters.

Finally, eicosanoids differ from other intracellular second messengers in one important way: unlike other messengers, the eicosanoids are able to leave the cell in which they are generated and act as first messengers on neighboring cells.[41] As a result, a metabolite of arachidonic acid might provide a diffusable extracellular signal from a postsynaptic cell to a presynaptic one. This type of signal could explain the operation of a Hebbian type of synapse of the kind recently postulated to be important for long-term potentiation (LTP) of pyramidal cells in the CA1 region of the hippocampus. In this region, a glutamate-induced depolarization of the postsynaptic pyramidal neurons in response to repetitive stimulation of afferent inputs leads to enhanced release of glutamate from the presynaptic region.[42,43] Bliss and co-workers have recently tested the possible involvement of arachidonate metabolites and have found that NDGA, the lipoxygenase inhibitor, blocks selectively the induction of long-term potentiation in the hippocampal dentate gyrus as well as in the CA1 region.[44] Moreover, as reported by Wolfe et al. in this volume,[45] glutamate, acting through NMDA receptors, is able to generate 12-lipoxygenase metabolites in rat cortex. As the NMDA receptors play a critical role in induction of LTP,[46,47] the eicosanoids are becoming even more attractive candidates as mediators for at least some aspects of LTP. As kinase C activation also appears to play an important role in LTP,[48,49] future experiments studying the interactions of the various second-messenger cascades seem worthwhile.

ACKNOWLEDGMENTS

The authors would like to thank Kathrin Hilten and Louise Katz for preparing the figures and Drs. F. Belardetti, E. R. Kandel, J. H. Schwartz, D. Piomelli, and N. Dale, who collaborated with us on the earlier research reviewed here.

REFERENCES

1. MACKEY, S. L., D. L. GLANZMAN, S. A. SMALL, A. M. DYKE, E. R. KANDEL & R. D. HAWKINS. 1987. Proc. Natl. Acad. Sci. USA **84:** 8730–8734.

2. KLEIN, M., J. S. CAMARDO & E. R. KANDEL. 1982. Proc. Natl. Acad. Sci. USA **79:** 5713–5717.
3. BAYLEY, C. H. & M. J. CHEN. 1988. J. Neurosci. In press.
4. HOCHNER, B., M. KLEIN, S. SCHACHER & E. R. KANDEL. 1986. Proc. Natl. Acad. Sci. USA **83:** 8794–8798.
5. GINGRICH, K. J. & J. H. BYRNE. 1985. J. Neurophysiol. **53:** 652–669.
6. COTTRELL, G. A., N. W. DAVIES & K. A. GREEN. 1984. J. Physiol. **356:** 315–333.
7. RUBEN, P., J. W. JOHNSON & S. THOMPSON. 1986. J. Neurosci. **6:** 252–259.
8. ERXLEBEN, C., V. BREZINA & R. ECKERT. 1985. Soc. Neurosci. Abstr. **11:** 170.
9. COLOMBAIONI, L., D. PAUPARDIN-TRITDCH, P. P. VIDAL & H. M. GERSCHENFELD. 1985. J. Neurosci. **5:** 2533–2538.
10. OCORR, K. A. & J. H. BYRNE. 1985. Neurosci. Lett. **55:** 113–118.
11. BREZINA, V., R. ECKERT & C. ERXLEBEN. 1987. J. Physiol. **382:** 267–290.
12. BREZINA, V., R. ECKERT & C. ERXLEBEN. 1987. J. Physiol. **388:** 565–596.
13. EDMONDS, B., E. R. KANDEL & M. KLEIN. 1988. Soc. Neurosci. Abstr. **14:** 1206.
14. KRETZ, R., E. SHAPIRO & E. R. KANDEL. 1986. J. Neurophysiol. **55:** 113–130.
15. SIEGELBAUM, S. A., J. S. CAMARDO & E. R. KANDEL. 1982. Nature **299:** 413–417.
16. CASTELLUCCI, V. F., S. SCHACHER, P. G. MONTAROLO, S. MACKEY, D. L. GLANZMAN, R. D. HAWKINS, T. W. ABRAMS, P. GOELET & E. R. KANDEL. 1986. In Coexistence of Neuronal Messengers: A New Principle in Chemical Transmission. Progress in Brain Research, Vol. 68. T. Hokfelt, K. Fuxe & P. Pernow, Eds: 83–102. Elsevier. Amsterdam.
17. CASTELLUCCI, V. F., E. R. KANDEL, J. H. SCHWARTZ, F. D. WILSON, A. C. NAIRN & P. GREENGARD. 1980. Proc. Natl. Acad. Sci. USA **77:** 7492–7496.
18. SHUSTER, M. J., J. S. CAMARDO, S. A. SIEGELBAUM & E. R. KANDEL. 1985. Nature **313:** 392–395.
19. PIOMELLI, D., E. SHAPIRO, S. J. FEINMARK & J. H. SCHWARTZ. 1987. J. Neurosci. **7:** 3675–3686.
20. PIOMELLI, D., A. VOLTERRA, N. DALE, S. A. SIEGELBAUM, E. R. KANDEL, J. H. SCHWARTZ & F. BELARDETTI. 1987. Nature **328:** 38–43.
21. PACE-ASCIAK, C. R., E. GRANSTROM & B. SAMUELSSON. 1983. J. Biol. Chem. **258:** 6835–6840.
22. PIOMELLI, D., S. J. FEINMARK & J. H. SCHWARTZ. 1987. Soc. Neurosci. Abstr. **13:** 598.
23. GILMAN, A. G. 1987. Annu. Rev. Biochem. **56:** 615–649.
24. OCORR, K. A., M. TABATA & J. H. BYRNE. 1985. Soc. Neurosci. Abstr. **11:** 481.
25. AXELROD, J., R. M. BURCH & C. L. JELSEMA. 1988. Trends Neurosci. **11:** 117–123.
26. SWEATT, J. D., T. M. CONNOLLY, E. J. CRAGOE & L. E. LIMBIRD. 1986. J. Biol Chem. **261:** 8667–8673.
27. NAKASHIMA, S., T. TOHMATSU, H. HATTORI, A. SUGANUMA & Y. NOZAWA. 1987. J. Biochem. **101:** 1055–1058.
28. BLUMENFELD, H., B. BUG, N. BUTTNER, J. D. SWEATT & S. A. SIEGELBAUM. 1988. Soc. Neurosci. Abstr. **14:** 1206.
29. VOLTERRA, A., J. D. SWEATT & S. A. SIEGELBAUM. 1987. Soc. Neurosci. Abstr. **13:** 1440.
30. VOLTERRA, A. & S. A. SIEGELBAUM. 1988. Proc. Natl. Acad. Sci. USA. **85:** 7810–7814.
31. PFEUFFER, T. & J. M. HELMREICH. 1975. J. Biol. Chem. **250:** 867–876.
32. UI, M. 1984. Trends Pharmacol. Sci. **5:** 277–279.
33. ECKSTEIN, F., D. CASSEL, H. LEVKOVITZ, M. LOWE & Z. SELINGER. 1979. J. Biol. Chem. **254:** 9829–9834.
34. SCHWARTZ, J. H., L. BERNIER, V. F. CASTELLUCCI, M. PALAZZOLO, T. SAITOH, A. STAPLETON & E. R. KANDEL. 1983. In Cold Spring Harbor Symposia on Quantitative Biology, Vol. **48**: 811–819. Cold Spring Harbor, NY.
35. JAKOBS, K. H., K. AKTORIES, M. MINUTH & G. SCHULTZ. 1985. In Advances in Cyclic Nucleotide and Protein Phosphorylation Research, Vol. 19. D.M.F. Cooper & K.B. Seamon, Eds.: 137–150. Raven Press. New York, NY.
36. MACKEY, S. L., N. LALEVIC, R. D. HAWKINS & E. R. KANDEL. 1988. Soc. Neurosci. Abstr. **14:** 842.
37. ABRAMS, T. W., V. F. CASTELLUCCI, J. S. CAMARDO, E. R. KANDEL & P. E. LLOYD. 1984. Proc. Natl. Acad. Sci. USA **81:** 7956–7960.

38. KRETZ, R., E. SHAPIRO, C. H. BAYLEY, M. CHEN & E. R. KANDEL. 1986. J. Neurophysiol. **55:** 131–146.
39. NORTH, R. A. 1986. Trends Neurosci. **9:** 114–117.
40. HOLZ, G. G., S. G. RANE & K. DUNLAP. 1986. Nature **319:** 670–672.
41. HEDQVIST, P. 1977. Annu. Rev. Pharmacol. Toxicol. **17:** 259–279.
42. WIGSTROM, H., B. GUSTAFSON, Y. Y. HUANG & W. D. ABRAHAM. 1986. Acta. Physiol. Scand. **126:** 317–319.
43. BLISS, T. V. P., R. M. DOUGLAS, M. C. ERRINGTON & M. A. LYNCH. 1986. J. Physiol. **377:** 391–408.
44. WILLIAMS, J. H. & T. V. P. BLISS. 1988. Neurosci. Lett. **88:** 81–85.
45. WOLFE, L. S. & L. PELLERIN. 1989. Ann. N.Y. Acad. Sci. This volume.
46. SMITH, S. J. 1987. Trends in Neurosci. **10:** 142–144.
47. AKERS, R. F., D. M. LOVINGER, P. A. COLLEY, D. LINDEN & A. ROUTTENBERG. 1986. Science **231:** 587–589.
48. MALINOW, R., D. V. MADISON & R. W. TSIEN. 1988. Biophys. J. **53:** 429a.

PART IV. THE ROLE OF CEREBRAL BLOOD FLOW AND
ARACHIDONIC ACID METABOLISM IN BRAIN INJURY AND
ISCHEMIC DAMAGE

The Role of Arachidonic Acid and Oxygen Radical Metabolites in the Pathogenesis of Vasogenic Brain Edema and Astrocytic Swelling[a]

PAK H. CHAN,[b] SUSAN LONGAR, SYLVIA CHEN,
ALBERT C. H. YU, LARS HILLERED, LILLIAN CHU,
SHIGEKI IMAIZUMI, BRYAN PEREIRA, KI MOORE,
VICKI WOOLWORTH, AND ROBERT A. FISHMAN

Neurochemistry Laboratory
Brain Edema Research Center
Department of Neurology
School of Medicine
University of California
San Francisco, California 94143

INTRODUCTION

Alterations of membrane phospholipids and the acyl fatty acid moieties of brain cells have been related to various pathological disorders of the brain, including brain ischemia, hypoxia, blood-brain barrier (BBB) dysfunction, and epileptic seizures. In most cases, the polyunsaturated fatty acids (PUFA), arachidonic acid (AA) (20:4), and docosahexaenoic acid (22:6) are rapidly released from cellular membrane phospholipids as a result of these pathological insults.[1-11]

Using single rat brain cortical slices as an *in vitro* bioassay system, our laboratory has demonstrated that free PUFA could induce cellular edema.[12] Further studies have indicated that the transient formation of free radicals and lipid peroxides are also involved in PUFA-induced swelling of brain slices and of cultured brain cells.[13-15] The mechanism of cellular swelling in these systems is related to altered membrane functions, since both neurotransmitter uptake and Na^+, K^+-ATPase activity in synaptic membranes are significantly reduced.[16] We have further studied the local effects of arachidonic acid on vasogenic edema in rats *in vivo*. Animals were infused with 0.05 mmol of saturated, monounsaturated, or PUFA into the thalamus, and the edema and cation levels were studied at 24 hours following the injection. Among the fatty acids, AA was the most potent fatty acid in inducing cerebral edema concomitant with the increase in sodium and decrease in potassium contents. Palmitic acid (16:0)

---

[a]This work was supported by National Institutes of Health Grants NS-14543 (R.A.F., P.H.C.) and NS-25372 (P.H.C.).

[b]Address for correspondence: Pak H. Chan, Ph.D., Neurochemistry Laboratory, Brain Edema Research Center, Department of Neurology, Box 0114, University of California, San Francisco, California 94143.

was ineffective in inducing brain edema and cation change.[17] Furthermore, AA and linolenic acid caused 3-fold and 2-fold increases, respectively in [^{125}-I] albumin space at 24 hours in the injected hemisphere when compared with Krebs Ringer. Oleic acid (18:1), palmitic acid (16:0), and nonanoic acid (9:0) were not effective in altering blood-brain barrier permeability.[17] Preliminary studies obtained from our laboratory suggest that superoxide radicals are involved in PUFA-mediated BBB permeability changes and the development of vasogenic edema, since coinjection of AA and liposome-entrapped superoxide dismutase (SOD) intracerebrally inhibited the AA-induced vasogenic edema and BBB permeability changes.[18]

The aims of our present studies are several. First, we would like to elucidate the cause-and-effect relationship between oxygen free radicals and the development of vasogenic edema. Second, the question arises as to whether brain cells like astroglia will produce superoxide radicals in the presence of AA. Third, the mode of action of AA and superoxide radicals on astrocytic swelling (cellular edema) and metabolism is unknown, and is the subject of the present study.

METHODS: COLD-INJURY MODEL

We used a cold-induced brain injury model, which is characterized by the breakdown of blood-brain-barrier permeability, focal brain necrosis, and development of vasogenic brain edema. Rats weighing 200 to 250 g were anesthetized with pentobarbital (50 mg/kg) and placed in a stereotaxic apparatus. A probe with 0.5-cm diameter, attached to a brass cup (20 cm^2) filled with dry ice and acetone (-50 °C), was applied directly to the right side of the bony skull for 1 minute. This cold-injury model is a highly reproducible method of inducing brain edema.[19,20] The injury is characterized by early changes; within minutes, an increase in BBB permeability is detected, followed by an increase in brain edema, which is maximal at 24 hours. Our time-course studies have shown that brain water content following a 1-minute freezing lesion was increased from a control value of 79.6% ± 0.3 to 81.9% ± 0.5 at 30 minutes, 82.9% ± 0.4 at 2 hours, and 85.1% ± 0.4 at 24 hours. Furthermore, AA was increased by 266%, 476%, and 485% at 1 minute, 30 minutes, and 24 hours, respectively, following the cold injury.[19]

PRIMARY CELL CULTURE OF ASTROCYTES

Primary cultures of cerebral cortical astrocytes were prepared from newborn Sprague-Dawley rats as described previously.[21–23] Cerebral hemispheres were removed aseptically from the skulls and freed of the meninges. The neopallia were removed and were cut into small cubes (1 mm^3) in a modified Eagle's minimum essential tissue culture medium (MEM) containing fetal calf serum (FCS). The tissue was disrupted by vortex mixing for one minute, and the suspension was passed through two sterile nylon Nitex sieves with pore sizes of 80 μm (first sieving) and 10 μm (second sieving). A volume of cell suspension equivalent to one-thirtieth of the brain was placed in a 60-mm Falcon tissue dish. Fresh MEM supplemented with 10% FCS was added to the dish to a final volume of 3 ml. All cultures were incubated at 37 °C in a 95%:5% (vol/vol) mixture of atmospheric air and carbon dioxide with 95% humidity. The culture medium was changed after 3 days of seeding and subsequently two times per week. After 2 weeks, the cultures reached confluency and were grown in the additional presence of 0.25 mM dibutyryl cyclic AMP. The cultures were used for experiments between the ages of 28 and 35 days *in vitro*.

PREPARATION OF LIPOSOMES AND LIPOSOME-ENTRAPPED Cu/Zn–SUPEROXIDE DISMUTASE

The procedures for the preparation of positively charged unilamellar liposomes, with a large internal aqueous space and high capture by reverse-phase evaporation, are based on the method of Szoka and Papahadjopoulos[24] and have been adopted by our laboratory (see FIG. 1). The lipids contain L-alpha-dipalmitoyl phosphatidylcholine, cholesterol, and stearylamine with a molar ratio of 14:7:4. The lipids were dissolved in chloroform, followed by the addition of ether and phosphate buffer (0.4 mM), and then sonicated for 5 minutes at 45 °C (bath type, Branson Instruments, St. Louis, MO). The solvent was removed by rotary evaporation at 45 °C, and the unilamellar liposomes were suspended in phosphate-buffered saline. The preparation of liposome-entrapped Cu/Zn-SOD is essentially the same as that for the liposomes.[19,25] Electrophoretically purified Cu/Zn-SOD, bovine blood 20,000 units/mg (Pharmacia, Uppsala, Sweden),

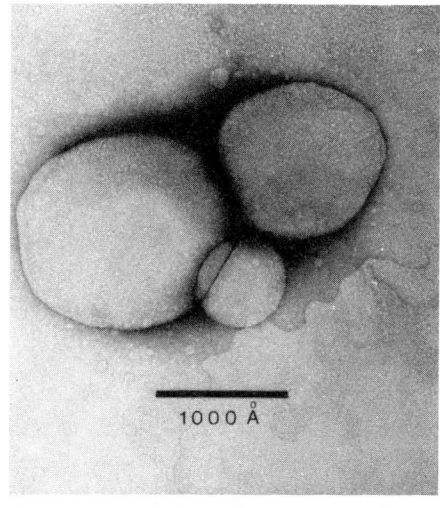

FIGURE 1. Negative-stain electron micrograph of unilamellar liposomes prepared by reverse-phase evaporation technique. The liposomes' size ranged from 800–4,000 Å.

or human Cu/Zn-SOD produced by genetic engineering method (2,000 units/mg, Chiron Company, Emeryville, CA) at a concentration of 2×10^5 units was first dissolved in 0.4 mM phosphate buffer and then added to the lipid film (400 μmol phospholipids) before sonication. The yield of liposome-entrapped Cu/Zn-SOD ranged from 25% to 40% and had a value of 2×10^2 of SOD units/μmol phospholipid. Prior to the enzyme assay, the liposome-SOD (20 μl) was sonicated in the presence of 20 μl of 1% Triton X-100 and diluted with phosphate-buffered saline.

EFFECTS OF LIPOSOME-ENTRAPPED Cu/Zn–SUPEROXIDE DISMUTASE ON SUPEROXIDE RADICAL FORMATION IN THE COLD-INJURED BRAIN

The brain level of nitroblue formazan (NBF), a reduction product of superoxide radical and nitroblue tetrazolium (NBT), was increased from a control value of 0.69 ±

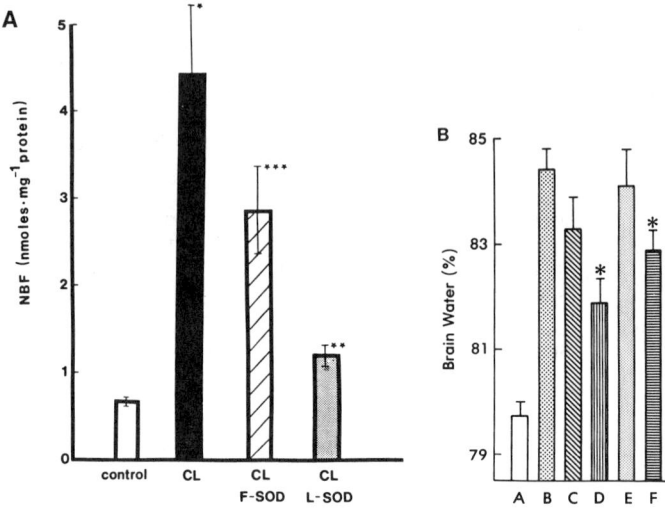

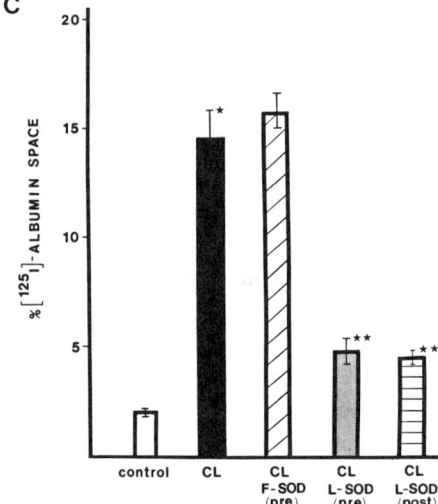

FIGURE 2. Effects of Cu/Zn-SOD on superoxide radical formation, vasogenic edema, and blood-brain barrier permeability. (**A**) Control = contralateral cortex (sham operated); CL = cold lesion; F-SOD = free SOD; L-SOD = liposome-entrapped SOD; * = significance as compared to control; ** = significance as compared to cold lesion; *** = significance as compared to control. (**B**) A = control brain; B = brain with lesion; C = brain with cold lesion after 5 minutes of pretreatment with free Cu/Zn-SOD; D = brain with cold lesion after 5 minutes of pretreatment with liposome-entrapped Cu/Zn-SOD; E = brain with cold lesion 5 minutes after treatment with free Cu/Zn-SOD; F = brain with cold lesion 5 minutes after treatment with liposome-entrapped Cu/Zn-SOD; * = significance at 0.05 as compared with the group with cold lesions. (**C**) Effects of liposome-entrapped Cu/Zn-SOD on blood-brain barrier permeability to ^{125}I-bovine serum albumin. Control = contralateral hemisphere; CL = hemisphere with cold lesion; F-SOD (pre) = animals were pretreated with free SOD; L-SOD (pre) = animals were pretreated with liposome-entrapped SOD; L-SOD (post) = animals were posttreated with liposome-entrapped SOD; * = significance as compared to the contralateral control hemisphere; ** significance as compared to cortex with the cold lesion.

0.04 to 4.44 ± 0.88 nmol per mg of protein at 1 hour following the cold injury (FIG. 2A). The intravenous injection of liposome-entrapped Cu/Zn-SOD (10,000 units) 5 minutes prior to the cold injury significantly reduced the level of superoxide radicals to 1.21 ± 0.14 nmol per mg of protein (FIG. 2A). Both pretreatment (5 minutes prior to the injury) and posttreatment (5 minutes after the injury) of cold-injured animals with liposome-entrapped Cu/Zn SOD also effectively reduced brain water content from 85.15% ± 0.4 and 82.9% ± 0.4, respectively (FIG. 2B).

Furthermore, cold injury caused a seven-fold increase in BBB permeability, as indicated by ^{125}I-BSA space 24 hours following injury (FIG. 2C; control ^{125}I-BSA space = 2.04% ± 0.10). Intravenous injection of liposome-entrapped Cu/Zn SOD 5 minutes prior to or 5 minutes after the traumatic injury reduced the level of ^{125}I-BSA space from 14.05% ± 1.3 to 4.69% ± 0.82 and 4.36% ± 0.37, respectively. Pretreatment or posttreatment with free Cu/Zn-SOD did not change the level of superoxide radicals, the degree of brain edema, and the ^{125}I-BSA space, indicating that only the liposome-entrapped Cu/Zn-SOD was effective in reducing the level of superoxide radical, brain edema, and BBB permeability dysfunction induced by traumatic injury.

EFFECTS OF ARACHIDONIC ACID ON NITROBLUE TETRAZOLIUM REDUCTION, O_2^-, LIPID PEROXIDATION, LACTATE PRODUCTION, AND SWELLING IN PRIMARY CELL CULTURE OF ASTROCYTES

We studied the time-and dose-dependent effects of AA on the NBT reduction in intact cultured astrocytes (FIG. 3). The formation of NBF in control astrocytes increased gradually with time. AA at concentrations of 0.1 and 0.5 mM significantly increased the rate of NBF formation to 1.33 ± 0.1 and to 1.93 ± 0.2 nmole per minute per mg protein, respectively, in astrocytes. The levels of NBF increased linearly within the 30 minutes of incubation with AA and reached a plateau at 60 minutes. Furthermore, other PUFA, including 22:6, linolenic acid (18:3), and linoleic acid (18:2), also increased significantly the level of NBT reduction in intact cultured astrocytes. The increase in NBT reduction was closely associated with the degree of unsaturation, with 22:6 the most effective. Both saturated palmitic acid (16:0) and mono-unsaturated oleic acid (18:1) were not effective. The stimulating effects of PUFA on the level of malondialdehyde (MDA) in astrocytes are shown in FIGURE 4B. The PUFA 18:3, 20:4, and 22:6 at 0.1-mM concentration increased the formation of MDA by 70%, 100%, and 95%, respectively. FIGURE 4C shows the effects of various

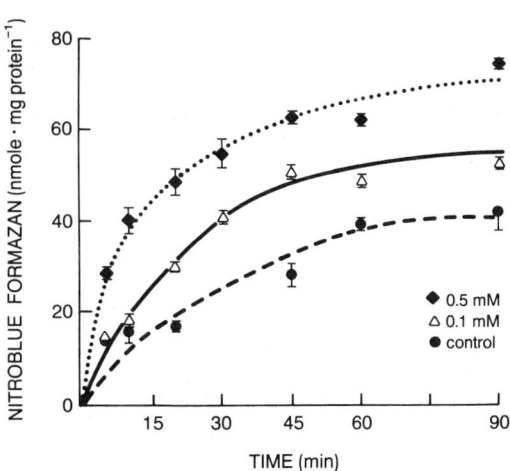

FIGURE 3. Stimulation of nitroblue formazan (NBF) formation by arachidonic acid (AA) in intact cultured astrocytes. Cultured astrocytes were incubated with 1.0 mM nitroblue tetrazolium in the presence of AA (0.1 mM or 0.5 mM) for various times. The extracted NBF was read at 515 nm. Results are means of four different experiments with duplication assays for each experiment. *Vertical bars* indicate SD.

fatty acids on the lactic acid production in intact astrocytes. PUFAs 20:4, 18:3 and 18:2 at 0.1 mM caused increases in lactate production by 240%, 160%, and 60%, respectively, in incubation medium. Both 16:0 and 18:1 were ineffective. Furthermore, AA (0.5 mM) caused a 3-fold increase in intracellular water space, as measured by the uptake of [^{14}C]-3-0-methyl glucose (Chan et al., unpublished data).

EFFECTS OF LIPOSOME-ENTRAPPED SUPEROXIDE DISMUTASE ON O_2^- AND ON LACTATE ACID PRODUCTION

TABLE 1 shows that when cultured astrocytes were incubated with liposome-entrapped SOD (100 units/ml), the levels of 20:4-induced NBF formation and lactic acid production were reduced significantly. Empty liposome or free SOD (100 units/ml) was not effective in reducing the increased cellular level of NBF or the lactate content in the incubation medium. Our preliminary data also showed that

TABLE 1. Effects of Liposome-Entrapped CuZn-SOD on AA-Induced O_2^- Formation and Lactate Production in Astrocytes

Incubation Medium	Nitroblue Formazan (% Control)	Lactate (% Control)
Control	100 ± 16	100 ± 11
20:4	199 ± 15[a]	183 ± 4[a]
+ Empty Liposomes	180 ± 17	177 ± 10
+ Free SOD (100 units/dish)	185 ± 13	190 ± 15
+ Liposome-SOD (100 units/dish)	93 ± 9[b]	92 ± 9[b]

NOTE: Astrocytes were preincubated with empty liposomes, free SOD, or liposome-entrapped SOD in MEM (serum-free) for 24 hours prior to the addition of 20:4 (0.1 mM) for another hour. Cell pellets were used for nitroblue formazan (NBF) assay, whereas incubation medium was assayed for lactate content. The control values of NBF and lactate were 54.3 ± 10.4 nmol/mg protein/h and 0.35 ± 0.04 μmol/mg protein/h, respectively. Values are the means ± SD of three different experiments.
[a]$p < 0.01$, compared to control group.
[b]$p < 0.01$, compared to 20:4 group, using analysis of variance.

liposome-entrapped SOD significantly reduced the astrocytic swelling concomitant with the release of lactate dehydrogenase in the medium (Chan et al., unpublished data). These data clearly indicated the involvement of intracellular superoxide radicals in AA-induced swelling in primary cell culture of astrocytes.

DISCUSSION

The present *in vivo* studies demonstrate that Cu/Zn-SOD, when entrapped in liposomes and injected intravenously before or immediately after the induction of cold injury, significantly reduced the level of superoxide radicals and ameliorated brain edema and BBB permeability changes. However, the intravenous injection of free SOD was not effective. There are many reasons for the failure of free SOD to reduce brain edema. First, Cu/Zn-SOD, a negative-charge protein (isoelectric point = 4.2) with a molecular weight of 31,000, is almost completely excluded by endothelial cells and fails to pass through the normal BBB. Second, even if the free SOD reaches the extracellular space in the injured brain, the brain cells are unable to take up the free enzyme, as was recently shown by our studies using both primary neuronal and astrocytic cultures.[23] Third, the half-life of SOD in plasma is short (about 6 minutes), as indicated from the pharmacokinetic studies of plasma clearance of SOD. By contrast, Cu/Zn-SOD, when entrapped with positively charged sterylamine liposomes, readily was taken up by primary cultures of neurons and astrocytes. The half-life of Cu/Zn-SOD in liposomes is increased from 6 minutes to 4.2 hours. Our data further demonstrated that a single intravenous injection of liposome-entrapped Cu/Zn-SOD caused a twofold increase in the SOD level in the injured brain at 30 minutes and for up to 2 hours thereafter. The level of Cu/Zn-SOD in the contralateral control brain at various time points followed a pattern similar to that of the injured brain, although it was significantly lower than the level in the injured brain, suggesting that liposomes facilitate the transport of SOD into uninjured brain compartments.[20] Furthermore, the transport of Cu/Zn-SOD into endothelial cells also was highly facilitated by liposomes, indicating that the breakdown of the BBB may allow a high degree of transport of Cu/Zn-SOD into the extracellular space of the injured brain.[20]

Although the direct involvement of superoxide radicals in the AA cascade in the cold-injured rat brain is not clear at present, the significant increases in AA following cold injury should provide an adequate source of substrate for oxygen radical formation via both cyclooxygenase and lipoxygenase.[19,26] Furthermore, AA can also co-oxidize with endothelial xanthine oxidase to form superoxide radicals.[27] Thus AA (and other PUFA) are likely to be involved in superoxide radical formation, vasogenic brain edema development, and BBB permeability changes.

Direct evidence of AA-mediated superoxide radical formation comes from our *in vitro* studies using primary cell cultures of astrocytes. The rate of NBF formation, induced by AA in intact cells, is both time- and dose-dependent. Our data further show that the stimulation of NBF formation is not specific for AA, since other PUFA, including linoleic acid (18:2), linolenic acid (18:3), and docosahexaenoic acid (22:6) were also effective (FIG. 4A). These data indicate that PUFA induce oxidative perturbations in cultured astrocytes and support our early observations in brain slices. The oxidative stress in astrocytes induced by PUFA was further demonstrated by the measurement of lipid peroxidation. Our data have shown that fatty acids that have three or more double bonds (18:3, 20:4, and 22:6) significantly increased the MDA content in astrocytes (FIG. 4B).

We have suggested previously that the O_2^- formation and subsequent lipid peroxidation via AA cascades cause the membrane perturbation.[28,29] The initial rate of uptake of glutamate in astrocytes was severely inhibited with 20:4 (concentrations ranged from 0.025–0.1 mM). We have suggested that the perturbation of membrane integrity induced by AA may be responsible for its inhibitory effect on glutamate uptake.[22,30] Furthermore, our preliminary data also show that AA severely inhibits the $(Na^+ + K^+)$-ATPase activity in astrocytes (unpublished data), further indicating the membrane perturbation induced by AA. It is likely that increased level of O_2^- and lipid peroxides are involved in these membrane injuries.

The mechanisms underlying the stimulation of lactate production in astrocytes are not clear at present, and several plausible explanations may be entertained. First, the various enzyme activities of the glycolytic pathway may be enhanced by AA and/or by its oxygen radical intermediates. Second, the normal mitochondrial respiratory activities and metabolic function are affected by AA and/or by oxygen radicals. For example, the enzymes of mitochondrial TCA cycle that are responsible for pyruvate flux and oxidation may be affected by AA. Free fatty acids, particularly PUFA, are potent uncouplers of mitochondrial phosphorylation. Our studies have found that

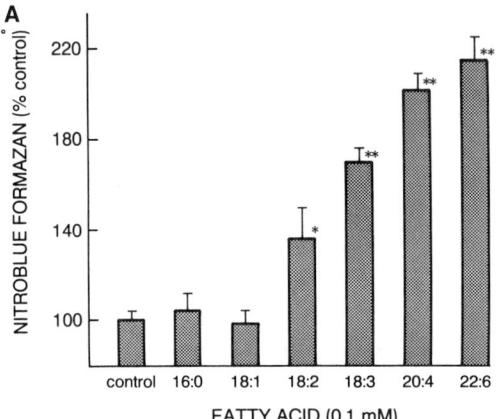
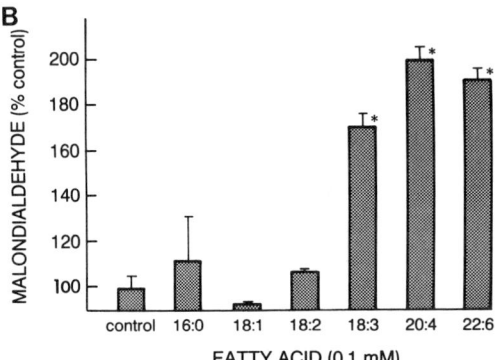
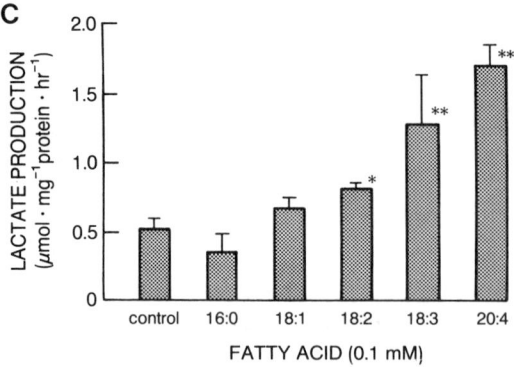

FIGURE 4. Effects of free fatty acids on the levels of nitroblue formazan (NBF), malondialdehyde (MDA) and lactic acid in astrocytes. **(A)** NBF formation in intact cultured astrocytes. Astrocytes were incubated with nitroblue tetrazolium in the presence of fatty acid (0.1 mM) for 10 min at 37 °C. Results are expressed as percentage of the rate of NBF formation of the control ± SD. The control rate of NBF formation in astrocytes is 0.61 ± 0.02 nmol/min/mg protein. Results are averages of three experiments. $* = p < 0.01$; $** = p < 0.001$. **(B)** MDA formation in cultured astrocytes. Astrocytes were incubated with thiobarbituric acid and free fatty acid for 1 h at 37 °C. Results are expressed as percentage of rate of MDA formation of the control ± SD. The control rate of MDA formation is 1.78 ± 0.06 nmol/mg protein/h. Results are averaged from four different experiments. $* = p < 0.01$. **(C)** Lactic acid production in astrocytes. Cultured astrocytes were incubated with individual fatty acid (0.1 mM) for 1 h at 37 °C. The incubation medium was used to assay for the lactic acid content. Values are means ± SD of four experiments. $* = p < 0.05$, $** = p < 0.001$, compared to control.

respiration was inhibited in isolated brain mitochondria with a relatively low concentration of 20:4 (13 nmoles/mg mitochondrial protein), suggesting that the normal mitochondrial function is altered by AA.[31]

Siesjo and his colleagues studied the influence of acidosis on O_2^- formation and lipid peroxidation, and have demonstrated that acidic pH in the range of pH 6.0–6.5 significantly induced free radical formation and lipid peroxidation in brain homogenates.[32] These investigators proposed that the effect of acidosis on brain homogenates may involve increased formation of the protonated form of O_2^-. Our data have shown that AA caused a dose-dependent increase in lactic acid content in astrocytes. Since the increase in lactic acid content will lower the pH and create acidosis, the nature of O_2^- induced by AA may be a hydroperoxyl radical ($\cdot OOH$), as suggested by Siesjo et al.[32]

The mechanisms underlying the AA-induced NBF formation in astrocytes are not clear at present. Various free radical scavengers and enzyme inhibitors have failed to reduce the level of NBF in astrocytes. Egan et al. found that the EPR signal detected during metabolism of arachidonate or prostaglandin G_2 by microsomal fractions and oxygenase was due to the oxidation of adventitious material that was isolated together with microsomal fractions. Their data suggest that the hydroperoxidase rather than the oxygenase of cyclooxygenase can release a reactive oxidant $[O_x] \cdot$ into solution to initiate a radical chain.[33] Our studies have demonstrated that the addition of NADH or NADPH stimulates the NBF production in cultured astrocytes.[23] These data again confirm our previous observation that NADPH-dependent, AA-stimulated oxidases (peroxidases) are involved in O_2^- formation in astrocytes. Kukreja et al.[34] identified the mechanism by which arachidonate and linoleate metabolism via prostaglandin H synthase produced O_2^-. This mechanism involves the oxygenation of NADH or NADPH to the radicals of NAD or NADP, which then react with oxygen to produce O_2^-. Our data support this mechanistic scheme, because NADPH or NADH enhances the 20:4-stimulated NBF formation in intact astrocytes. We speculate that the elevated level of NADH and lactic acidosis in the ischemic brain may provide a suitable environment favoring the formation of O_2^-.

Once it is taken up by the cells, 20:4 is localized primarily in the fluid domains of membranes with preferential incorporation into endoplasmic reticulum or plasma and of mitochondrial membranes.[35,36] These studies, together with the fact that the hydrophobic lipid environment is preferable for O_2^- and its protonated form ($\cdot OOH$),[37] suggest that the O_2^- or $\cdot OOH$ may be formed or localized in membrane fluid domains. Further studies of O_2^- distribution using a cytochemical approach,[38] as well as morphological and immunocytochemical studies of the distribution of encapsulated SOD in astrocytes may provide additional information to strengthen this argument. Nevertheless, our studies demonstrate the beneficial effects of liposome-entrapped antioxidative enzymes in ameliorating O_2^- formation and lactate production in AA-injured astrocytes.[23] Liposome-entrapped antioxidative enzymes have been shown to be effective in ameliorating CNS O_2^- toxicity in vivo[39] and in preventing oxygen injury in cultured endothelial cells in vitro.[40] Furthermore, it is noteworthy that vitamin E liposomes have been shown to have beneficial effects in reducing lipid peroxidation and augmenting reactive gliosis in reaggregate cultures of fetal rat brain.[41] Therefore, the present studies provide support for further study of the therapeutic potential of these liposome-entrapped antioxidative enzymes in CNS injury.

ACKNOWLEDGMENT

We thank Dianne Esson for her editorial assistance.

REFERENCES

1. BAZAN, N. G. 1970. Effects of ischemia and electroconvulsive shock on free fatty acid pool in the brain. Biochim. Biophys. Acta **218:** 1–10.
2. BAZAN, N. G., H. E. P. BAZAN, W. G. KENNEDY & C. D. JOEL. 1971. Regional distribution and rate of production of free fatty acids in rat brain. J. Neurochem. **18:** 1387–1393.
3. BAZAN, N. G. & E. B. R. TURCO. 1980. Membrane lipids in the pathogenesis of brain edema phospholipids and arachidonic acid, the earliest membrane components changed at the onset of ischemia. Adv. Neurol. **28:** 197–205.
4. REDDY, T. S. & N. G. BAZAN. 1987. Arachidonic acid, stearic acid, and diacylglycerol accumulation correlates with the loss of phosphatidylinositol 4,-5-bisphosphate in cerebrum 2 seconds after electroconvulsive shock: Complete reversion of changes 5 minutes after stimulation. J. Neurosci. Res. **18:** 449–455.
5. MARION, J. & L. S. WOLFE. 1979. Origin of the arachidonic acid released post-mortem in rat forebrain. Biochim. Biophys. Acta **574:** 25–32.
6. REHNCRONA, S., E. WESTERBERG, B. AKESSON & B. K. SIESJO. 1982. Brain cortical fatty acids and phospholipids during and following complete and severe incomplete ischemia. J. Neurochem. **38:** 84–93.
7. TANG, W. & G. SUN. 1982. Factors affecting the free fatty acids in rat brain cortex. Neurochem. Int. **4:** 269–273.
8. EDGAR, A. D., J. STROSZNAJDAR & L. A. HORROCKS. 1982. Activation of ethanolamine phospholipase A_2 in brain during ischemia. J. Neurochem. **39:** 1111–1116.
9. YOSHIDA, S., K. ABE, R. BUSTO, B. D. WATSON, K. KOGURE & M. D. GINSBERG. 1982. Influence of transient ischemia on lipid-soluble antioxidants, free fatty acids and energy metabolites in rat brain. Brain Res. **245:** 307–316.
10. YASUDA, H., K. KISHIRO, N. IZAMI & M. NAKASHI. 1985. Biphasic liberation of arachidonic and stearic acids during cerebral ischemia. J. Neurochem. **45:** 168–172.
11. SHIU, G. K., J. P. NEMMER & E. M. NEMOTO. 1983. Reassessment of brain free fatty acid liberation during global ischemia and its attenuation by barbiturate anesthesia. J. Neurochem. **40:** 880–884.
12. CHAN, P. H. & R. A. FISHMAN. 1978. Brain edema: Induction in cortical slices by polyunsaturated fatty acids. Science **201:** 358–360.
13. CHAN, P. H. & R. A. FISHMAN. 1980. Transient formation of superoxide radicals in polyunsaturated fatty acid–induced brain swelling. J. Neurochem. **35:** 1004–1007.
14. CHAN, P. H., R. A. FISHMAN, J. L. LEE & S. C. QUAN. 1980. Arachidonic acid–induced swelling in incubated rat brain cortical slices: Effect of bovine serum albumin. Neurochem. Res. **5:** 629–640.
15. CHAN, P. H., R. KERLAN & R. A. FISHMAN. 1982. Alterations of membrane integrity and cellular constituents by arachidonic acid in neuroblastoma and glioma cells. Brain Res. **248:** 151–157.
16. CHAN, P. H., R. KERLAN & R. A. FISHMAN. 1983. Reductions of GABA and glutamate uptake and Na^+, K^+-ATPase activity in brain slices and synaptosomes by arachidonic acid. J. Neurochem. **40:** 309–316.
17. CHAN, P. H., R. A. FISHMAN, J. CARONNA, J. W. SCHMIDLEY, G. PRIOLEAU & J. LEE. 1983. Induction of brain edema following intracerebral injection of arachidonic acid. Ann. Neurol. **13:** 625–632.
18. CHAN, P. H., S. LONGAR & S. F. CHEN. Unpublished observations.
19. CHAN, P. H., S. LONGAR & R. A. FISHMAN. 1983. Phospholipid degradation and edema development in cold-injured rat brain. Brain Res. **277:** 329–337.
20. CHAN, P. H., S. LONGAR & R. A. FISHMAN. 1987. Protective effects of liposome-entrapped superoxide dismutase on post-traumatic brain edema. Ann. Neurol. **21:** 540–547.
21. YU, A. C. H., A. SCHOUSBOE & L. HERTZ. 1982. Metabolic fate of ^{14}C-labeled glutamate in astrocytes in primary cultures. J. Neurochem. **39:** 954–960.
22. YU, A. C. H., P. H. CHAN & R. A. FISHMAN. 1986. Effects of arachidonic acid on glutamate and gamma-aminobutyric acid uptake in primary cultures of rat cerebral cortical astrocytes and neurons. J. Neurochem. **47:** 1181–1189.
23. CHAN, P. H., S. F. CHEN & A. C. H. YU. 1988. Induction of intracellular superoxide radical

formation by arachidonic acid and by polyunsaturated fatty acids in primary astrocytic cultures. J. Neurochem. **50:** 1185–1193.
24. SZOKA, F. & D. PAPAHADJOPOULOS. 1978. Procedure for preparation of liposomes with large internal aqueous space and high capture by reverse-phase evaporation. Proc. Natl. Acad. Sci. USA **75:** 4194–4198.
25. TURRENS, J. F., J. D. CRAPO & B. A. FREEMAN. 1984. Protection against oxygen toxicity by intravenous injection of liposome-entrapped catalase and superoxide dismutase. J. Clin. Invest. **73:** 83–95.
26. SAMUELSSON, B., S. HAMMARSTROM & P. BOGEAT. 1979. Pathway of arachidonic acid metabolism. Adv. Inflamm. Res. **1:** 405–411.
27. FRIDOVICH, S. E. & N. A. PORTER. 1981. Oxidation of arachidonic acid in micelles by superoxide and hydrogen peroxide. J. Biol. Chem. **250:** 8812–8817.
28. CHAN, P. H. & R. A. FISHMAN. 1984. The role of arachidonic acid in vasogenic brain edema. Fed. Proc. **43:** 210–213.
29. CHAN, P. H. & R. A. FISHMAN. 1985. Free fatty acids, oxygen free radicals and membrane alterations in brain ischemia and injury. *In* Cerebrovascular Diseases. F. Plum & W. Pulsinelli, Eds.: 161–171. Raven Press. New York, NY.
30. CHAN, P. H., A. C. H. YU & R. A. FISHMAN. 1988. Free fatty acids and excitatory neurotransmitter amino acids as determinants of pathological swelling of astrocytes in primary culture. *In* Biochemical Pathology of Astrocytes. M. D. Norenberg, L. Hertz & A. Schousboe, Eds.: 327–335. Alan R. Liss. New York, NY.
31. HILLERED, L. & P. H. CHAN. 1988. Effects of arachidonic acid on respiratory activities in isolated brain mitochondria. J. Neurosci. Res. **19:** 94–100.
32. SIESJO, B. K., G. BENDEK, T. KOIDE, E. WESTERBERG & T. WIELOCH. 1985. Influence of acidosis on lipid peroxidation in brain tissues *in vitro*. J. Cereb. Blood Flow Metab. **5:** 253–258.
33. EGAN, R. W., P. H. GALE, E. M. BAPTISTA, K. L. KENNICOTT, W. J. A. VANDENHEUVEL, R. W. WALKER, P. E. FAGERNESS & F. A. KUEHL. 1981. Oxidation reactions by prostaglandin cyclooxygenase-hydroperoxidase. J. Biol. Chem. **256:** 7354–7361.
34. KUKREJA, R. C., H. A. KONTOS, M. HESS & E. F. ELLIS. 1986. PGH synthase and lipoxygenase generate superoxide in the presence of NADH or NADPH. Circ. Res. **59:** 612–619.
35. KLAUSNER, R. D., A. M. KLEINFELD, R. L. HOOVER & M. J. KARNOVKSY. 1980. Lipid domains in membranes: Evidence derived from structural perturbations induced by free fatty acids and life time heterogeneity analysis. J. Biol. Chem. **255:** 1286–1295.
36. NEUFELD, E. J., P. W. MAJERUS, C. M. KRUEGER & J. E. SAFFITZ. 1985. Uptake and subcellular distribution of [^{3}H]arachidonic acid in murine fibrosarcoma cells measured by electron microscope autoradiography. J. Cell Biol. **101:** 573–581.
37. FRIDOVICH, I. 1986. Biological effects of the superoxide radical. Arch. Biochem. Biophys. **247:** 1–11.
38. BRIGGS, R. T., J. M. ROBINSON, M. L. KARNOVSKY & M. J. KARNOVSKY. 1986. Superoxide production by polymorphonuclear leukocytes, a cytochemical approach. Histochemistry **84:** 371–378.
39. YUSA, T., J. D. CRAPO & B. A. FREEMAN. 1984. Liposome-mediated augmentation of brain SOD and catalase inhibits CNS O_2 toxicity. J. Appl. Physiol. **57:** 1674–1681.
40. FREEMAN, B. A., S. L. YOUNG & J. D. CRAPO. 1983. Liposome-mediated augmentation of superoxide dismutase in endothelial cells prevents oxygen injury. J. Biol. Chem. **258:** 12534–12542.
41. HALKS-MILLER, M., M. HENDERSON & L. F. ENG. 1986. Alpha-tocopherol decreases lipid peroxidation, neuronal necrosis, and reactive gliosis in reaggregate cultures of fetal rat brain. J. Neuropathol. Exp. Neurol. **45:** 471–484.

Ischemia Stress and Arachidonic Acid Metabolites in the Fetal Brain[a]

E. YAVIN,[b,c] E. GOLDIN,[c] E. MAGAL,[c]
A. TOMER,[d] AND S. HAREL[d]

[c]Department of Neurobiology
Weizmann Institute of Science
Rehovot, Israel

[d]Pediatrics Neurology Unit
Tel Aviv Medical Center
Tel Aviv University
Tel Aviv, Israel

CEREBRAL ISCHEMIA AND FATTY ACID METABOLISM

It is generally recognized that obstruction of the cerebral blood flow and/or deprivation of tissue oxygen are responsible for the uncontrolled release of free fatty acids from membrane phospholipids[1] by yet-to-be-elucidated mechanisms. Accumulation of free fatty acids, particularly of multiple double bonds (i.e., arachidonic and docosahexaenoic acids), following insults such as ischemia, trauma, or electroconvulsive shocks[2-4] may produce damage at cellular and subcellular levels.[5]

Ample evidence suggests that the deleterious effect of the released polyunsaturated fatty acids (PUFA) is due to oxygen reappearance during the reflow period.[5-7] Oxygen is necessary for the synthesis of vasoactive prostanoids, which may play a modulatory role in cerebral blood flow.[8-11] Oxygen is also a major driving force for the generation of free radicals,[11-14] which are strongly believed to cause fragmentation of both esterified and unesterified polyenoic acids in the bilayer.[15] Therefore, prevention of tissue damage following injury or ischemia requires a complete understanding of both the molecular mechanism that causes fatty acid deesterification under stress and, subsequently, the metabolic fate such fatty acids undergo once they are released from the phospholipids.

IMPAIRED PLACENTA VASCULAR FLOW AND FETAL BRAIN ISCHEMIA

Placental insufficiency and persisting periods of oxygen depletion are believed today to be leading factors in generating perinatal damage.[16] These conditions, which commonly occur during late pregnancy or are generated as complications around birth, are considered to be major causes for the high incidence of neonatal mortality, neurological morbidity, and intellectual impairment seen, for example, in humans.[16-18]

In order to study the effects of placental vascular flow obstruction on the

---

[a]This work was supported in part by grants from the Gulton Foundation, New York, New York and the Israel Academy of Sciences and Humanities, Jerusalem.
[b]To whom correspondence should be addressed.

developing embryo, a number of experimental animal models have been devised. In his pioneering work, Wigglesworth[19] was able to obtain growth-retarded pups by occluding the uterine artery in the pregnant rat. These small-for-gestational-age newborns exhibited massive losses in body weight because of skeletal, muscular, hepatic, and adrenal growth impairment. Their brains appeared macroscopically (as determined by weight) protected and relatively spared.[19] In the fetal rabbit model, however, normal metabolism and postnatal neurological functions were also impaired.[20]

The potential sensitivity of the fetal brain to adverse conditions is not surprising, as it is considered to be vulnerable at periods of accelerated growth, known as "growth spurts."[21] The timing of the "brain growth spurt" in relation to birth has been established for a variety of animal species, including humans.[22] The fact that mammalian species exhibit substantial differences with respect to this timing has enabled classification of mammals into prenatal, perinatal, and postnatal brain developers.

The rabbit, for example, which is considered to be a perinatal brain developer, is believed to be vulnerable to placental insufficiency around birth.[23] The rat, on the other hand, which is a classical example of a postnatal brain developer, may also be vulnerable to placental insufficiency and ischemic insults,[24] since the active growth spurt of the neuronal cells is essentially a prenatal event.[25]

There is currently no information concerning the extent of damage and the adverse consequences to the development of the fetal brain that follow short or long periods of vascular occlusion. The relative resistance after periods of ischemia[26,27] may, however, be greater in the fetal brain than that found in the adult brain, due to the hypoxic conditions to which the brain is usually subject in the fetal state. Unlike the brain in its postnatal phase of development, the prenatal developing brain is almost exclusively dependent on maternal circulation. Furthermore, the fetal brain has no refined mechanism to prevent metabolites or toxic substances from reaching it because of its lack of a blood-brain barrier. Therefore, the placenta, a very elaborate and metabolically active tissue that is largely subject to environmental influences,[28] is the apparent barrier to the brain. When ischemic stress conditions prevail, an elevation of prostaglandins in the placenta is evident.[29] Concomitantly, increased concentration of free fatty acids and prostanoids in the amniotic fluid and maternal blood plasma are detected.[30–33] Some of these metabolites obviously may reach the brain through the fetal circulation and exert a physiological effect on brain vasculature.

Needless to say, the fetal brain of most mammal species is known to metabolize arachidonic acid into prostaglandins and leukotrienes.[34,35] Little is known about the appearance of these products under normal and stress conditions.

CONVERSION OF [^{14}C] ARACHIDONIC ACID INTO EICOSANOIDS BY FETAL RABBIT BRAIN AND PLACENTA PREPARATIONS

To further our understanding of the pathophysiology of placenta insufficiency and its adverse effects on the developing brain, we set up preliminary studies to examine eicosanoid metabolism during the normal course of intrauterine life of the rabbit.[36] Using particulate and cytosolic fractions of both placenta and brain tissue, we were able to demonstrate the rapid conversion of [^{14}C] arachidonic acid into a substantial number of radiolabeled products. As is apparent from the TLC autoradiogram (FIG. 1), the soluble ($10^5 \times g$ supernatant) placenta (Ps) and brain (Bs) fractions are by far more active than the particulate ($10^5 \times g$ pellet) fractions, respectively. The major products formed by either tissue are 12-HETE (hydroxyeicosatetraenoic acid) and 15-HETE lipoxygenase metabolites (bands 13–15). Further separation of these

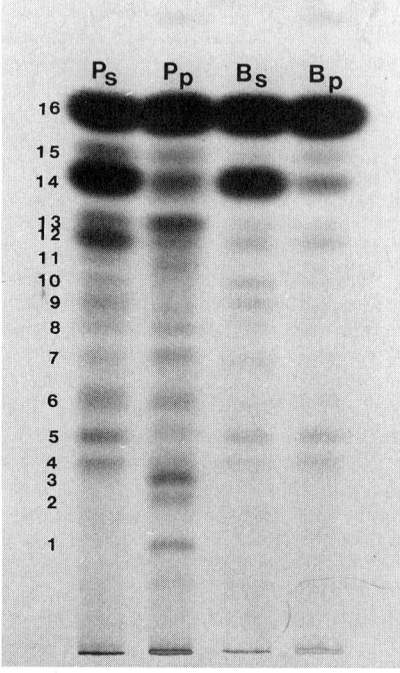

FIGURE 1. Autoradiography of ^{14}C arachidonic acid products after separation by TLC. The $100,000 \times g$ supernatant (s) and $100,000 \times g$ pellet (p) of fetal rabbit brain (B) and placenta (P) tissue at 27 days' gestation were prepared as described in Reference 36. Aliquots corresponding to 50 mg wet weight tissue were incubated with ^{14}C arachidonic acid (0.8 Ci/ml) in 0.5 ml of 50 mM Na phosphate buffer, pH 7.4, augmented with 0.1% gelatin, 1 mM EDTA, and 2 mM $CaCl_2$. After 30 min of incubation at 37 °C under vigorous shaking, the reaction was terminated by an acidic methanol/chloroform mixture and products were extracted and chromatographed on silica gel G, using a solvent system consisting of the organic layer of ethylacetate:isooctane:acetic acid:water (100:50:20:100 by vol.) mixture. Radioactive bands 1–12 belong mostly to the cyclooxygenase family, whereas 13–15 belong to the lipooxygenase family. Band 16 is free arachidonic acid.

two products can be attained by HPLC. As shown in FIGURE 2, in addition to the lipoxygenase pathway, brain and placenta cytosolic fractions convert [^{14}C] arachidonic acid into two distinct products identified with PGE_2 (peak 4) and 12-L-hydroxyheptadecatrienic acid (HHT, peak 7), indicating the existence of an effective cyclooxygenase pathway.

Compared to data reported on the fetal human brain,[34] the amount of [^{14}C] arachidonic acid converted into eicosanoid products by the fetal rabbit brain preparations is very extensive. Thus, by 40 min incubation more than 36% and 7% of the added radioactivity is converted by the soluble fraction into 12-HETE/15-HETE and PGE_2 eicosanoids, respectively[36] (see also FIG. 1).

The relatively high rates of *in vitro* formation of PGE_2 by fetal brain preparations prompted us to study the content of this prostanoid in greater detail. The interest in PGE_2 stems also from the wide spectra of nervous tissue related activities attributed to this particular compound,[11] its vasodilating properties in fetal circulation,[37] and abortive properties in pregnancy.[38]

In a recent report,[36] we have indicated that in the rabbit the activity converting ^{14}C arachidonic acid into PGE_2 resides predominantly in the soluble brain fraction. To extend these studies, we set up experiments to determine the subcellular content of PGE_2 using the more sensitive radioimmunoassay (RIA) technique. The values of PGE_2 in brain, liver, and placenta preparations taken from fetuses after 22 days' gestation or at birth are summarized in TABLE 1. The data clearly indicate that there are equal amounts of PGE_2 present in the soluble and particulate brain fractions at both ages. For comparison, the adult rabbit contains 321 ± 80 ng/g and 94.5 ± 7.6 ng/g of PGE_2 in the soluble and particulate compartments, respectively. The total content of PGE_2 in the newborn brain is more than twice as high as that observed in the fetal brain. The distribution of PGE_2 between the soluble and particulate fractions may indicate that these are at least two operationally defined subcellular compartments. Whether the compartmentation of PGE_2 occurs *in vivo* or is an *in vitro* artifact of PGE_2 partition following tissue disruption remains to be resolved.

A similar distribution pattern emerges when the PGE_2 content in the fetal liver is measured (TABLE 1). Like the situation in the brain, an almost equal amount of PGE_2 is found in the soluble and particulate liver fractions. In contrast, there is more PGE_2 in the newborn liver supernatant than in the particulate fraction. Also noticeable is a 6-fold increase in the total PGE_2 content in the newborn liver as compared to the fetal liver. TABLE 1 also documents the PGE_2 in the placenta, which, as expected, contains much higher levels than brain tissue. A limited PGE_2 compartmentation, more pronounced in the 22-day-old placenta, is also evident.

The changes in the subcellular distribution of PGE_2 prompted us to examine the ability of the soluble and particulate fractions to synthesize PGE_2. To achieve this, nonradioactive arachidonic acid was incubated with either soluble or particulate brain fractions at different gestation ages. Incubations were carried out at 4°C and 37°C for specified time periods, and the net accumulation of PGE_2 due to incubation at 37°C was determined by a RIA technique. As shown in FIGURE 3, a marked difference between the abilities of the soluble and the particulate fractions to synthesize PGE_2 is evident during the course of fetal brain development. This difference is even more pronounced in the postnatal brain. Thus, at the end of the second trimester of gestation (day 19), the capacity for PGE_2 synthesis is equally distributed between the soluble and the particulate fractions. In contrast, most of the activity during the third trimester

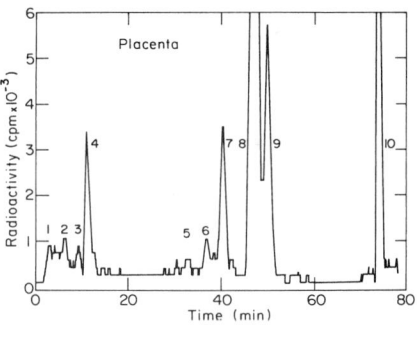
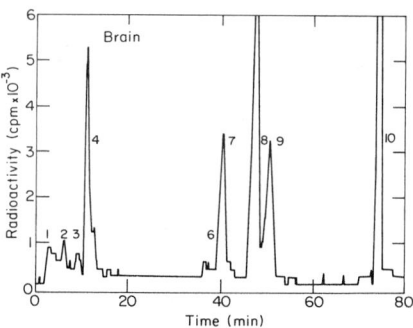

FIGURE 2. HPLC profile of ^{14}C arachidonic acid labeled products after incubation with placenta (*upper panel*) and brain (*lower panel*) 100,000 × g supernatants. Incubation and extraction of products were carried out in conditions essentially similar to those described in FIGURE 1. HPLC procedure was as described in Reference 36. The following peaks were positively identified with known standards: PGE_2 (4), HHT (7), 15-HETE (8), 12-HETE (9), and arachidonic acid (10).

TABLE 1. Distribution of PGE_2 in Subcellular Fractions of Various Rabbit Tissues

	PGE_2 Level (ng/g Tissue)			
	Fetal		Newborn	
Tissue	Soluble	Particulate	Soluble	Particulate
Brain	19.1 ± 2.9	23.6 ± 0.9	55.5 ± 4.1	49.9 ± 5.9
Liver	13.3 ± 3.8	16.7 ± 12.5	135.0 ± 9.5	61.6 ± 6.5
Placenta	5200.0 ± 400.0	2300.0 ± 300.0	9500.0 ± 1000.0	1900.0 ± 100.0

NOTE: Frozen samples (50–100 mg wet weight) homogenized in 10 volumes of 0.05 M phosphate buffer containing 1 mM EDTA and 0.1% gelatin were subjected to high-speed centrifugation at 100000 g for 1 h. The resulting pellet was reconstituted to the original volume with buffer, and aliquots were taken for RIA, after treating samples with formic acid and isopropanol followed by extraction with ether. The ether layer was collected and dried by flushing with nitrogen. The dry residue, dissolved in PBS containing 0.1% BSA, was then incubated for 1 h before assaying. Tissue samples were incubated overnight together with the antibody and the tracer, and unbound material was precipitated using dextran-coated charcoal. Aliquots were transferred to scintillation vials and counted by a Packard tricarb scintillation counter. The RIA enabled us to detect cyclooxygenase and lipoxygenase products present in less than nM levels. Antibodies were obtained from Dr. F. Cohen, of the Hormone Research Department.

resides in the supernatant fraction. After birth, activity in the brain supernatant is drastically reduced, whereas that in the particulate fraction gradually increases, to become in the adult state the main source for PGE_2 synthesis, (as has also been shown by others[39]). Thus, while the adult brain particulate fraction contains little over 20% of the PGE_2, it has most of the PGE_2-synthesizing capability. The most attractive possibility to account for these findings is that the appearance of the PGE_2-synthesizing capacity in the soluble fraction is a very characteristic feature, unique to the developing brain. As the rabbit brain at this stage is subject to an active phase of growth spurt, particularly of the neuronal elements, it is proposed that such an enzymatic activity may be related to a specific cell population that may secrete PGE_2. Evidence for the possible neurohumoral role of PGE_2 in the adult brain has been presented.[40,41] The physiological implication of this novel observation is at present not well understood and requires further investigation.

The current studies emphasize that the remarkable capacity of the fetal brain to generate its own eicosanoids is an important aspect of the regulation of fetal cerebral circulation. Some of these eicosanoids may fulfill important roles at particular stages of brain organogenesis, as they do in the adult brain.[11] In this context, the distinct

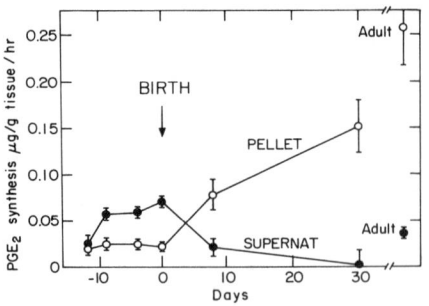

FIGURE 3. PGE_2 synthesis in the developing rabbit brain. Measurements were done with 100,000 × g supernatant and pellet fractions by RIA. Subcellular fractionation of brain tissue at different ages was done as described in the text. Samples equivalent to 2 mg tissue were incubated in phosphate buffer containing 0.1% BSA and 10^{-4} M arachidonic acid for 1 h, and the reaction was stopped by 35-sec microwave irradiation. Aliquots were taken for RIA, and the amount of PGE_2 measured was subtracted from duplicate time 0 samples. Values represent the levels ± SEM.

compartmentation of the enzymes involved in eicosanoid metabolism in the fetal brain could be one aspect of this regulation.

FETAL RABBIT BRAIN EICOSANOIDS DURING PLACENTAL INSUFFICIENCY

The levels and production of various prostaglandins in uterine tissues and fetal membranes, including the umbilical cord and placenta, were measured for most mammalian species and humans.[42] Recently, it was suggested by several investigators that normal prostaglandin production, especially of thromboxane A_2 and prostacyclin, is not adequately maintained in certain pregnancy complications of vascular origin.[43] Despite this, little or no data are available on the appearance of prostanoids in the fetal

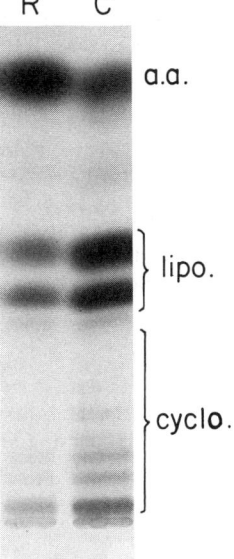

FIGURE 4. Autoradiography of ^{14}C arachidonic acid products incubated with restricted (R) and control (C) brain 100,000 × g preparations. Experimental conditions were similar to those described in FIGURE 1. Restriction was done for a period of 12 h.

brain during periods of placental insufficiency. To examine this question in some detail, we used pregnant rabbits between 23 and 28 days of gestation. The experimental outline included anesthesia of the rabbit by ketamine, followed by laparatomy and exposure of the uterine horns and the placental vessels. Then, embryos in one uterine horn were ligated by occluding one out of three-to-four blood vessels.[36] Embryos in the second uterine horn was considered to be sham animals. The rabbits were maintained for designated time periods ranging from hours to several days before being sacrificed by Nembutal anesthesia or CO_2 inhalation. Both techniques gave similar results. Brain, placenta, and liver from individual fetuses were dissected and frozen immediately in liquid nitrogen. Matched tissues were taken only from fetuses that survived the entire surgical procedure. Evaluation of the degree of restriction of fetuses after long-lasting placental insufficiency was established by body and brain weight measurements.[44]

TABLE 2. Eicosanoid Levels in the Fetal Rabbit and Placenta Tissue after 3 Hours of Restriction

Tissue	Eicosanoid	Eicosanoid Level (ng/g Tissue)		Change (-fold)
		Naive	Restricted	
Fetal brain	PGE_2	48.0 ± 16	90.8 ± 3.9	1.9
	TxB_2	0.4 ± 0.11	1.9 ± 0.45	4.5
	$6k\text{-}PGF_{1\alpha}$	7.9 ± 0.8	19.7 ± 2.5	2.5
Placenta	PGE_2	4330.0 ± 780.0	4760.0 ± 885.0	1.1
	TxB_2	5.8 ± 0.6	10.0 ± 2.5	1.7
	$6k\text{-}PGF_{1\alpha}$	148.0 ± 19.0	134.0 ± 1.9	0.9

NOTE: Experimental conditions were similar to those described under Figure 1.

The capacity of particulate and soluble brain fractions of embryos maintained for 24 h under placental insufficiency to convert ^{14}C arachidonic acid into other eicosanoids were examined. As shown in FIGURE 4, there is little or no conversion of the label into 12-HETE/15-HETE or other eicosanoids.

The quantitative evaluation of the prostanoid content in control and restricted fetuses was accomplished by the RIA technique. As shown in TABLE 2, brain tissue from fetuses exposed for 3 h to placental insufficiency, achieved by vascular ligation, contains twice as much PGE_2 as brain tissue from naive (unanesthetized and nonrestricted) animals. RIA analysis of the thromboxane B_2 and 6-keto $PGF_{1\alpha}$ content reveals 4.5- and 2.5-fold increases, respectively, over the values obtained in control fetuses. The content of these metabolites, which are the stable products of thromboxane A_2 and prostacyclin eicosanoids, respectively, in placenta tissue is by far greater than that of brain tissue. Nevertheless, apart from thromboxane B_2, little or no change in the steady state levels is seen in the placenta after 3 h of vascular restriction. After 20 h of restriction, the elevated levels of PGE_2 and 6-keto $PGF_1\alpha$, both known as vasodilating agents, are greatly diminished, reaching in the brain tissue a value similar to the steady state levels (FIG. 5). Thromboxane B_2, on the other hand, is still high (2.5-fold) in the brain but not in the placenta 20 h following surgery. The possibility that normal prostaglandin production, especially of thromboxane A_2 and prostacyclin, is different in the brain of the restricted fetuses prompted us to examine changes in the levels of these metabolites in the fetal rabbit brain at designated times over periods up to 48 h.

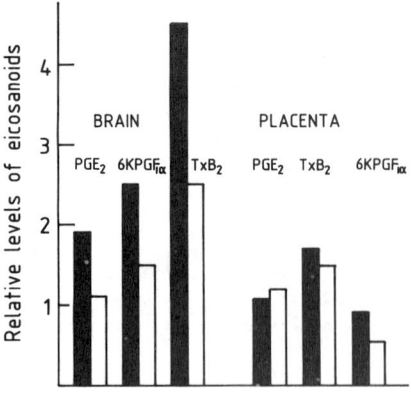

FIGURE 5. Relative steady state levels of eicosanoids determined by RIA. Brain and placenta samples, homogenized in phosphate buffer containing indomethacin, were acidified with formic acid and extracted by ether. The organic phase was dried by nitrogen flushing and the dry residue dissolved in PBS containing 0.1% BSA. Aliquots were subjected to RIA with the appropriate antibody and tracer, as described in the text. Values represent the relative change in eicosanoids levels in restricted animals after 3-h (*black bars*) and 20-h (*open bars*) restriction.

As shown in FIGURE 6, the content of thromboxane B_2 and 6-keto $PGF_{1\alpha}$ in the restricted animals attains a statistically significant ($p < 0.02$) maximum level 1.5 h following surgery, a level that gradually declines after 48 h. Surprisingly, the levels of the two metabolites in sham fetuses exhibit a substantial elevation that almost matches (as in the case of 6-keto $PGF_{1\alpha}$) that of the restricted counterparts. This observation would most likely suggest that production of eicosanoids under these experimental conditions is not entirely confined to the site of the vessel clamping, and that ischemic conditions may be induced via maternal circulation.

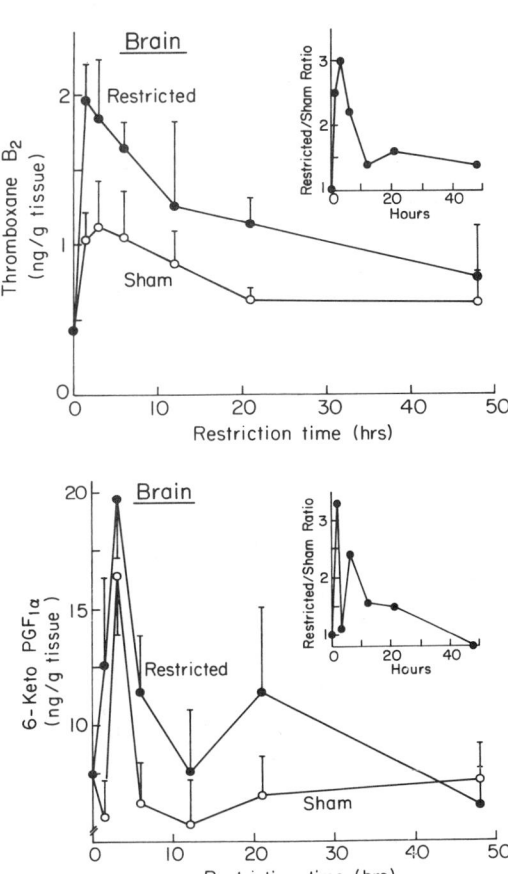

FIGURE 6. The effect of restriction time on thromboxane B_2 (*upper panel*) and 6-keto $PGF_{1\alpha}$ (*lower panel*) levels in the fetal brain. Prostaglandin levels assessed by RIA were obtained from 8–17 restricted or sham embryos from 3–4 mothers at each time point. The *bars* represent the standard error for each time point. The *insets* depict the change in prostaglandin levels in restricted over sham brains.

When the 6-keto $PGF_{1\alpha}$ values of the restricted fetuses are normalized to these of their sham counterparts, the apparent net consequence of the placental insufficiency is most pronounced within the first hour following surgery (FIG. 6, inset). The increase in the content of 6-keto $PGF_{1\alpha}$ may be indicative of a compensatory mechanism following the ischemic insult. The persisting high levels of thromboxane B_2 may, on the other hand, cause exacerbation of the damage over longer periods of time. When the thromboxane B_2 and 6-keto $PGF_{1\alpha}$ ratios in the restricted animals are compared (FIG.

7), it would appear that the thromboxane B_2 levels, compared to the 6-keto $PGF_{1\alpha}$ levels, are significantly higher in the restricted brain and placenta tissues.

The validity of vascular ligation as a model for examining eicosanoid metabolism in brain embryos after intrauterine placental insufficiency is well established.[24,36] In the present study, we provide biochemical evidence that following vascular ligation, the placenta and the fetal brain cease to metabolize exogenously added arachidonic acid into eicosanoids. The loss of the enzymatic activity is accompanied by the early accumulation of a number of prostanoids, including PGE_2, thromboxane B_2, and 6-keto $PGF_{1\alpha}$. Whether these metabolites exert product inhibition properties by preventing further conversion of free arachidonic acid into eicosanoids is not clear. Accumulation of a specific inhibitor[45] or excess formation of a prostanoid may explain the lack of enzymatic activity converting arachidonic acid. Alternatively, generation of free radicals may bring about enzyme inactivation.[46]

Studies in these directions should provide clues as to the biochemical basis of eicosanoid enzyme inactivation during intrauterine life, and should help determine whether such inactivation may have a consequence of adult brain function.

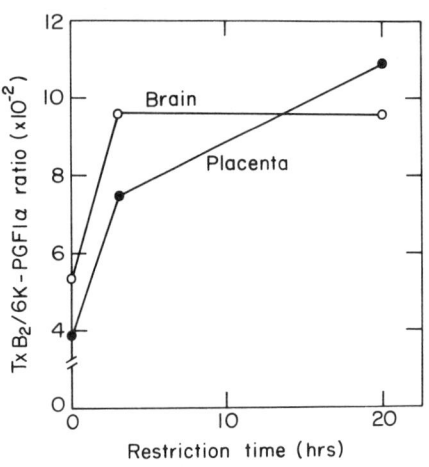

FIGURE 7. Thromboxane B_2 and 6-keto $PGF_{1\alpha}$ ratios in restricted rabbit brain and placenta tissue. Values were redrawn from FIGURE 6.

SUMMARY

Hypoxic-ischemic insults caused by placental insufficiency in perinatal life are today considered a major cause for neuronal injury and impaired postnatal development. A major consequence of placental insufficiency and ischemia is the change in metabolism of arachidonic acid and its oxidation products. A burst of postischemic production of prostaglandins, unequivocally shown in many systems, is documented in the fetal rabbit brain as well as in placenta tissue soon after vascular restriction. PGE_2, a most abundant prostaglandin of the fetal brain, is particularly elevated. Similarly, thromboxane B_2 and 6-keto $PGF_{1\alpha}$, the stable metabolites of thromboxane A_2 and prostacyclin, are both increased over the control values. However, after 48 h of restriction, the levels of these eicosanoids are restored to near-normal values. The metabolic machinery responsible for the conversion of arachidonic acid into eicosanoids in brain and placenta tissues appears to be impaired following a period of placental insufficiency. This inhibition can be accounted for by excessive production of eicosanoids and also by formation of an endogenous inhibitor or free radicals. Studies are in progress to test these possibilities.

REFERENCES

1. BAZAN, N. G. 1976. Adv. Exp. Med. Biol. **72:** 317–335.
2. GARDINER, M., B. NILSSON, S. REHNCRONA & B. K. SIESJO. 1981. J. Neurochem. **36:** 1500–1505.
3. REHNCRONA, S., E. WESTERBERG, B. AKESON & B. K. SIESJO. 1982. J. Neurochem. **38:** 84–93.
4. YOSHIDA, S., M. IKEDA, R. BUSTO, M. SANTISO, E. MARTINEZ &. M. D. GINSBERG. 1986. J. Neurochem. **47:** 744–757.
5. CHAN, P. H. & R. A. FISHMAN. 1978. Science **201:** 358–360.
6. WHITE, B. C., J. G. WIEGENSTEIN & C. D. WINEGAR. 1984. J. Am. Med. Assoc. **25:** 1586–1590.
7. PUSINELLI, W. A., J. B. BRIERLEY & F. PLUM. 1982. Ann. Neurol. **11:** 491–498.
8. GAUDET, R. J., I. ALAM & L. LEVINE. 1980. J. Neurochem. **35:** 653–658.
9. SIESJO, B. K. & B. NILSSON. 1982. Prostaglandins and cerebral circulation. In Prostaglandins and the Cardiovascular System. J. A. Oates, Ed.: 367–379. Raven Press. New York, NY.
10. MOSKOWITZ, M. A., K. J. KIWAK, K. HEKIMIAN & L. LEVINE. 1984. Science **224:** 886–889.
11. WOLFE, L. S. 1982. J. Neurochem. **38:** 1–14.
12. DEMOPOULOS, H. B., E. S. FLAMM, M. L. SELIGMAN & D. D. PIETRONIGRO. 1982. Oxygen free radicals in central nervous system ischemia and trauma. In Pathology of Oxygen. A. P. Autor, Ed.: 127–155. Academic Press. London.
13. CHAN, P. H., J. W. SCHMIEDLEY, R. A. FISHMAN & S. M. LONGAR. 1984. Neurology **34:** 315–320.
14. MCCORD, J. M. 1985. N. Engl. J. Med. **312:** 159–163.
15. MEAD, F. J. 1976. Free radical mechanisms of lipid damage and consequences for cellular membranes. In Free Radicals in Biology. W. A. Pryor, Ed.: 51–68. Academic Press. New York, NY.
16. GOTTFRIED, A. W. 1973. Psychol. Bull. **80:** 231–242.
17. MEIER, G. W. 1971. Hypoxia. In Pharmacological and Biophysical Agents and Behaviour. E. Furchgott, Ed.: 99–142. Academic Press. New York, NY.
18. SECHZER, J. A. 1969. Exp. Neurol. **24:** 497–507.
19. WIGGLESWORTH, J. S. 1964. J. Pathol. Bacteriol. **88:** 1–14.
20. VAN MARTHENS, E., S. HAREL & S. ZAMENHOF. 1975. Biol. Neonate **26:** 221–231.
21. DOBBING, J. 1968. Vulnerable periods in developing brain. In Applied Neurochemistry. A. Davison & J. Dobbing, Eds.: 287–316. Blackwell. Oxford.
22. DOBBING, J. & J. SANDS. 1963. Arch. Dis. Child. **48:** 757–767.
23. HAREL, S., K. WATANABE, I. LINKE & R. J. SCHAIN. 1972. Biol. Neonate **21:** 381–399.
24. MAGAL, E., E. GOLDIN, S. HAREL & E. YAVIN. 1988. J. Neurochem. **51:** 75–80.
25. ALTMAN, J. 1969. In Handbook of Neurochemistry. E. Lajhta, Ed.: 137. Plenum Press. New York, NY.
26. HOSSMANN, K.-A. 1985. Prog. Brain Res. **63:** 3–17.
27. NORDSTROM, C.-H., S. REHNCRONA & B. K. SIESJO. 1978. J. Neurochem. **30:** 479–486.
28. WINICK, M., 1967. J. Pediatr. **71:** 390–395.
29. DRAY, F. & R. FRYDMAN. 1976. Am. J. Obstet. Gynecol. **126:** 13–19.
30. KEIRSE, K. J. N., A. P. F. FLINT & A. C. TURNBULL. 1974. Br. J. Obstet. Gynaecol. **83:** 131–135.
31. RUDOLPH, A. M. 1977. Effects of prostaglandin and synthetase inhibitor on fetal circulation. Proceedings of the Fifth Symposium of the Royal College on Obstetrics and Gynaecology: 231–242. Royal College, London.
32. WILLMAN, E. A. & W. P. COLLINS. 1976. Br. J. Obstet. Gynaecol. **83:** 786–789.

33. URBAN, J. & A. IWASZKIEWICZ-PAWLOWSKA. 1986. J. Perinat. Med. **14:** 259–262.
34. SAEED, A. S. & M. D. MITCHELL. 1983. Biochem. Med. **30:** 322–327.
35. PACE-ASCIAK, C. R. & G. RANGARPU. 1976. J. Biol. Chem. **251:** 3381–3385.
36. GOLDIN, E., HAREL, S., TOMER, A. & E. YAVIN. 1987. J. Neurochem. **48:** 696–701.
37. CASSIN, S. 1980. Semin. Perinat. **4:** 101–106.
38. KARIN, S. M., M. K. HILLIER, R. R. TRUSSELL & R. C. PATEL. 1970. J. Obstet. Gynaecol. Br. Common. **77:** 200–210.
39. LYSZ, T. W. & P. NEEDLEMAN. 1982. J. Neurochem. **38:** 1111–1117.
40. OJEDA, S. R., Z. NAOR & S. M. MCCANN. 1978. Brain Res. **149:** 274–277.
41. PARTINGTON, C. R., M. W. EDWARDS & J. W. DALY. 1980. Proc. Natl. Acad. Sci. USA **77:** 3024–3028.
42. MITCHELL, M. D., S. P. BRENNEKE, S. A. SAEED & D. M. STRICKLAND. 1985. Arachidonic acid metabolism in the fetus and neonate. *In* Biological Protection with Prostaglandins, Vol. 1. M. M. Cohen, Ed.: 27–44. CRC Press. Boca Raton, FL.
43. STUART, M. J., D. A. CLARK, S. G. SUNDERJI, J. B. ALLEN, T. YAMBO & H. ELRAD. 1981. Lancet **1:** 1126–1128.
44. HAREL, S., E. YAVIN, A. TOMER, Y. BARAK & I. BINDERMAN. 1985. Brain Dev. **7:** 575–579.
45. SAEED, S. A., M. DREW & H. O. J. COLLIER. 1980. Eur. J. Pharmacol. **67:** 169–170.
46. LANDS, W. E. M., R. J. KULMACZ & P. J. MARSHALL. 1984. Lipid peroxide actions in the regulation of prostaglandin biosynthesis. *In* Free Radicals in Biology, Vol. 6. W. A. Pryor, Ed.: 39–61. Academic Press. San Diego, CA.

Arachidonic Acid Metabolism in Ischemic Neuronal Damage

KOJI ABE, MIKIO YOSHIDOMI, AND KYUYA KOGURE

Department of Neurology
Institute of Brain Diseases
Tohoku University School of Medicine
Sendai 980, Japan

INTRODUCTION

Polyphosphoinositides (PPIs) are generally thought to be the main source of the increase in free arachidonic acid (AA) during ischemia, especially in the early stage of ischemia.[1,2] This liberation of AA from PPIs is suspected to be the result of the transneuronal breakdown of PPIs triggered mainly by the release of glutamate in the synaptic cleft during ischemia.[3,4] A coupling of inositol phospholipid metabolism with excitatory amino acid receptors has recently been reported in the rat hippocampus.[5]

Transient global ischemia (even if for 5 min) is known to induce neuronal death in hippocampal CA1 pyramidal cells long after reperfusion, whereas parietal cortical neurons remain alive; this phenomenon is known as delayed neuronal death.[6,7] This type of neuronal damage may be the result mainly of excitatory neurotransmission caused by glutamate without energy failure,[8-11] although other causes have been proposed.[12,13]

A different type of release of AA in rat hippocampal CA1 and CA3 regions during cerebral ischemia has been reported.[13] The CA1 cells are selectively vulnerable after reperfusion, and the CA3 cells are resistant. Because the difference in the level of AA in these two areas seems to be very small, it seems that peroxidative derivatives of these AAs may not lead to a different prognosis between these two areas long after reperfusion. With regard to the regional differences in AA release, we are interested in these differences from the view points of both agonist-operated breakdown of PPIs and calcium-activated phospholipase activities. Therefore, we have investigated regional AA and PPI metabolism during transient ischemia and long after reperfusion in the parietal cortex (an area resistant to delayed neuronal damage) and the hippocampal CA1 subfield (a vulnerable area) using a forebrain ischemia model of mongolian gerbils. We have obtained positive results that indicate a close relationship between AA release and excitatory neurotransmission.

METHODS

Mongolian gerbils (*Meriones unguiculatus*) of both sexes, aged 8–10 weeks and weighing 60–80 g, were used for this study. The animals were anesthetized by inhalation of a nitrous oxide/oxygen/halothane (70%:30%:1%) mixture during the preparation of sampling. After the anesthesia was stopped and the animals regained consciousness, the brains were frozen *in situ*,[14] either immediately (in the case of sham control) or at various times after bilateral carotid ligation (ischemia for 5 min and reperfusion for 30 min, 1 day, 2 days, and 7 days). Parietal cortexes and CA1 subfields were dissected (FIG. 1), and the amounts of free fatty acids (FFAs) and PPIs were measured according to previously reported methods.[1]

A newly synthesized inhibitor of protein kinase C—K252a or K252b[15,16]—kindly donated by the Kyowa Hakko Company (Tokyo, Japan)—was dissolved in DMSO (dimethylsulfoxide)/physiological saline (1:20). One μl of 10^{-4} M of the above K252a or b solution was topically injected into the unilateral CA1 subfield (0.1 μl/min, 10 min) just before the induction of 5 min of ischemia. After 2 days and 7 days of reperfusion, histopathological examinations were performed[7] on the CA1 subfield in order to determine the ability of K252 to prevent delayed neuronal death of CA1 cells.

Statistical analyses were performed using Student's t-test.

RESULTS

As shown in FIGURE 2, the amount of PPIs in the cortex rapidly recovered during reperfusion periods. However, those in the CA1 area did not recover after 30 min of reperfusion. Only the amount of triphosphoinositide (TPI) in CA1 showed a partial recovery at 30 min of reperfusion.

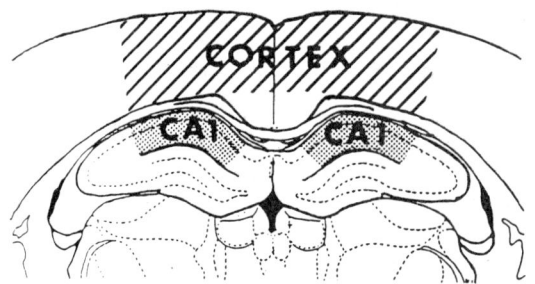

FIGURE 1. Areas dissected for the measurement of free fatty acids and polyphosphoinositides. Parietel cortex and hippocampal CA1 subfield were dissected at -20 °C without any contamination of white matter.

FIGURES 3 and 4 show changes in FFAs and AA. Although the amount of total FFAs in the cortex recovered during 30 min of reperfusion, this amount slowly increased again until 2 days after reperfusion and recovered to the control level at 7 days. On the other hand, the amount of total FFAs in the CA1 area continued to increase during the first day of reperfusion, precipitated on the second day, and finally increased again on the seventh day. The pattern of changes of AA in the cortex and the CA1 area seem to be almost the same as that of changes of total FFAs.

Compositions of total esterified fatty acids (TEFA) are rich in palmitic acid, stearic acid, and docosahexaenoic acid both in the cortex and the CA1 area (FIGS. 5 and 6). On the other hand, fatty acid compositions of FFAs that increase during 5 min of ischemia are rich in stearic acid and AA, rather different from the composition of TEFA and similar to that of PPIs. However, compositions of FFAs during reperfusion, especially when the total amounts of FFAs are increasing (for example, 1 day and 7 days in the CA1 area; 1 day and 2 days in the cortex), are very similar to those seen for TEFA (FIGS. 5 and 6).

Table 1 shows the effects of K252a and K252b on preventing delayed neuronal death of CA1 pyramidal cells. Although the experiment was too small in number of samples to perform a statistical analysis, both K252a and K252b seem to have positive protective effects.

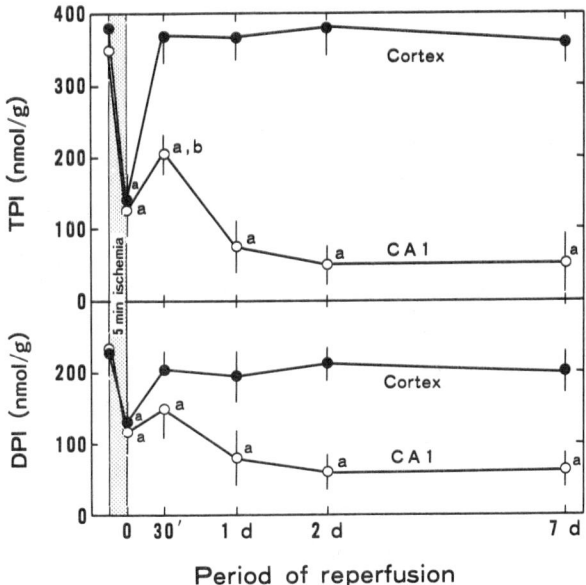

FIGURE 2. Changes in the amount of tri- and diphosphoinositides (TPI and DPI) during and after 5 min of forebrain ischemia in the parietal cortex (Cortex) or CA1 subfield (CA1). Open and closed *circles* represent mean ± SD expressed as nmol/g wet weight. $n = 6$. a: $p < 0.01$ different from the case of sham control; b: $p < 0.05$ different from the case treated with 5 min of ischemia.

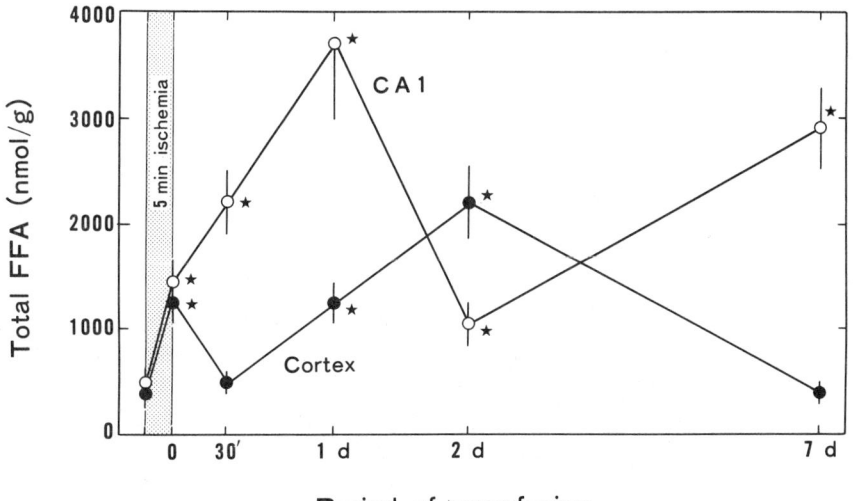

FIGURE 3. Changes in the amount of total free fatty acids during and after 5 min of forebrain ischemia in the parietal cortex (Cortex) or CA1 subfields (CA1). Open and closed *circles* represent mean ± SD expressed as nmol/g wet weight. $N = 6$. *Stars*: $p < 0.01$ different from the case of sham control.

DISCUSSION

Phosphatidyl inositol (PI) *response* has been understood to be stimulated mainly by cholinergic or noradrenergic stimulation. This response induces PI breakdown and produces both diacylglycerol (DG) and inositol-triphosphate (IP_3). IP_3 can increase cytosolic calcium concentration by releasing calcium from the intracellular calcium store;[17] and a part of IP_3 is converted by IP_3 kinase to IP_4, which can potentiate calcium influx from extracellular space,[18] also resulting in an increase in cytosolic calcium concentration. DG can activate protein kinase C (C-kinase) if both phosphatidylserin and calcium exist.[19] Thus, PI response involving the production of DG and IP_3 from triphosphoinositides may result in the activation of C-kinase.

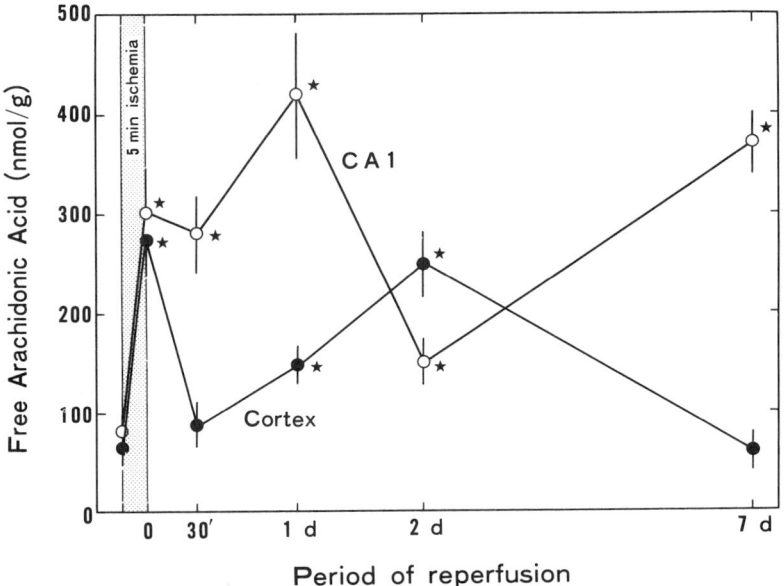

FIGURE 4. Changes in the amount of free arachidonic acid during and after 5 min of forebrain ischemia. All symbols and bars represent the same values shown in the legend to FIG. 3.

A breakdown of PPIs and an increase in the amount of DG are also seen in the model of brain ischemia,[20] and AA may be released from this increased DG by DG lipase in the early stage of ischemia.[1,2] Thus AA release is closely related to the breakdown of PPIs in the model of brain ischemia. There was no significant change in the amount of both total FFAs and AA in the cortex and the CA1 area during ischemia (FIGS. 3 and 4). However, the change might be different if the period of ischemia were of longer duration, as was seen in the CA1 and CA3 areas in the model of rat forebrain ischemia.[13] On the other hand, the changes in FFAs in the cortex and the CA1 area during reperfusion periods are remarkably different (FIGS. 3 and 4). The amount of FFAs and AA transiently recovered in the cortex, slowly reincreased until the end of the second day, and finally recovered to the control level (FIGS. 3 and 4), although there was no histological change during these periods (FIG. 8). Of interest were the

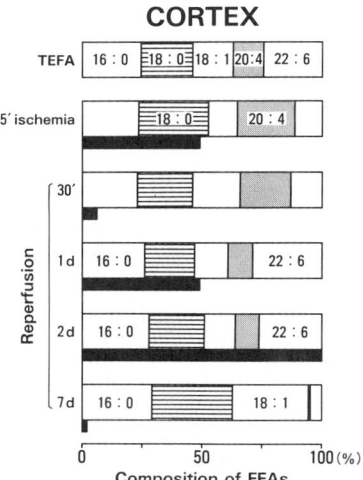

FIGURE 5. Fatty acid compositions of total esterified fatty acids (TEFA) and free fatty acids (5 min ischemia and reperfusion) in the parietal cortex. *Solid bars* represent total amounts of free fatty acids expressed as percent of the amount of free fatty acids seen in the case of reperfusion for 2 days. TEFA is rich in palmitic acid (16:0), stearic acid (18:0), and docosahexaenoic acid (22:6), the composition resembling that of free fatty acids seen on the first and second days of reperfusion. On the other hand, free fatty acids seen with 5 min of ischemia are rich in stearic acid and arachidonic acid (20:4).

changes in the composition of FFAs in the cortex (FIG. 5). FFAs, which increased during 5 min of ischemia, contained much stearic acid and AA, suggesting that they were liberated predominantly from inositol phospholipids.[1,2,20] On the other hand, the compositions of FFAs at the end of the first and second days approximated that of TEFA (FIG. 5). Therefore, this delayed increase in FFAs in the cortex seems to represent a reintegration of membrane lipids after possible disturbance induced by ischemic insults.

The amounts of FFAs and AA in CA1 continued to increase until after 1 day of reperfusion (FIGS. 3 and 4), which is compatible with the continuous electrophysiological firing of CA1 neurons (FIG. 7), and the amounts precipitated at 2 days, when no electroactivity was found in the CA1 area (FIG. 7). The continuous firing of CA1 cells

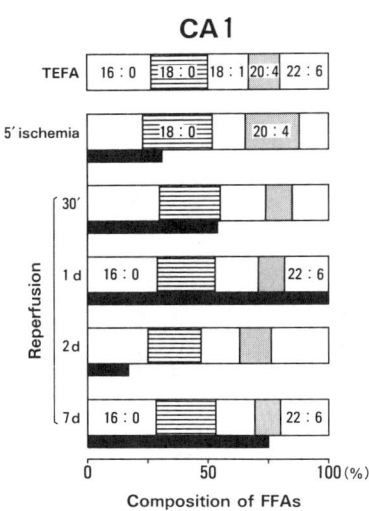

FIGURE 6. Fatty acid compositions of total esterified fatty acids (TEFA) and free fatty acids (5 min ischemia and reperfusion) in the CA1 subfields. *Solid bars* represent total amount of free fatty acids expressed as percent of the amount seen in the case of reperfusion for 1 day. Fatty acid compositions of free fatty acids seen on the first and seventh days of reperfusion are very similar to that of TEFA.

TABLE 1. Effects of the Topical Injection of K252a and K252b on Delayed Neuronal Necrosis of CA1 Pyramidal Cells

| | Total Number of CA1 Neurons | | | |
| | Sham Operation | | Ischemia | |
Drug	Left	Right	Left	Right
K252a	882	872	336	563
	780	813	279	548
	799	764	606	613
K252b	837	658	164	717
	800	818	439	364
	712	719	ND	ND

NOTE: Left = left hippocampus treated with vehicle; Right = right hippocampus treated with drug; ND = not determined.

has been understood to be the result of glutamatergic excitation.[9-11] Therefore, our results indicate a close relationship between AA release and excitatory neurotransmission. The amounts also increased again at the end of 7 days, which suggests active gliosis (FIG. 8). Changes in the composition of FFAs were also of interest in the CA1 area (FIG. 6). Composition of FFAs, which increased during 5 min of ischemia, was also similar to that of inositol phospholipids. However, the composition ratio of AA decreased and that of docosahexaenoic acid increased during 30 min and 1 day of reperfusion, which is very similar to the composition of TEFA (FIG. 6). The similarity of the fatty acid composition of FFAs to that of TEFA may represent the result of nonspecific activation of various phospholipases rather than specific activation of a phospholipase such as phospholipase A_2, or of the phospholipase C and DG lipase

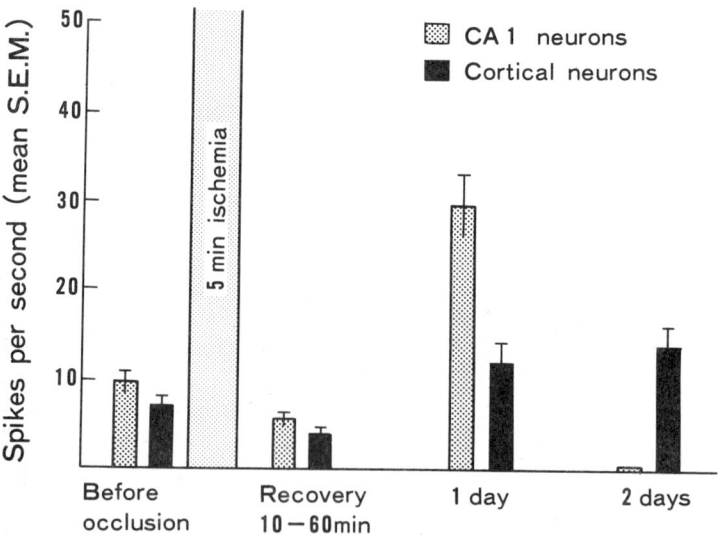

FIGURE 7. Histogram of frequency of action potentials in cortical and CA1 neurons at various periods after 5 min of forebrain ischemia. (Modified with permission from Suzuki *et al.*[32])

system. In the activation of phospholipases, PI-specific phospholipase C is far more sensitive to the calcium concentration than is phospholipase A_2. Therefore, a specific activation of phospholipase C may occur if an increase in the calcium concentration remained at the lower level. However, a massive influx of calcium due to glutamatergic excitation may induce nonspecific activation of phospholipases during these periods (from 30 min to 1 day of reperfusion in the CA1 area), when PPIs have already

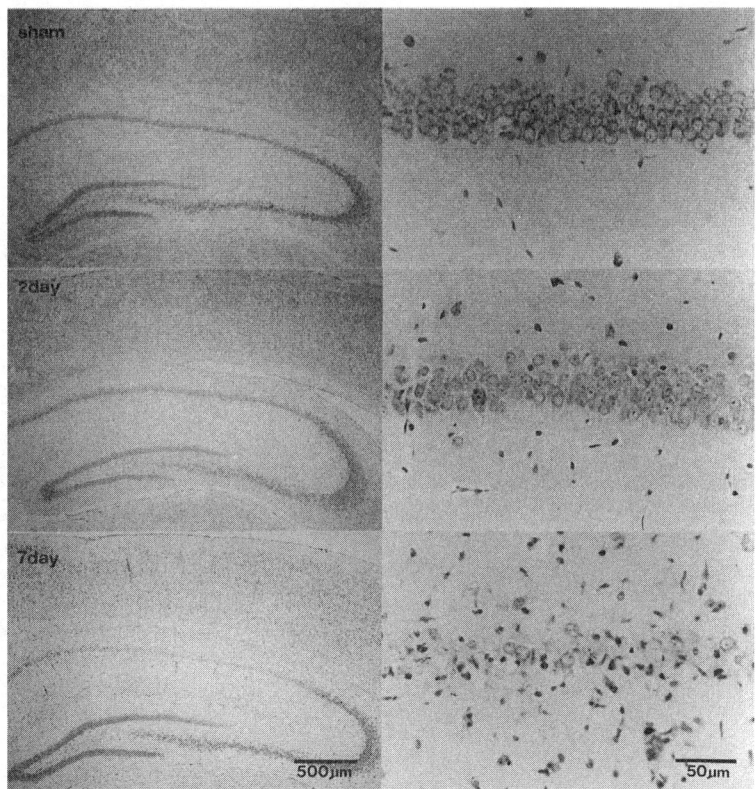

FIGURE 8. Histopathological demonstration of the CA1 area and the parietal cortex stained by cresyl violet. *Top:* sham control; *middle:* case 2 days after 5 min of forebrain ischemia; *bottom:* case 7 days after 5 min of forebrain ischemia. Note that the CA1 cells seem to show normal staining at 2 days, and a marked gliosis occurs at 7 days in the CA1 area; whereas the parietal cortical area seems to show normal staining during 7 days after the reperfusion.

precipitated and no longer have sufficient fatty acids to be liberated in the CA1 area (FIG. 2).

Excitability of hippocampal CA1 pyramidal cells is regulated mainly by potassium currents—that is, a calcium-activated potassium current (Ik(Ca)) and a second potassium conductance (Im), both of which normally serve to limit CA1 excitability[21] in what is known as *spike accommodation.* Muscarinic agonists and phorbol esters excite CA1 neurons by inhibiting both Ik(Ca) and Im, or Ik(Ca), respectively, under normal conditions. Muscarinic agonists are typical neurotransmitters that hydrolyze inositol phospholipids (especially triphosphoinositides) and result in activation of C-kinase. Muscarinic receptors exist more abundantly in the CA1 subfield than in the cerebral cortex (FIG 9); and C-kinase is also richer in the CA1 area than in the cerebral cortex.[22] Hippocampal pyramidal cells in rats have a voltage-dependent chloride current, which is active at resting potential, and are inhibited either by membrane depolarization or by activation of C-kinase by phorbol esters. Thus, blockade of this chloride current by activation of C-kinase potentiates the transmission of dendritic excitatory events by increasing dendritic membrane resistance.[23] Furthermore, C-kinase may play a major role in the long term potentiation of hippocampal pyramidal cells.[24,25] These results indicate that C-kinase may play a key role in the regulation of neuronal excitability of CA1 cells under normal conditions.[26]

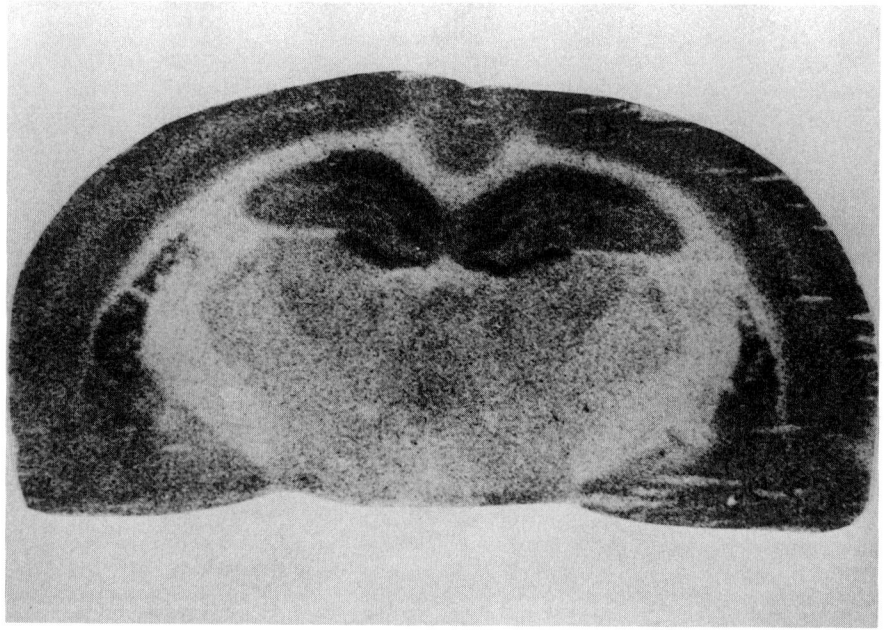

FIGURE 9. Topographical demonstration of muscarinic cholinergic receptors in rat brain, obtained using the method of Onodera et al.[33]

It has been thought that glutamatergic agonists can phospholylate A-kinase and G-kinase by activating adenylate cyclase or guanylate cyclase, respectively. However, it has recently been elucidated that a coupling of inositol phospholipid metabolism with excitatory amino acid receptors exists,[5] and glutamatergic agonists also inhibit the chloride channel, as was seen in the case of phorbol esters, by potentiating the PI response.[27] On the other hand, topographical techniques have demonstrated that glutamate receptors in the brain are richer in the CA1 area than in the cerebral cortex,[11] as was seen in the muscarinic cholinergic receptors (FIG. 9). However, receptors of inhibitory neurotransmitters such as γ-aminobutyric acid (GABA) and benzodiazepine seem richer in the cerebral cortex than in the CA1 area.[31] These imbalances in the distribution among various receptors of excitatory and inhibitory neurotransmitters may provide a background of excitotoxic vulnerability of the CA1 cells. Therefore, an excitotoxic mechanism has been indicated to be involved in postischemic delayed neuronal damage of CA1 cells.[9-11] Receptors of C-kinase and IP_3 are also richer in the CA1 area than in the cerebral cortex.[22] C-kinase is recognized as a key regulator of neuronal excitability of CA1 cells under normal conditions.[26] However, a relationship between the postischemic excitotoxic neurotransmission and a second messenger system, such as DG, IP_3, and C-kinase, has not been fully elucidated. To test the pathogenetic role of C-kinase in this delayed neuronal death of CA1 cells, we have tried to examine if a selective inhibitor of C-kinase (K252a or K252b) possibly helps to prevent CA1 cell death. K252a and K252b are newly synthesized specific inhibitors of C-kinase.[15,16] K252b has more specificity to C-kinase than does K252a. Although it remains to be studied further, treatment with K252a or K252b seems to protect the delayed neuronal loss of the CA1 cells (TABLE 1). These results suggest the possibility that C-kinase may play a certain pathogenetic role in this type of delayed neuronal damage of CA1 cells.

Previous reports have indicated that an excessive influx of calcium caused by an abnormal release of glutamate during ischemia may cause delayed neuronal death of CA1 cells.[4,11,28-30] This hypothesis can be tested using a few selective glutamate receptor antagonists[28,29] or an inhibitor of glutamate-operated calcium channels.[30] Although we did not measure the changes in the amount of DG that can activate C-kinase, our results suggest that glutamate-induced breakdown of PPIs may occur during and after transient ischemia; our results also suggest that activation of C-kinase may potentiate CA1 excitability and may exacerbate glutamate-induced excitotoxicity of these neurons.

REFERENCES

1. ABE, K., K. KOGURE, H. YAMAMOTO, M. IMAZAWA & K. MIYAMOTO. 1987. Mechanism of arachidonic acid liberation during ischemia in gerbil cerebral cortex. J. Neurochem. **48:** 503–509.
2. IKEDA, M., S. YOSHIDA, R. BUSTO, M. SANTISO & M. D. GINSBERG. 1986. Polyphosphoinositides as a probable source of brain free fatty acids at the onset of ischemia. J. Neurochem. **47:** 123–132.
3. WESTERBERG, E. & T. WIELOCH. 1986. Lesions to the corticostriatal pathways ameliorate hypoglycemia-induced arachidonic acid release. J. Neurochem. **47:** 1507–1511.
4. BENVENISTE, H., J. DREJER, A. SCHOUSBOE & N. H. DIEMER. 1984. Elevation of the extracellular concentrations of glutamate and aspartate in rat hippocampus during transient cerebral ischemia monitored by intracerebral microdialysis. J. Neurochem. **43:** 1369–1374.
5. NICOLLETI, F., J. L. MEEK, M. J. IADAROLA, D. M. CHUANG, B. L. ROTH & E. COSTA. 1986. Coupling of inositol phospholipid metabolism with excitatory amino acid recognition sites in rat hippocampus. J. Neurochem. **46:** 40–46.
6. KIRINO, T. 1982. Delayed neuronal death in the gerbil hippocampus following ischemia. Brain Res. **239:** 57–69.
7. PULSINELLI, W. A., J. B. BRIELEY & F. C. PLUM. 1982. Temporal profile of neuronal damage in a model of transient forebrain ischemia. Ann. Neurol. **11:** 491–498.
8. ARAI, H., W. D. LUST & J. V. PASSONNEAU. 1982. Delayed metabolic changes induced 5 min of ischemia in gerbil brain. Trans. Am. Soc. Neurochem. **13:** 177.
9. ROTHMAN, S. M. & J. W. OLNEY. 1986. Glutamate and pathophysiology of hypoxic-ischemic brain damage. Ann. Neurol. **19:** 105–111.
10. WIELOCH, T. 1985. Neurochemical correlates to selective neuronal vulnerability. Prog. Brain Res. **63:** 69–85.

11. ONODERA, H., G. SATO & K. KOGURE. 1986. Lesions to Schaffer collaterals prevent ischemic death of CA1 pyramidal cells. Neurosci. Lett. **68:** 169–174.
12. IMDALL, A. & K. A. HOSSMANN. 1986. Morphometric evaluation of postischemic capillary perfusion in selectively vulnerable areas of gerbil brain. Acta Neuropathol. (Berlin) **69:** 267–271.
13. WESTERBERG, E., J. K. DESHPANDE & T. WIELOCH. 1987. Regional differences in arachidonic acid release in rat hippocampal CA1 and CA3 regions during cerebral ischemia. J. Cereb. Blood Flow Metab. **7:** 189–192.
14. PONTEN, U., R. A. RATCHESON, L. G. SALFORD & B. K. SIESJÖ. 1973. Optimal freezing conditions for cerebral metabolites in rats. J. Neurochem. **21:** 1127–1138.
15. KASE, H., K. IWAHASHI & Y. MATSUDA. 1986. K252a, a potent inhibitor of protein kinase C from microbial origin. J. Antibiot. **39**(8): 1059–1065.
16. YAMADA, K., K. IWAHASHI & H. KASE. 1987. K252a, a new inhibitor of protein kinase C, concomitantly inhibits 40k protein phospholylation and serotonin secretion in phorbol ester-stimulated platelets. Biochem. Biophys. Res. Commun. **144**(1): 35–40.
17. BERRIDGE, M. J. & R. F. IRVINE. 1984. Inositol triphosphate, a novel second messenger in cellular signal transduction. Nature **312:** 315–321.
18. IRVINE, R. F., A. J. LETCHER, J. P. HESLOP & M. J. BERRIDGE. 1986. The inositol tris/tetrakisphosphate pathway—demonstration of Ins(1,4,5)P3 3-kinase activity in animal tissues. Nature **320:** 631–634.
19. NISHIZUKA, Y. 1984. Turnover of inositol phospholipids and signal transduction. Science **225:** 1365–1370.
20. ABE, K. & K. KOGURE. 1986. Accurate evaluation of 1,2-diacylglycerol in gerbil forebrain using HPLC and in situ freezing technique. J. Neurochem. **47:** 577–582.
21. ADAMS, P. R., D. A. BROWN & A. CONSTANTI. 1982. Pharmacological inhibition of the M-current. J. Physiol. (London) **332:** 223–262.
22. WORLEY, P. F., J. M. BARABAN & S. H. SNYDER. 1987. Beyond receptors: Multiple second-messenger systems in brain. Ann. Neurol. **21:** 217–229.
23. MADISON, D. V., R. C. MALENKA & R. A. NICOLL. 1986. Phorbol esters block a voltage-sensitive chloride current in hippocampal pyramidal cells. Nature **321:** 695–697.
24. LYNCH, G. & M. BAUDRY. 1984. The biochemistry of memory: A new and specific hypothesis. Science **224:** 1057–1063.
25. HU, G. Y., O. HVALBY, S. I. WALAAS, K. A. ALBERT, P. SKJEFLO, P. ANDERSON & P. GREENGARD. 1987. Protein kinase C injection into hippocampal pyramidal cells elicits features of long term potentiation. Nature **328:** 426–429.
26. MILLER, R. J. 1986. Protein kinase C: A key regulator of neuronal excitability? Trends Neurosci. **9:** 538–541.
27. SUGIYAMA, H., I. ITO & C. HIRONO. 1987. A new type of glutamate receptor linked to inositol phospholipid metabolism. Nature **325:** 531–533.
28. SIMON, R. P., J. H. SWAN, T. GRIFFITHS & B. S. MELDRUM. 1987. Blockade of N-methyl-D-aspartate receptors may protect against ischemic damage in the brain. Science **226:** 850–852.
29. GILL, R., A. C. FOSTER, I. L. IVERSEN & G. N. WOODRUFF. 1987. Ischemia-induced degeneration of hippocampal neurons in gerbils is prevented by systemic administration of MK801. J. Cereb. Blood Flow Metab. **7**(Suppl.1): s153.
30. IZUMIYAMA, K., T. HAYASHI & K. KOGURE. 1986. Possible cause of hypermetabolism of glucose and neuronal damage after brain ischemia. Abstracts of the 10th International Congress of Neuropathology, Stockholm, Sweden: 121.
31. ONODERA, H., G. SATO & K. KOGURE. 1987. GABA and benzodiazepine receptors in the gerbil brain after transient ischemia: Demonstration by quantitative receptor autoradiography. J. Cereb. Blood Flow Metab. **7:** 82–88.
32. SUZUKI, R., T. YAMAGUCHI, C. LI & I. KLAZO. 1983. The effects of 5-minute ischemia in Mongolian gerbils: II. Changes of spontaneous neuronal activity in cerebral cortex and CA1 sector of hippocampus. Acta Neuropathol. **60:** 217–222.
33. ONODERA, H., G. SATO & K. KOGURE. 1987. Quantitative autoradiographic analysis of muscarinic cholinergic and adenosine A1 binding sites after transient forebrain ischemia in the gerbil. Brain Res. **415:** 309–322.

Ischemic Injury in the Brain

Role of Oxygen Radical–Mediated Processes[a]

BRANT D. WATSON AND MYRON D. GINSBERG

*Cerebral Vascular Disease Research Center
and
Department of Neurology
University of Miami School of Medicine
Miami, Florida 33101*

OXYGEN FREE RADICALS AND LIPID PEROXIDATION

Free radicals are short-lived molecular species, produced under certain conditions, that are believed to initiate toxic effects in biological systems.[1-3] A free radical is chemically unstable, and thus potentially reactive, because one or more of its valence electron orbitals is half-filled, with just one electron instead of the usual pair of electrons. The reactivity of free radicals results from their propensity to acquire thermodynamic stability in the stable, opposite-spin configuration by abstracting electrons or hydrogen atoms from adjacent molecules. Perhaps the most familiar clinical expression of free radical injury in tissues is that induced by ionizing radiation. For example, the oxygen effect[4] of radiobiology, in which radiation damage leading to cell death is enhanced in the presence of molecular oxygen, is substantially mediated by reduced forms of the oxygen molecule resulting from the stepwise addition of electrons. These reduced forms, called "oxygen radicals" or "active oxygens," include the superoxide anion radical (O_2^-) and its protonated form the perhydroxyl radical ($HO_2\cdot$) produced at low pH (both singly reduced), hydrogen peroxide (doubly reduced), and hydroxyl radical ($OH\cdot$).[1-3,5-7] *In vivo,* hydrogen peroxide is produced by dismutation of superoxide anions, a reaction catalyzed by the enzyme superoxide dismutase.[8] Hydroxyl radical is derived by single electron reduction of hydrogen peroxide. When catalyzed by ferrous ion, this reaction is known as the Fenton reaction. Because ferrous ion is released from iron-binding sites by the interaction of superoxide anion with (ferri)proteins,[9] the reaction is "site specific," and is designated as the iron-catalyzed, superoxide-driven Fenton reaction.[10] (Without the redox participation of iron ions, the process is known as the Haber-Weiss reaction.)

The perhydroxyl radical,[11] and especially the hydroxyl radical,[12] can vigorously abstract hydrogen atoms from unsaturated fatty acids to form lipid radicals; this is the initial step in the chain process of lipid peroxidation. Lipid peroxidation is also known as lipid autoxidation, because in the presence of oxygen the lipid radical is spontaneously peroxidized (molecular oxygen is added directly). The resultant peroxy radical is capable of abstracting a hydrogen atom from a neighboring molecule, thus transferring radical character to this target molecule while transforming itself into a neutral hydroperoxide molecule.[1-3,5,13,14] The new radical can then reinitiate and propagate the cycle in chain fashion. The product hydroperoxides can be dissociated by ferrous ion into alkoxyl free radicals, in a manner analogous to the Fenton reaction.

---

[a]This work was supported by USPHS grants NS05820 and NS23244. Myron Ginsberg is a recipient of a Jacob Javits Neuroscience Investigatorship.

Both peroxyl[12] and alkoxyl[15] radicals are highly reactive with (and selectively induce conjugated diene formation in) unsaturated fatty acid molecules. Therefore, the "toxicities" of superoxide anion and hydrogen peroxide are explained largely by their participation at iron binding sites in yielding the much more reactive hydroxyl radical. Superoxide anion can enter the extravascular space through membrane anion channels,[16] as can hydrogen peroxide, a neutral species that can diffuse directly through cell membranes.[7] Thus, the potential for injury can be exported from a given cell to others, possibly over considerable distances if the target cells are endothelial.

Radical chain processes continue until termination by hydrogen atom donation from "antioxidant" molecules, such as alpha-tocopherol (vitamin E).[13,17] The products of antioxidant neutralization are the same hydroperoxides that arise during the chain process, but propagation is quenched because the resultant tocopherol radicals, owing to charge delocalization, are much less reactive with potential substrate molecules. The product hydroperoxides serve as substrates for enzymatic detoxification by glutathione peroxidase. In synergy with superoxide dismutase, glutathione peroxidase reduces hydrogen peroxide and lipid peroxides into water and alpha-hydroxy fatty acids, respectively, at the expense of reduced glutathione.[17] These enzymatic defense mechanisms are primarily intracellular, however, and will be less likely to suppress extracellular reactions mediated by active oxygen species.[7,18] Among the damaging effects of lipid peroxidation are unimolecular inactivation or polymerization of membrane lipids and proteins, owing to formation of abnormal intra- or intermolecular cross-links.[1-3,5-7,13,17] These bonds are mediated by direct radical combination or by bifunctional species, such as aldehydes, that result from peroxide decomposition mediated by ferrous ion. Accordingly, the structural integrity of cellular membranes is compromised owing to the formation of microscopically visible fissures or holes.[19-23]

DETECTION TECHNIQUES FOR LIPID PEROXIDATION AND THEIR SIGNIFICANCE TO *IN VIVO* ANALYSIS

Commonly used techniques for the detection of lipid peroxidation in the brain and spinal cord have included observation of vitamin E consumption, disappearance of ascorbyl radical or of unsaturated fatty acid content, and synthesis of oxidized glutathione (GSSG) at the expense of reduced glutathione.[5,6,24] Spectroscopic assays include detection of aldehyde decomposition products as a result of their reactivity with thiobarbituric acid (TBA) to form a green-absorbing chromophore; or detection of conjugated diene structures (resulting from double bond rearrangement after hydrogen atom abstraction) absorbing in the ultraviolet region of 235 nm.[5,24] These assays have been criticized owing to lack of specificity, especially the test for TBA reactants (in which a complex of reactions involving further tissue peroxidation is induced).[10] More recently, histochemical localization of aldehydic groups has been employed to assess the distribution of peroxidized products in tissue.[25]

However, the question of just what *in vivo* conditions are minimally sufficient to initiate processes leading to cell death by any means, including free radical processes, is still open. Certainly membrane permeability is enhanced upon exposure to superoxide anions,[26] and indicators of cell morbidity such as vacuolation are increased to the point of irreversibility during prolonged exposure[27,28] or during shorter, direct exposure to hydroxyl radical.[27] Despite these effects it has not yet been possible to induce, by oxygen radical attack, detectable lipid peroxidation *in vivo* that *precedes* any acutely observable signs of membrane destruction to a degree sufficient for cell death.[1,29] This calls into question whether lipid peroxidation *in vivo* necessarily expands the area of initial membrane damage after oxygen radical attack. Alternatively, it is possible that the degree of cellular morbidity is proportional to the density of pores formed by oxygen radical injury to the surface membrane, but that the levels of presumed product lipid peroxides are too low to detect by existing methods. Indeed, the formation of pores followed by development of lethal edema in target cells has recently been revealed as at least one strategy employed by cytotoxic T (killer) cells.[30] As membrane breakdown proceeds concomitant with a profusion of degradative responses (such as calcium ion influx[31] and consumption of energy stores), the chain process of lipid peroxidation may proceed to detectable levels provided that the radical intermediates are not diluted. At this point, however, the cell is likely metabolically quiescent and may well be dying or already dead.[1,29] By this scenario, the disorder engendered by primary oxygen radical processes is sufficient to sever any directly observable connection of oxygen radicals to *induction* of cell death by the lipid peroxidation pathway.

Contributing to this difficulty of interpretation is the fact that it has not been possible to attain overlap of the corresponding complementary methodologies for oxygen radical detection or lipid peroxidation in either time or space (i.e., regional specificity of tissue damage). At present, oxygen radicals are usually detected indirectly by means of (usually) preadministered scavenger molecules, either through formation of specific products or by suppression of structural or functional deficits attributed to oxygen radical attack. On the other hand, lipid peroxides, as we have seen, result from derivative events that may be delayed in their onset. Detection methods for superoxide anion include its reaction with nitroblue tetrazolium to yield an insoluble formazan precipitate,[32] scavenging of superoxide by exogenous superoxide dismutase,[32,33] or inhibition with allopurinol of its enzymatic formation (cf. next section). Molecular scavengers[33] of hydroxyl radical (mannitol or dimethylurea) or of ferric ion[34] (deferoxamine) have also been used to protect membranes from the initial assault of hydrogen atom abstraction. Direct detection in real time by electron spin resonance of superoxide radical has been reported recently in reoxygenated endothelium,[35] but in view of the amounts of tissue required it is unlikely that these measurements can be correlated with the development of pathology in specific tissue regions.

BIOLOGICAL PRODUCTION OF THE PRIMARY OXYGEN RADICAL, SUPEROXIDE ANION (O_2^-)

With the realization that oxygen radicals were the likeliest candidates to induce lipid peroxidation, efforts to identify their normal modes of production *in vivo*, and their amplification under conditions of metabolic stress, were begun and still continue. Because it is believed that the process of free radical–induced tissue degradation begins with the superoxide anion, some major pathways for its production are presented.

Purine metabolism: This pathway is potentiated by ischemia, during which ATP is degraded stepwise to its purine substrates and endothelial xanthine dehydrogenase is transformed to xanthine oxidase.[36,37] During reperfusion (reoxygenation), xanthine oxidase catalyzes O_2^- production from the purine substrates xanthine and hypoxanthine.[37]

Prostaglandin (PG) synthesis: The conversion of PGG_2 to PGH_2 by prostaglandin synthase is accomplished by the enzyme operating as a classical (hydro)peroxidase; that is, the enzyme itself assumes a free radical character through Compound I and II–type configurations.[38] (The leukotriene-producing lipoxygenases exhibit a similar character.) Concomitantly, the enzyme radicals can abstract hydrogen atoms from nucleotides (NAD(P)H), and their resultant radical forms (NAD(P)·) can be oxidized by molecular oxygen to yield O_2^-. Although this process occurs normally, it is presently conjectured that any type of tissue trauma (including ischemia) leading to arachidonic acid release can amplify this pathway; ischemia further potentiates this reaction via enhanced accumulation of reduced nucleotides, which then facilitates O_2^- production during reperfusion.[38]

Respiration: Oxidation of ubisemiquinone radical,[39] the diffusible electron transfer agent in the mitochondrial respiratory chain, yields O_2^-. This pathway operates during normal metabolism, but its enhancement (following reoxygenation) is likely potentiated by the reducing conditions present during ischemia.[7]

Neutrophil activation: Phagocytosis stimulates O_2^- synthesis by NADH oxidase during the respiratory burst.[40] Neutrophils responding to tissue injury (as signaled chemotactically by O_2^- release) may inappropriately enhance local, or possibly remote, destruction of tissue by releasing a flood of active oxygen species.[37,40]

ORIGINS OF CELLULAR TOXICITY INDUCED BY OXYGEN RADICALS

It has been proposed that certain oxygen radical processes are by themselves sufficient to precipitate subtle but determining metabolic changes leading to cell death. During efforts to repair single strand DNA breakage induced by hydrogen peroxide[41] (derived from neutrophils, for example), ATP and NAD(P)H are consumed by poly(ADP)ribose polymerase activation. If the influx of hydrogen peroxide is sufficiently intense, cell integrity will be diminished owing to inability to maintain energy-dependent membrane barriers.[42] In the setting of ischemia, replenishment of energy stores will be inactivated, as will successful operation of the enzymatic defense system, because glutathione peroxidase activity is dependent on the pentose phosphate pathway.[17,41] To further illustrate the critical dependence of cell viability on maintenance of sufficient metabolic potential via glucose utilization, neurons starved in culture produce superoxide anions at a rate that markedly increases when cell death is imminent.[43] It thus appears that tissue injury by any means leading to metabolic dysfunction may result in exacerbation of conditions for free radical generation, enhancement of local tissue injury, and possible export of injurious factors to outlying tissue regions.

Because superoxide anion is known to enhance intravascular permeability, the development of edema is a likely consequence. A cycle of interactions results that can exacerbate local tissue damage and provide for involvement of adjacent tissues as well.[37] At a locus of developing ischemia, superoxide anions produced by any of the pathways described can elicit an inflammatory response; the resultant influx of neutrophils will likely respond by secreting oxygen radicals of their own, and by forming vascular plugs. The edematous zone is thus increased, and this increase can in turn accentuate the severity of ischemia.[37] These conditions are representative of oxidative stress, defined as the potentiation of cellular injury by facilitation of superoxide anion formation, oxygen radical–induced membrane barrier breakdown, release of iron ions from tissue stores, consequent acceleration of local tissue destruction, and saturation of protective mechanisms against oxygen radicals. Oxidative stress is amplified during reperfusion following ischemia, owing to the interaction of oxygen with a preponderance of reduced species.[7] This contributes to the possibility of reperfusion injury; that is, attempted tissue resuscitation is concomitant with transformation of reversible ischemic cellular injury into an *irreversible* state.[44] It thus appears that the transition from developing cell morbidity to frank mortality during ischemia and its aftermath is not distinct, but is conditioned by tissue and neutrophil responses of various degrees of exaggeration and mutual reinforcement.

SPECIFIC EVIDENCE FOR CENTRAL NERVOUS SYSTEM TISSUE DAMAGE ATTRIBUTED TO FREE RADICAL ACTIVATION

Most of the original analyses concerning *in vivo* lipid peroxidation in the central nervous system were based on the derivative methods described previously.[24] Efforts to detect lipid peroxidation in terms of loss of reduced glutathione,[45,46] ascorbic acid,[46] TBA reactants,[45,47] or unsaturated fatty acids[48] following recirculation of globally ischemic rat brain were unsuccessful, even though analogous *in vitro* experiments yielded the expected positive results.[45,48] This particular problem was solved by monitoring conjugated diene content in small (less than 1 mg) tissue samples taken from rat brain coronal sections; it was shown that approximately 15% of the samples exhibited resolvable spectra indicative of the conjugated diene structure.[49] These results could be related to the previous work by computer-averaging all the spectra accumulated from each animal, thus simulating the large amounts of tissue used for those assays. When this was done, the small-scale positive effect was diluted so as to be indistinguishable from control samples. Recently, cerebral samples taken from rats subjected to reversible middle cerebral artery (MCA) territory stroke revealed conjugated dienes only infrequently in the ipsilateral region, even though this region is known to proceed to infarction.[50] The focality of conjugated diene concentration seen in these experiments, was also observed histochemically in the livers of bromobenzene-poisoned mice.[25]

Several observations follow from these examples. Because tissue regions exhibiting peroxidation cannot be localized beforehand, it will be difficult to correlate lipid peroxidation with early morphologic changes by ultrastructural analysis. This reservation also applies to experiments in which the development of lipid peroxidation can be actively monitored *in vivo,* as exemplified by the detection of pentane, a lipid peroxidation decomposition product, exhaled from gerbils breathing pure oxygen following global brain ischemia.[51] Further, the lack of correlation of infarction with lipid peroxidation suggests that irreversible tissue damage precedes lipid peroxidation and may well facilitate it, rather than vice versa.[1,3,42]

In recent work the emphasis has shifted from detection of lipid peroxidation to assessments of the participation of oxygen radical cascade components in the expression of CNS injury. Tissue edema and TBA reactants were produced in rat brain slices by the addition of polyunsaturated fatty acids; these effects were accompanied by superoxide anion production and were eliminated by the addition of superoxide dismutase.[52] Subsequent application of a hydroxyl radical–generating system (xanthine or hypoxanthine reacting with xanthine oxidase and chelated ferric ion) to rat brain preparations *in vitro* facilitated release of free fatty acids, tissue swelling, degradation of membrane phospholipids, and production of TBA reactants.[53] *In vivo,* infusion of a mixture of hydroxyl radical–generating components into rat brain induced blood-brain barrier breakdown leading to edema and neuronal death.[54] Finally, permanent middle cerebral artery occlusion in the rat precipitated superoxide anion production, which increased in time and was mitigated by topical superoxide dismutase (SOD); further, liposome-entrapped SOD injected intravenously just after occlusion attenuated the severity of edema observed 24 hr after the ictus.[55] These results may have as a common basis the accelerated operation (owing to an excess of substrate fatty acid) of the hydroperoxidase component of the cyclooxygenase or lipoxygenase pathways.[38]

It is tacitly assumed in these studies that the bulk of tissue damage is initiated by hydroxyl radical or lipid alkoxyl radicals, following their production by Fenton chemistry: ferrous ion interacting with hydrogen peroxide or with lipid hydroperoxides, respectively. Accordingly, the ferric iron chelator deferoxamine has been utilized frequently to inhibit the production of ferrous ion during superoxide-driven biochemical damage. Administration of deferoxamine and superoxide dismutase facilitated partial recovery of somatosensory evoked potentials (SEP) and normalization of cerebral blood flow profiles in dogs resuscitated for 1 hr following 7-min ischemia induced by cardiac arrest.[56] Similarly, the brains of dogs subjected to 15-min cardiac arrest followed by 2 hr of resuscitation accumulated thiobarbituric acid reactants; this accumulation was mitigated by deferoxamine administration.[57] In addition to their likely involvement in stroke and in CNS trauma, iron-catalyzed degradation reactions are thus conjectured to contribute to the high incidence of central nervous system injury observed following resuscitation.[58] New agents exhibiting less systemic toxicity and enhanced potency compared to deferoxamine are being developed. Members of the 21-aminosteroid series are believed to inhibit iron-dependent lipid peroxidation by several mechanisms, including chelation, and have been recently found to reverse the severity of postischemic blood flow decreases in the cat spinal cord following contusion injury.[59]

Direct scavenging or suppression of oxygen radicals per se in models of reversible cerebral ischemia has been widely employed in studies of reperfusion injury, as shown in the following descriptions. Administration of liposome-entrapped superoxide dismutase reduced the magnitude of brain edema[60] in rats subjected to 2-hr MCA occlusion and 2 hr of recirculation. The dilation of cat cerebral arterioles induced by 1 hr of recirculation following 15-min cerebral ischemia was associated with superoxide anion production, and was mitigated by topical SOD and catalase or deferoxamine.[61] In rats subjected to 90 min of focal ischemia by ligation of the MCA and both common carotid arteries (CCA), a 30% reduction in infarct volume was observed as a result of pretreatment with PEG (polyethylene glycol)-conjugated SOD and PEG-catalase.[62] After 3 hr of recirculation, the conversion of xanthine dehydrogenase to the oxidase form was confirmed as well. In other work, the hydrogen peroxide content and the extent of edema in the brains of gerbils subjected 3- or 6-hour unilateral carotid artery ligation followed by 3 hr of reperfusion were inversely related to the amount of dietary tungstate administered over several weeks;[63] tungstate inactivates xanthine oxidase and thereby suppresses postischemic superoxide production. Similar results were obtained following administration of dimethylthiourea (a hydroxyl radical scavenger) just before reperfusion.[63] The extent of edema development, sodium influx, and potassium efflux seen at 1 hr of recirculation in spontaneously hypertensive rats with 4-hr bilateral CCA ligation were mitigated in animals pretreated with the xanthine oxidase inhibitor allopurinol.[64] In cats in which 30-min MCA ligation was followed by 15 to 120 min of recirculation,[65] SOD improved cerebral blood flow (CBF) and SEP response. In addition, *in vivo* evidence for an ischemia/oxygen radical/neutrophil interrelationship has been presented; following 1-hr internal carotid artery occlusion in dogs,[66] cerebral granulocyte clusters were seen at 1 and 4 hr afterward. Also, in rats subjected to 15-min bilateral CCA occlusion and 1 hr of recirculation,[67] neutrophil depletion by antiserum injection decreased the magnitude of postischemic hypoperfusion.

VASCULAR DAMAGE INCITED BY REACTIONS INVOLVING PHOTOCHEMICALLY MEDIATED ACTIVE OXYGEN SPECIES

In the previous sections the contribution of oxygen radical–mediated intravascular damage was addressed in terms of neutrophil responses to ischemia per se. Recently, studies of such intravascular effects have been broadened to include the responses of other blood elements such as platelets and erythrocytes, in consideration of their involvement in stroke. Although stroke and cardiac arrest are certainly the leading instigators of cerebral ischemia, the participation of oxygen radicals or lipid peroxidation in the pathogenesis and development of stroke (in contrast to cerebral ischemia) has been studied infrequently, owing mainly to difficulties with experimental models. For example, embolic stroke initiated by intracarotid injection of homologous blood clots is liable to induce ischemia at foci that are variable in location and volume. In large infarcts that could be located and analyzed following regional ischemia induced by intracarotid injection of microspheres, lipid peroxides expressed as conjugated dienes were observed at 4 and 24 hours after the ictus—that is, after the onset of necrosis.[68] It is thus unlikely, either by product measurements or by application of radical scavengers, that radical processes could be implicated convincingly in the *acute* development of the resultant embolus-induced infarcts.

In an effort to determine the participation of oxygen-centered radicals in the context of reproducible experimental stroke, we invented several models of thrombotic stroke in which cerebrovascular thrombosis is produced by a photochemical reaction initiated by intravenously injected rose bengal, a potent photosensitizing dye. Initially this technique involved irradiation with 560-nm light (filtered xenon arc) of the exposed, but intact, translucent calvarium of rose bengal–injected rats; occlusion of the underlying microvasculature results in a reproducible cortical infarct.[69] Subsequently, we were able to obtain middle cerebral artery–territory strokes in rose bengal–injected rats following MCA occlusion; the MCA is photothrombosed by irradiation for several minutes with either a 514.5-nm argon laser[70] or a 543.5-nm He-Ne laser.[71] In this approach, the stimuli to clot formation likely include physical damage to the endothelial luminal surface, observable in the form of membrane discontinuities and focal defects.[69,72,73] Inasmuch as the sole photoreaction product, singlet molecular oxygen, is known to peroxidize unsaturated fatty acids[74,75] and proteins[76] directly, the likely mechanism of endothelial injury is direct peroxidation of these luminal membrane constituents.[77] Chain peroxidative processes will not be activated initially by this mechanism, because singlet oxygen is *not* a free radical and thus cannot be a chain initiator.

Despite the apparently artificial nature of membrane photochemical injury platelet adhesion, degranulation and aggregation are all expressed physiologically to the point of vascular occlusion. Both the microvascular[69,72,73] and MCA thrombi[70,71] appear ultrastructurally to be tightly packed networks consisting almost entirely of platelets, with very little intercalated fibrin. Fluorescent antibody analysis for Factor VIII and fibrinogen in MCA thrombi showed that these alpha-granule components stained very brightly compared to blood clotted in air (unpublished observations). This suggests that platelet agglutination is mediated by fibrinogen linkages between glycoprotein (GP) IIb/IIIa receptor molecules on different platelets.[78] The GP receptor–linked thrombus is likely to be clinically significant, because it was shown recently in dogs to be responsible for inducing reocclusion in previously thrombosed coronary arteries recanalized with tissue plasminogen activator.[79]

As observed through an operating microscope during laser irradiation of the MCA,[70,71] vasoconstriction is the immediate consequence of rose bengal–mediated, singlet oxygen–induced endothelial peroxidation. Vasoconstriction in conjunction with platelet deposition has also been observed in cerebral arterioles following arc-lamp irradiation of rose bengal–injected rats,[73] and in corneal new vessels of rabbits treated with rose bengal and 514.5-nm argon irradiation.[80,81] The enhancement of vasoconstriction throughout irradiation may be due to platelet-derived thromboxane and serotonin, and to the destruction of prostacyclin synthase by fatty acids peroxidized by singlet oxygen.[69] Consistent with these reports, vascular smooth muscle cells also constrict under singlet oxygen attack mediated by erythrosin B or rose bengal.[82] The contractile response was attributed to Ca^{2+} influx through the acutely photodamaged muscle membrane. The fast rate of response noted is in agreement with our observations on irradiated arteries.

On the other hand, MCA vasodilation is observed during irradiation with an argon laser operating at 488 nm in conjunction with intravenous flavin mononucleotide (FMN) utilized as a photostimulator of free radical chain processes (unpublished observations). An unstable red clot forms slowly in the dilating vessel, with little visual evidence of gross platelet accumulation; increasing the irradiation intensity to facilitate occlusion results in a white (platelet) clot forming just distally in a region of relative vessel constriction. The red portion responded negatively to fluorescent antibody analysis for Factor VIII and fibrinogen, indicating consumption of these components during coagulation cascade activation.

The fact that vasoconstriction or vasodilation can be induced, respectively, by singlet oxygen attack (Type II photochemistry[83]) or by free radical chain reactions (Type I photochemistry[83]) may yield mechanistic information relevant to cerebral vascular diseases. Originating from endothelial-bound rose bengal, singlet oxygen directly peroxidizes membrane lipids and proteins *in situ* consistent with its very short half-life (less than 2 μsec). Both conjugated and nonconjugated diene hydroperoxides of unsaturated fatty acids are formed.[74,75] In contrast, photoexcited FMN triplet states can abstract hydrogen atoms from endothelial lipids: either directly, leading to photoreduction of the triplet state; or indirectly, in which the photoreduced FMN triplet state interacts with molecular oxygen to produce superoxide anion. Thus, the latter pathway can initiate an oxygen radical cascade, although singlet oxygen may be produced, depending on solution conditions.[74] Consequently, hydroxyl radical produced by the Fenton reaction (reduction of hydrogen peroxide) at iron binding sites can then initiate endothelial damage by hydrogen atom abstraction, resulting in more lipid autoxidation. Either autoxidation pathway yields only conjugated diene hydroperoxides, and enables molecular damage to continue to be propagated in space via diffusible (oxygen radical) species or migrating (autoxidative) processes. Inasmuch as the fraction of nonconjugated dienes resulting from Type II photooxidation is only about 10% of the total diene amount,[84] the differences in vascular response between Type I and Type II photoreactions are likely not explained by the presence of these isomeric forms.

Several consequences result from the Type I and Type II schemes. The highly localized singlet oxygen reactions result in intensely expressed, overt structural damage to the endothelium, which damage is unlikely to be mitigated acutely by any naturally occurring scavenger compound or by attempts by the cell at repair. In contrast, the oxygen radical cascade through its diffusible components superoxide anion and hydrogen peroxide is capable of spreading damage far beyond its points of origin, but at the price of dilution and quenching by membrane-bound tocopherols. Thus, endothelial damage per unit area per membrane-bound photosensitizer molecule is likely to be much less for Type I sensitizers compared to those of Type II, and is further lessened by concomitant vasodilation.

RELATIONSHIP OF PHOTOCHEMICAL MECHANISMS TO OXYGEN RADICAL–MEDIATED RESPONSES *IN VIVO*

These mechanisms may be applied to explain the effects of certain clinically relevant states on cerebral tissue. To illustrate, the vasoconstrictive response of cerebral vessels to subarachnoid hemorrhage (SAH) or hemorrhagic trauma may be understood by analogy to the photochemical scheme of Type II. In cats, experimental SAH induced by injection of blood clotted *in situ* resulted in basilar artery constriction, and was associated with severe damage to smooth muscle cells and endothelium.[85] For expression of these effects, erythrocytes were necessary and sufficient. Similar evidence of vascular damage, and platelet deposition as well, was presented in another cat model of SAH induced by MCA rupture,[86] and during incubation *in vivo* of canine basilar artery with 15-hydroperoxy arachidonic acid (15-HPAA).[87] It is plausible that the experimental SAH results, including continuation of constriction over time, might originate from site-specific reactions and focal lipid peroxidation derived from local concentrations of reactive iron from hemoglobin released during clot degeneration. Vessel contraction elicited and sustained by topical 15-HPAA is dose-dependent,[87] suggesting that sufficiently intense site-specific production of fatty acid hydroperoxides will induce the same responses. These vascular changes, which resemble those seen during direct focal peroxidation by singlet oxygen, are related mechanistically inasmuch as the damaging reactions originate from relatively fixed sites. This analogy is supported by observations of erythrocyte deposition[85] in adventitia during SAH, thus potentiating microfocal expression of iron-catalyzed Fenton reactions.

On the other hand, recent work establishing that dispersible components of the oxygen radical cascade act as facilitators of vasodilation is consistent with the vascular effects of Type I photochemistry. Dilation of pial vasculature in cats has been observed following topical application of prostaglandin synthase substrates such as arachidonic acid (processed by the cyclooxygenase function) and 15-hydroperoxy arachidonic acid or prostaglandin G_2 (processed by the hydroperoxidase form).[32] Activation of the hydroperoxidase form stimulates superoxide anion production through a side reaction in which molecular oxygen is reduced by nucleotide radicals.[38] Topical superperfusion with the superoxide-generating combination of xanthine and xanthine oxidase, or the hydroxyl radical–generating combination of ferrous iron and hydrogen peroxide, engenders pial vasodilation.[33] Vasodilation and/or accompanying morphological signs of tissue damage (e.g., endothelial vacuolation), can be prevented by administration of quenching agents—such as deferoxamine[34] (to chelate free iron), superoxide dismutase and/or catalase,[32,33] and mannitol[33] (hydroxyl scavenger)—or inhibitors of the anion channel[16] (to prevent superoxide anion diffusion). These observations suggest that the ultimate mediator of oxygen radical cascade–induced vasodilation is the hydroxyl radical. Vascular damage elicited in this fashion by topical excitation of the oxygen radical cascade is not accompanied by platelet aggregation, however.

Vasodilation and many of the accompanying morphological changes in endothelium described above have been observed following pial vascular injury mediated photochemically in cats by sodium fluorescein.[88] (Vasodilation is not observed in mice, however.) An important difference is that platelet aggregation occurs routinely in this system, following the development of similar mild endothelial defects in the absence of denudation. The concomitance of platelet deposition in the presence of vasodilation indicates that both singlet oxygen and superoxide anion are produced during fluorescein activation. Because both oxygen species result from direct interaction of molecular oxygen with the photoexcited dye triplet state, fluorescein by definition is a Type II photosensitizer even though the superoxide-producing mode elicits Type I effects on vasculature. In support of this dual mechanism is the fact that the effects of intravascular fluorescein photoreactions can be mitigated by scavengers of either singlet oxygen[89] or superoxide anion.[90]

Further, relaxation of vascular tissue apparently can occur via activation, by hydrogen peroxide[91] or fatty acid hydroperoxides,[92] of soluble guanylate cyclase in smooth muscle. This mode of vasodilation is expressed without affecting the relaxant response to acetylcholine; damage to endothelial function induced by superoxide anion or hydroxyl radical is not present. In contrast, endothelial damage due to oxygen radical attack can be revealed operationally if the vasodilator effect of acetylcholine is converted to vasoconstriction. This damage may be mediated either by direct destruction of endothelial-derived relaxing factor (EDRF), or by inactivation of EDRF release. In the first case, the vasoconstrictor effect of acetylcholine on pial vessels can be reversed by oxygen radical scavengers following induction of relatively mild endothelial damage by fluorescein photochemistry, or following trauma induced by fluid-percussion injury or acute hypertension.[34] In the second case, endothelial damage is mediated by the hydroxyl radical following topical application of arachidonate. The resultant vasoconstrictor response to acetylcholine is not reversed by oxygen radical scavengers, suggesting that the severity of endothelial damage is sufficient to inhibit EDRF release.[34] The clinical development of SAH may be related significantly to these results. For example, topical administration of oxy(ferrous)hemoglobin, or of cerebrospinal fluid from patients with SAH, to the canine basilar artery destroys the EDRF-mediated response to dilation by the calcium ionophore A23187.[93]

Although to this point the induction of vascular phenomena has been discussed in terms of two distinct pathways of active oxygen chemistry, both features can occur in complementary fashion in the same system while separated in time or space, or the expression of one feature can be mimicked by the other. For example, the cortical infarct that develops following singlet oxygen–mediated (Type II) cerebral photothrombosis is surrounded by a progressively expanding border, owing to blood-brain barrier breakdown and vasogenic edema;[94,95] the extent of peripheral expansion is diminished by preadministration of superoxide dismutase (unpublished observations). Another example is the vasoconstrictor effect stimulated by erythrocyte[85] or oxyhemoglobin[93] deposition in vessel walls. Although mediated by hydrogen peroxide decomposition by ferrous iron—a process normally considered to be in the domain of diffusible lipid peroxidation chains—the intensity and focality of vascular damage following hydroxyl radical attack is comparable to that displayed by photosensitized singlet oxygen attack (as described previously).

Complementarity is also expressed in other ways: while superoxide anion activates platelets to aggregate and release their granules,[96] the endothelium in the presence of superoxide-induced vasodilation does not become thrombogenic. On the other hand, singlet oxygen attack renders the endothelium thrombogenic, but inhibits platelet degranulation and aggregation.[97] Evidently the platelets incorporated into a singlet oxygen–mediated thrombus have responded positively to the photodamaged endothelium much before the onset of photochemical inactivation. Inasmuch as fundamental responses of platelets and endothelium can be controlled by a given activated oxygen pathway, which in turn can be stimulated selectively by a simple photochemical mechanism, we anticipate further progress in understanding cerebral vascular responses to injury mediated by processes involving the oxygen radical cascade.

In view of the contribution of intravascular processes to the generation of oxygen radicals, an unresolved question remains: whether there is any significant parenchymal contribution to reperfusion-induced brain injury either due to oxygen radicals themselves, or to reactions initiated by them leading to lipid peroxidation. This question is important inasmuch as organic antioxidants or enzymes included in the reperfusate are not likely to gain uniform access to all ischemic zones.[18] Determination of the relative contributions of these scenarios requires a technique that can detect the earliest appearance of oxygen radicals and their reaction products in ischemic or reperfused tissue. With such a test, the association of morphologic signs of preischemic and postischemic brain damage might be correlated with oxygen radical–induced events and, possibly, early lipid peroxidation. Finally, the question of the development in time of oxygen radical–induced molecular injury or of lipid autoxidation, its microscopic heterogeneity or homogeneity, and its location vis-à-vis the vascular or parenchymal space may finally be addressed and perhaps resolved.

ACKNOWLEDGMENTS

We thank our colleagues S. Yoshida, W. D. Dietrich, R. Prado, and R. Busto for their research collaborations in the Cerebral Vascular Disease Research Center.

REFERENCES

1. SLATER, T. F. 1984. Biochem. J. **222:** 1–15.
2. HALLIWELL, B. & J. M. C. GUTTERIDGE. 1986. Arch. Biochem. Biophys. **246:** 501–514.
3. HALLIWELL, B. & J. M. C. GUTTERIDGE. 1984. Biochem. J. **219:** 1–14.
4. LIVESEY, J. C. & D. J. REED. 1987. Adv. Rad. Biol. **13:** 285–353.
5. SIESJO, B. K. 1981. J. Cerebr. Blood Flow Metabol. **1:** 155–185.
6. HALLIWELL, B. & J. M. C. GUTTERIDGE. 1985. TINS **8:** 22–26.
7. FREEMAN, B. A. & J. D. CRAPO. 1982. Circ. Res. **47:** 412–425.
8. FRIDOVICH, I. 1978. Science **201:** 875–880.
9. THOMAS, C. E., L. A. MOREHOUSE & S. J. AUST. 1985. J. Biol. Chem. **260:** 3275–3280.
10. GUTTERIDGE, J. M. C. 1988. In Oxygen Radicals and Tissue Injury Symposium (Proceedings). B. Halliwell, Ed.: 9–19. Federation of American Society for Experimental Biology. Bethesda, MD.
11. BIELSKI, B. H. J., R. L. ARUDI & M. W. SUTHERLAND. 1983. J. Biol. Chem. **258:** 4759–4761.
12. HASEGAWA, K. & L. K. PATTERSON. 1978. Photochem. Photobiol. **28:** 817–823.
13. TAPPEL, A. L. 1973. Federation Proc. **32:** 1870–1874.
14. SEVANIAN, A. & P. HOCHSTEIN. 1985. Ann. Rev. Nutr. **5:** 365–390.
15. SMALL, R. D., JR., J. C. SCAIANO & L. K. PATTERSON. 1979. Photochem. Photobiol. **29:** 49–51.
16. KONTOS, H. A., E. P. WEI, L. W. JENKINS, J. T. POVLISHOCK, G. T. ROWE & M. L. HESS. 1985. Circ. Res. **57:** 142–151.
17. TAPPEL, A. L. 1980. In Free Radicals in Biology, Vol. 4. W. A. Pryor, Ed.: 1–47. Academic Press. New York, NY.
18. KONTOS, H. A. 1988. Possible roles of superoxide anion in cerebrovascular pathology. In Cerebrovascular Diseases, Vol. 16. M. D. Ginsberg & W. D. Dietrich, Eds. Raven Press. New York, NY. In press.
19. NORONHA-DUTRA, A. A. & E. M. STEEN. 1982. Lab. Invest. **47:** 346–353.
20. DIETRICH, W. D., B. D. WATSON, R. BUSTO, M. D. GINSBERG & J. R. BETHEA. 1987. Acta Neuropath. **72:** 315–325.
21. YAGI, K., H. OHKAWA, N. OHISHI, M. YAMASHITA & T. NAKASHIMA. 1981. J. Appl. Biochem. **3:** 58–65.
22. ANDERSON, W. R., W. C. TAN, T. TAKATORI & O. S. PRIVETT. 1976. Arch. Path. Lab. Med. **100:** 154–162.
23. PASQUALI-RONCHETTI, I., A. BINI, B. BOTTI, G. DE ALOJSIO, C. FORNIERI & V. VANNINI. 1980. Lab. Invest. **42:** 457–468.
24. WATSON, B. D. & M. D. GINSBERG. 1988. In Oxygen Radicals and Tissue Injury Symposium (Proceedings). B. Halliwell, Ed.: 81–91. Federation of American Society for Experimental Biology. Bethesda, MD.
25. POMPELLA, A., E. MAELLARO, A. F. CASINI & M. COMPORTI. 1987. Am. J. Pathol. **129:** 295–301.
26. LEVY, K. & K.-E. ARFORS. 1982. Microvasc. Res. **24:** 25–33.
27. BURTON, K. P., J. M. MCCORD & G. GHAI. 1984. Am. J. Physiol. **246:** H776–H783.
28. THAW, H. H., H. HAMBERG & U. T. BRUNK. 1983. Eur. J. Cell. Biol. **31:** 46–54.
29. HALLIWELL, B. & J. M. C. GUTTERIDGE. 1984. Lancet **i:** 1396–1397.

30. YOUNG, J. D.-E. & Z. A. COHN. 1988. Sci. Am. **258:** 38–44.
31. CHEUNG, J. Y., J. V. BONVENTRE, C. D. MALIS & A. LEAF. 1986. New Engl. J. Med. **314:** 1670–1676.
32. KONTOS, H. A. 1985. Circ. Res. **57:** 508–516.
33. KONTOS, H. A. & M. L. HESS. 1983. Adv. Exp. Med. Biol. **161:** 365–375.
34. KONTOS, H. A., E. P. WEI, J. T. POVLISHOCK, R. C. KUKREJA & M. L. HESS. Am. J. Physiol. In press.
35. ZWEIER, J. L., P. KUPPUSAMY & G. A. LUTTY. 1988. Proc. Natl. Acad. Sci. USA **85:** 4046–4050.
36. BETZ, A. L. 1985. J. Neurochem. **44:** 574–579.
37. MCCORD, J. M. 1987. Federation Proc. **46:** 2402–2406.
38. KUKREJA, R. C., H. A. KONTOS, M. H. HESS & E. F. ELLIS. 1986. Circ. Res. **59:** 612–619.
39. TURRENS, J. F., A. ALEXANDRE & A. L. LEHNINGER. 1985. Arch. Biochem. Biophys. **237:** 408–414.
40. CLIFFORD, D. E. & J. E. REPINE. 1982. Mol. Cell. Biochem. **49:** 143–149.
41. SCHRAUFSTATTER, I. U., D. B. HINSHAW, P. A. HYSLOP, R. G. SPRAGG & C. G. COCHRANE. 1986. J. Clin. Invest. **77:** 1312–1320.
42. HALLIWELL, B. 1987. FASEB J. **1:** 358–364.
43. SAEZ, J. C., J. A. KESSLER, M. V. L. BENNETT & D. C. SPRAY. 1987. Proc. Natl. Acad. Sci. **84:** 3056–3059.
44. WHITE, B. C., J. G. WIEGENSTEIN & C. D. WINEGAR. 1984. J. Am. Med. Assoc. **251:** 1586–1590.
45. REHNCRONA, S., E. WESTERBERG, B. AKESSON & B. K. SIESJO. 1980. J. Neurochem. **34:** 477–486.
46. COOPER, A. J. L., W. A. PULSINELLI & T. E. DUFFY. 1980. J. Neurochem. **35:** 1242–1245.
47. MACMILLAN, V. 1982. J. Cerebr. Blood Flow Metabol. **2:** 457–465.
48. REHNCRONA, S., E. WESTERBERG, B. AKESSON & B. K. SIESJO. 1982. J. Neurochem. **38:** 84–93.
49. WATSON, B. D., R. BUSTO, W. J. GOLDBERG, M. SANTISO, S. YOSHIDA & M. D. GINSBERG. 1984. J Neurochem. **42:** 268–274.
50. WATSON, B. D., R. PRADO, H. NAKAYAMA, R. BUSTO, M. SANTISO & M. D. GINSBERG. 1987. J. Cerebr. Blood Flow Metabol. **7:** S11.
51. MICKEL, H. S., Y. S. VAISHNAV, O. KEMPSKI, D. VON LUBITZ, J. F. WIESS & G. FEUERSTEIN. 1987. Stroke **18:** 426–430.
52. CHAN, P. H. & R. A. FISHMAN. 1980. J. Neurochem. **35:** 1004–1007.
53. CHAN, P. H., M. YURKO & R. A. FISHMAN. 1982. J. Neurochem. **38:** 525–531.
54. CHAN, P. H., J. W. SCHMIDLEY, R. A. FISHMAN & S. M. LONGAR. 1984. Neurology **34:** 315–320.
55. CHAN, P. H., R. A. FISHMAN, M. A. WESLEY & S. LONGAR. 1988. In Proceedings of the 6th International Symposium on Brain Edema. In press.
56. CERCHIARI, E. L., T. M. HOEL, P. SAFAR & R. J. SCLABASSI. 1987. Stroke **18:** 869–878.
57. KOMARA, J. S., N. R. NAYINI, H. A. BIALICK, R. J. INDRIERI, A. T. EVANS, A. M. GARRITANO, T. J. HOEHNER, W. A. JACOBS, R. R. HUANG, G. S. KRAUSE, B. C. WHITE, S. A. AUST. 1986. Ann. Emerg. Med. **15:** 384–389.
58. BABBS, C. F. 1985. Ann. Emerg. Med. **14:** 777–783.
59. HALL, E. D. 1988. J. Neurosurg. **68:** 462–465.
60. PEREIRA, B. M., P. H. CHAN, P. R. WEINSTEIN & R. A. FISHMAN. 1988. In Proceedings of the 6th International Conference on Brain Ischemia. In press.
61. WEI, E. & H. A. KONTOS. 1987. Physiologist **30:** 122.
62. BECKMAN, J. S., T. H. LIU, E. L. HOGAN, B. A. FREEMAN & C. Y. HSU. 1987. Soc. Neurosci. Abst. **13**(Part 3): 1498.
63. PATT, A., A. H. HARKEN, L. K. BURTON, T. C. RODELL, D. PIERMATTEI, W. J. SCHORR, N. B. PARKER, E. M. BERGER, I. R. HORESH, L. S. TERADA, S. L. LINAS, J. C. CHERONIS & J. E. REPINE. 1988. J. Clin. Invest. **81:** 1556–1562.
64. ITOH, T., M. KAWAKAMI, Y. YAMAUCHI, S. SHIMIZU & M. NAKAMURA. 1986. Stroke **17:** 1284–1287.
65. DAVIS, R. J., G. B. BULKLEY & R. J. TRAYSTMAN. 1987. J. Cerebr. Blood Flow Metabol. **7:** S10.

66. HALLENBECK, J. M., A. J. DUTKA, T. TANISHIMA, P. M. KOCHANEK, K. K. KUMAROO, C. B. THOMPSON, T. P. OBRENOVITCH & T. J. CONTRERAS. 1986. Stroke **17:** 246–253.
67. SCHURER, L., B. GROGAARD, B. GERDIN, K.-E. ARFORS & A. BAETHMANN. 1987. J. Cerebr. Blood Flow Metabol. 7(Suppl 1): S72.
68. KOGURE, K., B. D. WATSON, R. BUSTO & K. ABE. 1982. Neurochem. Res. **7:** 437–454.
69. WATSON, B. D., W. D. DIETRICH, R. BUSTO, M. S. WACHTEL & M. D. GINSBERG. 1985. Ann. Neurol. **17:** 497–504.
70. WATSON, B. D., R. PRADO, W. D. DIETRICH, R. BUSTO, P. SCHEINBERG & M. D. GINSBERG. 1987. *In* Cerebrovascular Diseases, Vol. 15. M. E. Raichle & W. J. Powers, Eds.: 317–330. Raven Press. New York, NY.
71. NAKAYAMA, H., W. D. DIETRICH, B. D. WATSON, R. BUSTO & M. D. GINSBERG. 1988. J. Cerebr. Blood Flow Metabol. **8:** 357–366.
72. DIETRICH, W. D., M. D. GINSBERG, R. BUSTO, B. D. WATSON & S. YOSHIDA. 1986. Central Nervous System Trauma **3:** 265–280.
73. DIETRICH, W. D., B. D. WATSON, R. BUSTO, J. R. BETHEA, P. SCHEINBERG & M. D. GINSBERG. 1987. Acta Neuropath. (Berl.) **72:** 315–325.
74. CHACON, J. N., J. MCLEARIE & R. S. SINCLAIR. 1988. Photochem. Photobiol. **47:** 647–656.
75. CHAN, H. W.-S. 1977. J. Am. Oil Chem. Soc. **54:** 100–104.
76. SPIKES, J. D. & R. LIVINGSTON. 1969. Adv. Rad. Biol. **3:** 29–121.
77. VALENZENO, D. P. 1987. Photochem. Photobiol. **46:** 147–160.
78. LEUNG, L. & R. NACHMANN. 1986. Ann. Rev. Med. **37:** 179–186.
79. YASUDA, T., H. K. GOLD, J. T. FALLON, R. C. LEINBACH, J. L. GUERRERO, L. E. SCUDDER, M. KANKE, D. SHEALY, M. J. ROSS, D. COLLEN & B. S. COLLER. 1988. J. Clin. Invest. **81:** 1284–1291.
80. HUANG, A. J.-W., B. D. WATSON, E. HERNANDEZ & S. C.-G. TSENG. 1988. Ophthalmol. **95:** 228–235.
81. HUANG, A. J.-W., B. D. WATSON, E. HERNANDEZ & S. C.-G. TSENG. 1988. Arch. Opthalmol. **106:** 680–685.
82. MATHEWS, E. K. & D. E. MESLER. 1984. Br. J. Pharmacol. **83:** 555–566.
83. FOOTE, C. S. 1976. *In* Free Radicals in Biology, Vol. 2. W. A. Pryor, Ed.: 85–134. Academic Press. New York, NY.
84. TERAO, J. & S. MATSUSHITA. 1981. Agric. Biol. Chem. **45:** 595–599.
85. DUFF, T. A., J. LOUIE, J. A. FEILBACH & G. SCOTT. 1988. Stroke **19:** 68–72.
86. HAINING, J. L., B. R. CLOWER, Y. HONMA & R. R. SMITH. 1988. Stroke **19:** 898–902.
87. SASAKI, T., S. WAKAI, T. ASANO, T. WATANABE, T. KIRINO & K. SANO. 1981. J. Neurosurg. **54:** 357–365.
88. ROSENBLUM, W. I. 1986. Lab. Invest. **55:** 252–268.
89. HERMANN, K. S. 1983. Microvasc. Res. **26:** 238–249.
90. BEAUCHAMP, C. & I. FRIDOVICH. 1971. Analyt. Biochem. **44:** 276–287.
91. BURKE, T. M. & M. S. WOLIN. 1987. Am. J. Physiol. **252:** H721–732.
92. THOMAS, G. & P. RAMWELL. 1986. Biophys. Biochem. Res. Commun. **139:** 102–108.
93. KANAMARU, K., S. WAGA, T. KOJIMA, K. FUJIMOTO & S. NIWA. 1987. Stroke **18:** 938–943.
94. DIETRICH, W. D., B. D. WATSON, R. BUSTO, J. R. BETHEA, P. SCHEINBERG & M. D. GINSBERG. 1987. Acta Neuropathol. (Berl.) **72:** 326–334.
95. GROME, J. J., G. GOJOWCZYK, W. HOFMANN & D. I. GRAHAM. 1988. J. Cerebr. Blood Flow Metabol. **8:** 89–95.
96. HANDIN, R. I., R. KARABIN & G. J. BOXER. 1977. J. Clin. Invest. **59:** 959–965.
97. ZIEVE, P. D., H. M. SOLOMON & J. R. KREVANS. 1966. J. Cell Physiol. **67:** 271–280.

Arachidonic Acid and Its Metabolites in Cerebral Ischemia[a]

C. Y. HSU,[b] T. H. LIU,[b] J. XU,[b] E. L. HOGAN,[b]
J. CHAO,[b] G. SUN,[c] H. H. TAI,[d] J. S. BECKMAN[e]
AND B. A. FREEMAN[e]

[b]*Departments of Neurology and Pharmacology*
Medical University of South Carolina
Charleston, South Carolina 29425

[c]*Sinclair Research Farm and Department of Biochemistry*
University of Missouri
Columbia, Missouri 65203

[d]*College of Pharmacy*
University of Kentucky
Lexington, Kentucky 40536

[e]*Departments of Anesthesiology and Biochemistry*
University of Alabama Medical Center
Birmingham, Alabama 35233

INTRODUCTION

Among the therapeutic agents currently employed in the medical management of cerebral ischemia, only aspirin, an antiplatelet agent and an irreversible inhibitor of cyclooxygenase, has been proven in rigorous clinical trials to show a moderate efficacy in reducing stroke and death in patients with transient ischemic attacks (TIA).[1-2] The rationale for using antiplatelet agents in the prevention and treatment of cerebral ischemia is based on the recognition that platelets are involved in the development of atherosclerosis, the formation of thrombi on atherosclerotic plaques, and the pathogenesis of postischemic microvascular injury.[3] The possibility of pharmacological modification of platelet function in cerebral ischemia has been enhanced by new insights into the biochemical regulation of blood cell–vessel wall interactions, particularly those involving arachidonic acid (AA) metabolism. This paper will begin with a brief review of the formation of AA metabolites in cerebral ischemia. This will be followed by a summary of recent experimental findings from our laboratories concerning AA metabolism in relation to postischemic vascular changes and the effects of therapeutic intervention directed at AA metabolism.

ARACHIDONIC ACID METABOLITES IN CEREBRAL ISCHEMIA

In cerebral ischemia, AA metabolites may contribute to postischemic hypoperfusion, brain edema, and irreversible neuronal damage. Ischemia triggers an initial rise

---

[a]This work was supported by grants from the National Institutes of Health (NS-25545, 11066, 00792, 23700, 24275, 24338, and HL-29397), the American Cancer Society (BD556), and AHA South Carolina and Alabama Affiliates.

in intracellular calcium ions leading to activation of phospholipases, phospholipid breakdown, and release of fatty acids, including AA,[4] which is rapidly converted to prostaglandins (PGs), thromboxane (TX) A_2, and leukotrienes (LTs).[5-7]

Several reactions catalyze the conversion of AA to active metabolites. AA is metabolized to the labile endoperoxides PGG_2 and PGH_2 by fatty acid cyclooxygenase (prostaglandin endoperoxide synthase). Free oxygen radicals are generated in the conversion of PGG_2 to PGH_2, which is the precursor of PGD_2, PGE_2, PGF_2, PGI_2, and TXA_2 (FIG. 1).

With the notable exception of PGI_2, the formation of AA metabolites such as PGD_2, PGE_2, PGF_2, PGH_2, TXA_2, and leukotrienes may interfere with brain perfu

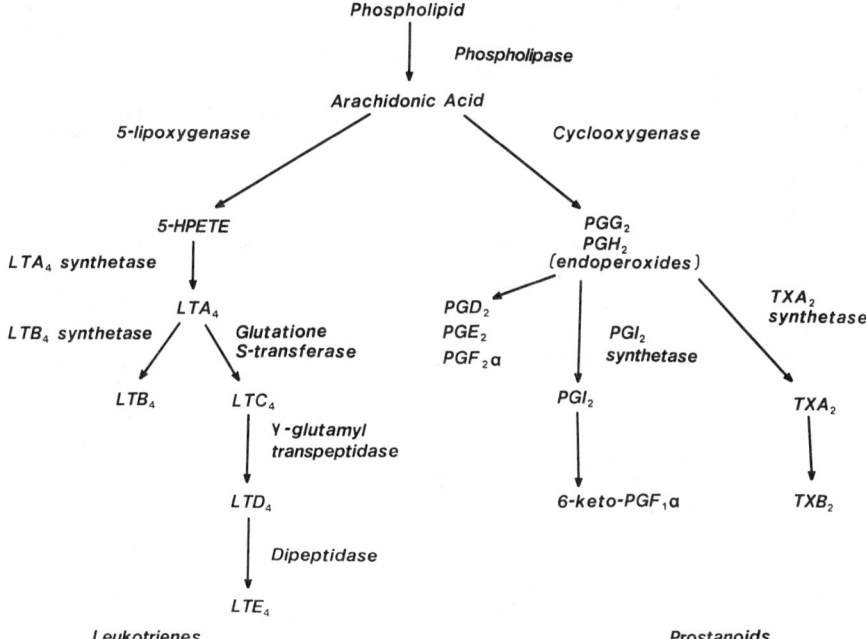

FIGURE 1. Biosynthetic pathways of thromboxane (TX), prostaglandins (PG), and leukotrienes (LT).

sion.[5,8] Of the vasoactive prostanoids, TXA_2 and PGI_2 are two of the most potent. They appear to affect hemostasis and vascular integrity in different diseases by modifying platelet–vessel wall interactions.[5,9] TXA_2 stimulates platelet aggregation and vasoconstriction. PGI_2, on the other hand, inhibits platelet aggregation and causes vasodilation. Although the pathophysiology of cerebral ischemia has not been fully elucidated, one intriguing hypothesis is that TXA_2-PGI_2 imbalance causes platelet activation and microcirculatory stasis that culminates in the "no reflow phenomenon."[10-13]

Lipoxygenase acts on AA to form hydroperoxy derivatives with concomitant generation of oxygen free radicals. Of the several known lipoxygenases, 5-lipoxygenase seems most important, converting AA to 5-hydroperoxyeicosatetraenoic acid (5-HPETE) and its metabolites, the LTs. The conversion of 5-HPETE to LTA_4 is catalyzed by LTA_4 synthase. LTA_4 reacts with water to form LTB_4 and is converted to LTC_4 by glutathione S-transferase. The subsequent formation of LTD_4 and LTE_4 is catalyzed by τ-glutamyl transpeptidase and a dipeptidase respectively (FIG. 1).[5,6]

The slow-reacting substances of anaphylaxis released during immune and allergic reactions are a mixture of LTC_4, LTD_4, and LTE_4. They stimulate contraction of smooth muscle and alter vascular permeability. LTB_4 also alters vascular permeability and has a potent chemotactic effect on polymorphonuclear leukocytes (PMNs) that may be necessary for plasma exudation.[5,6]

Two other 20-carbon polyunsaturated fatty acids give rise to PGs and lipoxygenase products. One is dihomo-τ-linolenic acid (DHLA), which is converted to the 1-series of PGs; the lack of a double bond in the 5 position, however, prevents the formation of the PGI analogue of DHLA. The other product is eicosapentaenoic acid (EPA), a fatty acid enriched in marine fishes, which gives rise to PGs of the 3-series, including PGI_3. PGI_3 is as potent an antiaggregating agent as PGI_2, whereas TXA_3 is a weak agonist for platelet aggregation and vasoconstriction. LTB_5 derived from EPA is only one-tenth as potent as LTB_4 as a chemoattractant. These fatty acids affect biosynthesis of eicosanoids. Dietary modification of fatty acid composition, including enrichment of EPA and reduction of AA content by fish oil supplementation, may alleviate athersclerosis-related disorders by modulating these mechanisms.[3,5]

ARACHIDONIC ACID METABOLISM AND POSTISCHEMIC VASCULAR INJURIES

Postischemic vascular injuries may contribute to progressive tissue damage, including effects of delayed hypoperfusion and vasogenic edema. The latter is the

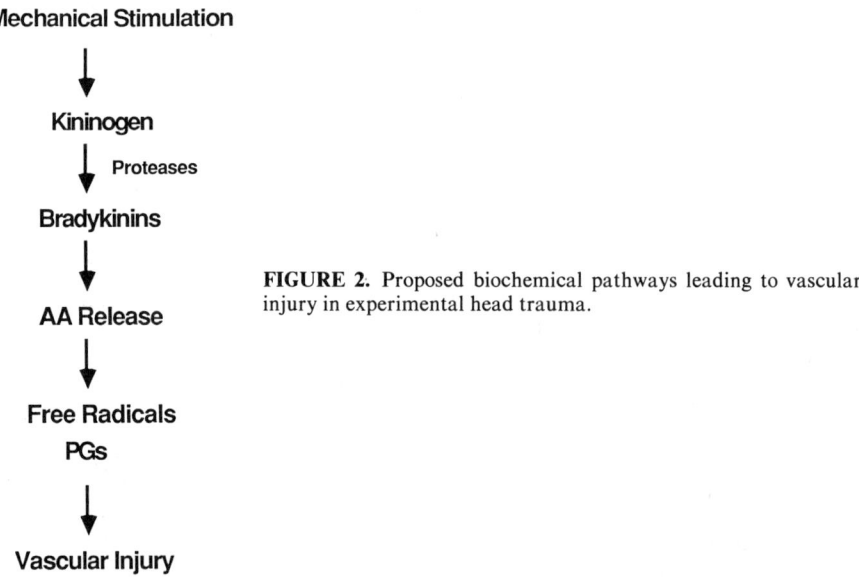

FIGURE 2. Proposed biochemical pathways leading to vascular injury in experimental head trauma.

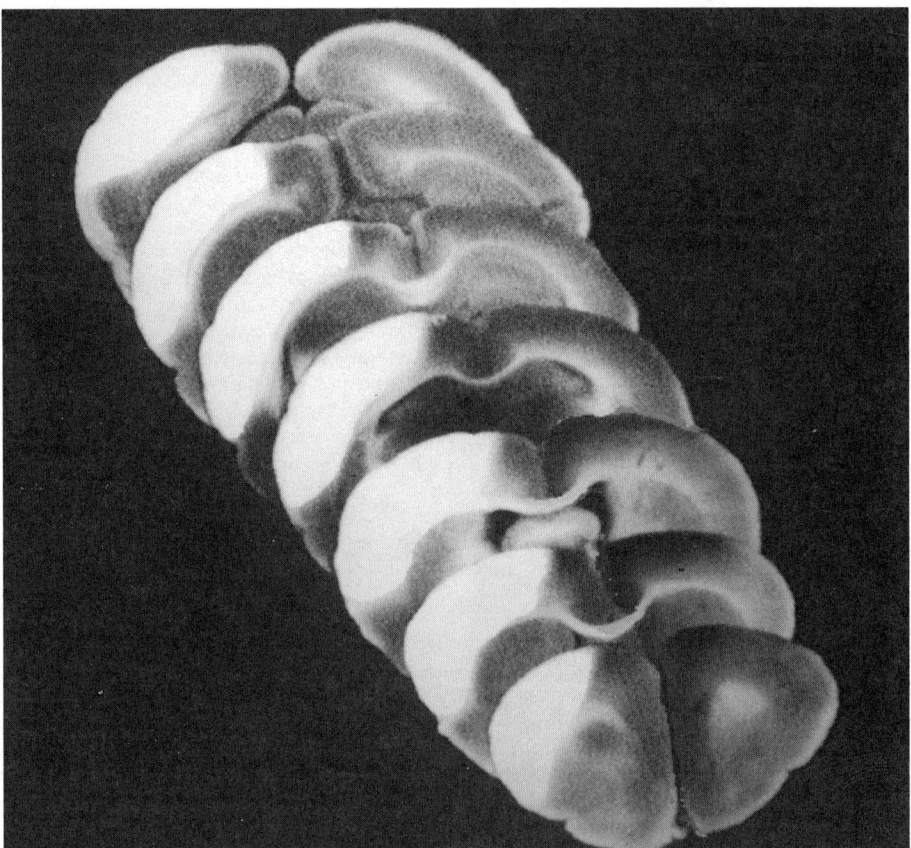

FIGURE 3. Delineation of infarct areas in the cerebral cortex of the middle-cerebral-artery territory by triphenyltetrazolium.

major cause of death among patients with ischemic stroke during the first month. AA and its metabolites play important roles in cerebrovascular injuries.[5,6] The potential roles of TXA_2, PGI_2, and LTs in vascular injuries have been summarized in the preceding section. Bradykinin may be a missing chemical link in vascular injuries involving AA.[14–16] Bradykinin activates AA metabolism by stimulating phospholipases.[15] Free radical–mediated vascular injuries[17–19] were thought to be a consequence of activation of AA metabolism that may depend on bradykinin[14–16] (FIG. 2). Bradykinin is released from its precursor, kininogen, by proteolytic enzymes, kallikreins.[20] Activation of the kallikrein-kinin system has recently been implicated in vasogenic brain edema.[21,22] Other proteolytic enzymes that may release kinins from kininogens are calcium-dependent neutral proteases (calpains)[23] and proteases released by PMNs. PMNs are a major factor in inflammatory vascular injury. Their involvement in cerebral ischemia is suggested by a postischemic inflammatory reaction dominated by PMN infiltration in the ischemic brain tissue.[24,25]

Using a focal ischemia model in the rat, we have studied the alteration of eicosanoid production in relation to postischemic vascular injuries. In the following section, our recent findings and results of therapeutic intervention directed at AA metabolism are summarized.

MATERIALS AND METHODS

Focal Cerebral Ischemia in the Rat

The animal model of focal cerebral ischemia in the rat has been fully described elsewhere.[26] In brief, Long-Evans rats (Charles River, weighing 250–300 g) were anesthetized with ketamine (100 mg/kg IP) plus xylazine (6 mg/kg, IM). Body temperature was maintained at 37 ± 1°C. Arterial blood pressures and blood gases were monitored through a PE-50 catheter in the right femoral artery. Both common carotid arteries (CCAs) were isolated after a midline cervical ventral incision. A 1.5-cm incision was made at the midpoint between the right eye and the right ear, the temporalis muscle separated, and a 2-mm burr hole drilled to expose the right middle cerebral artery (MCA) 1 mm rostral to the anterior junction of the zygoma and the squamosal bone. With the aid of a dissecting microscope, the MCA was ligated with 10-O silk. The common carotid arteries were then occluded for 90 min with atraumatic clamps. Rats were sacrificed at various intervals after release of the carotid clamps for measurement of eicosanoid content and parameters reflecting vascular injury (see below).

Morphometric Measurement of Infarct Volume

The extent of focal ischemic injury was quantitatively determined by morphometric analysis of infarct volume.[27] Infarct volume was calculated from the cross-sectional areas of eight 2-mm thick coronal sections that remained unstained after incubation with 2% triphenyltetrazolium chloride (TTC) in phosphate buffered saline (pH 7.4)[16] (FIG. 3). TTC-delineated infarct area closely corresponds with that determined histologically with hematoxylin-eosin and luxol fast blue ($r = 0.93, n = 70$).

Quantitative Determinations of Postischemic Vascular Changes

Brain water content in the cerebral cortex of the left and right MCA distribution was determined by wet and dry weight methods as previously described.[28] The postischemic increase in vascular permeability was determined by measurement of the amount of I-125 labeled human serum albumin (HSA) entering the extravascular space in the ischemic cortex[28] and spectrophotometric measurement of Evans blue in MCA cortex following intracardiac perfusion with normal saline (200 cc) 24 hours after intravenous administration of Evans blue (2%, 0.75 cc). The extent of PMN infiltration was determined by enzymatic assay of myeloperoxidase (MPO),[29] a marker enzyme of neutrophils. Kininogen content was determined by radioimmunoassay of kinin[30] following trypsin treatment. Western blot analysis of kininogens and HPLC separation of kinins were by the previously described procedures.[30-32]

Radioimmunoassays of Eicosanoids

For determination of cortical eicosanoid content, rat brains were frozen *in situ* by liquid nitrogen using the funnel technique. The dissected cortex in MCA territory was then homogenized and extracted with methanol. The supernatant was acidified to pH 3 with formic acid and the volume diluted with water to a 15% aqueous methanol concentration before application to a C18 Sep-Pak column (Waters) that was primed with 1 ml methanol and 15 ml 15% aqueous methanol containing 0.5% EDTA (pH adjusted to 3 with formic acid). The column was eluted in succession with 5 ml each of 15% and 30% aqueous methanol. TXB_2, 6-keto-$PGF_{1\alpha}$ (6KF), LTB_4, LTC_4, and LTD_4 were quantitatively eluted with 100% methanol. The 100% methanol fraction was evaporated to dryness and dissolved in mobile phase for HPLC or radioimmunoassay (RIA) buffer for RIA. Recovery rate was also monitored by exogenous PGB_2 (94–102%, $n=$ 12).

RIAs of TXB_2 and 6KF have been described in detail elsewhere.[33,34] RIA for LTC_4/D_4 was conducted using antisera kindly provided by Dr. E. Hayes of Merck Sharp and Dohme (Rahway, NJ). The antisera do not distinguish LTC_4 and LTD_4. The lack of specificity can be circumvented by HPLC separation of leukotrienes. LTB_4 RIA, which is similar to that of LTC_4/LTD_4, followed the procedure developed by H.H. Tai.[35] The authenticity of LTB_4, LTC_4, and LTD_4 was confirmed by HPLC.

Experiments with Fish Oil Supplement

Fish oil (FO) (12% eicosapentaenoic acid, Squibb, Princeton, NJ) or safflower oil (SO) (General Nutrition Center) to constitute 20% of total calorie intake were mixed with blended rat chow (Wayne Research Animal Diet, Chicago, IL) fresh every day for feeding. The dietary modification was begun at weaning and continued for approximately 7 weeks, at which age the animal weighed 300 grams. A third group of animals was fed with normal rat chow (NO) to serve as another control. Since no difference in infarct size was noted between the SO and NO groups, subsequent experiments were carried out comparing the FO and NO groups only. The animals were subjected to triple-vessel MCA ischemia as described above. Twenty-four hours following the ischemia, a blood sample was obtained for measurement of serum TXB_2. The blood sample was allowed to clot at room temperature for 60 min. Serum was diluted 100–200× for TXB_2 RIA.[33] Animals were then sacrificed by intracardiac perfusion with normal saline under anesthesia. Liver was removed for assay of AA and EPA in phospholipids. Phospholipids were extracted and separated by two-dimensional TLC. The fatty acid content of each phospholipid was determined by gas chromatography.[36,37] Infarct size, brain edema, and PMN infiltration were then determined as described above.

Therapeutic Trial With Free Radical Scavengers

Superoxide dismutase and catalase conjugated to polyethylene glycol (PEG) (average molecular mass of 5000 Da) were generously provided by Enzon, Inc. (South Plainfield, NJ). Polyethylene glycol–superoxide dismutase (PEG-SOD) was inactivated with alkaline hydrogen peroxide,[38] while PEG-catalase (PEG-CAT) was inactivated by treatment with aminotriazole and hydrogen peroxide.[39] These inactive proteins were used as placebos in control groups in order to separate free radical scavenging properties from nonspecific PEG-protein effects. The amount of inactive PEG-superoxide dismutase and PEG-catalase administered was equivalent to the active enzyme conjugate on a mg protein basis. The cytochrome c method of McCord and Fridovich[40] was used to assay superoxide dismutase, while catalase was assayed by the method of Bergmeyer.

Rats were randomly assigned to receive either PEG-superoxide dismutase (10,000

U/kg) plus PEG-catalase (10,000 U/kg) or equivalent amounts of inactive enzymes, and those performing the surgery or evaluating the outcome were blind to the treatment code. Plasma was collected 10 min after reperfusion for measurement of SOD activity. Infarct volume was determined 24 hours after reperfusion.

RESULTS

Ischemic Brain Edema and Eicosanoid Formation

Focal cerebral ischemia following the right MCA ligation and CCA clamping for 90 min consistently produced a large infarct in the cerebral cortex of the right MCA territory.[26,27] The infarct became apparent 6 hours after ischemia, and the infarct volume delineated by TTC staining (FIG. 3) remained unchanged in the period between 24 and 72 hours after ischemia.[41] Ischemic brain edema reflected by increased water content evolved in a time-dependent manner and peaked 24 hours after ischemia (TABLE 1). The vasogenic nature of the brain edema was supported by the corresponding increase in vascular permeability in the ischemic region determined by I-125 HSA and Evans blue (TABLE 1). TXB_2, 6KF, LTB_4, and LTC_4/LTD_4 production in the ischemic cortex increased for at least 3 days after ischemia. With the exception of LTC_4/LTD_4, eicosanoid production peaked 24 hours after ischemia (TABLE 2).

Kininogen Accumulation in Ischemic Cortex

Following focal ischemia, progressive accumulation of kininogen in the ischemic cortex was also noted. However, the time course of kininogen increase did not

TABLE 1. Brain Edema and Vascular Injury Following Cerebral Ischemia

Time	% H$_2$O Lt	% H$_2$O Rt	HSA Lt	HSA Rt	Evans Blue Lt	Evans Blue Rt	MPO Lt	MPO Rt
2 h	78.71 ± 0.26	81.95 ± 0.17	—	—	—	—	ND	0.02 ± 0.01
4 h	78.69 ± 0.15	83.26 ± 0.11	—	—	—	—	ND	0.06 ± 0.02
6 h	78.67 ± 0.21	84.45 ± 0.17	—	—	—	—	ND	0.03 ± 0.02
24 h	78.67 ± 0.37	89.41 ± 0.24	0.21 ± 0.07	4.24 ± 0.4	ND	0.136 ± 0.031	ND	0.46 ± 0.11
48 h	78.71 ± 0.51	88.47 ± 0.31	0.15 ± 0.01	3.13 ± 0.21	ND	0.088 ± 0.016	ND	0.63 ± 0.10
72 h	78.77 ± 0.38	85.30 ± 0.50	0.21 ± 0.07	3.22 ± 0.92	ND	0.038 ± 0.010	ND	0.59 ± 0.09
96 h	79.73 ± 0.62	83.10 ± 0.65	0.11 ± 0.03	2.7 ± 0.79	—	—	ND	0.28 ± 0.04
168 h	78.99 ± 0.42	83.01 ± 0.36	0.1 ± 0.03	1.29 ± 0.37	—	—	ND	0.09 ± 0.03

NOTE: Percent H$_2$O was determined by wet-dry weight method. I-125 HSA (human serum albumin) denotes extent of extravasation of I-125 HSA (cpm in middle cerebral artery [MCA] cortex/dry weight/radioactivity in 100 μl plasma). Evans Blue denotes extent of extravasation of Evans blue (μl plasma/mg wet weight). Data shown are mean ± SEM from cortex of the left MCA (Lt) and right MCA (Rt) territories, respectively. $n \geq 4$. — denotes experiments not done. ND denotes Evans blue or MPO (myeloperoxidase) activity were not detectable.

correspond to that of the edema or eicosanoid production. The former did not peak in 72 hours after ischemia (TABLE 3). Western blot analysis of kininogen in the ischemic cortex showed a single band with an approximate molecular weight of 66,000 comigrating with T-kininogen or low-molecular-weight kininogen. HPLC separation of kinins derived from trypsin treatment of kininogens in the ischemic cortex revealed two peaks, corresponding to bradykinin and T-kinin, respectively. No increase in kallikrein activity was detected in the ischemic cortex (data not shown).

Postischemic Neutrophil Accumulation

A preliminary morphological study showed that PMN infiltration peaked 48 hours after ischemia. This finding was confirmed by quantitative measurement of neutrophil accumulation employing MPO assay. The time course of PMN infiltration also did not correspond with that of vasogenic edema, eicosanoid formation, or kininogen accumulation (TABLE 1).

Effects of Fish Oil Supplement on Postischemic Vascular Changes

Dietary fish oil supplementation produced an increase in EPA and decrease in AA content in hepatic phospholipids except for the phosphoinositol fraction (TABLE 4). Decreased platelet activity in fish-oil-fed rats was suggested by the significant reduction in the serum TXB_2 level. However, brain edema and postischemic neutrophil accumulation were not less in rats fed fish oil. Infarct volume did not differ among rats treated with fish oil, vegetable oil, or regular chow (TABLE 4).

Effects of PEG-SOD and PEG-CAT Pretreatment on Infarct Volume

Plasma SOD activity was 235 ± 15 U/ml in the treatment group, compared to 14 ± 2 in the placebo group. PEG-SOD and PEG-CAT treatment did not affect cardiopulmonary function or body temperature. As shown in FIGURE 4, infarct volume was reduced by approximately 30% in the treatment group. Infarct volume in the placebo group did not differ from that without treatment.

TABLE 2. Eicosanoid Content following Focal Cerebral Ischemia

Time	TXB_2		6KF		LTB_4		LTC_4/LTD_4	
	Lt	Rt	Lt	Rt	Lt	Rt	Lt	Rt
15 min	25 ± 2	164 ± 35[a]	82 ± 5	112 ± 17	33 ± 11	31 ± 5	45 ± 6	47 ± 3
60 min	29 ± 4	126 ± 3[a]	64 ± 3	174 ± 17[a]	25 ± 3	47 ± 12	36 ± 3	78 ± 14[a]
6 h	18 ± 1	90 ± 16[a]	64 ± 3	165 ± 27[a]	17 ± 2	49 ± 14	38 ± 3	89 ± 17[a]
24 h	19 ± 3	379 ± 90[a]	40 ± 5	221 ± 25[a]	21 ± 3	423 ± 45[a]	36 ± 6	168 ± 26[a]
48 h	25 ± 4	163 ± 40[a]	64 ± 9	204 ± 20[a]	35 ± 4	277 ± 44[a]	57 ± 3	294 ± 40[a]
72 h	35 ± 4	160 ± 28[a]	59 ± 7	179 ± 11[a]	50 ± 6	233 ± 22[a]	55 ± 5	272 ± 18[a]

NOTE: Data shown are eicosanoids in pg/mg protein (mean ± SEM, $n \geq 6$) from cerebral cortex of the left (Lt) and right (Rt) middle cerebral artery territory. TX = thromboxane; 6KF = 6-keto-prostaglandin $F_{1\alpha}$; LT = leukotriene.

[a]Denotes difference between Lt and Rt is significant (t test, $p < 0.05$).

TABLE 3. Accumulation of Kininogen in the Ischemic Cortex

	Left MCA	Right MCA
Normal	0.01 ± 0.01	0.01 ± 0.01
Sham, day 3	0.02 ± 0.01	0.04 ± 0.02
Ischemia		
Day 1	0.05 ± 0.02	6.06 ± 3.02
Day 2	0.04 ± 0.04	12.21 ± 1.52
Day 3	0.18 ± 0.06	16.53 ± 1.55

NOTE: Kininogen content is expressed as ng kinin equivalent/mg protein. MCA = middle cerebral artery.

DISCUSSION

Creation of an anatomically discrete infarct confined to the cerebral cortex in the right MCA territory makes our model suitable for biochemical study. The vasogenic edema evolves to peak approximately 24 hr after ischemia, and this is analogous to human stroke. It is distinctly different from the short-lived increase in brain water content in animal models subjected to brief ischemia and subsequent reperfusion.[42,43] Except for LTC_4/LTD_4, the time course of eicosanoid formation corresponded approximately with the evolution of brain edema, indicating an intimate relationship between AA metabolism and the pathogenesis of brain edema.[44,45] The eicosanoid profile noted contrasts with those found in studies of brief ischemia in which an increase in eicosanoid production was only transient.[42,43] The molecular mechanism of the sustained activation of AA found here is unknown and intriguing. Since bradykinin stimulates AA metabolism,[15,46,47] increases blood-brain barrier permeability,[48] and causes brain edema, it may be the missing link in trauma-induced and free radical–mediated vascular injury involving AA.[14-19] The progressive accumulation of T-kininogen (which contains bradykinin) during the development of brain edema suggests that conversion of T-kininogen to bradykinin contributes to postischemic brain edema. Surprisingly, the activity of kallikreins, the proteases converting kinino-

TABLE 4. Effects of Fish Oil Supplementation

	Regular Diet	Fish Oil	Vegetable Oil
Serum TXB_2 (ng/ml)	222 ± 16	102 ± 12	—
Phosphatidylcholine			
AA (mg FA/mg protein)	14.4 ± 2.5	6.2 ± 0.7	—
EPA (mg FA/mg protein)	0.6 ± 0.4	3.1 ± 0.4	—
Phosphatidylethanolamine			
AA (mg FA/mg protein)	15.2 ± 3.7	7.9 ± 2.1	—
EPA (mg FA/mg protein)	0.9 ± 0.3	4.1 ± 1.1	—
Phosphatidylinositol			
AA (mg FA/mg protein)	19.2 ± 3.1	19.0 ± 3.8	—
EPA (mg FA/mg protein)	0.6 ± 0.3	1.6 ± 0.6	—
Phosphatidylserine			
AA (mg FA/mg protein)	15.0 ± 3.6	5.2 ± 1.4	—
EPA (mg FA/mg protein)	1.8 ± 0.6	4.1 ± 1.3	—
Edema (% H_2O)	87.56 ± 0.22	88.75 ± 0.22	—
MPO activity (unit/gm)	0.35 ± 0.08	0.37 ± 0.12	—
Infarct volume (mm³)	127 ± 9	137 ± 8	140 ± 2

NOTE: TX = thromboxane; AA = arachidonic acid; FA = fatty acid; EPA = eicosapentaenoic acid; MPO = myeloperoxidase.

gens to kinins, was not increased in the ischemic cortex. Other proteolytic enzymes, including calpains and proteases released by neutrophils, may participate in the bradykinin release. We have previously reported an increase in tissue calcium content paralleling increased neurofilament protein degradation in the ischemic cortex.[49] Neurofilament proteins are the best substrates for calpains, and this suggests calpain activation in the ischemic cortex. At this point, however, there is no direct evidence that calpain catalyzes release of bradykinin from kininogens following ischemic injury.

Postischemic PMN infiltration indicates that proteases released by neutrophils may also contribute to bradykinin-related edema formation. Neutrophils play an important role in the acute inflammation that features vascular injury and plasma exudation. Free radicals, LTs, and TXA_2 released by activated neutrophils contribute to these. The exact roles of neutrophils in postischemic edema have not been characterized, but since their infiltration became apparent only after infarction had fully developed, it is unlikely that neutrophils mediate acute ischemic injury. Recently,

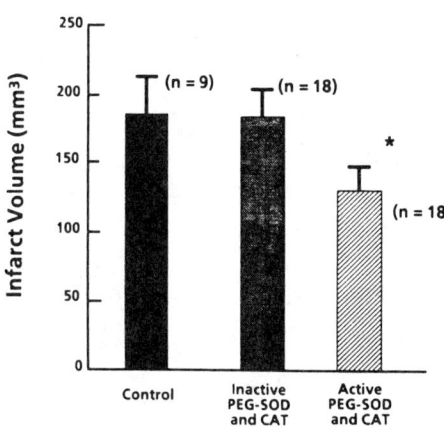

FIGURE 4. Effects of active and inactive polyethylene glycol–superoxide dismutase/ polyethylene glycol–catalase (PEG-SOD/ PEG-CAT) on infarct volume. *Asterisk:* difference from control (untreated) and inactive enzyme groups are significant ($p < 0.05$, t test).

the interaction of platelets, neutrophils, and endothelial cells in the amplification of vascular injury has drawn increasing attention. This interest stems partly from studies of AA metabolites released by these three cell types and from the identification of such other mediators as platelet-activating factor (PAF) (50) and interleukin-1(IL-1). AA metabolites (including HETEs, LTs, PGs, and TXA_2) and PAF and IL-1 may interact in complex ways to amplify cellular reaction to ischemia and subsequent vascular injuries.

Postischemic activation of AA metabolism and the potent vascular effects of eicosanoids have prompted experimental therapies directed at inhibiting formation of AA metabolites or moderating eicosanoid actions. Pharmacological modification of AA metabolism has, so far, been unsuccessful in reducing ischemic brain injury. The discrepancies in the evolution of edema, eicosanoids, kininogens, and PMN infiltration, which peak at different times following ischemia, suggest that the pathogenesis of vasogenic edema involves multiple mediators. This complexity may well explain the failure of a single therapeutic agent to reduce ischemic brain edema.

The antithrombotic and anti-inflammatory profile of EPA metabolites (the favorable effect of TXA_3/PGI_3 and the weak chemotactic potency of LTB_5)[4,5] makes EPA enrichment an attractive regimen because multiple eicosanoids are affected in a desirable way. Our studies of fish oil supplementation showed that despite an apparent reduction in platelet activity as reflected by a significant reduction in serum TXB_2, no beneficial effects on edema and PMN infiltration were observed. This finding contrasted with an earlier report of a favorable effect of EPA upon acute cerebral ischemia.[51,52] In view of the increased stroke incidence reported in Eskimos, who consume a great quantity of marine fish rich in EPA, the usefulness of such a supplement in preventing or limiting ischemic brain injury must be considered questionable.

Quantitative measurement of the discrete cortical infarct delineated by TTC allows objective determination of the extent of ischemic brain injury in our model. Using infarct volume as an index, we found that the magnitude of ischemic brain injury did not differ among rats fed fish oil, vegetable oil, or ordinary rat chow; we concluded that EPA used as sole therapy lacks efficacy.

Reperfusion of ischemic tissue can exacerbate injury due to the excess production of the partially reduced cytotoxic species of oxygen-superoxide, hydrogen peroxide, and hydroxyl radicals.[53] Activation of AA metabolism and neutrophils, and conversion of xanthine dehydrogenase to xanthine oxidase by calpains are the major pathways producing free radicals. Superoxide and hydrogen peroxide are efficiently scavenged by the enzymes superoxide dismutase and catalase. The high substrate specificity of superoxide dismutase and catalase fits these enzymes well as a putative means of implicating oxygen radicals in biological processes. The experimental and therapeutic potential of native superoxide dismutase and catalase is constrained by their circulatory half-lives, which are only 6–10 min following intravenous administration. Furthermore, partially reduced oxygen species can diffuse only short distances before reacting with cellular components, and neither superoxide dismutase nor catalase can penetrate cell membranes to gain access to intracellular sites of free radical generation.

Covalent coupling of the lysine amino groups of superoxide dismutase and catalase to PEG increases the circulatory half-lives of these proteins to 40 hr in the rat and to 5 days in humans, while also reducing enzyme immunogenicity and catabolism.[54] We have shown that PEG-conjugation of superoxide dismutase and catalase augments intracellular antioxidant enzyme activities in cultured endothelial cells and that prior incubation of cells with these enzyme conjugates provides greater resistance to oxidant stress than that afforded by the native enzymes.[55] Thus, PEG-conjugation increases the plasma circulating half-lives of superoxide dismutase and catalase and reduces the dose of antioxidant needed; increases the duration of catalytic effectiveness; and facilitates intracellular delivery to cellular sites of free radical generation.

The contribution of the partially reduced oxygen species to cerebral ischemic injury is of more importance now that treatment with tissue plasminogen activator enables reperfusion of the ischemic brain.

In the present studies, we provide evidence that scavenging of partially reduced oxygen species reduces the extent of cerebral ischemic infarction, and we corroborate earlier findings regarding the roles of free radicals in CNS injuries.[56-58] The reduction of this lasting brain injury by free radical scavengers emphasizes the importance of superoxide and hydrogen peroxide in cerebral ischemia and opens new avenues for therapeutic intervention directed at free radical–mediated mechanisms, including activation of AA metabolism and neutrophils.

REFERENCES

1. THE CANADIAN COOPERATIVE STUDY GROUP. 1978. A randomized trial of aspirin and sulfinpyrazone in threatened stroke. N. Engl. J. Med. **299:** 53–59.

2. FIELDS, W. S., N. A. LEMAK, R. F. FRANKOWSKI & R. J. HARDY. 1977. Controlled trial of aspirin in cerebral ischemia. Stroke **8**: 301–316.
3. HSU, C. Y. & E. L. HOGAN. 1989. Antiplatelet agents in acute cerebral ischemia. *In* Medical Therapy of Acute Stroke. M. Fisher, Ed. Marcel Dekker. New York, NY. In press.
4. BAZAN, N. G. 1970. Effects of ischemia and electroconvulsive shock on free fatty acids pool in the brain. Biochim. Biophys. Acta **218**: 1–10.
5. CHEN, S. T., C. Y. HSU, E. L. HOGAN, P. V. HALUSHKA, O. I. LINET & F. M. YATSU. 1986. Thromboxane, prostacyclin and leukotrienes in cerebral ischemia. Neurology **36**: 466–470.
6. WOLFE, L. S. 1982. Eicosanoids: Prostaglandins, thromboxane, leukotrienes, and other derivatives of carbon-20 unsaturated fatty acids. J. Neurochem. **38**: 1–14.
7. MOSKOWITZ, M. A. & S. R. COUGHLIN. 1981. Basic properties of the prostaglandins. Stroke **12**: 696–701.
8. HSU, C. Y., R. E. FAUGHT, A. J. FURLAN, B. M. COULL, D. C. HUANG, E. L. HOGAN, O. I. LINET & F. M. YATSU for Prostacyclin Study Group. 1987. Intravenous prostacyclin in acute non-hemorrhagic stroke: A placebo-controlled double blind study. Stroke **18**: 353–358.
9. MONCADA, S. & J. R. VANE. 1979. Arachidonic acid metabolites and their interactions between platelets and blood vessel walls. N. Engl. J. Med. **300**: 1142–1147.
10. HALLENBECK, J. M. 1977. Prevention of postischemic impairment of microvascular perfusion. Neurology **27**: 3–10.
11. CROWELL, R. M. & Y. OLSSON. 1972. Impaired microvascular filing after focal cerebral ischemia in monkeys. J. Neurosurg. **36**: 303–309.
12. GINSBERG, M. D. & R. E. MYERS. 1972. The topography of impaired microvascular perfusion in the primate brain following total circulatory arrest. Neurology **22**: 998–1011.
13. AMES, A., R. L. WRIGHT, M. KOWADA, J. M. THURSTON & G. MAJINO. 1968. Cerebral ischemia: II. The no-reflow phenomenon. Am. J. Pathol. **52**: 437–453.
14. ELLIS, E. F., S. A. HOLT, E. P. WEI & H. A. KONTOS. 1988. Kinins induced vascular reactivity. Am. J. Physiol. **255**(2 Pt. 2): H397–400.
15. KAMITANI, T., M. H. LITTLE & E. F. ELLIS. 1985. Evidence for a possible role of the brain kallikrein-kinin system in the modulation of the cerebral circulation. Circ. Res. **57**(4): 545–552.
16. KONTOS, H. A., E. P. WEI, J. T. POVLISHOCK & C. W. CHRISTMAN. 1984. Oxygen radicals mediate the cerebral arteriolar dilatation from arachidonate and bradykinin. Circ. Res. **55**: 295–303.
17. KONTOS, H. A. & E. P. WEI. 1986. Superoxide production in experimental brain injury. J. Neurosurg. **64**: 803–807.
18. KONTOS, H. A., E. P. WEI, J. T. POVLISHOCK & E. F. ELLIS. 1980. Cerebral arteriolar damage by arachidonic acid and prostaglandin G2. Science **209**: 1242–1244.
19. KONTOS, H. A. 1985. Oxygen radicals in cerebral vascular injury. Circ. Res. **57**(4): 508–516.
20. MULLER-ESTERL, W., S. IWANAGA & S. NAKANISKI. 1986. Kininogens revisited. Trends Biochem. Sci. **11**: 336–339.
21. UNTERBERG, A. & A. J. BAETHMANN. 1984. The kallikrein-kinin system as mediator in vasogenic brain edema. Part 1: Cerebral exposure to bradykinin and plasma. J. Neurosurg. **61**: 87–96.
22. UNTERBERG, A., C. DAUTERMANN, A. J. BAETHMANN & W. MULLER-ESTERL. 1986. The kallikrein-kinin system as mediator in vasogenic brain edema. Part 3: Inhibition of the kallikrein-kinin system in traumatic brain swelling. J. Neurosurg. **64**: 269–276.
23. HIGASHIYAMA, S., H. ISHIGURO, I. OHKUBO, S. FUJIMOTO, T. MATSUDA & M. SASAKI. 1986. Kinin release from kininogens by calpains. Life Sci. **39**: 1639–1644.
24. HALLENBECK, J. M., A. J. DUTKA, T. TANISHIMA, P. M. KOCHANEK, K. K. KUMAROO, C. B. THOMPSON, T. P. OBRENOVITCH & T. J. CONTRERAS. 1986. Polymorphonuclear leukocyte accumulation in brain regions with low blood flow during the early post-ischemic period. Stroke **17**(2): 246–253.
25. GARCIA, J. H. & Y. KAMIJYO. 1974. Cerebral infarction. Evolution of histopathological

changes after occlusion of a middle cerebral artery in primates. J. Neuropathol. Exp. Neurol. **33:** 456–460.
26. CHEN, S. T., C. Y. HSU, E. L. HOGAN, H. MARICQ & J. D. BALENTINE. 1986. A rat stroke model with consistent large cortical infarct. Stroke **17:** 738–743.
27. CHEN, S. T., C. Y. HSU, E. L. HOGAN, N. L. BANIK & J. D. BALENTINE. 1987. Brain calcium content in ischemic infarction. Neurology **37:** 1227–1229.
28. HSU, C. Y., E. L. HOGAN, R. H. GADSDEN, SR., R. D. COX, K. M. SPICER & M. P. SHI. 1985. Vascular permeability in experimental spinal cord injury. J. Neurol. Sci. **70:** 275–280.
29. BRADLEY, P. P., D. A. PRIEBAT, R. D. CHRISTENSEN & G. ROTHSTEIN. 1982. Measurement of cutaneous inflammation: Estimation of neutrophil content with an enzyme marker. J. Invest. Dermatol. **78:** 206.
30. CHAO, J., C. C. SWAIN, S. CHAO, W. XIONG & L. CHAO. 1988. Analyses of kininogen induction and tissue distribution with a kinin-directed monoclonal antibody. Biochim. Biophys. Acta **964:** 329–339.
31. CHAO, J., S. CHAO, W. XIONG, L. CHEN, C. SWAIN & L. CHAO. 1988. Sex dimorphism and estrogen regulation of kininogens in rat serum, adrenal gland and kidney. Kinins V. Adv. Exp. Biol. Med. In press.
32. LU, H. S., F. K. LIN, L. CHAO & J. CHAO. 1988. Human urinary kallikrein: Complete amino acid sequence and sites of glycosylation. Int. J. Proteins Peptides. In press.
33. HSU, C. Y., P. V. HALUSHKA, E. L. HOGAN, N. L. BANIK, W. A. LEE & P. L. PEROT, JR. 1985. Increased production of arachidonate metabolites following spinal cord injury. Neurology **35:** 1003–1008.
34. HSU, C. Y., P. V. HALUSHKA, E. L. HOGAN & R. D. COX. 1986. Thromboxane-prostacyclin imbalance and vascular injury in experimental spinal cord injury. J. Neurol. Sci. **74:** 289–295.
35. DEMPSEY, R. J., M. W. ROY, K. MEYER, D. E. COWEN & H. H. TAI. 1986. The development of cyclooxygenase metabolites and lipoxygenase metabolites of arachidonic acid after transient cerebral ischemia. J. Neurosurg. **64:** 118–124.
36. TANG, W. & G. Y. SUN. 1982. Factors affecting free fatty acids in rat brain cortex. Neurochem. Int. **4:** 269–273.
37. SUN, G. Y., H.-M. HUANG, J. A. KELLEHER, E. B. STUBB, JR. & A. Y. SUN. 1988. Marker enzymes, phospholipids and acyl group composition of a small plasma membrane fraction isolated from rat cerebral cortex: A comparison with microsomes and synaptic plasma membranes. Neurochem. Int. **12:** 69–77.
38. HODGSON, E. K. & I. FRIDOVICH. 1975. The interaction of bovine erythrocyte superoxide dismutase with hydrogen peroxide: Inactivation of the enzyme. Biochemistry **14:** 5294–5299.
39. MARGOLIASH, E., A. NOVOGRODSKY & A. SCHEJTER. 1960. Irreversible reaction of 3-amino-1:2,4-triazole and related inhibitors with the protein of catalase. J. Biochem. **74:** 339–348.
40. MCCORD, J. M. & I. FRIDOVICH. 1969. Superoxide dismutase: An enzymatic function for erythrocuprein. J. Biol. Chem. **244:** 6049–6055.
41. TAYLOR, R., Y. O. LUK, S. T. CHEN, J. D. BALENTINE, E. L. HOGAN & C. Y. HSU. 1987. Quantitation of infarct area by triphenyl tetrazolium chloride in a rat stroke model. Neurology **37**(Suppl. 1): 82.
42. MINAMISAWA, H., A. TERASHI, Y. KATAYAMA, Y. KANDA, J. SHIMIZU, T. SHIRATORI, K. INAMURA, H. KASEKI & Y. YOSHINO. 1988. Eicosanoid levels in spontaneously hypertensive rats after ischemia with reperfusion: Leukotriene C_4 as a possible cause of cerebral edema. Stroke **19:** 372–377.
43. MOSKOWITZ, M. A., K. J. KIWAK, K. HEKIMIAN & L. LAWRENCE. 1984. Synthesis of compounds with properties of leukotrienes C_4 and D_4 in gerbil brains after ischemia and reperfusion. Science **224:** 886–889.
44. CHAN, P. H. & R. A. FISHMAN. 1978. Brain edema: Induction in cortical slices by polyunsaturated fatty acids. Science **201:** 358.
45. CHAN, P. H., R. A. FISHMAN, J. CARONNA, J. W. SCHMIDLEY, G. PIROLEAU & J. LEE. 1983. Induction of brain edema following intracerebral injection of arachidonic acid. Ann. Neurol. **13:** 625–632.

46. BRAZY, P. C., D. R. TRELLIS & P. E. KLOTMAN. 1985. Bradykinin stimulation of oxidative metabolism in renal cortical tubules from rabbit: Possible role of arachidonic acid. J. Clin Invest. **76**(5): 1812–1818.
47. WONG, P. Y., P. WESTLUND, M. HAMBERG, E. GRANSTROM & P. H.-W. CHAO. 1985. 15-Lipoxygenase in human platelets. J. Biol. Chem. **260**(16): 9162–9165.
48. RAYMOND, J. J., D. M. ROBERTSON & H. B. DINSDALE. 1986. Pharmacological modification of bradykinin induced breakdown of the blood-brain barrier. Can. J. Neurol. Sci. **13**: 214–220.
49. HSU, C. Y., Y. O. LUK, S. T. CHEN & E. L. HOGAN. 1988. Pathophysiology of focal cerebral ischemia. *In* Cerebrovascular Diseases. H. Lechner, Ed.: 247–252. Elsevier. Amsterdam.
50. BUSSOLINO, F. & A. P. BIFFIGNANDI. 1986. Platelet-activating factor-A powerful lipid eutacoid possibly involved in microangiopathy. Acta Haematol. **75**: 129–140.
51. BLACK, K. L., B. CULP, P. MADISON, O. S. RANDALL & W. E. M. LANDS. 1979. The protective effects of dietary fish oil on focal cerebral infarction. Prostaglandins Med. **3**: 257.
52. BLACK, K. L., J. T. HOFF, N. S. RADIN & G. D. DESHMUKH. 1984. Eicosapentaenoic acid: Effect on brain prostaglandins, cerebral blood flow and edema in ischemic gerbils. Stroke **15**: 64.
53. MCCORD, J. M. 1985. Oxygen-derived free radicals in postischemic tissue injury. N. Engl. J. Med. **312**: 159–163.
54. PYATAK, P. S., A. ABUCHOWSKI & F. F. DAVIS. 1976. Preparation of a polyethylene glycol:superoxide dismutase adduct and an examination of its blood circulating life and anti-inflammatory activity. Res. Commun. Chem. Pathol. Pharmacol. **29**: 113–127.
55. BECKMAN, J. S., R. L. MINOR, JR., C. W. WHITE, J. E. REPINE, R. M. ROSEN & B. A. FREEMAN. 1988. Superoxide dismutase and catalase conjugated to polyethylene glycol increases endothelial enzyme activity and oxidant resistance. J. Biol. Chem. **263**: 6884–6890.
56. TANSWELL, A. K. & B. A. FREEMAN. 1987. Liposome-entrapped antioxidant enzymes prevent lethal O_2 toxicity in the newborn rat. J Appl. Physiol. **63**: 347–352.
57. CHAN, P. H., S. LONGAR & R. A. FISHMAN. 1986. Protective effects of lipsome-entrapped superoxide dismutase on post-traumatic brain edema. Ann. Neurol. **21**: 540–547.
58. KONTOS, H. A. 1989. Free radicals in CNS injuries. *In* Cerebrovascular Diseases: 16th Princeton Conference. M.D. Ginsburg. Ed. Raven Press, New York, NY. In press.

The Role of Platelet-Activating Factor in Cerebral Ischemia and Related Disorders

P. BRAQUET,[a] B. SPINNEWYN,[a] C. DEMERLE,[a]
D. HOSFORD,[a] V. MARCHESELLI,[b] M. ROSSOWSKA,[b]
AND N. G. BAZAN[b]

[a]*Institut Henri Beaufour*
Le Plessis-Robinson
Paris, France

[b]*Louisiana State University Eye Center*
Louisiana State University School of Medicine
New Orleans, Louisiana 70112

INTRODUCTION

Platelet-activating factor (PAF) is a potent autacoid mediator implicated in a diverse range of human pathologies, including asthma, shock, cardiac and systemic anaphylaxis, ulceration, psoriasis, immune and renal disorders, and a variety of inflammatory conditions (reviewed in References 1,2). There is also considerable evidence suggesting the involvement of PAF in central nervous system (CNS) functions and ischemic diseases (reviewed in Reference 1).

Originally isolated from antigen-stimulated rabbit basophils and characterized structurally is 1-O-alkyl-2(R)-acetyl-glycero-3-phosphocholine, the alkyl phospholipid is now known to be produced by, and act on, a variety of cell types, including neutrophils, eosinophils, monocytes, macrophages, platelets, and endothelial cells (reviewed in References 1,2). The synthesis of PAF upon cell stimulation is generally accepted as involving a deacylation of the precursor molecule, 1-alkyl-2-acyl-glycero-3-phosphocholine (1-alkyl-2-acyl-GPC) by a phospholipase A_2 (PLA_2) and a subsequent acetylation of the 2-lyso-PAF to the active PAF molecule by a specific acetyltransferase (reviewed in References 1,3).

Studies on the pathophysiological role of PAF have been facilitated by a variety of synthetic and natural compounds that can specifically antagonize the mediator. Synthetic antagonists (reviewed in Reference 4)—for example, CV-6209 (Takeda), SRI 63-441 (Sandoz), and Ro 19-3704 (Hoffman-LaRoche)—are derived mainly from the PAF framework; although the structurally unrelated RP 55270 (Rhone-Poulenc), WEB 2086, and WEB 2170 (Boehringer) are also potent inhibitors. The largest group of specific PAF antagonists derive from natural sources and comprise: (i) the ginkgolides (i.e., BN 52021; Institut Henri Beaufour), unique twenty-carbon cage molecules from the leaves of *Ginkgo biloba* (reviewed in Reference 5); (ii) lignans such as kadsurenone isolated from *Piper futokadsurae* and the related synthetic furanoid frameworks L-652,731 and L-659,989 (Merck); and (iii) some gliotoxin-related compounds (i.e., FR-900452; Fusijawa) produced by various fungi and bacteria. In this review we will consider the role of PAF and the effects of some of the above antagonists in ischemic conditions.

At the onset of brain ischemia, the activation of phospholipases A and C leads to the accumulation of free fatty acids and diacylglycerols.[6] Since free polyunsaturated fatty acids are the predominant components of the enlarged free fatty acid pool,[7] the hydrolysis of phospholipids of excitable membranes from phospholipase A_2 is thought to be a major event early in ischemia.[8] The accumulation of diacylglycerol may reflect the breakdown of inositol lipids by phospholipase C activation, since the prevailing molecular species is 1-stearoyl-2-arachidonoyl-sn-glycerol.[9]

After ischemia, reperfusion activates the arachidonic acid (AA) cascade, utilizing the enhanced pool of free AA for the synthesis of cyclooxygenase and lipoxygenase reaction products such as thromboxane A_2[10] hydroxyeicosatetraenoic acids[11] and leukotrienes.[12]

Recent studies indicate that alkyl acyl-GPC, the precursor of PAF, contains largely AA in the acyl position and is an important source of PLA_2-derived AA (reviewed in References 1,3). Thus, a single parent molecule could serve as a major source of both eicosanoid and PAF production during reperfusion after cerebral ischemia. Indeed, PAF itself is known as a highly potent mediator of injury responses in a variety of tissues, including gastric intestinal and cardiac ischemia (reviewed in Reference 1a). In the brain, the effects of PAF are still not well-defined, but there is indirect evidence that PAF is an important mediator of brain injury responses.

PRESENCE OF SPECIFIC BINDING SITES FOR PLATELET-ACTIVATING FACTOR IN THE BRAIN

The existence of specific binding sites for [^{3}H]-labeled PAF ([^{3}H]-PAF) has been demonstrated in both the gerbil[13] and the rat[14] brain. In gerbils, binding assays of [^{3}H]-PAF showed specific, saturable, reversible, and time-dependent binding. Scatchard analysis indicated the presence of two apparent populations of binding sites, with $K_{d_1} = 3.66 \pm 0.92$ nM and $K_{d_2} = 20.4 \pm 0.50$ nM corresponding, respectively, to a maximum number of binding sites: $Bmax_1 = 0.83 \pm 0.23$ pmol/mg protein, $Bmax_2 = 1.1 \pm 0.32$ pmol/mg protein. Distribution of [^{3}H]-PAF specific binding revealed a maximum amount of binding in the midbrain and hippocampus.[13]

In similar studies using rats, Junier et al.[14] have found two specific sites for [^{3}H]-PAF binding, with $K_{d_1} = 0.35 \pm 0.03$ nM and $K_{d_2} = 11.45 \pm 0.95$ nM corresponding respectively to a maximum number of binding sites: $Bmax_1 = 7.8 \pm 2.7$ fmol/mg protein, $Bmax_2 = 68.6 \pm 25.9$ fmol/mg protein. Here again, the binding of [^{3}H]-PAF was fully displaced by cold PAF and partially inhibited by PAF antagonists.[9]

Using different subcellular fractions obtained from the rat brain cortex, we found[15] the highest specific binding in the microsomal fraction; and the kinetic studies showed a best-fit two binding sites model with apparent $K_{d_1} = 28.4$ pmol and a $K_{d_2} = 81.8$ nmol with correlatives $Bmax_1 = 74$ fmol/mg protein and $Bmax_2 = 32.9$ pmol/mg protein.[15] [^{3}H]-PAF was displaced by cold PAF and PAF antagonists such as CV 3988, CV 6209, BN 52111, BN 52115, and L652,731.[15]

PRODUCTION OF PLATELET-ACTIVATING FACTOR BY BRAIN TISSUE

More than 4% of phospholipids of brain tissues are etherlipids such as alkyl acyl GPC, the precursor of PAF.[16] About 50% of these etherlipids have a phosphatidylcholine moiety, as does PAF.[16] Under the action of phospholipase A_2, alkyl glycerophosphorylcholine (GPC) is converted into lyso-PAF, a small fraction of the latter yielding PAF after transfer of an acetyl group by acetyl transferase (reviewed in Reference 1). PAF and various analogues have thus been detected in bovine brain tissue,[17-19] and preliminary data from our laboratories have shown that large amounts of PAF are produced by CNS after cerebral ischemia/reperfusion in Mongolian gerbils. At the same time as PAF is produced, free fatty acids are released from the C-2 position of the glycerol framework of alkyl acyl GPC—among them, AA, which is a major component of the acyl position of alkyl acyl GPC.[20] Phosphatidylcholine-derived phospholipids may constitute the major source of both AA and PAF released after brain ischemia/reperfusion.[21]

EFFECT OF PLATELET-ACTIVATING FACTOR ON CEREBRAL BLOOD FLOW

Decreased cerebral blood flow (CBF) and increased metabolism are classical features of the delayed postischemic hypoperfusion occurring in the brain after stroke.[22,23] Interestingly, two independent teams, Bourgain et al.[24] and Kochanek et al.,[25] have shown that PAF infusion in rabbits and Wistar rats, respectively, induced a similar pattern of effects: CBF decreased by 25–30%, while the cerebral metabolic rate for oxygen ($CMRO_2$) increased by 15–25%. This drop in CBF occurred despite maintenance of mean arterial pressure well above the lower limit of CBF autoregulation in the rat.[26] The same pattern of CBF impairment and increased cerebral metabolism has been recorded after administration of endotoxin in dogs.[27] In further experiments, the same group showed that endotoxin increased blood-brain barrier permeability and suggested that plasma catechols increased during endotoxin-induced hypotension and crossed and damaged blood-brain barrier, producing cerebral hypermetabolism.[28] In addition, we have shown that brain mitochondria respiratory control ratios (RCR, see STROKE INDEX AND RESPIRATORY CONTROL RATIO, below, for details) were significantly depressed in endotoxemia, a phenomenon prevented by BN 52021 and other PAF antagonists (B. Spinnewyn and P. Braquet, unpublished). Since (i) PAF administration produces a similar effect on RCR and (ii) PAF antagonists of various chemical frameworks antagonize endotoxin-induced hemodynamic impairments (reviewed in Reference 1), the effects of endotoxin on mitochondrial respiration, CBF, and metabolism may partly be attributed to the effects of PAF on the brain microvessels.

EFFECTS OF PLATELET-ACTIVATING FACTOR ANTAGONISTS IN MODELS OF CEREBRAL ISCHEMIA

Ischemia/Reperfusion in Gerbils

The absence of posterior communicating arteries is the reason most often quoted for the unique susceptibility of the gerbil to carotid ligation.[29–31] Ten minutes of clamping and recirculation produce consequent behavioral disturbances due to brain damage localized chiefly in the cortex and hippocampus.[32,34] Drastic changes in cerebral metabolism linked to mitochondrial dysfunction have been reported.[35] PAF antagonists given before, during, or after clamping have been shown to improve significantly the stroke index, RCR, and CBF, the levels of FFA being significantly reduced at the same time.

Stroke Index and Respiratory Control Ratio

The stroke index evaluates morbidity according to the index chart defined by McGraw,[36] which assigns a numerical value for various behavioral impairments:

decrease in alertness and movement, ptosis, cocked head, circling behavior, hind-limb splaying and rotation, seizure behavior, piloerection, tremor, coma, and death. The respiratory control ratio is an index of mitochondrial respiration and is given by the ratio of state-3 over state-4 respiratory rates.[37] In gerbils, after bilateral clamping and recirculation, the stroke index indicates a severe behavioral disturbance, together with a drop in RCR values.[38]

Interestingly, when PAF antagonists are administered preventively, the initial value of the stroke index is identical to that of the controls. In contrast, stroke index evolution over time differs greatly according to the treatment administered: in ligatured control gerbils, this parameter remains high throughout the four hours of measurement.[38] Conversely, in animals treated with BN 52021, the most active PAF-antagonist of the ginkgolide series ([^{3}H]-PAF binding assay on rabbit platelet membrane: $IC_{50} = 2.5 \times 10^{-7}$ M),[5] a progressive and significant trend towards normalization is recorded. On the contrary, BN 52024, which is practically devoid of activity on the PAF receptor ($IC_{50} = 7.3 \times 10^{-5}$ M), is ineffective. The other antagonists (BN 52020 and BN 52022) give intermediate values; this agrees with their capacity to inhibit PAF binding to its receptor ($IC_{50} = 8.4 \times 10^{-7}$ M and 8.1×10^{-6}

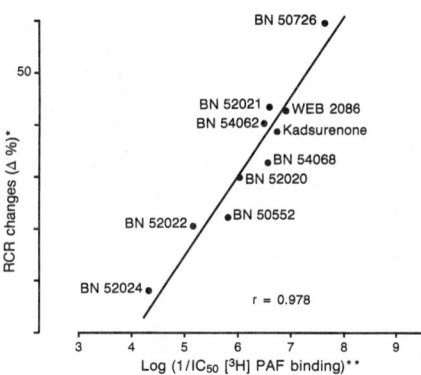

FIGURE 1. Correlation between antagonistic activity ([^{3}H] binding assay) and the change in respiratory control ratio after cerebral ischemia in Mongolian gerbils. * = in comparison with ischemic group; ** = rabbit platelet membrane preparation.

M, respectively).[38] These data are corroborated by the RCR values obtained at the end of the experiment, which display a coefficient correlation equal to 0.978 between RCR values and the capacity of the antagonist to inhibit PAF binding to platelets (FIG. 1).[38] These findings clearly show that treatment with PAF antagonists does not modify the initial cerebral impairment, but does improve the postischemic phase.

When the compounds were administered upon clamping, the same order of beneficial effect was observed: BN 52021 > BN 52020 > BN 52022 > BN 52024, both on the stroke index and on RCR measurements.[38] Furthermore, administered one hour after recirculation, BN 52021 was able to reverse the trend in cerebral impairment, as assessed by the improved RCR value observed at the end of the experiment.

In order to obtain final proof that this protection was due to a PAF antagonistic effect, we used several other chemically unrelated PAF antagonists: a lignan, kadsurenone ([^{3}H]-PAF binding assay rabbit platelet membrane $IC_{50} = 1.9 \times 10^{-7}$ M),[39] and some triazolobenzodiazepines, WEB 2086 (IC_{50} ca. 10^{-7} M)[40] and BN 50726 ($IC_{50} = 8.10^{-8}$ M). These products led to similar recovery.[38] Thus PAF appears to play an important role in the postischemic phase after bilateral ligation in Mongolian gerbils; this assumption is supported by the data obtained with both CBF and biochemical parameters.

Cerebral Blood Flow

Blood flow is drastically reduced during ischemia. When carotid blood flow is restored at the termination of ischemia, CBF initially overshoots the preischemic value (reactive hyperemia). Then CBF falls, reaching markedly subnormal values (delayed hypoperfusion).[41,42]

In animals treated with the PAF antagonist BN 52021, no delayed hypoperfusion is recorded, although the reactive hyperemia is not improved by the drug.[42] After 90 minutes of reperfusion, there is a complete recovery of CBF to close to baseline levels in both midbrain and forebrain. This improvement is unrelated to changes in systemic blood pressure. This effect of BN 52021 may be related to the inhibition of vasospasm and cerebral edema resulting from hypertensive disruption of the blood-brain barrier; these phenomena are known to decrease CBF.[41]

Lipid Peroxidation and Phospholipid Metabolism

Lipid peroxidation due to free radical formation contributes to brain cell damage in ischemia.[43] In addition, there is an activation of the cyclooxygenation and lipoxygenation of the accumulated arachidonic acid upon recirculation.[6] The *in vitro* formation of superoxide anion $O_2^{\cdot-}$, as well as the elevated levels of free fatty acids (FFA), impairs mitochondrial function.[44] PAF potently amplifies the respiratory burst in leukocytes; at very low doses ($10^{-11} \rightarrow 10^{-6}$ M), it dramatically potentiates the release of $O_2^{\cdot-}$ from polymorphonuclear cells induced by various stimuli.[45] These results may explain why BN 52021 and other PAF antagonists, which are not free radical scavengers per se, inhibit lipid peroxidation in the postischemic phase of cerebral ischemia.[38]

Such an indirect effect of PAF antagonists on lipid peroxidation is reinforced by the blockade of FFA accumulation during reperfusion. Indeed, total FFA content in control animals are 10 times and 3 times greater in the forebrain and midbrain, respectively, than in sham controls.[42] BN 52021 significantly reduces the content of FFA in both brain areas except for 16:0 in midbrain (FIG 2).[42] Diacylglycerol (DG) content is also consistently lower in BN 52021-treated gerbils, although the difference is not statistically significant in comparison with controls.[42] In addition, the changes in inositol lipids are not affected by BN 52021 except in phosphatidylinositol-4', 5'-biphosphate (PIP_2), which is increased in both the forebrain and midbrain of BN 52021-treated animals, this increase mainly comprising the arachidonoyl groups (FIG. 3).[42]

Edema

Brain edema is one of the most important clinical complications in ischemic brain damage. Classical features of cerebral edema are an increase in tissue water and sodium contents and loss of potassium.[46] In the gerbil model, BN 52021 antagonizes the hydroelectrolytic impairments;[38] this confirms the protective effect, as indicated by the other parameters. This finding is not surprising, since it is well established that PAF increases vascular permeability in various circulatory beds, including cerebral arteries—a phenomenon inhibited by PAF antagonists.[47] PAF injection directly into the brain perenchyma induces a dramatic edema in rats.[48] Such impairment is also significantly reduced by oral administration of ginkgolides 30 min prior to PAF injection.[48] These results suggest that PAF might be a major factor in promoting brain edema.

Electroconvulsive Shock and Postdecapitation Ischemia

Similar improvement of cerebral metabolism by PAF antagonists is also recorded in other types of cerebral impairments, such as electroconvulsive shock (ECS) and postdecapitation ischemia. Like ischemic reperfusion, ECS causes a loss mainly of stearic (18:0) and arachidonic acid (20:4) acids from phosphatidylinositol -4',5'-bisphosphate (PIP_2).[49] Pretreatment of ECS-treated mice with the PAF antagonist BN 52021 decreases the accumulation of palmitic acid (16:0), 18:0, 20:4 and docosahexaenoic acid (22:6) in the FFA pool, with no effect on the content or composition of fatty acids in DG, or the loss of PIP_2; BN 52021 per se has no effect on basal levels of 18:0 or 20:4 in FFA, DG, or PIP_2.[49]

Similarly, one minute after decapitation, ischemia induces a loss of PIP_2 and an accumulation of FFA and DG in the mouse brain.[49] Pretreatment with BN 52021

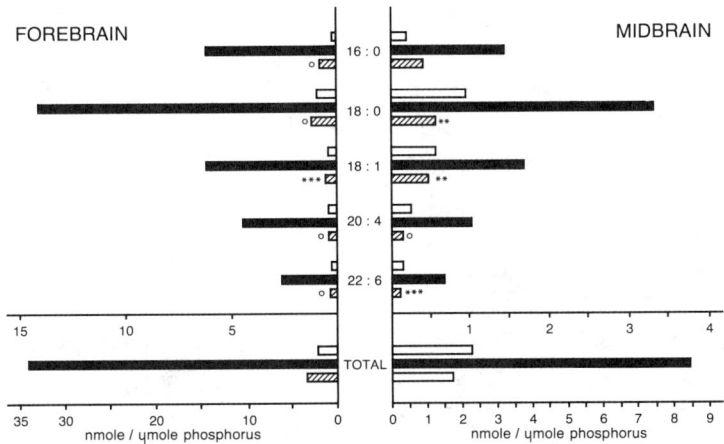

FIGURE 2. Effect of platelet-activating factor antagonist BN 52021 on free fatty acid pool in two different gerbil brain regions. After 10 min of bilateral carotid occlusion, the animals were subjected to 90 min of reperfusion and killed. *White bars* = sham-operated mice; *black bars* = DMSO control (ischemia reperfusion and vehicle); *hatched bars* = ischemia reperfusion and antagonist BN 52021. Values are averages ± SEM for seven animals. BN 52021 treated v. DMSO control: * = $p < 0.05$; ** = $p < 0.005$; *** = $p < 0.0025$; ° = $p < 0.0001$.

attenuates the accumulation of free 20:4 and 22:6 in DG but has no effect on the loss of PIP_2.[49] These data indicate that BN 52021 attenuates the injury-induced activation of phospholipase A_2, which mediates the release of polyunsaturated fatty acids in the brain while having little or no effect on phospholipase C–mediated degradation of PIP_2.

Other Models of Cerebral Ischemia

These results are in accordance with those of Kochanek *et al.*,[50] who demonstrated the beneficial action of kadsurenone on multifocal ischemia in the dog. In these studies, the right internal carotid of anesthetized dogs was injected repeatedly with small doses

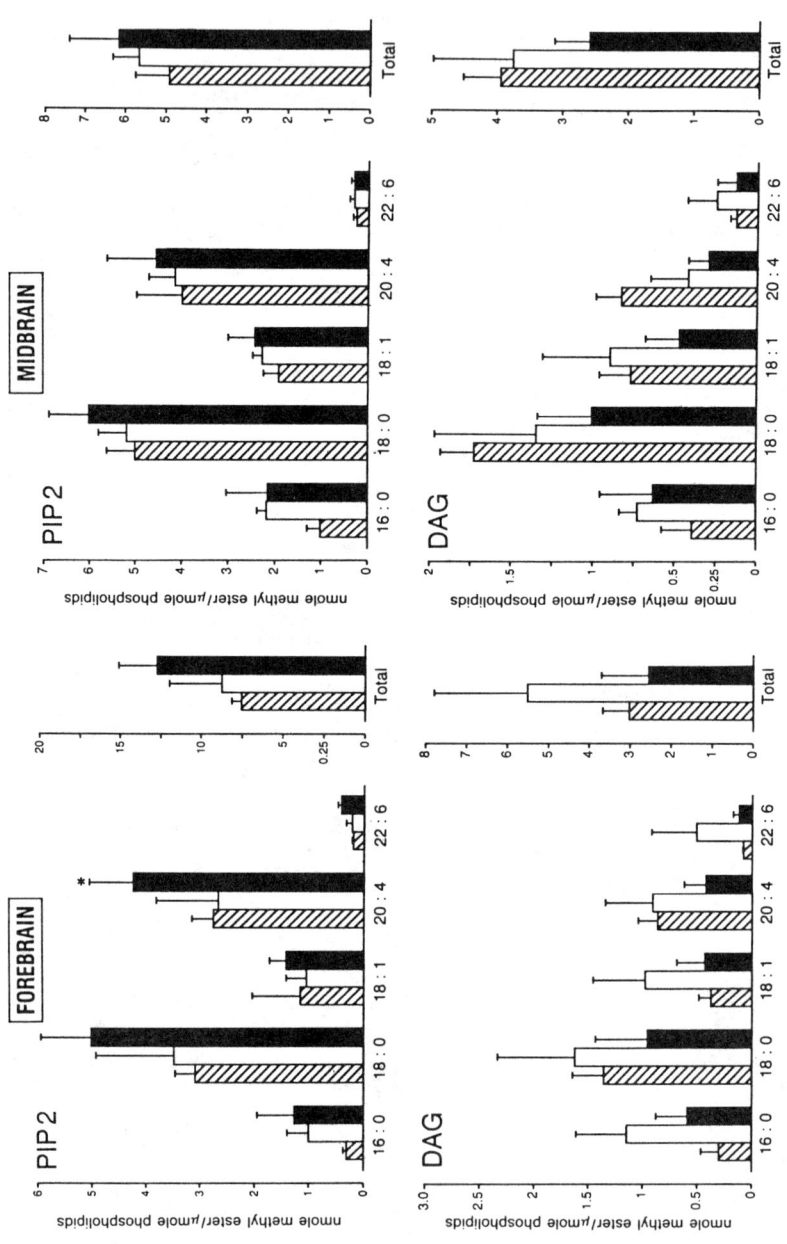

FIGURE 3. The effects of a platelet-activating factor antagonist (BN 52021) on brain diacylglycerols after ischemia-reperfusion in gerbils. PIP2 = phosphatidylinositol-4',5'-bisphosphate; DAG = diacylglycerol; *hatched columns* = sham-operated; *white columns* = DMSO control; *black columns* = BN 52021; * = $p < 0.05$.

of air for 1 h to produce multifocal ischemia, then infused with autologous ^{111}In-labeled platelets. The dogs then received kadsurenone (3 mg/kg bolus and a 1 mg/kg/h infusion) beginning 5 min prior to ischemia. Control animals received the same dose of DMSO/saline drug vehicle. After 1 h of reperfusion, kadsurenone markedly enhanced neuronal recovery as measured by cortical somatosensory evoked potential (36.0 ± 6.0 treated, 15.5 ± 2.8 control). However, platelet accumulation, estimated by right-left cerebral hemisphere difference in ^{111}In activity, was the same in both groups; thus, this antagonist seems to enhance early postischemia recovery, but not via inhibition of platelet accumulation.[50] Furthermore, D. Gilboe and colleagues at the University of Wisconsin have also recently observed the beneficial effect of PAF antagonists on energy metabolism in isolated, perfused dog brains subjected to ischemia/reperfusion. While the N-methyl-D-aspartate receptor antagonist MK-801 was effective only at higher doses, ischemic brains treated curatively after reperfusion with PAF antagonists were found to have significantly improved auditory potentials, higher ATP and phosphocreatine levels, and significantly lower creatine levels than did the ischemic controls (D. Gilboe, personal, communication).

In a study by Buchanan et al.[51] halothane-anesthetized Wistar rats were catheterized to monitor and control temperature, mean arterial pressure, blood gases, and intracranial pressure (ICP). A craniotomy was performed over the right parietal cortex, and the rats were subjected to a 50- or 100-g/cm^2 traumatic insult. Groups of rats were treated with BN 52021 (10 mg/kg) or vehicle immediately prior to trauma. After 2 hours, the animals were decapitated, and the percent brain water was determined.

Although there were no differences in any of the controlled parameters or ICP before or after trauma, BN 52021 significantly decreased edema formation (hemispheric right-left difference in percent brain water) in rats subjected to a 50-g/cm^2 insult. Buchanan et al.[51] concluded that treatment with BN 52021 attenuates the development of early posttraumatic cerebral edema and speculated that PAF may be involved in the pathogenesis of posttraumatic cerebral edema.

In a photochemically induced middle cerebral artery thrombosis model, acute blood-brain barrier alterations take place.[52] A thrombus is formed from platelets that aggregate in response to damaged endothelium. Bilateral blood-brain barrier breakdown to the ultrastructural protein tracer horseradish peroxidase can be seen 15 min following thrombosis. The degree of barrier alterations seems to be directly related to periods of irradiation; less thrombotic material produced only mild barrier alterations. Preliminary studies using BN 52021 demonstrated a trend towards inhibition of the barrier alterations (D. Dietrich and N. G. Bazan, unpublished).

ISCHEMIA-AGGRAVATING EFFECTS OF PLATELET-ACTIVATING FACTOR

Unilateral Carotid Ligation in Mice

The gravity of the neurological consequences of carotid artery ligation is known to differ among various species of rodents. Mice have an efficient collateral circulation system that prevents the induction of extensive, reliable brain ischemia resulting from occlusion of the carotid artery. Hence the unilateral ligation of this artery does not induce any neurological signs. Injection of 0.5% bovine serum albumin to control nonischemic and ischemic mice does not result in significant changes in the stroke index.[53] In addition, PAF given in normal mice at doses of 0.5 and 1 μg./g induces a small increase in the stroke index but no change in the water content in the

TABLE 1. Effect of Platelet-Activating Factor (PAF) on Unilateral Carotid Artery Ligation in Mice

Treatment[a]	Stroke Index[b]		Water Content (%)[c]	
	Before Treatment	After Treatment	Right Hemisphere	Left Hemisphere
Sham-operated mice[d]				
Saline + BSA	0	0	77.51 ± 0.080	77.59 ± 0.092
0.5 µg PAF/kg, iv	0	2.4 ± 1.12	77.46 ± 0.081	77.73 ± 0.194
1.0 µg PAF/kg, iv	0	2.2 ± 1.15	77.63 ± 0.054	77.44 ± 0.080
Ligatured mice				
Saline + BSA	0	1.43 ± 1.02	77.45 ± 0.100	77.63 ± 0.068
0.5 µg PAF/kg, iv	0	6.71 ± 1.76	77.58 ± 0.124	78.92 ± 0.919[e]
1.0 µg PAF/kg, iv	0	12.7 ± 0.89	77.46 ± 0.109	78.16 ± 0.167[e]

[a] Given 1 hour after ligation.
[b] Recorded immediately before and 2 hours after treatment.
[c] Measured 24 hours after the induction of unilateral ischemia.
[d] Surgery was the same as for ligatured mice except for clamping.
[e] Significant increase relative to right hemisphere and to both hemispheres in sham-operated treated mice.

sham-operated mice. In contrast, the same doses of PAF given to ischemic mice induce the appearance of typical signs of neurological ischemic disorders, such as cocked head, ptosis, extreme rotation in hind limbs, and circling behavior. In accordance with these results, 24 hours later the water content of the left hemisphere increases significantly relative to that of the right hemisphere in these animnals and to both hemispheres in sham-operated treated mice (TABLE 1).[53]

Transient Ischemia in Gerbils

Occlusion of the common carotids for 5 min followed by recirculation induces neurological impairments, while the stroke index decreases from the 4th until the 24th hour. Intravenous administration of low doses of PAF one hour after recirculation aggravates the development of cerebral ischemia.[53] Twenty-four hours after clamping, the stroke index of PAF-treated gerbils is three times higher than the control (FIG. 4).[53]

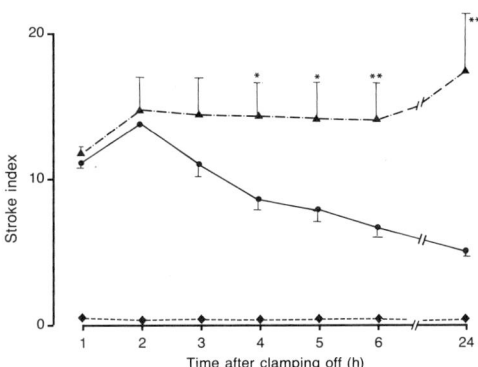

FIGURE 4. Evolution of the stroke index recorded after 5-min ischemia and recirculation in conscious Mongolian gerbils: the effect of platelet-activating factor (PAF) (1.25 μg · kg^{-1}) given 1 hour after clamping off. Values for stroke index are mean ± SEM ($n = 10$); stroke index score is expressed according to McGraw.[36] *Diamonds:* sham operated; $* = p < 0.05$; $** = p < 0.01$ v. ligatured gerbils. *Circles:* ligatured controls; for all points $p < 0.001$ v. sham-operated gerbils. *Triangles:* PAF-treated (1.25 μg · kg^{-1}) ligatured gerbils.

THE ROLE OF PLATELETS AND LEUKOCYTES IN CEREBRAL EDEMA

Incomplete return of blood flow ("no-reflow") in the brain after periods of ischemia has been reported.[54] The no-reflow phenomenon is assumed to be a pathophysiologic disorder involving the capillaries or feeding arterioles. When perfusion pressure is reduced, white blood cells and platelets may induce major disturbances in microvascular flow. It is well known that PAF is produced by, and acts on, various cell types, such as platelets,[55] monocytes,[56] neutrophils,[57] eosinophils,[57] and endothelial cells.[58] The "cross talk" involving PAF between platelets/leukocytes and endothelial cells could play a major role in the breakdown of the blood-brain barrier during cerebral ischemia (reviewed in Reference 1a).

Beneficial Effects of Platelet and Leukocyte Depletion on Cerebral Ischemia

Ischemic reperfusion in gerbils, as described above, is accompanied by a significant decrease in platelet and leukocyte counts in comparison with sham-operated controls.

These phenomena are prevented if the animals are treated with the PAF antagonist BN 52021.[59] In addition, platelet depletion by treatment with an anti-platelet antiserum improves both the stroke index and the RCR values.

In order to determine whether this decrease in the number of circulating platelets was due to the presence of platelet aggregates, we calculated the percent of circulating aggregates, using the method described by Wu and Hoak.[60] A significant number of platelet aggregates was not detected in circulating blood during reperfusion. These results suggest that the decrease in circulating platelets may reflect platelet activation and adherence to the microvascular wall, resulting in the formation of platelet microthrombi in the cerebral hemispheres. Platelet accumulation in the brain during incomplete ischemia is a well-established phenomenon, initially described by Dougherty et al.,[61] who used the unilateral carotid artery ligation model in the gerbil. Subsequently, Obrenovitch and Hallenbeck[62] demonstrated that platelets are accumulated in the dog brain as early as 5 min after embolic ischemia and that a second wave of platelet accumulation occurs in areas of low blood flow by 4 h after ischemia. In cats, platelet activation was observed in cerebral venous blood after experimental occlusion of the middle cerebral artery.[63] Platelet thrombi in the cerebral microcirculation were similarly observed through a cortical window after occlusion of the middle cerebral

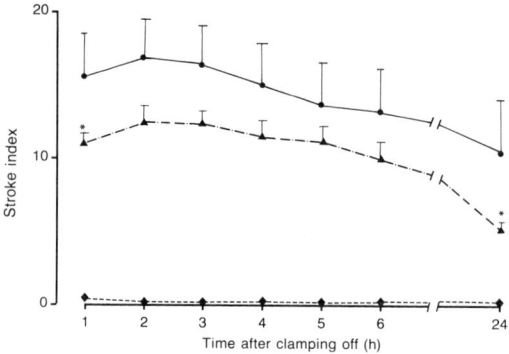

FIGURE 5. Evolution of the stroke index recorded after 10-min ischemia and recirculation in control and neutropenic gerbils. Values for stroke index are mean ± SEM ($n = 10$); stroke index score is expressed according to McGraw.[36] *Diamonds:* sham operated; $* = p < 0.05$ v. ligatured gerbils. *Circles:* ligatured control (WBC = 10200 ± 780); for all points $p < 0.001$ v. sham-operated gerbils. *Triangles:* neutropenic gerbils (WBC = 3400 ± 470).

artery in the squirrel monkey.[64] Finally, platelet microvascular aggregates have recently been found in cerebral infarcts in human autopsies.[65] The increase of platelet factor IV and β-thromboglobulin levels following thromboembolic cerebral infarction, also recorded in humans,[66] could reflect platelet activation in brain microvessels. Because (i) platelet activation can occur in stroke even though the platelet cyclooxygenase pathway is suppressed and (ii) PAF releases platelet factor 4 and β-thromboglobulin from platelets, the generation of these mediators in cerebral ischemia may result from PAF production.

In gerbils, pretreatment with nitrogen mustard induces a significant decrease in white blood cells (ca. 70% decrease), with no effect on red blood cells or platelets.[59] When animals pretreated in this way are subjected to brain ischemia/reperfusion, the stroke index and RCR values show less impairment than in the control ischemic group (FIGURE 5).[59] These results suggest that leukocytes could participate in the cerebral impairments, corroborating previous data by Schurer et al.,[67] who demonstrated that depletion of polymorphonuclear leukocytes by antineutrophil antiserum in the peripheral blood was effective in attenuating postischemic hypoperfusion following a 15-min period of cerebral ischemia. In addition, recent work by Hallenbeck et al.[68]

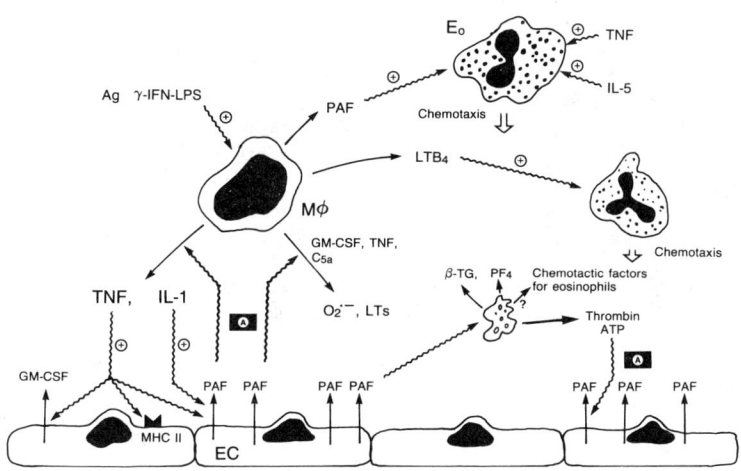

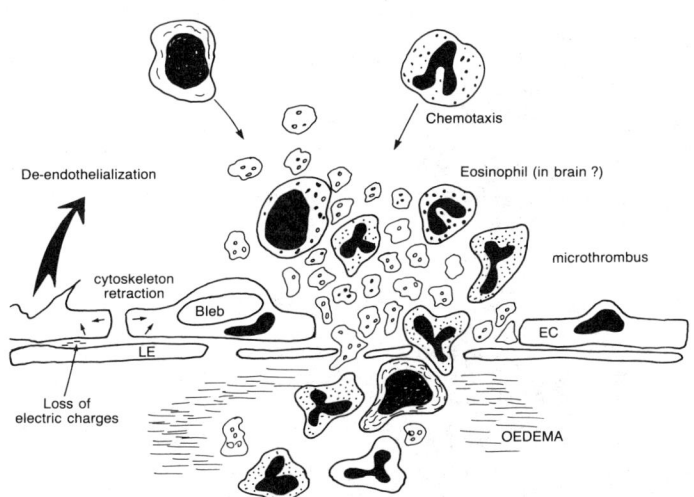

FIGURE 6. The platelet-activating factor (PAF)–generated amplification cycles (*upper panel*) and the resultant endothelial damage (*lower panel*) in microvascular injury. A = amplification induced by PAF; Ag = antigen; Eo = eosinophil; EC = endothelial cells; IL-1 = interleukin-1; Mϕ = macrophage; LPS = endotoxin; LTB$_4$ = leukotriene B$_4$; PF$_4$ = platelet factor 4; β-TG = beta thromboglobulin; TNF = tumor necrosis factor; LTs = leukotrienes; IL-5 = interleukin-5; GM-CSF = granulocyte-monocyte colony stimulating factor; MHC II = major histocompatibility complex II.

has revealed that granulocytes progressively accumulate during the first 4 hours of reperfusion after cerebral ischemia in dogs subjected to intracarotid air embolism.[68] In this model, the amount of granulocyte accumulation observed during early reperfusion occurred in proportion to the severity of ischemia and predominantly in areas of low blood flow.[68,69] Furthermore, an epidemiological study identified the total white cell count as a predictor for cerebral infarction during a two-year observation period.[70]

Eosinophil infiltration may also be an important feature of the late phase following cerebral ischemia, since eosinophilic cationic proteins have been detected in the cerebrospinal fluid of patients following cerebral infarction.[71] Moreover, it has been postulated that eosinophilic cationic proteins may account for the cerebral impairments observed after brain ischemia.[72]

The Priming Role of Platelet-Activating Factor in Blood Cell/Endothelial Cell "Cross Talk"

PAF is a potent amplifier of platelet and leukocyte responses (FIG. 6): at low concentrations ($10^{-16} \rightarrow 10^{-11}$ M), it dramatically potentiates not only the release of interleukin-1 (IL-1) and tumor necrosis factor (TNF) by monocytes/macrophages, but also the production of leukotrienes (M. Braquet, in preparation) and free radicals (O_2^-, $OH^.$)[45] from stimulated polymorphonuclear cells. Similarly, PAF activates platelets to form thrombin and ATP, which in turn, as IL-1 and TNF, act on endothelial cells to produce more PAF.[73] This amplification results in the formation of a large, dense platelet thrombus, which is surrounded and invaded by neutrophils and subsequently by eosinophils and macrophages, and which spreads over the adjoining vacuolized endothelium.[74] Indeed, PAF alters the molecular organization of the cytoskeletal proteins that control endothelial permeability.[75] Human endothelial cells stimulated by PAF retract and separate, while stress fibers disappear or become less regular, causing bleb formation. Such sequences of events may lead to cerebral edema when they occur in brain microvessels; therefore, PAF antagonists may counteract the amplification processes and improve cerebral metabolism by inhibiting the various positive feedback mechanisms. (See Reference 1a for review of mechanisms.)

REFERENCES

1. BRAQUET, P., L. TOUQUI, T. Y. SHEN & B. B. VARGAFTIG. 1987. Perspective in platelet-activating factor research. Pharmacol. Rev. **39**: 97.
1a. BRAQUET, P., M. PAUBERT-BRAQUET, M. KOLTAI, R. BOURGAIN, F. BUSSOLINO & D. HOSFORD. 1989. Is there a case for PAF antagonists in the treatment of ischemic states? Trends Pharmacol. Sci. **10**: 23.
2. MENCIA-HUERTA, J. M. & M. BENHAMOU. 1986. Platelet-activating factor (PAF-acether): An update. *In* Asthma: Clinical Pharmacology and Therapeutic Progress. A. B. Kay, Ed.: 237. Blackwell Scientific Publications. Oxford.
3. SNYDER, F. 1985. Chemical and biochemical aspects of platelet activating factor: A novel class of acetylated ether-linked choline-phospholipids. Med. Res. Rev. **5**: 107.
4. BRAQUET, P., P. E. CHABRIER & J. M. MENCIA-HUERTA. 1988. The promise of PAF antagonists. *In* Advances in Inflammation Research, Vol. 12. A. Lewis, Ed.: 135. Raven Press. New York, N.Y.
5. BRAQUET, P. 1987. The Ginkgolides: Potent platelet-activating factor antagonists isolated from *Ginkgo biloba L.:* Chemistry, pharmacology and clinical applications. Drugs of the Future **12**: 643.
6. BAZAN, N. G. 1970. Effects of ischemia and electroconvulsive shock on free fatty acid pool in brain. Biochem. Biophys. Acta **218**: 10.

7. BAZAN, N. G., H. E. P. BAZAN, W. G. KENNEDY & C. D. JOEL. 1971. Regional distribution and rate of production of free fatty acids in rat brain. J. Neurochem. **18:** 1387.
8. AVELDANO, M. I. & N. G. BAZAN. 1975. Rapid production of diacylglycerols enriched in arachidonate and stearate during early brain ischemia. J. Neurochem. **25:** 919.
9. PANETTA, T., V. L. MARCHESELLI, P. BRAQUET, B. SPINNEWYN & N. G. BAZAN. 1987. Effects of a platelet activating factor antagonist (BN 52021) on free fatty acids, diacylglycerols, polyphosphoinositides and blood flow in the gerbil brain: Inhibition of ischemia-reperfusion induced cerebral injury. Biochem. Biophys. Res. Commun. **149:** 580.
10. GAUDET, R. J., I. ALAM & L. LEVINE. 1980. Accumulation of cyclooxygenase products of arachidonic acid metabolism in gerbil brain during reperfusion after bilateral common carotid artery occlusion. J. Neurochem. **35:** 653.
11. KEMPSEY, R. J., M. W. ROY, K. MEYER, D. E. COWEN, H. H. TAL. 1986. Development of cyclooxygenase and lipoxygenase metabolites of arachidonic acid after transient cerebral ischemia. J. Neurosurg. **64:** 118.
12. MOSKOWITZ, M. A., K. J. KIWAK, K. HEKIMIAN & L. LEVINE. 1984. Synthesis of compounds with properties of leukotrienes C_4 and B_4 in gerbil brains after ischemia and reperfusion. Science **224:** 836.
13. DOMINGO, M. T., B. SPINNEWYN, P. E. CHABRIER & P. BRAQUET. 1988. Presence of specific binding sites for platelet-activating factor (PAF) in brain. Biochem. Biophys. Res. Commun. **151:** 730.
14. JUNIER, M. P., C. TIBERGHIEN, C. ROUGEOT, V. FASEUR & F. DRAY. 1988. Inhibitory effect of platelet-activating factor on LHRH and somatostatin release on rat medial eminence *in vitro* correlated with the characterization of specific PAF receptor sites in rat hypothalamus. Endocrinol. **123:** 72.
15. MARCHESELLI, V. L., M. ROSSOWSKA, M. T. DOMINGO, P. BRAQUET & N. BAZAN. 1989. In preparation.
16. CLARKE, N. G. & R. M. C. DAWSON. 1981. Alkaline O → N transcylation. Biochem. J. **195:** 201.
17. YOSHIDA, J. I., A. TOKUMURA, K. FUKUZAWA, M. TERAO, K. TAKAUCHI & H. TSUKATANI. 1986. A platelet-aggregating and hypotensive phospholipid isolated from bovine brain. J. Pharm. Pharmacol. **38:** 878.
18. TOKUMURA, A. & H. TSUKATANI. 1986. Determination of molecular species of platelet-activating factor in bovine brain lipid extract. Proceedings from the Second International Conference on Platelet-activating Factor and Structurally Related Alkyl Ether Lipids. October 1986. Gatlinburg, TN.: 121.
19. TOKUMURA, A., K. KAMIYASU, K. TAKAUCHI & H. TSUKATANI. 1987. Evidence for existence of various homologues and analogues of platelet activating factor in a lipid extract of bovine brain. Biochem. Biophys. Res. Commun. **154:** 415.
20. LEE, T. C. & F. SNYDER. 1985. Function, metabolism, and regulation of platelet activating factor and related ether lipids. *In* Phospholipids and Cellular Regulation. CRC Press. Bacon Raton, FL.: 1.
21. MARION, J. & L. S. WOLFE. 1979. Origin of the arachidonic acid released post-mortem in rat forebrain. Biochim. Biophys. Acta **574:** 25.
22. HOSSMANN, K. A. 1982. Treatment of experimental cerebral ischemia. J. Cereb. Blood Flow Metab. **2:** 275.
23. NEMOTO, E. M., K. A. HOSSMAN & H. K. COOPER. 1981. Postischemic hypermetabolism in cat brain. Stroke **12:** 666.
24. BOURGAIN, R. H. & R. ANDRIES. In preparation.
25. KOCHANEK, P. M., E. M. NEMOTO, J. M. MELICK, R. W. EVANS & D. F. BURKE. 1987. Platelet activating factor alters cerebral blood flow and metabolism in rats (abstract). Circulation **75**(Suppl. 4): 53.
26. BARRY, D. I., S. STRADGAARD, D. I. GRAHAM, U. G. SVENDSEN, O. BRAENDSTRUP & O. B. PAULSON. 1984. Cerebral blood flow during dihydralazine-induced hypotension in hypertensive rats. Stroke **15:** 102.
27. EKSTROM-JODAL, B., E. HAGGENDAL & L. E. LARSSON. 1982. Cerebral blood flow and oxygen uptake in endotoxic shock: An experimental study in dogs. Acta Anaesthesiol. Scand. **26:** 163.

28. EKSTROM-JODAL, B., J. HAGGENDAL, L. E. LARSSON & A. WESTERLIND. Cerebral hemodynamics, oxygen and cerebral arteriovenous differences of catecholamines following *E. coli* endotoxin in dogs. Acta Anaesthesiol. Scand. **26:** 446.
29. KAHN, K. 1972. The natural course of experimental cerebral infarction in the gerbil. Neurology **22:** 510.
30. LEVINE, S. & H. PAYAN. 1966. Effects of ischemia and other procedures on the brain and retina of the gerbil (*Meriones unguiculatus*). Exp. Neurol. **16:** 255.
31. BERRY, K., H. M. WISNIEWSKI, L. SVARZBEIN & S. BAEZ. 1975. On the relationship of brain vasculature to production of neurological deficit and morphological changes following acute unilateral common carotid artery ligation in gerbils. J. Neurol. Sci. **25:** 75.
32. ITO, U., M. SPATZ, J. T. WALKER & I. KLATZO. 1975. Experimental cerebral ischemia in Mongolian gerbils I. Light microscopic observations. Acta Neuropathol. **32:** 209.
33. KIRINO, T., A. TAMURA & K. SANO. 1986. A reversible type of neuronal injury following ischemia in the gerbil hippocampus. Stroke **17:** 455.
34. YAMOMOTO, K., K. MORIMOTO & T. YANAGIHARA. 1986. Cerebral ischemia in the gerbil: Transmission electron microscopic and immunoelectron microscopic investigation. Brain Res. **384:** 1.
35. NORDSTRÖM, C. H., S. REHNCRONA & B. K. SIESJÖ. 1978. Effects of phenobarbital in cerebral ischemia. Part II: Restitution of cerebral energy state, as well as of glycolytic metabolites, citric acid cycle intermediates and associated amino acids after pronounced incomplete ischemia. Stroke **9:** 3.
36. MCGRAW, C. P. 1977. Experimental cerebral infarction effects of pentobarbital in Mongolian gerbils. Arch. Neurol. **34:** 334.
37. CHANCE, B. & G. R. WILLIAMS. 1955. The respiratory chain and oxidative phosphorylation. Nature **175:** 1120.
38. SPINNEWYN, B., N. BLAVET, F. CLOSTRE, N. BAZAN & P. BRAQUET. 1987. Involvement of platelet-activating factor (PAF) in cerebral post-ischemic phase in Mongolian gerbils. Prostaglandins **34:** 337.
39. SHEN, T. Y., S. B. HWANG, M. N. CHANG, T. W. DOEBBER, M. H. LAM, M. S. WU, X. WANG, G. Q. HANG & R. Z. LI. 1985. Characterization of a platelet-activating factor receptor antagonist isolated from haifenteng (*Piper futokadsura*): specific inhibition of *in vitro* and *in vivo* platelet-activating factor-induced effects. Proc. Natl. Acad. Sci. USA **82:** 672.
40. WEBER, R. H. 1988. WEB 2086. Drugs Future **13:** 242.
41. SIESJÖ, B. K. 1981. Cell damage in the brain; a speculative synthesis. J. Cereb. Blood Flow Metab. **12:** 155.
42. MARCHESELLI, V. L., T. PANETTA, P. BRAQUET, K. T. THIBODEAUX & N. G. BAZAN. 1989. Effects of a platelet activating factor antagonist (BN 52021) on cerebral lipid metabolism following ischemia reperfusion in the gerbil. Ann. N.Y. Acad. Sci. This volume.
43. DEMOPOULOS, H., M. SELIGMAN, M. SCHWARTZ, J. TOMASULA & E. FLAMM. 1984. Molecular pathology of regional cerebral ischemia. *In* Cerebral Ischemia. Excerpta Medica International Congress Series 654. A. Bes, P. Braquet, R. Paoletti & B. Siesip, Eds.: 259. Elsevier. New York, NY.
44. HILLERED, L. & L. ERNSTER. 1983. Respiratory activity of isolated rat brain mitochondria following *in vitro* exposure to oxygen radicals. J. Cereb. Blood Flow Metab. **3:** 207.
45. VERCELLOTI, G. M., P. W. HUH, H. Q. YIN, R. D. NELSON & H. S. JACOB. 1986. Enhancement of PMN-mediated endothelial damage by platelet-activating factor (PAF): PAF primes PMN responses to activating stimuli. Clin. Res. **34:** 917.
46. FUJIMOTO, T., J. T. WALKER, M. SPATZ & I. KLATZO. 1976. Pathophysiological aspects of ischemic edema. *In* Dynamics of Brain Edema. H. M. Pappius & W. Feindel, Eds.: 171. Springer-Verlag. Heidelberg.
47. BRAQUET, P., R. F. VIDAL, M. BRAQUET, H. HAMARD & B. B. VARGAFTIG. 1984. Involvement of platelet-activating factor and lipoxygenase products in the increased microvascular permeability of rabbit retina. Agents Actions. **15:** 82.
48. PLOTKINE, M., L. MASSAD, M. ALLIX, C. CAPDEVILLE & R. G. BOULU. 1986. Cerebral effects of PAF-acether in rats. 6th International Conference on Prostaglandins and Related Compounds. Florence. Abstr. 300.

49. BIRKLE, D. L., P. KURIAN, P. BRAQUET & N. G. BAZAN. 1988. Inhibition of free polyunsaturated fatty acid accumulation in mouse brain during ischemia and electroconvulsive shock by specific PAF antagonist, BN 52021. J. Neurochem. **51**: 1900.
50. KOCHANEK, P. M., A. J. DUTKA, K. K. KUMAROO & J. M. HALLENBECK. 1987. Platelet-activating factor receptor blockade enhances early neuronal recovery after multifocal brain ischemia in dogs. Life Sci. **41**: 2639.
51. BUCHANAN, D. C., P. M. KOCHANEK, E. M. NEMOTO, J. A. MELICK & R. J. SCHOETTLE. 1989. Platelet-activating factor receptor blockade decreases early posttraumatic cerebral edema in rats. Ann. N. Y. Acad. Sci. This volume.
52. GROME, J. J., G. GOJOWCZYCK, W. HOFMANN & D. I. GRAHAM. 1988. Quantitation of photochemically induced focal cerebral ischemia in the rat. J. Cereb. Blood Flow Metab. **8**: 89.
53. SPINNEWYN, B., N. CARVAL, E. PIROTZY & P. BRAQUET. 1988. Cerebral ischemia aggravating effect of platelet-activating factor. Abstr. 2nd International Symposium on Pharmacology of Cerebral Ischemia, Marburg, F.R.G., October 3–5: E11.
54. AMES, A., R. L. WRIGHT, M. KOWADA, J. M. THURSTON & G. MAJNO. 1968. Cerebral Ischemia II. The no reflow phenomenon. Am. J. Pathol. **52**: 437.
55. CHIGNARD, M., J. P. LE COUEDIC, B. B. VARGAFTIG & J. BENVENISTE. Platelet-activating factor (PAF-acether) secretion from platelets: Effect of aggregating agents. Br. J. Haematol. **46**: 455.
56. CAMUSSI, G., M. AGLIETTA, F. MALAVASI, C. TETTA, W. PIACIBELLO, F. SANAVIO & F. BUSSOLINO. 1983. The release of platelet-activating factor from human endothelial cells in culture. J. Immunol. **131**: 2397.
57. LEE, T. C., B. MALONE, S. I. WASSERMAN, V. FITZGERALD & F. SNYDER. 1982. Activities of enzymes that metabolize platelet-activating factor (1-Alkyl-2-acetyl-sn-glycero-3-phosphocholine) in neutrophils and eosinophils from humans and the effect of a calcium ionophore. Biochem. Biophys. Res. Commun. **105**: 1303.
58. BUSSOLINO, F., F. BREVIARIO, C. TETTA, M. AGLIETTA, A. MANTOVANI & E. DEJANA. 1986. Interleukin 1 stimulates platelet-activating factor production in cultured human endothelial cells. J. Clin. Invest. **77**: 2027.
59. SPINNEWYN, B., N. CARVAL, E. PIROTZKY & P. BRAQUET. Beneficial effect of leukocyte depletion on cerebral ischemia. In preparation.
60. WU, K. K. & J. C. HOAK. 1974. A new method for the quantitative detection of platelet aggregates. Lancet **2**: 924.
61. DOUGHERTY, J. H., D. E. LEVY & B. B. WEKSLER. 1979. Experimental cerebral ischemia produces platelet aggregates. Neurology **29**: 1460.
62. OBRENOVITCH, T. P. & J. M. HALLENBECK. 1985. Platelet accumulation in region of low blood flow during the postischemic period. Stroke. **16**: 224.
63. DENTON, I. C., J. T. ROBERTSON & M. DUGDALE. 1971. An assessment of early platelet activity in experimental subarachnoid hemorrhage and middle cerebral artery thrombosis in the cat. Stroke **2**: 268.
64. WALTZ, A. G. & T. M. SUNDT. 1967. The microvasculature and microcirculation of the cerebral cortex after arterial occlusion. Brain **90**: 681.
65. ROMANUL, F. C. A. & A. ABRAMOWICZ. 1964. Changes in brain and pial vessels in arterial border zones. Arch. Neurol. **11**: 40.
66. SHAM, A. B., N. BEARMER & B. M. COULL. 1985. Enhanced *in vivo* platelet-activation in subtypes of ischemic stroke. Stroke **16**: 643.
67. SCHURER, L., B. GROGAARD, B. GERBIN, K. E. ARFORS & A. BAETHMANN. 1987. Effects of antineutrophil serum and superoxide dismutase on postischemic hypoperfusion of the brain in rats. J. Cereb. Blood Flow Metab. 7(Suppl. 1): S72.
68. HALLENBECK, J. M., A. J. DUTKA, T. TANISHIMA, P. M. KOCHANEK, K. K. KUMARRO, C. B. THOMPSON, T. P. OBRENOVITCH & T. J. CONTRERAS. 1986. Polymorphonuclear leukocyte accumulation in brain regions with low blood flow during the early post-ischemic period. Stroke **17**: 246.
69. KOCHANEK, P. M., A. J. DUTKA & J. M. HALLENBECK. 1987. Indomethacin, prostacyclin and heparin improve postischemic cerebral blood flow without affecting early post-ischemic granulocyte accumulation. Stroke **18**: 634.

70. PRENTICE, R. L., T. P. SZATROWSKI, H. KATO & M. W. MASON. 1982. Leucocyte counts and cerebrovascular disease. J. Chronic Dis. **35:** 703.
71. HALLGREN, R., A. TERENT & P. VENGE. 1983. Eosinophil cationic protein (ECP) in the cerebrospinal fluid. J. Neurosci. **58:** 57.
72. DURACK, D. T., S. M. SUMI & S. J. KLEBANOFF. 1979. Neurotoxicity of human eosinophils. Proc. Natl. Acad. Sci. USA **76:** 1443.
73. BUSSOLINO, F., G. CAMUSSI, F. BREVARIO, F. BERTOCCHI, D. GHIGO, G. PASCARMONA, M. AGLIETTA, G. GARBARINO, A. BOSIA & E. DEJANA. 1988. Endothelial cells and inflammation: The role of platelet-activating factor, Interleukin 1, tumor necrosis factor and circulating neutrophils. *In* Platelet Activating Factor and Cell Immunology. New Trends in Lipid Mediators Research, Vol. 1. P. Braquet, Ed.: 135. Karger. Basel.
74. BOURGAIN, R. M., L. MAES, P. BRAQUET, R. ANDRIES, L. TOUQUI & P. BRAQUET. 1985. The effect of 1-O-alkyl-2-acetyl-sn-glycero-3-phosphocholine (PAF-acether) on the arterial wall. Prostaglandins **30:** 185.
75. BUSSOLINO, F., G. CAMUSSI, M. AGLIETTA, P. BRAQUET, A. BOSIA, G. PESCARMONA, F. SANAVIO, N. D'URSO & P. C. MARCHISIO. 1987. Human endothelial cells are target for platelet activating factor (PAF) I. PAF induces changes in cytoskeleton structures. J. Immunol. **139:** 2439.

Eicosanoids in Deteriorating Stroke

Review of Studies on the Rabbit Spinal Cord Ischemia and Reperfusion Model[a,b]

GIORA FEUERSTEIN[c]

Department of Neurology
Uniformed Services University of the Health Sciences
Bethesda, Maryland 20814

INTRODUCTION

Injury to the central nervous system (CNS)—such as ischemia, electroconvulsive shock, chemically induced convulsions, or various forms of trauma[1-6]—has been shown to result in tissue accumulation of free fatty acids, including the polyunsaturated fatty acid arachidonate. The fatty acids accumulated in the injured tissue are believed to be a source of potential additional damage by direct action on membrane-bound enzymes,[7] by lipid peroxidation,[8] or by serving as substrates for various enzymatic pathways that lead to production of potent vasoactive substances. This latter event has been shown to result in the production of numerous arachidonate metabolites of both the cyclooxygenase and lipoxygenase pathways (FIG. 1). In fact, all major prostaglandins—PGD_2, PGE_2, $PGF_{2\alpha}$, TXB_2 (a nonactive metabolite of TXA_2), and 6-keto-$PGF_{1\alpha}$ (a nonactive metabolite of prostacyclin, PGI_2); leukotrienes—LTC_4 and LTD_4; and other lipoxygenase metabolites—5-HETE and 12-HETE—were identified in large quantities in the brain exposed to ischemia[9-12] or other forms of injury.[13-16]

The significance of excessive eicosanoid production in damaged brain tissue has been the subject of many debates. For example, some eicosanoids (e.g., leukotrienes, PGE_2, $PGF_{2\alpha}$, TXA_2) can modify cerebral blood vessel tone and blood-brain barrier (BBB) permeability,[17,18] while others (TXA_2-prothrombotic and PGI_2-antithrombotic) are potent modulators of blood cell aggregation. In addition, prostaglandins and leukotrienes have been suggested to play a modulatory role in neuronal excitability and glial function.[20,21] Furthermore, selective prostanoids were shown to prevent impairment of dog brain function during postischemic reperfusion,[22,23] while inhibition of cyclooxygenase products was found to increase seizure susceptibility in convulsion-prone gerbils.[24] These data taken together strongly favor a role for arachidonate products in mediating CNS injury.

While numerous studies (of which only a small part have been cited above) have implicated the eicosanoids in a variety of acute pathological processes in the CNS, little is known about the relationships of eicosanoid production to chronic or delayed brain damage in response to injury. Delayed CNS injury has been recognized both experimentally and clinically. Clinical progression of motor deficits hours or days after

---

[a]This work was supported in part by USUHS Grants GM9229, AHA G19218, and ONR G19219 to Dr. G. Feuerstein.

[b]The opinions or assertions contained herein are the private ones of the author and are not to be construed as official or reflecting the view of the Department of Defense or the Uniformed Services University of the Health Sciences.

[c]Address for correspondence: Dr. G. Feuerstein, Department of Neurology, USUHS, 4301 Jones Bridge Road, Bethesda, Maryland 20814.

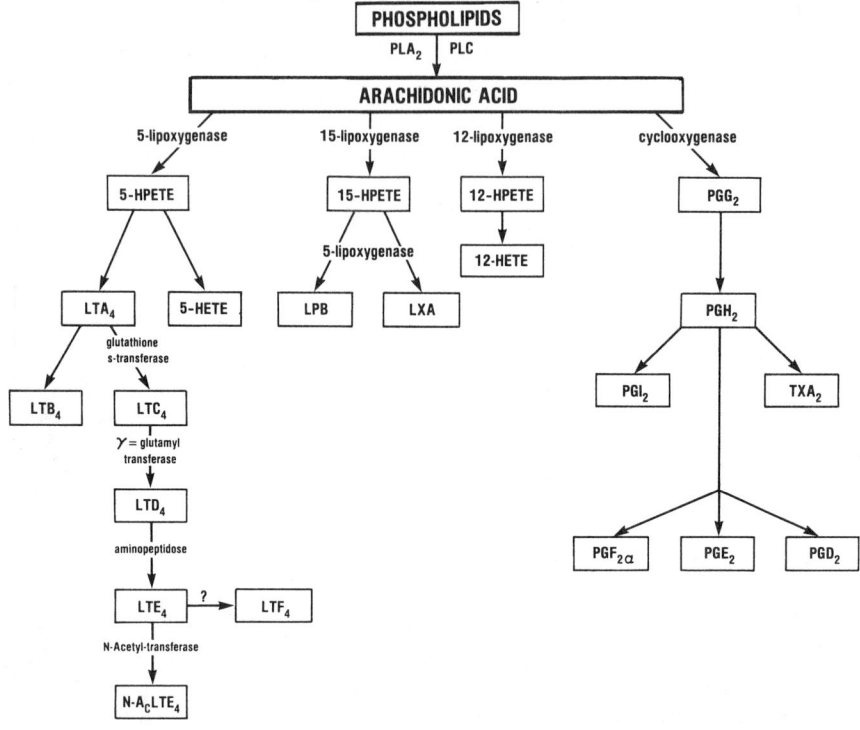

FIGURE 1. Arachidonate metabolism by lipoxygenase and cyclooxygenase pathways. LT = leukotrienes; LXA = lipoxin A; LPB = lipoxin B; PL = phospholipase; PG = prostaglandin.

an ischemic episode in the CNS has been termed "deteriorating stroke" or "stroke in evolution."[25] The pathophysiological and biochemical processes underlying this phenomenon are largely unknown, and only few attempts have been made to explore the mechanisms underlying delayed CNS deterioration after ischemia.

In recent years, a new model has been introduced, which allows us to study motor function in conscious animals exposed to spinal cord ischemia and reperfusion. This model features complete paralysis during the ischemia, which is followed by substantial recovery of hind limb motor function for several hours; then, a secondary deterioration phenomenon emerges with a progressive course of between 4 and 48 hrs after reperfusion. This model is reproducible and well characterized.[26,27] The purpose of the present review is to highlight the evidence raised in support of a role eicosanoids might have in mediation of some of the pathological consequences associated with delayed deterioration of motor function after spinal cord ischemia and reperfusion.

MATERIAL AND METHODS

Surgical Preparation

Male New Zealand albino rabbits (Hazleton Labs, York, PA) are anesthetized with 50 mg/kg im ketamine hydrochloride and 40 mg/kg iv sodium pentobarbital.

Under aseptic technique, a transperitoneal incision is made to expose the abdominal aorta, and 0.75-mm o.d. polyethylene tubing is placed around the aorta distal to the renal arteries and threaded through two 6.0-mm diameter plastic buttons dorsal and ventral to the aorta, to produce a snare ligature (FIG. 2). To prevent movement through the incision site, the ligature is passed through a 6.25-mm o.d. vinyl guide tube that is sutured to the abdominal muscles. A custom-made canvas jacket is then placed around the rabbit to protect the incision site and the externally accessible ligature.

Induction of Experimental Ischemia

Ischemia is induced in the spinal cord using a modification of the stroke model described by Zivin and De Girolami.[26] Approximately 18 hours after surgery, when the rabbits are awake, the aorta is occluded for 25 minutes by pulling on the snare ligature and clamping with a pair of hemostat forceps. Motor function is evaluated immediately after, and at 15 and 20 minutes after, occlusion. After occlusion, the ligature is released and removed with the guide tube through the surgical site. A retaining suture that was placed through the abdominal muscles at surgery is then secured. Neurologic scoring of hind limb motor function is performed at designated time points after reperfusion.[28]

Neurologic Examination

Hind limb motor function is graded at hourly intervals during the first 24 hours after occlusion. The following ordinal grading scale is used: 0, complete paralysis; 1, minimal functional movement, severe paresis; 2, functional movement, cannot hop; 3, hopping, ataxia, and paresis; 4, hopping, mild ataxia and/or paresis; and 5, normal.

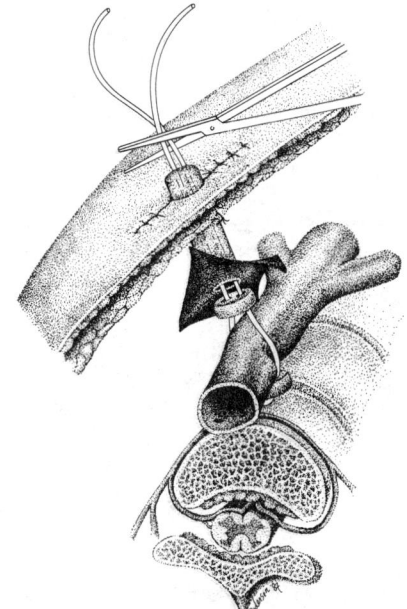

FIGURE 2. Schematic presentation of spinal cord ligature implantation for acute lumbar spinal cord occlusion.

Biochemical Measurements

At 5 and 30 minutes and 4, 18, and 24 hours after occlusion, rabbits were killed with 100 mg/kg i.v. sodium pentobarbital, and the spinal cord was rapidly (within 45 seconds) removed from the spinal canal. The lesion area was sliced and processed for eicosanoid analysis by freezing on dry ice and for analysis of edema by immersion in kerosene to prevent water evaporation.[29] The *de novo* release of the eicosanoids from the tissue was determined from 0.5–1.0 mm spinal cord slices incubated in oxygenated Krebs-Ringer (pH = 7.4). This method has previously been described in detail for brain tissue.[30,31] TXB_2 (the stable metabolite of TXA_2) and 6-keto-$PGF_{1\alpha}$ (the stable metabolite of PGI_2) were extracted from the spinal cord using a technique previously

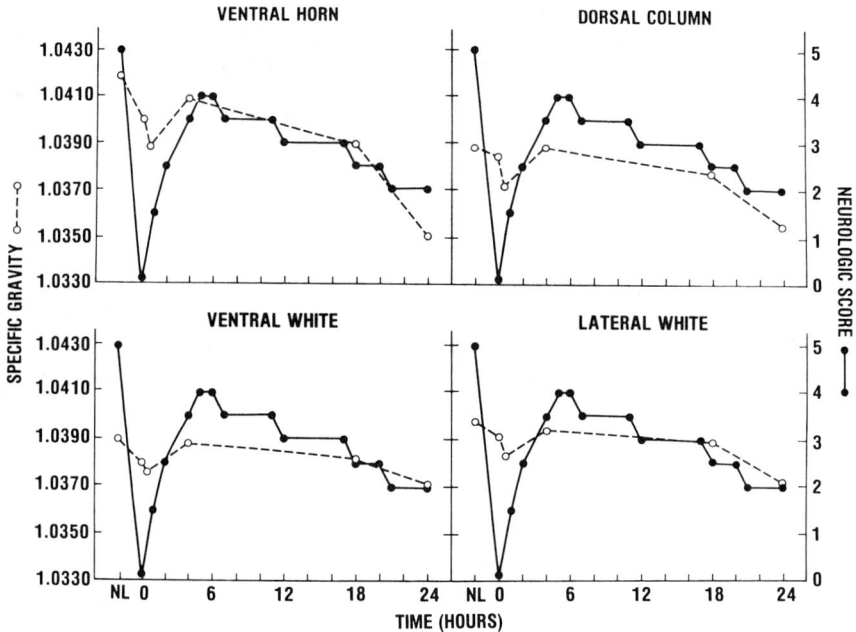

FIGURE 3. Motor function and tissue specific gravity in deteriorating stroke. O = edema; ● = motor function (neurological score); NL = normal. (From Jacobs *et al.*[28] Reprinted by permission from *Stroke*.)

described.[28] These metabolites, as well as 5-HETE released from *ex vivo* incubated spinal cord tissue were analyzed by RIA, as previously described in detail.[11,15,16,28] Tissue protein levels were determined by a standard Lowry method.

RESULTS

Motor Function

The functional results of 25 min of lumbar spinal cord ischemia followed by reperfusion are depicted in FIGURE 3. Soon after the onset of the ischemia, the hind

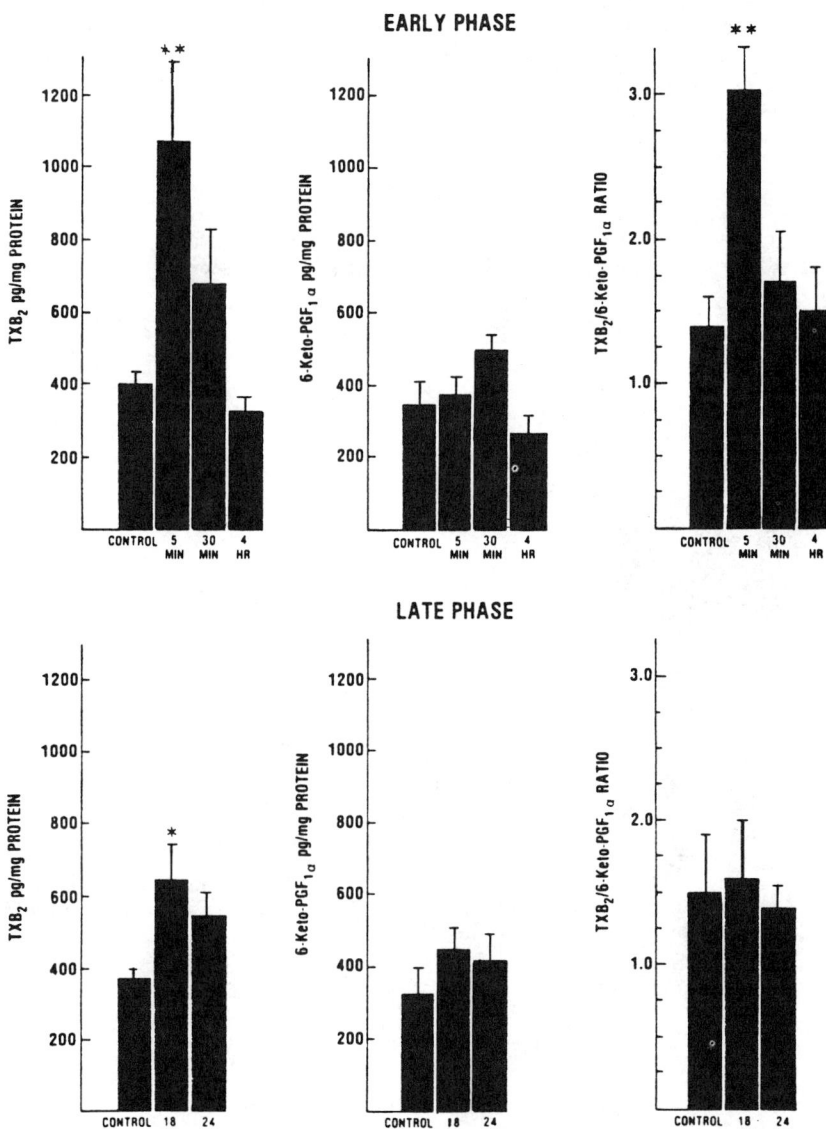

FIGURE 4. TXB_2 and 6-keto-$PGF_{1\alpha}$ in spinal cord tissue. The early phase represents the acute paralysis and recovery period. The late phase represents the secondary deterioration. *Asterisks* denote statistical significance by ANOVA and Dunnett's test. *: $p < 0.05$; **: $p < 0.01$. Six to eight animals were studied. (From Jacobs et al.[28] Reprinted by permission from *Stroke*.)

limb became completely paralyzed and remained so throughout the ischemia period. Upon reperfusion, progressive recovery of motor function is dependent on the duration of the ischemia; maximal recovery is stabilized 4–6 hrs after reperfusion. A secondary period of motor function deterioration then develops, with slow progression to final deficits, which are dependent on the duration of the initial insult. The prolonged ischemic period of 25 min results in a final complete paralysis 48 hrs after reperfusion.

Edema

The cascade of events seen in motor function are associated with similar changes in the spinal cord water content (FIG. 3). Edema formation was seen already 5 min after

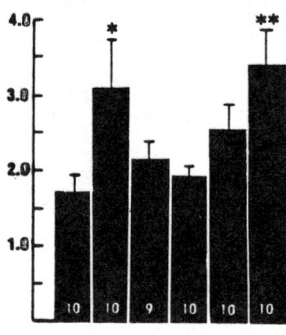

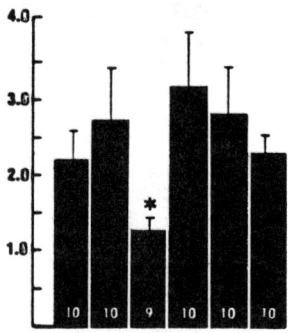

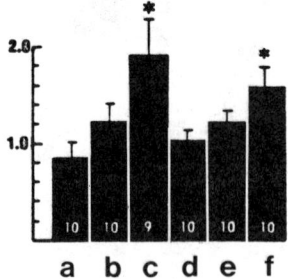

a b c d e f

FIGURE 5. Eicosanoid release from spinal cord slices *ex vivo* at (a) 0 min, (b) 5 min, (c) 30 min, (d) 4 h, (e) 18 h, and (f) 1 week after reperfusion. *Upper panel:* ng TXB_2/mg protein; *middle panel:* ng 6-keto $PGF_{1\alpha}$/mg protein; *lower panel:* ratio of TXB_2 to 6-keto $PGF_{1\alpha}$. Number of animals in each group is presented at the bottom of each column. *Asterisks* are as in FIGURE 4. (From Shohami *et al.*[15] Reprinted by permission from *Prostaglandin Leukotriene Medicine.*)

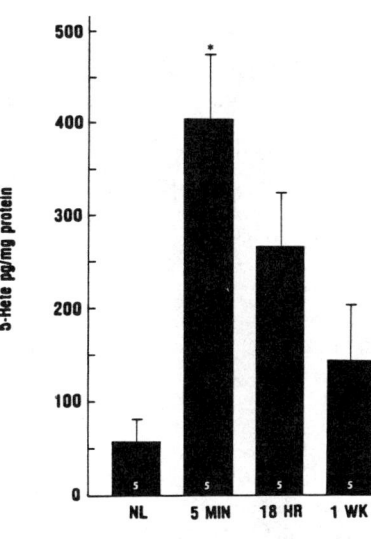

FIGURE 6. Release of 5-HETE from spinal cord slices incubated *ex vivo*. *Asterisks* denotes statistical significance at $p < 0.01$. Five rabbits were used in each time point. NL = normal. (From Shohami et al.[15] Reprinted by permission from *Prostaglandin Leukotriene Medicine*.)

reperfusion and was further developed at 30 min after reperfusion. Parallel to the functional recovery, the early water accumulation in the spinal cord regressed, and no significant edema was seen during the period of maximal recovery. The secondary motor deterioration was also accompanied by progressive development of a new phase of edema.

Eicosanoids in the Spinal Cord

FIGURE 4 demonstrates the levels of TXB_2 and 6-keto-$PGF_{1\alpha}$ extracted from the lumbar spinal cord at various time points after reperfusion. As early as 5 min after reperfusion, a large increase in tissue TXB_2 concentration was found; no change was observed in tissue 6-keto-$PGF_{1\alpha}$ at that time. Therefore, the ratio of TXB_2/6-keto-$PGF_{1\alpha}$ was greatly elevated at 5 min after reperfusion. During the later part of the reperfusion period (18 hrs after reperfusion), a second significant rise in the TXB_2 levels was found.

Eicosanoid release from spinal cord tissue incubated *ex vivo* is shown in FIGURE 5. Two major changes were clearly found: (1) marked increase in TXB_2, 5 min after reperfusion; (2) a late (18 hrs and 1 week later reperfusion) postreperfusion increase in TXB_2 release. A significant reduction in 6-keto-$PGF_{1\alpha}$ was also seen 30 min after reperfusion; overall, the TXB_2/6-keto-$PGF_{1\alpha}$ ratio was significantly elevated both early (30 min) and late (18 hrs and 1 week) after reperfusion. In addition, evidence for activation of the 5-lipoxygenase pathway immediately (5 min) and later (18 hrs) after reperfusion was also seen (FIG. 6).

DISCUSSION

The present review seeks to demonstrate that substantial perturbations in eicosanoid metabolism are not confined to the period immediately following reperfusion of ischemic CNS tissue, but are a complex and prolonged event.

Previous studies conducted in many species have shown that the rate of eicosanoid production within minutes of to a few hours after reperfusion of ischemic brain tissue is markedly elevated. However, only a few studies have examined eicosanoid metabolism after ischemia and reperfusion during subacute or chronic conditions. In gerbils, early increments in CNS eicosanoids shortly after reperfusion of the ischemic brain were reversed 24 hrs later; thus, the rates of PGD_2 and PGE_2 release (the two major prostanoids produced by the gerbil's brain) were markedly decreased (by more than 50%) in all brain areas examined (cortex, hypothalamus, striatum, and hippocampus). These changes seem to be selective for PGE_2 and PGD_2, since TXB_2 and 6-keto-$PGF_{1\alpha}$ did not change.[10]

In the present study 5-HETE and TXB_2 were found to be the major cyclooxygenase metabolites associated with spinal cord injury. Enhanced TXB_2 and 5-HETE production were found acutely after reperfusion of the spinal cord, subacutely (18 hrs later), and even at the chronic stage of the injury (1 week). The late changes in motor function, edema formation, and eicosanoid levels taken together support the hypothesis that these specific cylooxygenase metabolites of arachidonate might be involved in the propagation of spinal cord damage.

Although no cause-effect relationships can be drawn at the present time, the principal demonstration of lingering deranged eicosanoid metabolism deserves special attention. Of particular importance in this regard are the data obtained by the *ex vivo* incubation method. This method provides definite advantages over tissue level data for several reasons: (1) the *in situ* synthesis rate of the eicosanoids can be monitored in a discrete area; (2) tissue is prepared for incubation after several washes, which reduce the contribution of blood cells to eicosanoid production; (3) the eicosanoids and free arachidonate present in the tissue prior to incubation are washed out.

Therefore, the enhanced release of TXA_2 and 5-HETE indicates that a more permanent change in arachidonate metabolism—a change that is independent of the early accumulation of arachidonate during the ischemia—has been established after the ischemic insult. In which cellular element(s) the enhanced arachidonate metabolism takes place is unclear; it is also not known whether the early and late changes in arachidonate are derived from the same or different cell types. Yet, the distinct changes in 5-HETE and TXA_2 release could be associated with continuous proinflammatory processes underlying the late deterioration phenomenon.

REFERENCES

1. AVELDANO DE CALDISONI, M. I. & N. G. BAZAN. 1979. α-methyl-p-tyrosine inhibits the production of free arachidonic acid and diacylglycerols in brain after a single electroconvulsive shock. Neurochem. Res. **4:** 213–221.
2. BAZAN, N. G. 1970. Effect of ischemia and electroconvulsive shocks on free fatty acid pool in the brain. Biochim. Biophys. Acta **218:** 1–10.
3. BAZAN, N. G. 1971. Changes in free fatty acids of brain by drug induced convulsion, electroshock and anesthesia. J. Neurochem. **18:** 1379–1385.
4. BAZAN, N. G. & N. M. GIUSTO. 1983. Anoxia-induced production of methylated and free fatty acids in retina, cerebral cortex and white matter. Comparison with triglycerides and with other tissues. Neurochem. Pathol. **1:** 17–41.
5. REHNCRONA, S., E. WESTERNBERG, B. AKESSON & B. K. SIEJO. 1982. Brain cortical fatty acids and phospholipids during and following complete and severe incomplete ischemia. J. Neurochem. **38:** 84–93.
6. DEMEDIAK, P., R. D. SAUNDERS, D. K. ANDERSON, E. D. MEANS, & L. A. HORROCKS. 1985. Membrane lipid changes in laminectomized and traumatized cat spinal cord. Proc. Natl. Acad. Sci. USA **82:** 7071–7075.

7. RHOADS, D. E., L. D. OSBURN, N. A. PETERSON & E. RAGHUPATHY. 1983. Release of neurotransmitter amino-acids from synaptosomes: Enhancement of Ca^{+2}-independent afflux by oleic and arachidonic acid. J. Neurochem. **41:** 531–537.
8. YOSHIDA, S., K. ABE, R. BUSTO, B. D. WATSON, K. KOGURE & M. D. GINSBURG. 1982. Influence of transient ischemia on lipid-soluble antioxidants, free fatty acids and energy metabolites in rat brain. Brain Res. **245:** 307–316.
9. BAZAN, N. G., D. L. BIRKLE, W. TANG & T. SANJEEVA-REDDY. 1986. The accumulation of free arachidonic acid, diacylglyarols, prostaglandins and lipoxygenase reaction products in the brain during experimental epilepsy. Adv. Neurol. **44:** 879–902.
10. KEMPSKI, O., E. SHOHAMI, D. VON LUBITZ, J. M. HALLENBECK & G. FEUERSTEIN. 1987. Postischemic production of eicosanoids in Gerbil brain. Stroke **18:** 111–119.
11. GAUDET, R. J. & L. LEVINE. 1983. Transient cerebral ischemia and brain prostaglandins. Biochem. Biophys. Res. Commun. **86:** 893–901.
12. MOSKOVITZ, M., K. J. KIWAK, K. HEKIMIAN & L. LEVINE. 1986. Synthesis of compounds with properties of leukotriene C_4 and D_4 in gerbil brain after ischemia and reperfusion. Science **224:** 886–889.
13. WOLFE, L. S. & H. M. PAPPIUS. 1983. Involvement of arachidonic acid metabolites in functional disturbances following brain injury. Adv. Prostaglandins Thromboxane Leukotriene Res. **12:** 345–349.
14. ELLIS, E. F., K. F. WRIGHT, E. P. WEI & H. A. KONTOS. 1981. Hydrooxygenase products of arachidonic acid metabolism in cat cerebral cortex after experimental concussive brain injury. J. Neurochem. **37:** 892–896.
15. SHOHAMI, E., T. J. JACOBS, J. H. HALLENBECK & G. FEUERSTEIN. 1987. Increased thromboxane A_2 and 5-HETE production following spinal cord ischemia in the rabbit. Prostaglandin Leukotriene Med. **28:** 169–181.
16. JACOBS, T. P., E. SHOHAMI, W. BAZE, E. BURGARD, C. GUNDERSON, J. HALLENBECK & G. FEUERSTEIN. 1987. Thromboxane and 5-HETE increase after experimental spinal cord injury in rabbits. Cent. Nervous Syst. Trauma **4:** 95–117.
17. FEUERSTEIN, G. 1985. Autonomic pharmacology of leukotrienes. J. Autonomic Pharmacol. **5:** 149–168.
18. BLACK, K. L. 1984. Leukotriene C_4 induces vasogenic cerebral edema in rats. Prostaglandin Leukotriene Med. **14:** 339–340.
19. MONCADA, S. & J. P. VANE. 1979. Pharmacology and endogenous role of prostaglandin, thromboxane A_2 and prostacyclin. Pharmacol. Rev. **30:** 293–331.
20. KIMURA, H., K. OKAMOTO & Y. SAKAI. 1985. Modulatory effects of prostaglandins D_2, E_2, F_2 on the postsynaptic actions of inhibitory and excitatory amino-acid in cerebellar Purkinje cell dendrites in vitro. Brain Res. **330:** 235–244.
21. KELLER, M., R. JACKISCH, A. SEREGI & G. HERTTING. 1985. Comparison of prostanoid forming capacity of neuronal and astroglial cells in primary cultures. Biochem. Int. **7:** 655–665.
22. HALLENBECK, J. M. & T. W. FURLOW. 1979. Prostaglandin I_2 and indomethacin prevent impairment of post-ischemic brain reperfusion in the dog. Stroke **10:** 629–637.
23. AWAD, I., J. R. LITTLE, F. LUCAS, V. SHRINSKA, R. SLUGG & R. P. LESSER. 1983. Treatment of acute local cerebral ischemia with prostacyclin. Stroke **14:** 203–209.
24. SEREGI, A., U. FORSTERMANN & G. HERTTING. 1984. Decreased levels of brain cyclooxygenase products as a possible cause of increased seizure susceptibility in convulsion-prone gerbils. Brain Res. **305:** 393–395.
25. HACHINSKI, V. C. & J. W. NORRIS. 1980. The deteriorating stroke. In Cerebral Vascular Disease, Vol. 3. J. S. Meyer, H. Lechner, M. Reivich & A. Aranibar, Eds.: 113. Excerpta Medica. Amsterdam.
26. ZIVIN, J. A. & U. DE GIROLAMI. 1980. Spinal cord infarction: A highly reproducible stroke model. Stroke **11:** 200–202.
27. DE GIROLAMI, U. & J. A. ZIVIN. 1982. Neuropathology of experimental spinal cord ischemia in the rabbit. J. Neuropathol. Exp. Neurol. **41:** 129–149.
28. JACOBS, T., E. SHOHAMI, W. BAZE, E. BURGARD, C. GUNDERSON, J. M. HALLENBECK & G. FEUERSTEIN. 1987. Deteriorating stroke model: Histopathology, edema and eicosanoid changes following spinal-cord ischemia stroke. Stroke **18:** 741–750.

29. MARMAROU, A., W. POLL, K. SHULMAN & H. BHARGARAN. 1978. A simple gravimetric technique for measurement of cerebral edema. J. Neurosurg. **49:** 530–537.
30. SHOHAMI, E. & J. GROSS. 1985. An ex-vivo method for evaluating prostaglandin synthetase activity in cortical slices of mouse brain. J. Neurochem. **45:** 132–136.
31. WOLFE, L. S., K. LOSTOWOROWSKI & H. M. PAPPIUS. 1976. The endogenous biosynthesis of prostaglandins by brain tissue in vitro. Can. J. Biochem. **54:** 629–640.

PART V. ARACHIDONIC ACID METABOLISM
AND CONVULSIVE DISORDERS

Arachidonic Acid Metabolism in Seizures

BO K. SIESJÖ, CARL-DAVID AGARDH,
FINN BENGTSSON, AND MAJ-LIS SMITH

Laboratory for Experimental Brain Research
University of Lund
S-221 85 Lund, Sweden

It has been known for almost 20 years that seizures due to electroshock or convulsants are associated with an accumulation of free fatty acids (FFAs) in the brain, particularly of arachidonic (AA, 20:4) and stearic acid (18:0). The original work came from the laboratory of Nicolas Bazan,[1-4] who, as will be discussed later, is also responsible for a substantial part of the subsequent development in the field.

These early observations were soon confirmed and extended, and it was established that the accumulation of 20:4 was accompanied by the formation of its cyclooxygenase and lipoxygenase products[5-9] (for further literature, see Ref. 9). Other work showed that the FFAs and their oxidation products accumulated as a result of seizure activity per se, and not because of accompanying hypoxia.[10-12] Finally, it has become increasingly clear that a substantial part of the FFAs accumulating during seizures, particularly in the initial seizure period, emanates from inositol phospholipids enriched in 20:4 and 18:0. This was suspected on grounds that seizures caused the accumulation of diacylglycerol (DAG) with that FFA composition,[3,13] and more directly shown in experiments in which short-lasting seizures were found to cause rapid breakdown of phosphatidylinositol bisphosphate (PIP_2).[14] Although such findings suggest that activation of phospholipase C is a prominent cause of the accumulation of FFAs in seizures, a significant contribution from phospholipase A_2 cannot be excluded, particularly during more long-lasting seizures. This raises the questions of the extent to which the enhanced arachidonic acid metabolism reflects stimulation of receptors coupled to phospholipase C, and of the contribution of increased cytosolic calcium concentrations (Ca_i^{2+}).

In the present article we will begin by considering FFA accumulation during ischemia and hypoglycemia. The purpose of this comparison is to provide information on rates of FFA accumulation in situations in which receptor stimulation of phospholipase C and a rise in Ca_i^{2+} are coupled to ATP failure, the latter preventing reacylation of lysophospholipids and resynthesis of phospholipids. We will then turn to corresponding events during seizures, asking whether energy failure is at all involved and whether a rise in Ca_i^{2+} seems likely. This discussion leads to another question: what information is there on the role played by receptor stimulation? Furthermore, why are the FFA levels decreasing during continuous seizures following their abrupt accumulation at seizure onset? Finally, we will address the possibility that accumulation of AA and its continuous oxidation to potentially toxic substances contribute to the neuronal damage incurred after long-lasting seizures.

PHOSPHOLIPIDS AND FREE FATTY ACIDS DURING ISCHEMIA AND HYPOGLYCEMIA

Complete or near-complete ischemia leads to a progressive rise in brain FFA concentrations, with AA concentration showing the largest relative increase.[1,3] After 30 min of ischemia total FFA content is about 1.2 mM · kg^{-1} and AA concentration about 0.4 mM · kg^{-1}.[15,16] Three further points should be recalled. First, release of FFAs occur already within the first minute of anoxia, when 18:0 and 20:4 accumulate.[17] Second, although the concentrations of most phospholipids remain unchanged during even long-lasting ischemia,[16,18] the concentrations of PIP$_2$ and phosphatidylinositol phosphate (PIP) are reduced.[17,19] Third, recirculation is accompanied by a gradual but still relatively rapid disappearance of accumulated FFAs.[16,18,20,21]

Events during ischemia can be schematically illustrated as shown in FIGURE 1, which summarizes current knowledge on phospholipid turnover. Two major reactions are shown as causing phospholipid breakdown, catalyzed by phospholipase C and A$_2$, respectively. The first is shown as encompassing breakdown of phosphatidylinositols, exemplified by the breakdown of PIP$_2$ to DAG and inositol triphosphate (IP$_3$). The

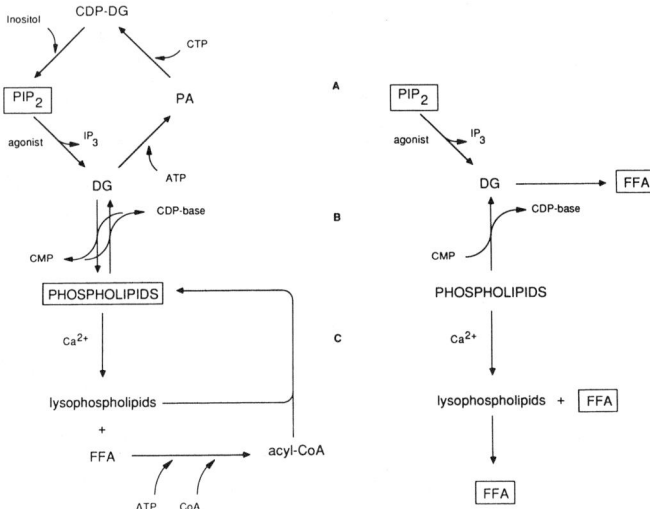

FIGURE 1. The main phospholipid turnover pathways in the brain under normal (*left*) and ischemic (*right*) conditions. *Left panel*, **A:** The agonist-stimulated breakdown of phosphatidylinositols, exemplified by the breakdown of phosphatidylinositol-4'-5'-bisphosphate (PIP$_2$) energy-dependent resynthesis by phosphorylation to phosphatidic acid (PA) and further to CDP-diglyceride (CDP-DG). IP$_3$ = inositol triphosphate. *Left panel*, **B:** The base exchange reaction. The direction of this reaction is highly dependent on the concentrations of the reactants CMP and CDP-bases. *Left panel*, **C:** The Ca^{2+}-triggered breakdown of phospholipids to lysophospholipids and free fatty acid (FFA), and the ATP-dependent reacylation of lysophospholipids. CDP, CMP = cytidine di- and monophosphate, respectively. *Right panel:* Under ischemic conditions, the anabolic pathways are inhibited. The release of transmitters will trigger PIP$_2$ breakdown to DG and FFA, and Ca^{2+} influx into cells causes phospholipid degradation to lysophospholipids and FFAs. In addition, the increased CMP levels will drive the base exchange reaction with phospholipid breakdown to DG and further to FFAs.

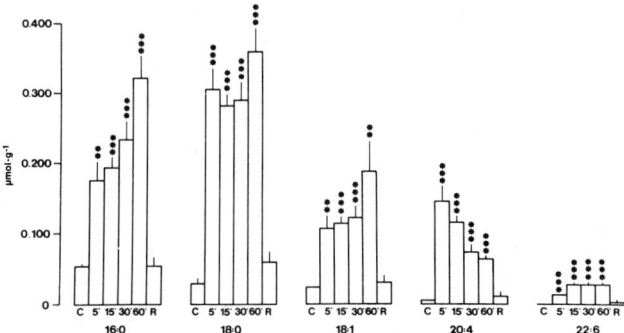

FIGURE 2. Cortical free fatty acid concentrations in hypoglycemia (16:0, palmitic acid; 18:0 stearic acid; 18:1, oleic acid; 20:4, arachidonic acid; 22:6, docosahexenoic acid) in control (C) and experimental groups with an isoelectric EEG for 5 to 60 min and after 90 min of recovery following an isoelectric period of 30 min (R). Values are means ± SEM, μmol · g^{-1} wet tissue weight. **, ***, significant increase in experimental group compared with control group ($p < 0.01$ and $p < 0.001$, respectively, Student's t-test). (From Agardh et al.[25] Reprinted by permission from *Journal of Neurochemistry*.)

second reaction is shown as causing hydrolysis of other phospholipids to the corresponding lysocompounds and FFAs. The two cycles are interconnected by a reversible reaction for base exchange that involves CMP/CDP. As the figure recalls, reacylation of lysophospholipids and resynthesis of the phospholipids require ATP, either as such or in the form of CTP. Clearly, when ischemia causes ATP depletion, it opens the loops and allows hydrolysis of phospholipids without a corresponding resynthesis. Thus, lack of ATP per se can cause FFAs to accumulate due to the continued activity of available lipases, which encompass DAG lipases and lysophospholipases. However, since phospholipase C is activated by a number of neurotransmitters, neuromodulators, and growth factors and requires calcium, and since phospholipase A_2 is activated by calcium, it seems likely that breakdown of phospholipids is enhanced. Thus, ischemia is accompanied by a massive release of transmitters from presynaptic endings (e.g., Ref. 22) and by cellular uptake of calcium (see Ref. 23). It should be emphasized, though, that the initial accumulation of FFAs (see Ref. 17) seems to occur before neurons depolarize and calcium disappears from extracellular fluid (ECF). Since ATP may be depleted at critical sites already within 30–60 sec of anoxia,[17,24] failure of reacylation of lysophospholipids and resynthesis of phospholipids due to ATP shortage may contribute substantially to the initial accumulation of FFAs.

Hypoglycemia also leads to marked accumulation of FFAs in brain tissues,[25] and this accumulation is known to occur when depolarization and energy failure mark the beginning of the period of "coma."[26] The pattern of changes observed in individual FFAs is shown in FIGURE 2. This pattern is not very different from that observed in ischemia. However, hypoglycemia differs from ischemia in three important respects, since (1) blood flow and, therefore, oxygen supply are upheld; (2) some ATP (about 15–25%) remains; and (3) glucose supply is critically reduced, forcing the tissue to oxidize endogenous compounds to maintain energy production.[25,27,28] Continued reacylation/resynthesis, oxidation, and transport may contribute to curtail the rise in FFA concentrations, to lower the AA concentration following the initial rise, and to lower

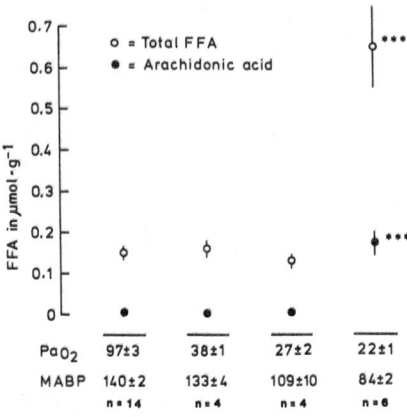

FIGURE 3. The effect of graded hypoxia (PaO_2; mm Hg) and hypotension (mean aortic blood pressure, MABP; mm Hg) upon total FFA content and AA concentration in cortical tissue. *** = $p < 0.05$. Values are means ± SEM.

the total phospholipid-bound FFA pool by 8–10%.[25] Thus, one may envisage that FFA concentrations in hypoglycemia remain lower than in ischemia either because FFAs are oxidized or leave the tissue via the blood, or because some reacylation/resynthesis occurs. One or several of these factors should be operating, since the decrease in Ca^{2+}_e is as extensive as in ischemia,[29,30] and since massive release of neurotransmitters occurs at the onset of coma onset.[31,32] Thus, stimulation of phospholipase activity is probably extensive.

The experiments quoted raise the question about the role energy failure plays in causing FFAs to accumulate. This issue is also pertinent to the question of whether hypoxia contributes to FFA accumulation during seizures. Gardiner et al.,[33] who gradually reduced arterial PO_2 in steps in ventilated animals, failed to record any increase in cerebral cortical FFA and AA concentrations unless a very low PO_2 level was combined with hypotension (FIG. 3). At that point, EEG showed a burst-suppression pattern or overt flattening, and tissue ATP values were reduced. Thus, in the absence of seizure discharges, marked perturbation of phospholipid metabolism and accumulation of FFAs are observed only in hypoxia/ischemia and hypoglycemia of sufficient severity to cause energy failure and membrane depolarization.

PHOSPHOLIPID AND FREE FATTY ACID METABOLISM IN SEIZURES

Changes in arachidonic acid metabolism have been extensively mapped in seizure states. Our discussion will be centered on long-lasting seizures induced in ventilated animals, and on brief seizures induced by electroshock.

Changes in Free Fatty Acids and Phospholipids during Seizures

FIGURE 4 illustrates changes in total FFA and AA concentrations in the neocortex of ventilated rats in which seizures were induced by an intravenous injection of bicuculline.[11] The results demonstrate (1) that total FFAs increase precipitously during the first 5 min of seizures, remain elevated for 20–30 min, and then decrease to a level of about 150% of control; (2) that 18:0 and 20:4 are responsible for the major share of the increase; and (3) that AA concentration peaks at 1 min, with a gradual return towards normal thereafter. However, as the figure shows, both total FFA content and AA concentration were elevated above normal after seizures for 2 hours.

In this context, we wish to recall some additional findings. First, the concentrations of total and individual phospholipid-bound fatty acids, and the phospholipid phosphorous, did not change at any time points during seizures.[11] Later it was shown that short-lasting seizures reduce the tissue content of a single phospholipid (PIP_2), suggesting that measurable changes in phospholipid content are observed only in polyphosphoinositides (see below). Second, the changes in FFAs seem related to the degree of increase of metabolic rate during seizures, since similar changes were observed in the neocortex and hippocampus—two hypermetabolic structures—and since very moderate changes were seen in the cerebellum, a structure that is electrically and metabolically relatively quiescent during seizures[11] (see also Ref. 34). Interestingly, only AA showed a significant (and transient) increase in the cerebellum. Third, similar changes in FFAs have been demonstrated in seizures induced by pentylenetetrazole, suggesting that it is the seizure discharges per se that are important, not the type of convulsant.[35]

As stated, early studies by Bazan and coworkers showed transient increases in FFAs and DAG after electroshock. Recent studies corroborate these findings, demonstrating increased lipolysis after only 5 s of seizure discharge, and establish that PIP_2

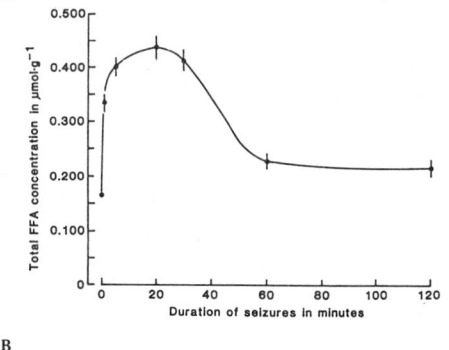
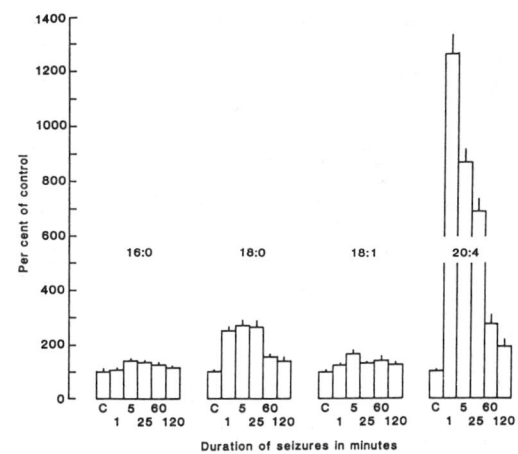

FIGURE 4. Time-dependent cortical changes in total FFA content (A) and individual FFA concentration (B) during continuous biculline-induced seizures of 1–120 min duration. The values are means ± SEM. C = control. (From Siesjö et al.[11] Reprinted by permission from *Journal of Neurochemistry*.)

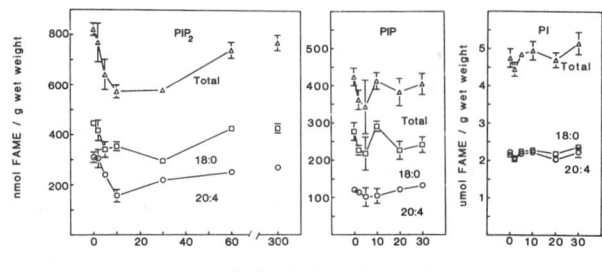

FIGURE 5. Changes in the total mass and in the levels of stearate and arachidonate in brain inositol phospholipids after electroconvulsive shock. FAME = fatty acid methyl esters. Data points are the average ± SD of 4 to 8 samples, each composed of one rat brain. For total PIP_2 in 18:0 and 20:4 at 5- and 10-s time points, $p < 0.05$ and < 0.01, respectively. (From Reddy and Bazan.[14] Reprinted by permission from *Neuroscience Research*.)

concentration falls as a result of seizure discharge (FIG. 5). The data emphasize the rapid breakdown and resynthesis of this phospholipid, and suggest that seizures cause rapid activation of phospholipase C (see below). In this context, it should be recalled that there is an endogenous asymmetry in FFA and DAG metabolism in the two hemispheres, both under normal conditions and during induced electroshock seizures.[36,37] Probably, such an asymmetrical behavior is related to differences in phospholipid composition and distribution, such differences probably correlating to lateralization of function.

Triggering Events

In discussing what triggers phospholipid hydrolysis during seizures, it seems justified to recall the density of energy failure during ischemia, hypoglycemia, and status epilepticus, and to relate the reduction in energy charge to the amounts of FFAs and AA accumulated (FIG. 6).

Changes in labile energy metabolites during seizures induced by bicuculline or other convulsants have been extensively characterized.[35,38–40] When animals are artificially ventilated, the initial perturbation in cerebral energy state is small (see FIG. 6). During continued seizures, the energy charge is maintained close to control, and the only conspicuous change is a sustained reduction in phosphocreatine (PCr) content to about 50–70% of control. However, this is probably caused by reduction in intracellular pH due to accumulation of lactate plus H^+, which shifts the creatine kinase reaction in the direction of PCr hydrolysis.[11,39]

Clearly, whole tissue analysis of labile metabolites cannot exclude the possibility of a larger fall in ATP content at critical loci. However, the very moderate perturbation of the overall energy state, the ongoing synthesis of glycogen and glutamine (see Ref. 39), and the paucity of damaged neurons after 2 hrs of continued seizures,[41] suggest that ATP failure is not at hand. It does not seem likely, therefore, that shortage of ATP (and CTP) can be responsible for the accumulation of FFAs during seizures. An explanation more likely than energy insufficiency, and probably than decreased elimination from the brain, is that FFAs accumulate because phospholipase A_2 and/or C are activated to an extent that is beyond the capacity of the reacylation/resynthesis pathways. One likely activator is calcium. Thus, electrical stimulation and induced seizure activity reduce Ca_e^{2+}, suggesting that voltage-dependent and/or agonist-activated calcium channels are opened, causing Ca_i^{2+} to rise.[42-44] This assumption is supported by results suggesting that sustained seizure activity causes sequestration of calcium in mitochondria of dendrites, among other structures.[45]

As discussed elsewhere,[14,34,46] seizures may cause accumulation of DAG and FFAs by one of two mechanisms. The first mechanism is a sequential series of reactions in which the phosphodiesteric cleavage of polyphosphoinositides is coupled to release of FFAs from DAG by diacyl- and monoacylglyceride lipases. This mechanism, which is very likely involved in the initial phases of the seizure discharge, would thus represent lipolysis caused by stimulation of receptors coupled to phospholipase C. The second mechanism is one in which phospholipase A_2 is activated as well. For example, one could envisage that intracellular release of Ca^{2+}, triggered by IP_3, leads to activation of phospholipase A_2, which then becomes responsible for at least part of the accumulation of FFAs. We recognize that with such activation some DAG may arise from a reversal of the reaction catalyzed by choline phosphotransferase.[47,48]

There is circumstantial evidence that seizures cause prompt stimulation of phospholipase C. As already mentioned, electroshock is accompanied by breakdown of PIP_2 and by accumulation of DAG and FFAs enriched in 20:4 and 18:0, the predominant fatty acids of phosphatidylinositols.[49] Other indirect evidence hints in the same direction. This evidence is based on the coupling of PIP_2 hydrolysis to DAG stimulation of protein kinase C and the subsequent activation of the Na^+/H^+ antiporter by the protein kinase.[50] As FIGURE 7 shows, the onset of seizure discharge is followed by a rapid reduction in extracellular pH (pH_e). Since this acidification is larger (and faster) than what can be accounted for by lactic acid production (FIG. 7)

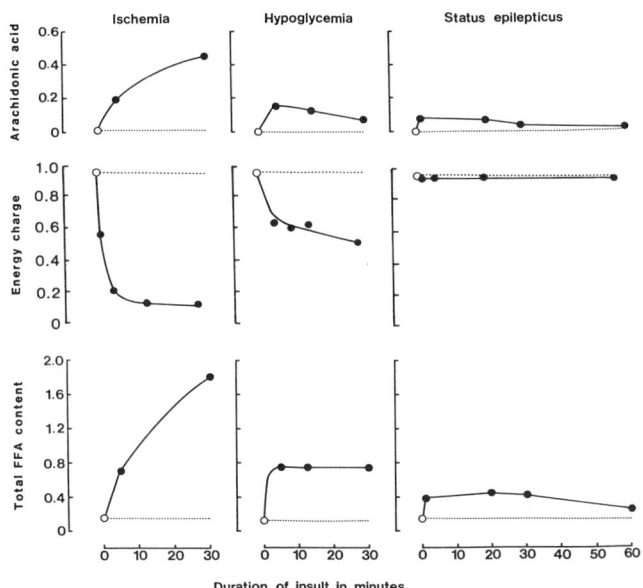

FIGURE 6. Changes in AA (μmol · g^{-1}) (top), energy charge ([ATP + 0.5 ADP]/[ATP + ADP + AMP]) (middle) and total FFA (μmol · g^{-1}) content (bottom) during 30 min of ischemia (left) and hypoglycemia (middle) and during 60 min of status epilepticus (right).

and transport, it seems likely that protein kinase C is activated. This conclusion is supported by results demonstrating that interruption of seizure discharge leads not only to a rapid return of pH_i to normal, but also to intracellular alkalinization.[51] It is tempting to speculate, therefore, that seizures lead to sustained stimulation of receptors coupled to phospholipase C and protein kinase C. However, it has become increasingly evident that receptor stimulation can cause activation of phospholipase A_2 as well.[52] Recognizing that seizures probably activate both phospholipase C and A_2, we will probe into seizure-related alterations in neuromodulators.

Seizures, Neuromodulators, and Arachidonic Acid

A rapidly increasing bulk of information on alterations in various neuromodulator concentrations, metabolism and/or release, and function concomitant with seizures is developing. This will briefly be commented upon, with particular focus on changes that could relate to arachidonic acid.

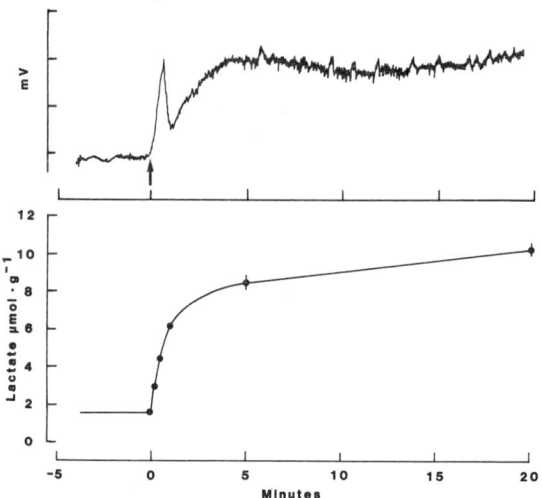

FIGURE 7. *Upper panel* shows one representative cortical extracellular pH recording during seizures of 20-min duration. Note the initial rapid acidification at the onset of seizures (*arrow*), followed by partial recovery and attainment of stable acidosis after 5 min. Scale on the left gives electrode output in mV (the distance between two bars is 10 mV or ~0.17 pH units). *Lower panel* gives the corresponding cortical lactate concentrations (values are means ± SEM).

It must be recalled that the amino acid neuromodulators are the most universal transmitters, as far as neurons or the terminals that release them in the brain are concerned.[53] In addition, they are most consistent in their postsynaptic effects: the neutral amino acid γ-aminobutyric acid (GABA), for example, is universally inhibitory,[54] and the dicarboxylic amino acids aspartate and glutamate are universally excitatory.[55] Conversely, the monoamines (serotonin; 5-HT, dopamine; DA and noradrenaline; NA) and acetylcholine (ACh), are restricted to a very limited number of neurons, where the postsynaptic effects vary with location and presence of other excitatory or inhibitory inputs.[56,57] It is likely that ACh, similarly with the excitatory amino acids and in contrast to the monoamines, is a transmitter used by a significant population of intrinsic cortical neurons.[58] The major transmitter of cortical neurons, however, is GABA, which accounts for at least 30% of the cortical neuronal population.[53] The broad class of mostly cortically localized neuropeptides (approximately 5-10% of the cortical neurons) might be interneuronlike and tentatively inhibitory,[53,59,60] but many of these peptidergic terminals appear to make nonconventional synapses. Their possible role of indirectly regulating "classical" transmitters over a wide brain area[61,62] might be important in seizures, but this as yet unproven.[63]

There is a large body of evidence suggesting that postsynaptic GABA-mediated inhibition plays an important role in epilepsy.[64] It has been suggested that a local decline in GABAergic cortical interneurons and/or of their axon terminals on pyramidal cells occurs,[65] and that intact, primarily cortical GABAergic inhibition is important in diminishing the effect of augmented afferent activity and preventing pathologically enhanced output in seizures.[64] (Antiseizure activity has been reported by treatment with liposome-entrapped GABA, whereas this effect was not observed for GABA itself or phosphatidylserine injections to isoniazid-induced epileptogenic bursts in rats.[66])

It seems likely that epileptic discharges could be maintained by an increased presynaptic release of excitatory transmitters such as aspartate and glutamate. In seizures, where the energy state and metabolic rate are sustained and increased 2- to 3-fold, respectively, the neurotransmitter metabolism and other energy-requiring events in neurotransmission are available. Taken together several lines of evidence suggest that excitatory transmission mediated by dicarboxylic amino acids appears to play a role in epileptiform activity in many animal models generated at different CNS levels, cortical to spinal.[64] One most likely mechanism in relation to GABA is that seizures induced by deficiency in GABA transmission result, at least in part, from the relative overactivity of excitatory amino acids on postsynaptic receptors in different brain regions.[67-69]

The ACh and choline levels in rat brain regions immediately increased greatly in status epilepticus induced by lithium and pilocarpine, and therefore increased ACh activity has been implicated in epileptogenesis.[70] While alterations in DAergic activity seems to be of minor importance in seizures, at least regional increases in 5-HT turnover and activity have been reported during the initial phase of bicuculline-induced seizures.[71] Multiple observations suggest that the NAergic system is involved in seizures, and there might be, as well, a possible connection to arachidonic acid. Repeated electroshock seizures are known to raise tissue NA levels and increase the turnover of the neurotransmitter.[72] Bicuculline-induced seizures lead to a sustained decrease in tissue NA content, and since the rate of tyrosine decarboxylation is increased, the NA turnover and release seem markedly enhanced.[71] This enhanced NA activity is probably important in controlling the spread of seizure activity.[73-75] These and other results suggest that epileptiform activity is curbed by NA, which exerts a cAMP-mediated inhibitory effect at β-adrenergic receptors (see Ref. 76). Experiments with lesions of the NA-system originating in the locus ceruleus demonstrate that at least part of the rise in cAMP during seizures, and the associated breakdown of glycogen, is due to activation of such receptors.[76]

The question early arose whether the accumulation of DAG and FFAs was related to enhanced activity at synapses such as the NA system originating in the locus ceruleus. Aveldano de Caldironi and Bazan[77] reported that α-methyl-p-tyrosine (α-MT) pretreatment of mice virtually prevented the increase in DAG and FFAs following a single electroshock seizure. A subsequent study on rats with bilateral locus ceruleus lesions showed that although tissue NA levels were reduced to <5% of control, the rise in FFA concentrations during bicuculline-induced seizures of 5 min duration was not reduced.[76] Similar results were reported by Rodriguez de Turco et al.[34] in rats pretreated with α-MT. However, these authors found that the drug inhibited the production of stearoyl- and arachidonoyl-DG in both the cerebrum and cerebellum. These results suggest that stimulation of adrenergic receptors could cause activation of phospholipase C, and could thus be responsible for at least part of the DAG production.

It is known that cholinergic agonists stimulate neuronal receptors coupled to phospholipase C[50,78]; now evidence hints that excitatory amino acids play a similar role.[79,80] However, there is no evidence at present that links these agonist-receptor interactions to changes in phospholipids and FFAs during seizures. This means that evidence for the very likely connection between receptor activation and phospholipase activity is circumstantial.

What Attenuates Accumulation of Free Fatty Acids during Sustained Seizures?

The results reviewed above (see Fig. 4) demonstrate that the total FFA content decreases after 20–30 min of seizure activity, while the AA concentration falls continuously after the first min of seizure activity. The reason for this adaptation is not known. Sustained bicuculline-induced seizures give rise to an equally sustained increase in cerebral oxygen and glucose consumption.[81-83] We will assume that brain-to-blood transport is not responsible. It is, therefore, necessary to postulate that the stimulus to FFA and AA release is attenuated in spite of the continued seizures, or that reacylation of lysocompounds is enhanced. A third alternative, that AA concentrations fall because the fatty acid is utilized by cyclooxygenase and lipoxygenase, appears less likely, since the maximal rates of these enzymes are small compared to the rate of AA disappearance.[11]

There is no evidence that allows us to decide which of these alternatives applies. It is tempting to speculate that one or several receptors, coupled to phospholipase A_2 or C, are down-regulated during continued seizures. Some evidence for this is provided by data on cAMP that demonstrate a precipitous rise of cAMP concentration at seizure onset, with subsequent normalization.[84] However, we do not know if the time course of changes in cAMP and FFA concentrations are closely related. It also seems clear from data on metabolic rate that down-regulation of other receptors may not occur, and it is of interest that cGMP concentrations remain elevated during sustained seizures. Evidently, it remains to be established why FFA concentrations fall during continued seizures, stabilizing at values of around 150% of control.

Epileptic Brain Damage and Arachidonic Acid Metabolism

Sustained seizures give rise to neuronal damage localized to selectively vulnerable regions such as the neocortex, the hippocampus, and the thalamus.[85,86] Evaluation of the density and localization of such damage was greatly facilitated by the advent of a long-term recovery model of status epilepticus in rats.[87] Data obtained with this model demonstrate that 2 hours of status epilepticus gives sparse damage to neurons in the neocortex (layers 3–4), hippocampus (CA1 sector), and thalamus (ventromedial nucleus), and, surprisingly, to dense necrosis in the substantia nigra, pars reticulata (SNPR), and globus pallidus.[87]

Previous studies of more localized epileptiform discharges,[88] or of long-term stimulation of pathways projecting to the hippocampus,[89] have clearly shown that continuous synaptic bombardment causes necrosis of postsynaptic neurons. It has been speculated that the lesions observed are caused by an excitotoxic mechanism in which release of glutamate or a related excitatory amino acid is involved.[45,88,90] Part of the evidence rests on the presence of dendrosomatic axon-sparing lesions, with early damage to dendritic structures that are presumed to contain a high density of

TABLE 1. Cerebral Cortical Concentrations of Reduced (GSH) and Oxidized (GSSG) Glutathione after 2 Hours of Bicuculline-induced Status Epilepticus

Experimental Group (n)	GSH μmol · g^{-1}	GSSG μmol · g^{-1}	% GSSG
Controls (6)	2.27 ± .02	0.0080 ± .0004	0.35 ± .02
Seizures (6)	2.29 ± .066	0.0086 ± .0003	0.38 ± .01

NOTE: The values are means ± SEM.

glutamate receptors, particularly of the N-methyl-D-aspartate (NMDA) type. It has recently been shown that the cortical and hippocampal lesions observed in fluorothyl-induced status epilepticus have similar characteristics, and it was speculated that the distribution of the lesions coincides with that of the NMDA receptors. It is also of interest that a similar distribution has been described for receptor sites coupled to IP$_3$ and protein kinase C.[91,92] However, since excitatory amino acids have been shown to stimulate receptors coupled to phospholipase C, it is tempting to speculate that epileptic neuronal necrosis occurs because overstimulation of such receptors causes breakdown of intracellular homeostasis. However, it is premature to speculate that such tight links exist between overstimulation of a particular type of receptor and epileptic cell damage. Furthermore, although the dense necrosis of the SNPR is preceded by gross swelling of dendrites, the lesion is not of the axon-sparing type, which suggests a somewhat different pathogenesis.[93,94]

It has been assumed that epileptic brain damage is caused by toxic breakdown products of AA.[3,46] In theory, such damage can be vascular, or it can affect neurons by mechanisms more related to functional than to circulatory aberrations. Some vascular damage seems likely following prolonged seizures, since flow rates decrease in spite of metabolic rates of sustained elevation.[81,83,95] However, the localization of epileptic brain damage to certain functional groups of neurons, with neighboring neurons being preserved, argues against vascular factors playing a decisive role. Furthermore, prolonged seizures do not give rise to deterioration of the cerebral energy state, hence oxygenation appears adequate to meet the functional demands. In fact, it has sometimes been emphasized that epileptic seizures represent an oxidative stress to the tissue, and the possibility remains that free radical reactions are involved. There is no indication, though, that products of free radical reactions accumulate and whole tissue (cortical) concentrations of reduced and oxidized glutathione (GSH and GSSG) remain unaltered (TABLE 1).

Why, then, does neuronal necrosis occur? It appears likely that the postsynaptic damage observed is the result of excessive and prolonged release of excitatory neurotransmitters (e.g., glutamate). FIGURE 8 illustrates the presumed ionic events that are triggered by glutamate at two types of receptors, selectively activated by

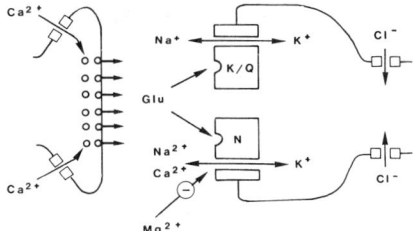

FIGURE 8. Schematic diagram illustrating agonist-operated channels. Presynaptic Ca^{2+} influx is followed by synaptic transmitter release. Postsynaptic agonist-operated channels are activated by either glutamate or a related amino acid. These channels have been assumed to be gated by kainate/quisqualate (K/Q) or by NMDA (N) receptors. Normally, only the latter is supposed to open a conductance for Ca^{2+}.

Kainate/Quisqualate and by NMDA. At the former receptor activation causes Na^+ influx, which, when coupled to Cl^- influx via separate conductance channels, leads to dendritic swelling.[96-98] The NMDA receptor, on the other hand, is believed to open a conductance for calcium (for literature and further discussion, see Refs. 99, 100). In support of this theory, qualitative visualization of calcium by the pyriantimonate technique demonstrates mitochondrial precipitates in dendrites during prolonged seizures.[45]

It has been shown *in vitro* that the toxic effects of glutamate and other NMDA agonists are mediated by calcium[101,102] (see also Ref. 98). It appears likely, therefore, that the dendritic damage and subsequent neuronal necrosis that are incurred after long periods of epileptic seizures are linked to a disturbed intracellular calcium homeostasis. The molecular mechanisms are unknown, however. As discussed elsewhere (see Refs. 28, 103), calcium can damage cells by overloading mitochondria, thereby interfering with oxidative phosphorylation; or by causing sustained overactivation of proteases and lipases. Overactivation of proteases could damage the cytoskeleton and its anchorage to the plasma membrane, or adversely alter the properties of membrane proteins. Sustained lipolysis carries the risk of causing membrane damage by products of arachidonic acid breakdown. Further exploration of the relationship between sustained arachidonic acid accumulation and epileptic cell damage is clearly justified.

REFERENCES

1. BAZAN, N. G. 1970. Effects of ischemia and electroconvulsive shock on free fatty acid pool in the brain. Biochim. Biophys. Acta **218:** 1–10.
2. BAZAN, N. G. 1971. Changes in free fatty acids of brain by drug-induced convulsions, electroshock and anesthesia. J. Neurochem. **18:** 1379–1385.
3. BAZAN, N. G. 1976. Free arachidonic acid and other lipids in the nervous system during early ischemia and after electroshock. Adv. Exp. Med. Biol. **72:** 317–335.
4. BAZAN, N. G. & H. RAKOWSKI. 1970. Increased levels of brain free fatty acids after electroconvulsive shock. Life Sci. **9:** 501–507.
5. ZATZ, M. & R. H. ROTH. 1975. Electroconvulsive shock raises prostaglandins F in rat cerebral cortex. Biochem. Pharmacol. **24:** 2101–2103.
6. FOLCO, G. C., D. LONGIAVE & E. BOSISIO. 1977. Relations between prostaglandin E_2, F_{2a} and cyclic nucleotide levels in rat brain and induction of convulsions. Prostaglandins **13:** 893–900.
7. MARION, J. & L. WOLFE. 1978. Increase *in vivo* of unesterified fatty acids, prostaglandin F_{2a} but not thromboxane B_2 in rat brain during drug-induced convulsions. Prostaglandins **16:** 99–110.
8. STEINHAUER, H. B., H. ANHUT & G. HERTTING. 1979. The synthesis of prostaglandins and thromboxane in the mouse brain *in vivo*. Influence of drug induced convulsions, hypoxia and the anticonvulsants trimethadione and diazepam. Naunyn Schmiedeberg's Arch. Pharmacol. **310:** 53–58.
9. WOLFE, L. S. 1982. Eicosanoids: Prostaglandins, thromboxanes, leukotrienes, and other derivatives of carbon-20 unsaturated fatty acids. J. Neurochem. **38:** 1–14.
10. CHAPMAN, A., M. INGVAR & B. K. SIESJÖ. 1980. Free fatty acids in the brain in bicuculline-induced status epilepticus. Acta Physiol. Scand. **110:** 335–336.
11. SIESJÖ, B. K., M. INGVAR & E. WESTERBERG. 1982. The influence of bicuculline-induced seizures on free fatty acid concentrations in cerebral cortex, hippocampus and cerebellum. J. Neurochem. **39:** 796–802.
12. FÖRSTERMANN, U., R. HELDT & G. HERTTING. 1983. Increase in brain prostaglandins during convulsions is due to increased neuronal activity and not to hypoxia. Arch. Int. Pharmacodyn. Ther. **263:** 180–188.
13. AVELDAÑO, M. I. & N. G. BAZAN. 1975. Differential lipid deacylation during brain

ischemia in a homeotherm and a poikilotherm. Content and composition of free fatty acids and triacylglycerols. Brain Res. **100:** 99–110.
14. REDDY, T. S. & N. G. BAZAN. 1987. Arachidonic acid, stearic acid, and diacylglycerol accumulation correlates with the loss of phosphatidylinositol 4,5-bisphosphate in cerebrum 2 seconds after electroconvulsive shock: Complete reversion of changes 5 minutes after stimulation. Neurosci. Res. **18:** 449–455.
15. YOSHIDA, S., K. ABE, R. BUSTO, B. D. WATSON, K. KOGURE & M. D. GINSBERG. 1982. Influence of transient ischemia on lipid-soluble antioxidant, free fatty acid and energy metabolites in rat brain. Brain Res. **245:** 307–316.
16. REHNCRONA, S., E. WESTERBERG, B. ÅKESSON & B. K. SIESJÖ. 1982. Brain cortical fatty acids and phospholipids during and following complete and incomplete ischemia. J. Neurochem. **38:** 84–93.
17. ABE, K., K. KOGURE, H. YAMAMOTO, M. IMAZAWA & K. MIYAMOTO. 1987. Mechanism of arachidonic acid liberation during ischemia in gerbil cerebral cortex. J. Neurochem. **48:** 503–509.
18. YOSHIDA, S., S. INOH, T. ASANO, K. SANO, M. KUBOTA, H. SHIMAZAKI & N. UETA. 1980. Effect of transient ischemia on free fatty acids and phospholipids in the gerbil brain. J. Neurosurg. **53:** 323–331.
19. YOSHIDA, S., M. IKEDA, R. BUSTO, M. SANTISO, E. MARTINEZ & M. D. GINSBERG. 1986. Cerebral phosphoinositide, triacylglycerol, and energy metabolism in reversible ischemia: Origin and fate of free fatty acids. J. Neurochem. **47:** 744–757.
20. REHNCRONA, S., D. S. SMITH, B. ÅKESSON & B. K. SIESJÖ. 1980. Peroxidative changes in brain cortical fatty acids and phospholipids, as characterized during Fe^{2+}- and ascorbic acid-stimulated lipid peroxidation *in vitro*. J. Neurochem. **34:** 1630–1638.
21. YOSHIDA, S., S. INOH, T. ASANO, K. SANO, H. SHIMAZAKI & N. UETA. 1983. Brain free fatty acids, edema, and mortality in gerbils subjected to transient, bilateral ischemia, and effect of barbiturate anesthesia. J. Neurochem. **40:** 1278–1286.
22. BENVENISTE, H., J. DREJER, A. SCHOUSBOE & N. H. DIEMER. 1984. Elevation of the extracellular concentrations of glutamate and aspartate in rat hippocampus during transient cerebral ischemia monitored by intracerebral microdialysis. J. Neurochem. **43:** 1369–1374.
23. HANSEN, A. J. 1985. Effects of anoxia on ion distribution in the brain. Physiol. Rev. **65(1):** 101–148.
24. NILSSON, B., K. NORBERG & B. K. SIESJÖ. 1975. Biochemical events in cerebral ischemia. Br. J. Anaesth. **47:** 751–760.
25. AGARDH, C.-D., A. G. CHAPMAN, B. NILSSON & B. K. SIESJÖ. 1981. Endogenous substrates utilized by rat brain in severe insulin-induced hypoglycemia. J. Neurochem. **36(2):** 490–500.
26. WIELOCH, T., R. J. HARRIS, L. SYMON & B. K. SIESJÖ. 1984. Influence of severe hypoglycemia on brain extracellular calcium and potassium activities, energy, and phospholipid metabolism. J. Neurochem. **43:** 160–168.
27. SIESJÖ, B. K. & C.-D. AGARDH. 1983. Hypoglycemia. *In* Handbook of Neurochemistry, Vol. 3. Metabolism in the nervous system. 2nd edit. A. Lajtha, Ed.: 353–379. Plenum, New York, NY.
28. SIESJÖ, B. K. 1988. Hypoglycemia, brain metabolism, and brain damage. Diabetes/Metabolism Rev. **4(2):** 113–144.
29. HARRIS, R. J., T. W. WIELOCH, L. SYMON & B. K. SIESJÖ. 1984. Cerebral extracellular calcium activity in severe hypoglycemia: Relation to extracellular potassium and energy state. J. Cereb. Blood Flow Metab. **4:** 187–193.
30. WIELOCH, T., R. J. HARRIS, L. SYMON & B. K. SIESJÖ. 1984. Influence of severe hypoglycemia on brain extracellular calcium and potassium activities, energy, and phospholipid metabolism. J. Neurochem. **43:** 160–168.
31. WIELOCH, T., B. ENGELSEN, E. WESTERBERG & R. AUER. 1985. Lesions of the glutamatergic cortico-striatal projections in the rat ameliorate hypoglycemic brain damage in the striatum. Neurosci. Lett. **58:** 25–30.
32. SANDBERG, M., S. P. BUTCHER & H. HAGBERG. 1986. Extracellular overflow of neuroactive amino acids during severe insulin-induced hypoglycemia: *In vivo* dialysis of the rat hippocampus. J. Neurochem. **47:** 178–185.

33. GARDINER, M., B. NILSSON, S. REHNCRONA & B. K. SIESJÖ. 1981. Free fatty acids in the rat brain in moderate and severe hypoxia. J. Neurochem. **36:** 1500–1505.
34. RODRIGUES DE TURCO, E. B., S. MORELLI DE LIBERTI & N. G. BAZAN. 1983. Stimulation of free fatty acid and diacylglycerol accumulation in cerebrum and cerebellum during bicuculline-induced status epilepticus. Effect of pretreatment with γ-methyl-p-tyrosine and p-chlorophenylalanine. J. Neurochem. **40:** 252–259.
35. INGVAR, M., B. SÖDERFELDT, J. FOLBERGROVÁ, H. KALIMO, Y. OLSSON & B. K. SIESJÖ. 1984. Metabolic, circulatory, and structural alterations in the rat brain induced by sustained pentylenetetrazole seizures. Epilepsia **25**(2): 191–204.
36. GINÓBILI DE MARTINÉZ, M. S. & E. B. RODRIGUEZ DE TURCO. 1985. Endogenous asymmetry of rat brain lipids and dominance of the right cerebral hemisphere in free fatty acid response to electroconvulsive shock. Brain Res. **339:** 315–321.
37. GINÓBILI DE MARTINÉZ, M. S., E. B. RODRIGUEZ DE TURCO & F. J. BARRANTES. 1986. Asymmetry of diacylglycerol metabolism in rat cerebral hemispheres. J. Neurochem. **46:** 1382–1386.
38. DUFFY, T. E., D. C. HOWSE & F. PLUM. 1975. Cerebral energy metabolism during experimental status epilepticus. J. Neurochem. **24:** 925–934.
39. CHAPMAN, A. G., B. S. MELDRUM & B. K. SIESJÖ. 1977. Cerebral metabolic changes during prolonged epileptic seizures in rats. J. Neurochem. **28:** 1025–1035.
40. FOLBERGROVÁ, J., M. INGVAR, G. NEVANDER & B. K. SIESJÖ. 1985. Cerebral metabolic changes during and following fluorothyl-induced seizures in ventilated rats. J. Neurochem. **44:** 1419–1426.
41. SÖDERFELDT, B., H. KALIMO, Y. OLSSON & B. K. SIESJÖ. 1983. Bicucullinie-induced brain injury: Transient and persistent changes in rat cerebral cortex in the early recovery period. Acta Neuropathol. **62:** 87–95.
42. HEINEMANN, U., H. D. LUX & M. J. GUTNICK. 1977. Extracellular free calcium and potassium during paroxysmal activity in the cerebral cortex of the cat. Exp. Brain Res. **27:** 237–243.
43. SOMJEN, G. C. 1980. Stimulus-evoked and seizure-related responses of extracellular calcium activity in spinal cord compared to those in cerebral cortex. J. Neurophysiol. **44:** 617–631.
44. PUMAIN, R. & U. HEINEMANN. 1985. Stimulus- and amino acid-induced calcium and potassium changes in rat neocortex. J. Neurophysiol. **53**(1): 1–16.
45. GRIFFITHS, T., M. C. EVANS & B. S. MELDRUM. 1983. Intracellular calcium accumulation in rat hippocampus during seizures induced by bicuculline or L-allylglycerine. Neurosci. **10:** 385–395.
46. BAZAN, N. G., D. L. BIRKLE, W. TANG & T. S. REDDY. 1986. The accumulation of free arachidonic acid, diacylglycerols, prostaglandins, and lipoxygenase reaction products in the brain during experimental epilepsy. *In* Advances in Neurology, Vol. 44. A. V. Delgado-Escueta, A. A. Ward, Jr., D. M. Woodbury & R. J. Porter, Eds.: 879–902. Raven Press. New York, NY.
47. GORACCI, G., E. FRANCESCANGELI, L. A. HORROCKS & G. PORCELLATI. 1981. The reverse reaction of cholinephosphotransferase in rat brain microsomes, a new pathway for degradation of phosphatidylcholine. Biochim. Biophys. Acta **664:** 373–379.
48. HORROCKS, L. A., R. V. DORMAN, Z. DARBROWIECKI, G. GORACCI & G. PORCELLATI. 1982. CDPcholine and CDPethanolamine prevent the release of free fatty acids during brain ischemia. Prog. Lipid Res. **20:** 531–534.
49. BAKER, R. & W. THOMPSON. 1972. Positional distribution and turnover of fatty acids in phosphatidic acid, phosphoinositides, phosphatidylcholine and phosphatidylethanolamine in rat brain *in vivo*. Biochim. Biophys. Acta **270:** 489–503.
50. BERRIDGE, M. J. 1984. Inositol triphosphate and diacylglycerol as second messengers. Biochem. J. **221:** 345–360.
51. SIESJÖ, B. K., R. VON HANWEHR, G. NERGELIUS, G. NEVANDER & M. INGVAR. 1985. Extra- and intracellular pH in the brain during seizures and in the recovery period following arrest of seizure activity. J. Cereb. Blood Flow Metab. **5:** 47–57.
52. BURGOYNE, R., T. R. CHEEK & A. J. SULLIVAN. 1987. Receptor-activation of phospholipase A_2 in cellular signalling. Trends Biochem. Sci. **12:** 332–333.
53. JONES, E. G. 1986. Neurotransmitters in the cerebral cortex. J. Neurosurg. **65:** 135–153.

54. MELDRUM, B. S. 1985. GABA and other amino acids. *In* Antiepileptic Drugs. H. H. Frey & D. Janz, Eds.: 153–188. Springer-Verlag. Berlin.
55. WATKINS, J. C. & R. H. EVANS. 1981. Excitatory amino acid transmitters. Annu. Rev. Pharmacol. Toxicol. **21:** 165–204.
56. MOORE, R. Y. & F. E. BLOOM. 1978. Central catecholamine neuron systems: Anatomy and physiology of the dopamine systems. Annu. Rev. Neurosci. **1:** 129–169.
57. MOORE, R. Y. & F. E. BLOOM. 1979. Central catecholamine neuron systems: Anatomy and physiology of the norepinephrine and epinephrine systems. Annu. Rev. Neurosci. **2:** 113–168.
58. HOUSER, C. R., G. D. CRAWFORD, P. M. SALVATERRA & J. E. VAUGN. 1985. Immunocytochemical localization of choline acetyltransferase in rat cerebral cortex: A study of cholinergic neurons and synapses. J. Comp. Neurol. **234:** 17–34.
59. HENDRY, S. C. H., E. G. JONES & M. C. BEINFELD. 1983. Cholecystokinin-immunoreactive neurons in rat and monkey cerebral cortex make symmetric synapses and have intimate relations with blood vessels. Proc. Natl. Acad. Sci. USA **80:** 2400–2404.
60. HENDRY, S. C. H., E. G. JONES & P. C. EMSON. 1984. Morphology, distribution, and synaptic relations of somatostatin- and neuropeptide Y-immunoreactive neurons in rat and monkey cortex. J. Neurosci. **4:** 2497–2517.
61. JAN, L. Y. & Y. N. JAN. 1982. Peptidergic transmission in sympathetic ganglia of the frog. J. Physiol. (London) **327:** 219–246.
62. CROUCHER, M. J., J. F. COLLINS & B. S. MELDRUM. 1982. Anticonvulsant action of excitatory amino acid antagonists. Science **216:** 899–901.
63. BAJOREK, J. G., R. J. LEE & P. LOMAX. 1986. Neuropeptides: Anticonvulsant and convulsant mechanisms in epileptic model systems and in humans. *In* Advances in Neurology, Vol. 44. A. V. Delgado-Escueta, A. A. Ward, Jr., D. M. Woodbury & R. J. Porter, Eds.: 489–500. Raven Press. New York, NY.
64. MELDRUM, B. S. 1986. Drugs acting on amino acid neurotransmitters. *In* Advances in Neurology, Vol. 43. S. Fahn, C. D. Marsden & M. H. Van Woert, Eds. 687–706. Raven Press. New York, NY.
65. RIBAK, C. E., R. M. BRADBURNE & A. B. HARRIS. 1982. A preferential loss of GABAergic, symmetric synapses in epileptic foci: A quantitative ultrastructural analysis of monkey neocortex. J. Neurosci. **2:** 1725–1735.
66. LOEB, C., G. BESIO, P. MAINARDI, P. SCOTTO, E. BENASSI & G. P. BO. 1986. Liposome-entrapped gamma-aminobutyric acid inhibits isoniazide-induced epileptogenic activity in rats. Epilepsia **27:** 98–102.
67. PATEL, S., M. H. MILLAN, L. M. MELLO & B. S. MELDRUM. 1986. 2-amino-7-phosphonoheptanoic acid (2-APH) infusion into entopenduncular nucleus protects against limbic seizures in rats. Neurosci. Lett. **64:** 226–230.
68. PIREDDA, S. & K. GALE. 1986. Anticonvulsant action of 2-amino-7-phosphonoheptanoic acid and muscimol in the deep prepiriform cortex. Eur. J. Pharmacol. **120:** 115–118.
69. ASHWOOD, T. J., B. LANCASTER & H. V. WHEAL. 1986. Intracellular electrophysiology of CA1 pyramidal neurones in slices of the kainic acid lesioned hippocampus of the rat. Exp. Brain Res. **62:** 189–198.
70. JOPE, R. S., M. SIMONATO & K. LALLY. 1987. Acetylcholine content in rat brain is elevated by status epilepticus induced by lithium and pilocarpine. J. Neurochem. **49:** 944–951.
71. CALDERINI, G., A. CARLSSON & C.-H. NORDSTRÖM. 1978. Monoamine metabolism during bicuculline-induced epileptic seizures in the rat. Brain Res. **157:** 295–302.
72. KETY, S. S., F. JAVOY, A. M. THIERRY, L. JULOU & J. GLOWINSKI. 1967. A sustained effect of electroconvulsive shock on norepinephrine in the central nervous system of the rat. Proc. Natl. Acad. Sci. USA **58:** 1249–1254.
73. MASON, S. T. & M. E. CORCORAN. 1979. Catecholamines and convulsions. Brain Res. **170:** 497–507.
74. EHLERS, C. L., D. K. CLIFTON & C. H. SAWYER. 1980. Facilitation of amygdala kindling in rat by transecting ascending noradrenergic pathways. Brain Res. **189:** 274–278.
75. MCINTYRE, D. C. & N. EDSON. 1981. Facilitation of amygdala kindling after norepinephrine depletion with 6-hydroxydopamine in rats. Exp. Neurol. **74:** 748–757.
76. INGVAR, M., O. LINDVALL, J. FOLBERGROVÁ & B. K. SIESJÖ. 1983. Influence of lesions of

the noradrenergic locus coeruleus system on the cerebral metabolic response to bicuculline-induced seizures. Brain Res. **264:** 225–231.
77. AVELDANO DE CALDIRONI, M. I. & N. G. BAZAN. 1979. Alphamethyl-p-tyrosine inhibits the production of free arachidonic acid and diacylglycerols in brain after a single electroconvulsive shock. Neurochem. Res. **4:** 213–221.
78. FISHER, S. K., C. A. BOAST & B. W. AGRANOFF. 1980. The muscarinic stimulation of phospholipid labelling in hippocampus is independent of its cholinergic input. Brain Res. **189:** 284–288.
79. SLADECZEK, F., J.-P. PIN, M. RÉCASENS, J. BOCKAERT & S. WEISS. 1985. Glutamate stimulates inositol phosphate formation in striatal neurones. Nature **317:** 717–719.
80. NICOLETTI, F., M. L. BARBACCIA, M. J. IADAROLA, O. POZZI & H. E. LAIRD, II. 1987. Arachidonic acid, stearic acid, and diacylglycerol accumulation correlates with the loss of phosphatidylinositol 4,5-bisphosphate in cerebrum 2 seconds after electroconvulsive shock: Complete reversion of changes 5 minutes after stimulation. Neurosci. Res. **18:** 449–455.
81. MELDRUM, B. & B. NILSSON. 1976. Cerebral blood flow and metabolic rate early and late in prolonged epileptic seizures induced in rats by bicuculline. Brain **99:** 523–542.
82. BORGSTRÖM, L., A. CHAPMAN & B. K. SIESJÖ. 1976. Glucose consumption in the cerebral cortex of rats during bicuculline-induced status epilepticus. J. Neurochem. **27:** 971–973.
83. INGVAR, M. & B. K. SIESJÖ. 1983. Local blood flow and glucose consumption in the rat brain during sustained bicuculline-induced seizures. Acta Neurol. Scand. **68:** 129–144.
84. FOLBERGROVÁ, J., M. INGVAR & B. K. SIESJÖ. 1981. Metabolic changes in cerebral cortex, hippocampus, and cerebellum during sustained bicuculline-induced seizures. J. Neurochem. **37:** 1228–1238.
85. CORSELLIS, J. A. N. & B. MELDRUM. 1976. Epilepsy. *In* Greenfield's Neuropathology. W. Blackwood & J. A. N. Corsellis, Eds.: 771–795. Edward Arnold. Edinburgh.
86. BLENNOW, G., J. B. BRIERLEY, B. S. MELDRUM & B. K. SIESJÖ. 1978. Epileptic brain damage. The role of systemic factors that modify cerebral energy metabolism. Brain **101:** 687–700.
87. NEVANDER, G., M. INGVAR, R. N. AUER & B. K. SIESJÖ. 1985. Status epilepticus in well-oxygenated rats causes neuronal necrosis. Ann. Neurol. **18:** 281–290.
88. COLLINS, R. C. & J. W. OLNEY. 1982. Focal cortical seizures cause distant thalamic lesions. Science **218:** 177–179.
89. SLOVITER, R. S. 1983. "Epileptic" brain damage in rats induced by sustained electrical stimulation of the perforant path. I. Acute electrophysiological and light microscopic studies. Brain Res. Bull. **10:** 675–697.
90. OLNEY, J. W., T. DE GUBAREFF & R. S. SLOVITER. 1983. "Epileptic" brain damage in rats induced by sustained electrical stimulation of the perforant path. II. Ultrastructural analysis of acute hippocampal pathology. Brain Res. Bull. **10:** 699–712.
91. WORLEY, P. F., J. M. BARABAN, J. S. COLVIN & S. H. SNYDER. 1987. Inositol trisphosphate receptor localization in brain: Variable stoichiometry with protein kinase C. Nature **325:** 159–161.
92. INGVAR, M., P. F. MORGAN & R. N. AUER. 1988. The nature and timing of excitotoxic neuronal necrosis in the cerebral cortex, hippocampus and thalamus due to fluorothyl-induced status epilepticus. Acta Neuropathol. (Berlin) **75:** 362–369.
93. AUER, R. N., M. INGVAR, G. NEVANDER, Y. OLSSON & B. K. SIESJÖ. 1986. Early axonal lesion and preserved microvasculature in epilepsy-induced hypermetabolic necrosis of the substantia nigra. Acta Neuropathol. (Berlin) **71:** 207–215.
94. INAMURA, K., Y. OLSSON & B. K. SIESJÖ. 1988. Substantia nigra damage induced by ischemia in hyperglycemic rats. Acta Neuropathol. (Berlin) **75:** 131–139.
95. HORTON, R. W., B. S. MELDRUM, T. A. PEDLEY & J. R. MCWILLIAM. 1980. Regional cerebral blood flow in the rat during prolonged seizure activity. Brain Res. **192:** 399–412.
96. VAN HARREVELD, A. 1966. Brain Tissue Electrolytes. Butterworths. London.
97. VAN HARREVELD, A. 1970. A mechanism for fluid shifts specific for the central nervous system. *In* Topical Problems of Psychiatry and Neurology, Vol. 10. H. T. Wycis, Ed.: 62–70. Karger. Basel.

98. ROTHMAN, S. M. & J. W. OLNEY. 1987. Excitotoxicity and the NMDA receptor. Trends Neurosci. **10:** 299–302.
99. FOSTER, A. C. & G. E. FAGG. 1987. Taking apart NMDA receptors. Nature **329:** 395–396.
100. MAYER, M. L. & G. L. WESTBROOK. 1987. The physiology of excitatory amino acids in the vertebrate central nervous system. Prog. Neurobiol. **28:** 197–276.
101. CHOI, D. W. 1985. Glutamate neurotoxicity in cortical cell culture is calcium dependent. Neurosci. Lett. **58:** 293–297.
102. CHOI, D. W. 1987. Ionic dependence of glutamate neurotoxicity. J. Neurosci. **7**(2): 369–379.
103. SIESJÖ, B. K. & T. WIELOCH. 1986. Epileptic brain damage: Pathophysiology and neurochemical pathology. *In* Advances in Neurology, Vol. 44. A. V. Delgado-Escueta, A. A. Ward, Jr., D. M. Woodbury & R. J. Porter, Eds.: 813–847. Raven Press. New York, NY.

Arachidonic Acid Metabolism and Cerebral Blood Flow in the Normal, Ischemic, and Reperfused Gerbil Brain

Inhibition of Ischemia-Reperfusion–Induced Cerebral Injury by a Platelet-Activating Factor Antagonist (BN 52021)

THOMAS PANETTA,[a] VICTOR L. MARCHESELLI,[b]
PIERRE BRAQUET,[c] AND NICOLAS G. BAZAN[b]

*Departments of [a]Surgery and [b]Ophthalmology
Louisiana State University School of Medicine
New Orleans, Louisiana 70112*

*[c]Institut Henri Beaufour
Le Plessis-Robinson, France*

INTRODUCTION

Ischemia and ischemia-reperfusion of the brain result in biochemical, structural, and functional changes that are integrally related to injury and recovery from an ischemic insult. Cerebral ischemia results in a rapid accumulation in the brain of free fatty acids (FFAs),[1] including arachidonic acid (AA), and diacylglycerols (DAG).[2] Reperfusion increases metabolites of AA, including cyclooxygenase[3,4] and lipoxygenase[5] reaction products and lipid peroxides.[6,7] In the resting state, low levels of FFAs reflect low levels of activity of phospholipases in conjunction with continuous reesterification by acyl transferases.[8] Ischemia results in disruption of the balance between acylation and deacylation, with increased phospholipidic deacylation and decreased reacylation resulting in the accumulation of FFAs.[2,9,10] Breakdown of neutral lipids cannot account for more than 20% of the liberated free fatty acids.[1] Ratios of saturated and unsaturated free fatty acids suggest that hydrolysis of phosphoinositides predominates as an early source of liberated stearate and arachidonate. It has been suggested that the predominant mechanism of release of arachidonic acid during the initial ischemic release of FFAs is the result of phospholipase C action on inositol phospholipids followed by diglyceride and monoglyceride lipases rather than initial activation of phospholipase A_2.[11]

Reperfusion results in rapid decrease in AA and gradual decrease in saturated fatty acids.[7] Free arachidonic acid is subject to reacylation through acyl-CoA[12] cyclooxygenase metabolism, lipoxygenase metabolism, or washout into the peripheral circulation or cerebrospinal fluid.

Ischemia results in increased activity of calcium-dependent phospholipases. Phospholipase A_1 and phospholipase A_2 have been isolated from several cell membranes in the rat brain.[13] Increased activity of phospholipases A_1 and A_2 have been documented during the first minute of cerebral ischemia in gerbils.[14] Increased phospholipase C activity specific for phosphatidylinositol (PI) during ischemic results in increased diacylglycerols enriched in stearate and arachidonate. Decreased levels of phosphatidylinositol-4'-5'-bisphosphate (PIP$_2$) and phosphatidylinositol-4'-phosphate (PIP) result from increased phospholipase activity.

We studied the *in vivo* time course of ^{14}AA incorporation and turnover in the gerbil whole brain and synaptoneurosome subcellular fraction. Experiments were designed to study patterns of incorporation into individual lipids during basal and ischemic conditions induced by bilateral carotid artery ligation.

Recently we have investigated the effects of a platelet-activating factor (PAF) antagonist (BN 52021) on free fatty acids, diacylglycerols, and polyphosphoinositides following ischemia-reperfusion induced cerebral injury.[15] Platelet activating factor (1-0 alkyl-2(R)-acetyl-sn-glycero-3-phosphocholine) was discovered by Benveniste in 1972.[16] Deacylation of 1-alkyl-2-acyl-GPC (glycerophosphorylcholine) by phospholipase A$_2$ results in the formation of lyso-paf (1-0-alkyl-GPC), which is acetylated to form PAF.[17] Since phospholipases A$_2$ and C are activated during cerebral ischemia, we investigated the role of a PAF antagonist (BN 52021) in an ischemia-reperfusion model of cerebral injury. BN 52021 is a terpene isolated from *Ginkgo biloba* extract (GBE 761). BN 52021 has been shown to inhibit leukotriene C$_4$ and free radical production in leukocytes[18] and to reduce the stroke index following unilateral carotid artery ligation in gerbils.[19] *Ginkgo biloba* extracts (GBE 761) have been shown to improve cerebral metabolism, protect against hypoxic brain damage, and prolong survival in rats.[20]

^{14}C ARACHIDONIC ACID INCORPORATION INTO THE WHOLE BRAIN

In all experiments, Mongolian gerbils (*Meriones unguiculatus;* 40–60 grams) were anesthetized with 0.05 cc of ketamine:acepromazine (1:1). Following scalp removal, bilateral burr holes were drilled over the lateral ventricles. A volume of 2 μl (1 μCi per side) of ^{14}C arachidonic acid, prepared as a sodium salt with 50 mM sodium bicarbonate, was injected intraventricularly at a depth of 3 mm bilaterally. Animals were sacrificed at 5, 10, 30, 60, and 120 minutes following intracerebral injection. Head-focused microwave irradiation (HFMI, 6.5 kW for 1.25 sec) was utilized for tissue enzyme inactivation. Forebrain, midbrain, and cerebellum were separated and homogenized in chloroform:methanol (2:1) (v/v). Lipids were extracted from tissue according to Folch.[21]

Following intraventricular injection of ^{14}C arachidonic acid, rapid incorporation into lipids parallels a rapid loss of radiolabeled fatty acid in the free pool (FIG. 1). Peak incorporation into lipids occurred at thirty minutes in the forebrain, midbrain, and cerebellum. Absolute levels of incorporation in the forebrain and midbrain were greatest in triglycerides, followed by phosphatidylcholine (PC) and PI. In the cerebellum, absolute levels of incorporation were similar in PI and PC, which were greater than in triglycerides. Phosphatidylethanolamine had low levels of incorporation, but greater than phosphatidic acid. Taking into consideration the relative amount of phosphatidylinositol in cerebral tissue (approximately 3.2% of total phospholipids[11]), incorporation of ^{14}C arachidonic acid was 22 times greater in PI than PC.

Rapid loss of labeled FFA results from rapid acylation of lysophospholipids, washout into the cerebrospinal fluid and the peripheral circulation, and metabolism by cyclooxygenase and lipoxygenase. We have looked at washout into the peripheral circulation. Significant amounts of ^{14}C arachidonic acid accumulate within 60 minutes in viscera (liver > spleen > heart > kidney > lung), with low levels of detectable radioactivity in the blood (unpublished data). Following peak incorporation into phospholipids and neutral lipids, loss of ^{14}C arachidonic acid in lipids results from

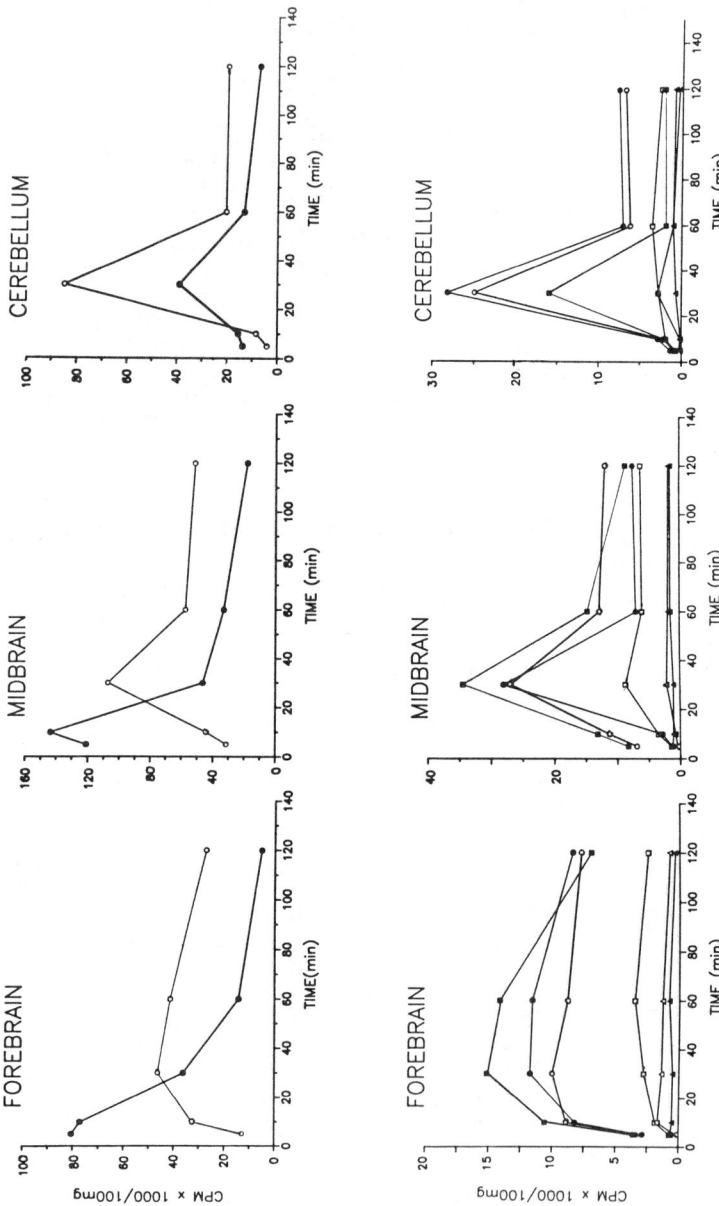

FIGURE 1. Time curve of ^{14}C arachidonic acid incorporation into the forebrain, midbrain, and cerebellum. Data are expressed as cpm/100 mg of protein. Each point represents an average from five animals. Standard errors (not shown) were less than 10% of total values. *Upper panels: open circles* = total; *solid circles* = free fatty acids. *Lower panels: solid triangles* = phosphatidic acid; *open triangles* = phosphatidylserine; *open circles* = phosphatidylinositol; *solid circles* = phosphatidylcholine; *open squares* = phosphatidylethanolamine; *solid squares* = triglycerides.

deacylation/reacylation with cold arachidonic acid, washout into the cerebrospinal fluid and peripheral circulation, and catabolism of lipids.

EFFECT OF BILATERAL CAROTID ARTERY LIGATION ON ^{14}C ARACHIDONIC ACID INCORPORATION INTO THE WHOLE BRAIN

Following peak incorporation (30 minutes) of ^{14}C arachidonic acid, animals underwent bilateral carotid artery ligation. Gerbils were sacrificed by head-focused microwave irradiation after 0, 30, 90, 180, and 300 seconds of ischemia. Forebrains and midbrains were separated and homogenized in chloroform:methanol (2:1) (v/v). Lipids were extracted from tissue according to Folch.[21]

Five minutes of bilateral carotid artery ligation resulted in decreased levels of incorporation into PI (FIG. 2). This decrease was more pronounced in the forebrain than in the midbrain, corresponding to the relative changes that occur in cerebral blood flow in the forebrain and midbrain by bilateral carotid artery ligation.[15] Triacylglycerols increased in the forebrain. Phosphatidylinositol-4'-phosphate decreased during the five minutes of ischemia. Phosphatidylinositol-4',5'-bisphosphate and diacylglycerols also demonstrated an overall decrease in early ischemia. Our findings suggest a possible correlation between cerebral blood flow and PI turnover.

The ratio of PI/PC fell from 0.92 to 0.52, representing greater activity for phsopholipases on phosphatidylinositol than on phosphatidylcholine. Phospholipase A_2 and phospholipase C may be involved in the decreased total levels of PI. Four animals died as a result of the experimental conditions. In each case brain enzymes were immediately inactivated by HFMI, and brain lipids were sampled. In these four gerbils, midbrain PI/PC < 0.4. Surviving gerbils all had midbrain PI/PC > 0.4.

^{14}C ARACHIDONIC ACID INCORPORATION INTO SYNAPTONEUROSOMES

Following intraventricular injection of ^{14}C arachidonic acid, gerbils were sacrificed at 15, 30, 60, and 120 minutes. Animals were sacrificed by decapitation, which was followed by immediate dissection at 4 °C. Forebrain, midbrain, and cerebellum were separated and homogenized with 7 ml of ice-cold Krebs-Henselheit buffer (pH = 7.4) per gm of fresh tissue. Synaptoneurosome fractions were isolated according to the method of E. B. Hollingsworth.[22] Synaptoneurosomes are intact synaptic clefts with surrounding resealed pre- and postsynaptic subcellular elements. This preparation reduces red blood cell, white blood cell, platelet, and endothelial cell contamination. Although this preparation is enriched with pre- and postsynaptic subcellular elements, some contamination with unidentified subcellular components exist.

Incorporation of ^{14}C AA into synaptoneurosomes was similar to that of the whole brain (FIG. 3). There was some delay in cerebellar incorporation, with the peak occurring at 60 minutes. However, similar ratios of incorporation into phospholipids occurred (PI > PC > PE). Triglyceride incorporation peaked earlier in the forebrain (15 min) and was lower than PI and PC from 30 to 120 minutes. Aside from these minor differences, ratios of incorporation of ^{14}C AA into phospholipids was paralleled in the whole brain and synpatoneurosomes. Bilateral common carotid ligation as in the whole brain resulted in a decreased ratio of PI/PC in synaptoneurosomes (data not shown).

EFFECTS OF BN 52021 ON CEREBRAL BLOOD FLOW, FREE FATTY ACIDS, DIACYLGLYCEROLS, AND POLYPHOSPHOINOSITIDES

Animals underwent ten minutes of bilateral carotid artery ligation and were then reperfused for 90 minutes. Following reperfusion, gerbils received intraperitoneal

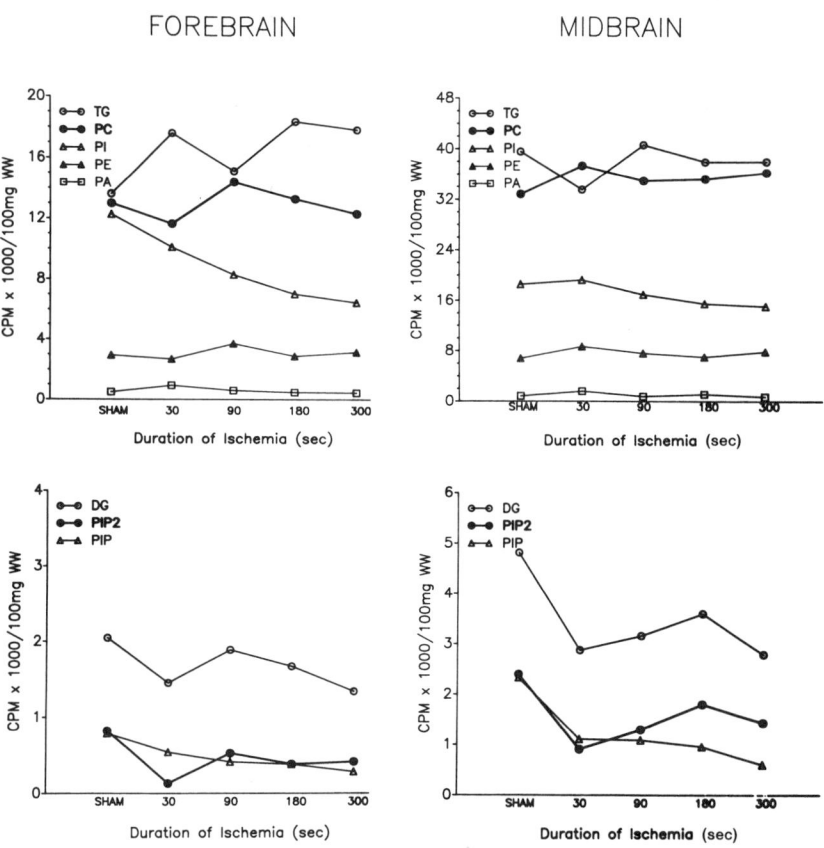

FIGURE 2. ^{14}C arachidonic acid metabolism during five minutes of bilateral carotid artery ligation. Ligation was performed following 30 min of incorporation. Data are expressed as cpm/100 mg wet weight (WW). Each point represents an average from three animals. Standard errors (not shown) were less than 10% of total values. *Upper panels: open circles* = triglycerides; *solid circles* = phosphatidylcholine; *open triangles* = phosphatidylinositol; *solid triangles* = phosphatidylethanolamine; *open squares* = phosphatidic acid. *Lower panels: open circles* = diacylglycerols; *solid circles* = phosphatidylinositol-4',5'-bisphosphate (PIP_2); *open triangles* = phosphatidylinositol-4'-phosphate (PIP).

injections of either BN 52021 (10 mg/kg) or the same volume of 50% DMSO vehicle. Cerebral blood flow (CBF) and systemic blood pressure were measured during ligation and at 5, 15, 30, 45, 60, and 90 minutes of reperfusion. Cerebral blood flow was determined using the hydrogen clearance technique[23] and initial slope calculation.[24] Intracerebral electrodes of Teflon-coated 0.005" platinum wire were inserted through

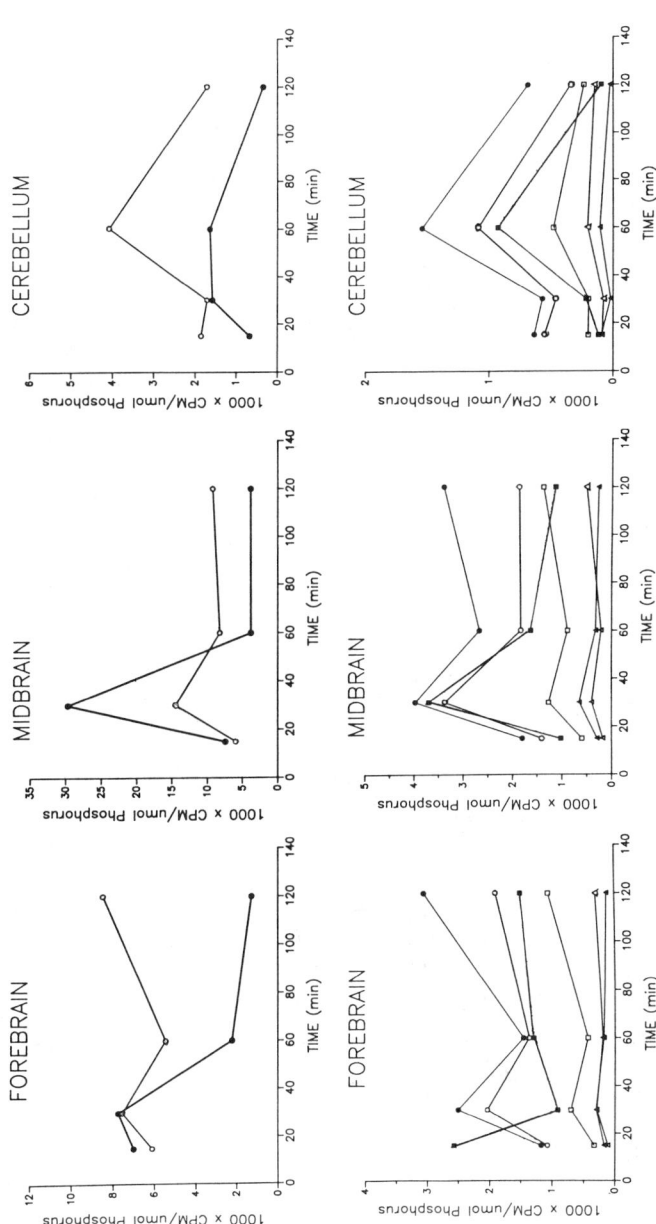

FIGURE 3. Time curve of ^{14}C arachidonic acid incorporation into synaptoneurosomal fractions of the forebrain, midbrain, and cerebellum. Data are expressed as cpm/μmoles of phospholipid. Each point represents an average from three animals. Standard errors (not shown) were less than 10% of total values. *Upper panels: open circles* = total; *solid circles* = free fatty acids. *Lower panels: solid triangles* =phosphatidic acid; *open triangles* = phosphatidylserine; *open circles* = phosphatidylinositol; *solid circles* =phosphatidylcholine; *open squares* = phosphatidylethanolamine; *solid squares* = triglycerides.

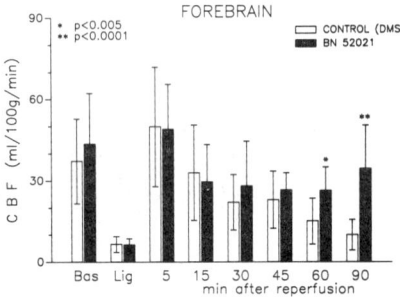
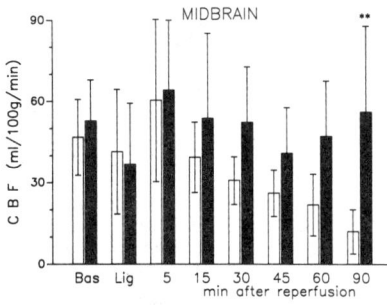

FIGURE 4. The effect of BN 52021 on cerebral blood flow (CBF) following ischemia-reperfusion of the gerbil brain. Platelet-activating factor antagonist (BN 52021) was injected at the onset of reperfusion. Values for CBF are averages ± standard errors of seven gerbils. Data are expressed as ml/100 gm/min, as determined by hydrogen clearance. Bas = baseline value; Lig = value at time of bilateral carotid artery ligation; * = $p < 0.005$; ** = $p < 0.0001$.

burr holes into the midbrain (2 electrodes) and superficial cortex (3 electrodes). All gerbils were sacrificed by HFMI following 90 minutes of reperfusion.

Following extraction of brain lipids,[25] free fatty acids and diacylglycerols were isolated by thin-layer chromatography (TLC). Fatty acid methyl esters were quantitated following methanolysis by capillary gas-liquid chromatography. Polyphosphoinositides were extracted with chloroform:methanol (2:1) (v:v) and 0.5% concentrated HCl,[26] separated by TLC, and quantitated following methanolysis by gas-liquid chromatography.

Bilateral carotid artery ligation in gerbils results in complete forebrain ischemia (CBF less than 7 ml/100 g/min) and a 20–50% reduction of midbrain CBR (FIG. 4). During ischemia, midbrain perfusion is maintained by the posterior circulation. Although midbrain ischemia is incomplete, complete forebrain ischemia in the gerbil is the result of an incomplete circle of Willis. During ligation, midbrain perfusion is also maintained by the profound hypertensive response that occurs. Reperfusion is associated with reactive hyperemia in both forebrain and midbrain, and an initial profound systemic hypotension. Post-reperfusion systemic hypotension was not inhibited by pretreatment of gerbils with BN 52021.[15] This was investigated because PAF is a potent mediator of anaphylaxis and hypotension.

Cerebral blood flow is directly proportional to systemic arterial pressure and inversely proportional to intracranial pressure. Bilateral carotid artery ligation in gerbils results in a profound hypertensive response. Complete forebrain ischemia is a direct result of occlusion proximal to the internal carotid arteries. However, a 20% to 50% decrease in midbrain CBF occurs even in the presence of patent posterior circulation and systemic hypertension. This may reflect an acute onset of increased intracranial pressure. Hypertension results in increased sensitivity to ischemic changes in the blood-brain barrier[27] and may contribute to cerebral injury.

Platelet activating factor antagonist (BN 52021) inhibited the maturation of ischemia-reperfusion induced cerebral injury resulting from 10 minutes of ischemia and 90 minutes of reperfusion. In DMSO controls, reperfusion resulted in progressive deterioration of cerebral blood flow after the initial reactive hyperemia. In this experimental model a combination of factors contributed to contain deterioration of cerebral blood flow. Gerbils were subjected to ischemia-reperfusion, cerebral injury from the trauma of drilling burr holes and implanting intracerebral electrodes, and 420-mV polarization current across cerebral tissue, with intermittent hydrogen inhalation required to measure CBF. Animals treated with BN 52021 at the onset of reperfusion had statistically increased CBF from 60 to 90 minutes of reperfusion in the forebrain and at 90 minutes of reperfusion in the midbrain. CBF in forebrain and midbrain returned to baseline levels at 90 minutes after reperfusion in treated animals. Improvement of CBF was not related to any changes in systemic blood pressure.

Animals were sacrificed at 90 minutes of reperfusion by head-focused microwave irradiation. Free fatty acids, diacylglycerols, and polyphosphoinositides were measured at this time to determine the involvement of platelet activating factor in ischemia-reperfusion induced cerebral injury and the involvement of PAF antagonist BN 52021 in inhibiting the maturation of cerebral injury as seen by improvement of CBF.

Free fatty acid content was significantly reduced by BN 52021 at 90 minutes of reperfusion (FIG. 5). This is likely due to inhibition of phospholipase A_2 activity. The total FFA pool was ten times greater in DMSO controls than in sham controls in the forebrain and three times greater in the midbrain. BN 52021 reduced FFA content, including arachidonic acid content, to sham-control levels in both brain parts. Activation of the arachidonic acid cascade with reperfusion is associated with the accumulation of cyclooxygenase and lipoxygenase reaction products that contribute to ischemic brain damage. Reduction of free arachidonic acid accumulation by BN 52021 reduces substrate availability for cyclooxygenase and lipoxygenase pathways. PAF may contribute directly to ischemic brain damage. PAF has been associated with

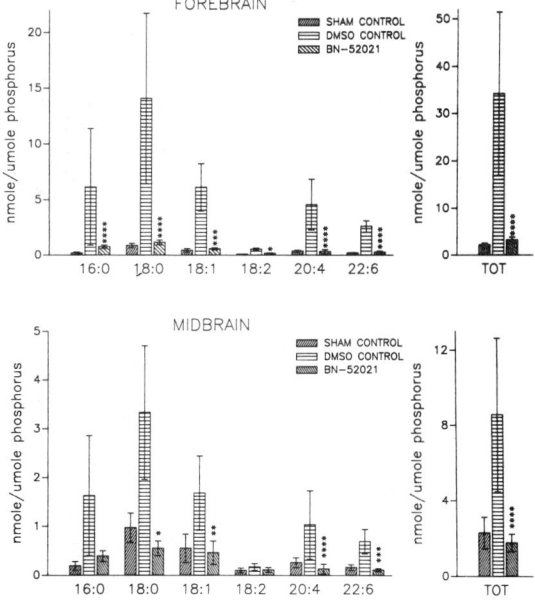

FIGURE 5. Effects of platelet-activating factor antagonist (BN 52021) on brain free fatty acid pools following 90 minutes of reperfusion. Data are expressed as nmole methyl ester/µmole phospholipids. Values are averages ± SEM of seven animals. * = $p < 0.05$; ** = $p < 0.005$; *** = $p < 0.0025$; **** = $p < 0.0001$.

vasoconstriction, endothelial cell injury, and leukotriene C_4-mediated release of norepinephrine and epinephrine.

The stable precursor of PAF, 1-alkyl-2-acyl-GPC, is composed of predominantly 18:0 or 16:0 bound by an ether union to the first glycerol carbon, and 20:4 acyl group in the second carbon. Phospholipase A_2 conversion of alkyl-acyl-GPC to lyso-PAF results in liberation of arachidonic acid. The contribution of arachidonic acid from alkyl-acyl-GPC to the accumulation of free fatty acids as a result of cerebral ischemia is undefined.

Although there was a trend of increased individual fatty acids esterified to PIP_2 and total PIP_2 pool (FIG. 6), and a trend of decreased individual and total fatty acids in diacylglycerols (FIG. 7), only the increased arachidonolyl pool in forebrain PIP_2 was significant. These changes suggest a possible coinhibition of phospholipase C that is calcium dependent.

Although FFA release as a result of cerebral ischemia has been shown to decrease during reperfusion in the gerbil, the elevated FFA in our DMSO controls may represent a secondary increase as a result of deteriorating cerebral blood flow. As a result of the previously described experimental design, untreated gerbils did not survive for more than two to six hours.[15] Therefore, reduced FFA levels in treated animals may represent a secondary effect of BN 52021 as a result of improved cerebral blood flow and recovery from the ischemia-reperfusion induced injury.

SUMMARY

Cerebral ischemia and ischemia-reperfusion induced cerebral injury results in the accumulation of free fatty acids and diacylglycerols as a result of increased activity of

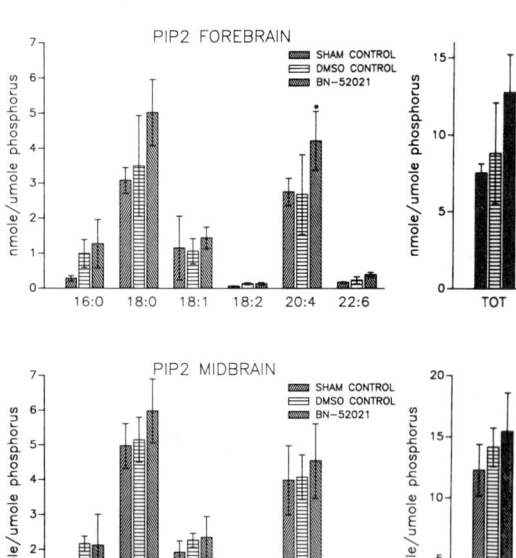

FIGURE 6. Effects of platelet-activating factor antagonist (BN 52021) on the fatty acid composition of phosphatidylinositol-4',5'-bisphosphate (PIP_2) pool following 90 minutes of reperfusion. Details as in FIGURE 5. * = $p < 0.05$.

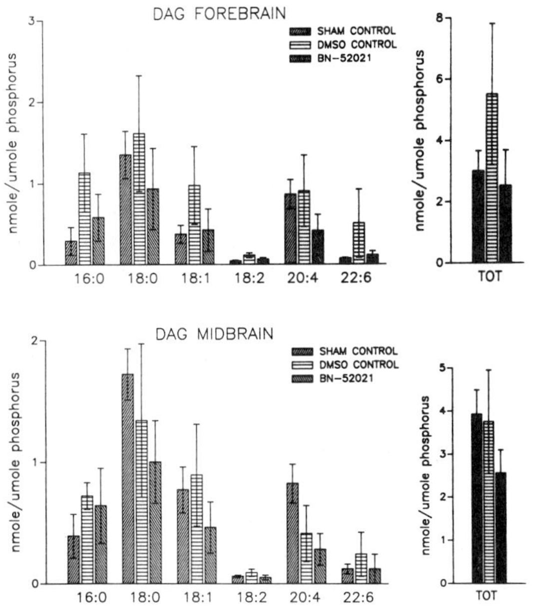

FIGURE 7. Effects of platelet-activating factor antagonist (BN 52021) on diacylglycerol (DAG) fatty acid composition following 90 minutes of reperfusion. Details as in FIGURE 5.

phospholipases A and C. We have evaluated the incorporation of ^{14}C arachidonic acid into the whole brain and synaptoneurosomes, the effect of cerebral ischemia on ^{14}C incorporation, and the effect of a PAF antagonist (BN 52021) on cerebral blood flow, free fatty acids, diacylglycerols, and polyphosphoinositides. Peak incorporation of ^{14}C arachidonic acid into the whole brain and synaptoneurosomal fractions occurred 30 minutes following intraventricular injection. Peak incorporation into cerebellar synaptoneurosomal fractions was at 60 minutes following intraventricular injection. Turnover in phospholipid pools was similar in the whole brain and synaptoneurosomes (PI > PC > PE). Considering phosphatidylinositol content in the gerbil brain, the specific activity of ^{14}C arachidonic acid was 22 times greater in PI than PC. Five minutes of bilateral carotid artery ligation resulted in decreased phosatidylinositol and polyphosphoinositols. Bilateral carotid artery ligation resulted in systemic arterial hypertension, complete forebrain ischemia (CBF less than 7 ml/100 gm/min) and a 20% to 50% reduction in midbrain CBF. Reperfusion resulted in cerebral reactive hyperemia and systemic hypotension.

BN 52021 inhibited the maturation of ischemia-reperfusion induced cerebral injury. Cerebral blood flow was improved. Free fatty acids were decreased, suggesting inhibition of phospholipase A activity. Decreased DAG pools with increased PIP$_2$ pools suggest a possible coinhibition of phospholipase C.

REFERENCES

1. BAZAN, N. G. 1970. Effects of ischemia and electroconvulsive shock on free fatty acid pool in the brain. Biochim. Biophys. Acta **218:** 1–10.
2. AVELDANO, M. I. & N. G. BAZAN. 1975. Rapid production of diacylglycerols enriched in arachidonate and stearate during early brain ischemia. J. Neurochem. **25:** 919–920.

3. GAUDET, R. J. & L. LEVINE. 1979. Transient cerebral ischemia and brain prostaglandins. Biochem. Biophys. Res. Commun. **86:** 893–901.
4. KEMPSKI, O., E. SHOHAMI, D. VON LUBITZ, J. M. HALLENBECK & G. FEUERSTEIN. 1987. Postischemic production of eicosanoids in gerbil brain. Stroke **18:** 111–119.
5. MOSKOWITZ, M. A., K. J. KIWAK, K. HEKIMIAN & L. LEVINE. 1984. Synthesis of compounds with properties of leukotrienes C4 and D4 in gerbil brains after ischemia and reperfusion. Science **244:** 886–889.
6. FLAMM, E. S., H. B. DEMOPOULOS, M. L. SELIGMAN, R. G. POSER & J. RANSOHOFF. 1978. Free radicals in cerebral ischemia. Stroke **9:** 445–447.
7. YOSHIDA, S., S. INOH, T. ASANO, K. SANO, M. KUBOTA, H. SHIMAZAKI & N. UETA. 1980. Effect of transient ischemia on free fatty acids and phospholipids in the gerbil brain. Lipid peroxidation as a possible cause of postischemic injury. J. Neurosurg. **53:** 323–331.
8. LANDS, W. E. M. & I. MERKEL. 1963. Reactivity of various acyl esters of coenzyme A with α acylglycerophosphocholine and positional specificities in lecithin synthesis. J. Biol. Chem. **238:** 898–904.
9. HUANG, S. F. L. & G. Y. SUN. 1986. Cerebral ischemia induced quantitative changes in brain membrane lipids involved in phosphoinositide metabolism. Neurochem. Int. **9:** 185–190.
10. YOSHIDA, S., M. IKEDA, R. BUSTO, M. SANTISO, E. MARTINEZ & M. D. GINSBERG. 1986. Cerebral phosphoinositide, triacylglycerol, and energy metabolism in reversible ischemia: Origin and fate of free fatty acids. J. Neurochem. **47:** 744–757.
11. ABE, K., K. KOGURE, H. YAMAMOTO, M. IMAZAWA & K. MIYAMOTO. 1987. Mechanism of arachidonic acid liberation during ischemia in gerbil cerebral cortex. J. Neurochem. **48:** 503–509.
12. TANG, W. & G. Y. SUN. 1985. Metabolic relationship between arachidonate activation and its transfer to lysophospholipids by brain microsomes. Neurochem. Res. **10:** 1343–1353.
13. BAZAN, N. G. & M. CUMMINGS. 1969. The turnover of brain fatty acids following decapitation or convulsions. In Proceedings of the 2nd International Meeting of the International Society of Neurochemistry. R. Paoletti, R. Fumagelli & C. Galli, Eds.: 83-84. Tamburini Editore. Milan.
14. EDGAR, A. D., J. STROSZNAJDER & L. A. HORROCKS. 1982. Activation of ethanolamine phospholipase A2 in brain during ischemia. J. Neurochem. **39:** 1111–1116.
15. PANETTA, T., V. L. MARCHESELLI, P. BRAQUET, B. SPINNEWYN & N. G. BAZAN. 1987. Effects of a platelet activating factor antagonist (BN 52021) on free fatty acids, diacylglycerols, polyphosphoinositides and blood flow in the gerbil brain: Inhibition of ischemia-reperfusion induced cerebral injury. Biochem. Biophys. Res. Commun. **149:** 580–587.
16. BENVENISTE, J., P. M. HENSON & C. G. COCHRANE. 1972. Leukocyte-dependent histamine release from rabbit platelets: The role of IgE, basophils, and platelet activating factor. J. Exp. Med. **136:** 1356–1377.
17. BENVENISTE, J., M. CHIGNARD, J. P. LECOUEDIC & B. VARGAFTIG. 1982. Biosynthesis of platelet activating factor (PAF-acether). II. Involvement of phospholipase A2 in the formation of PAF-acether and lyso-PAF-acether from rabbit platelets. Thromb. Res. **25:** 375–385.
18. WICKHAM, N. W. R., G. M. VERCELOTTI, H. Q. YIN, C. F. MOLDOW & H. S. JACOB. 1989. Neutrophils are primed to release toxic oxidants by contact with thrombin-stimulated endothelium: Role of endothelial cell-generated platelet activating factor. Fed. Proc. Fed. Am. Soc. Exp. Biol. In press.
19. BRAQUET, P., T. Y. SHEN, L. TOUQUI & B. B. VARGAFTIG. 1987. Perspectives in platelet-activating factor research. Pharmacol. Rev. **39:** 97–145.
20. KRIEGLSTEIN, J., T. BECK & A. SIEBERT. 1986. Influence of an extract of Ginkgo biloba on cerebral blood flow and metabolism. Life Sci. **39:** 2237–2334.
21. FOLCH, J., M. LEES & G. H. SLOANE-STANLEY. 1957. A simple method for the isolation and purification of total lipids from animal tissue. J. Biol. Chem. **226:** 497–509.
22. HOLLINGSWORTH, E. B., E. T. MCNEAL, J. L. BURTON, R. J. WILLIAMS, J. W. DALY & C. R. CREVELING. 1985. Biochemical characterization of a filtered synaptoneurosome preparation from guinea pig cerebral cortex: Cyclic adenosine 3':5'-monophosphate-generating systems, receptors, and enzymes. J. Neurosci. **5:** 2240–2253.

23. YOUNG, W. 1980. H2 clearance measurement of blood flow: A review of technique and polarographic principles. Stroke **11:** 552–564.
24. OLESEN, J., O. B. PAULSON & N. A. LASSEN. 1971. Regional cerebral blood flow in man determined by the initial slope of the clearance of intra-arterially injected 133Xe. Stroke **2:** 519–540.
25. MARCHESELLI, V. L., B. L. SCOTT, T. S. REDDY & N. G. BAZAN. 1988. Quantitative analysis of acyl group composition of brain. *In* Neuromethods, Vol. 7: 83–110. Humana Press. Clifton, NJ.
26. EICHBERG, J. & G. HAUSER. 1967. Concentrations and disappearance post mortem of polyphosphoinositides in developing rat brain. Biochem. Biophys. Acta **144:** 415–422.
27. ITO, U., K. OHNO, T. YAMAGUCHI, H. TAKEI, H. TOMITA & Y. INABA. 1980. Effect of hypertension on blood-brain barrier change after restoration of blood flow in postischemic gerbil brains. Stroke **11:** 606–611.

Arachidonic Acid and Its Metabolites during Cerebral Ischemia and Recirculation

Pharmacological Interventions[a]

CLAUDIO GALLI, ANNA PETRONI,
ANTONELLA BERTAZZO, AND SILVIA SARTI

Institute of Pharmacological Sciences
University of Milan
20133 Milan, Italy

INTRODUCTION

The metabolic characteristics of the nervous system—such as high blood flow and high rate of O_2 utilization with respect to other compartments, and the abundance of specialized membranes with an elevated concentration of lipids, rich in highly unsaturated long-chain fatty acids of both the n-6 and n-3 series—explain both the sensitivity of this tissue to hypoxia/ischemia and the involvement of lipid-derived metabolites in the biochemical processes occurring under these conditions. In addition to modulators and metabolites of the nature of lipids, other factors, such as enhanced H^+ concentration in the tissue, and mediators—for example, adenosine, serotonin, bradykinin, angiotensin II, acetylcholine, and especially the cytotoxic amino acid glutamate[1]—may be involved in the onset of functional and circulatory derangements in the ischemic tissue.

LIPID METABOLITES IN ISCHEMIA AND REPERFUSION

Polyunsaturated fatty acids (PUFA) are present in brain tissue in high concentrations, far exceeding those found in other organs, such as the liver. Both 20:4 n-6 (arachidonic acid, AA) and 22:6 n-3 are the major PUFA in the brain, but the concentration of 20:4 is much higher in the brain cortex than in the cerebellum; levels of 22:6 are comparable in both brain areas in the rat (TABLE 1).

Release of fatty acids, mainly AA, from complex lipids occurs during ischemia in the brain cortex more than in other areas and is followed by further transformations. Activation of various phospholipases (C, A_1, and A_2), which may be favored by the influx of calcium ions into ischemic neurons[2] stimulated by glutamate-like agonists[1] released during ischemia,[3] may be involved in this release of fatty acids. Release of arachidonate in the brain during ischemia in mice follows two phases,[4] and early hydrolysis of inositol-containing phospholipids[5] suggests that these complex lipids are the initial donors of this fatty acid.

---

[a]This work was supported in part by a contract of FIDIA Research Laboratories, Abano Terme, Italy.

It is not known whether phospholipid breakdown during brain ischemia generates other mediators as well, such as platelet activating factor (PAF). This product is formed through acetylation of 1-0-alkyl-GPC, which results from the action of phospholipase A_2 on 1-alkyl-2-acyl-GPC. PAF was found in baboon myocardium after ischemia but not in normal conditions.[6] The use of PAF antagonists may enhance neuronal recovery after brain ischemia[7] and prevent the generation of fatty acids and diacylglycerol (DAG).[8]

Products of oxygenated transformation of AA through the cyclooxygenases (CO) and lipoxygenases (LO) are subsequently generated in brain tissue. Problems, arise, however, in the correct measurement of these compounds due to the unspecific activation of lipolytic enzymes and the subsequent generation of eicosanoids following decapitation of the animals and manipulation of the brain tissue. However, the use of fixation techniques (rapid freezing, microwave fixation) allows some control of the early processes in eicosanoid production and, thus, measurement of the endogenous levels of the compounds. In addition, determinations of eicosanoid levels in whole tissue do not provide informations on changes in selected compartments.

AA, massively released in the brain, is not effectively converted by the CO and the LO to eicosanoids during complete ischemia, since no elevation of these products has

TABLE 1. Comparative Concentrations of 20:4 n-6 in Rat Brain and Liver, and of 20:4 n-6 and 22:6 n-3 in Brain Cortex and Cerebellum

Location (No. of Samples)	20:4 n-6	22:6 n-3
Brain (6)	5.1 ± 0.2^a	—
Liver (6)	3.4 ± 0.6^a	—
Brain cortex (4)	53.5 ± 0.3^b	61.6 ± 0.3^b
Cerebellum (4)	30.1 ± 0.2^b	58.2 ± 0.3^b

NOTE: Levels were measured by GLC analysis of methyl esters prepared from total lipids extracted from tissues, with C:19:0 used as internal standard.
^{a}Values are mg/g fw (mean ± SEM).
^{b}Values are µg/mg total lipids (mean ± SEM).

been described in the brain cortex after bilateral occlusion of common carotid arteries in the gerbil.[9,10] The lack of further metabolic conversion of AA through the oxygenases is attributed to the absence of oxygen in the tissue during complete ischemia. Instead, eicosanoids are accumulated in the brain in conditions of incomplete ischemia,[11-13] when the presence of blood and oxygen allows the oxygenated conversion of AA, and, possibly, also the formation of lipoperoxides. The accumulation of lipid products such as the cytotoxic free fatty acids and lipoperoxides,[14,15] DAG resulting from cleavage of phosphoinositides, and, possibly, PAF may exert detrimental effects on neuronal cells.

The *phase of reperfusion* after ischemia is characterized by further aggravation of the ischemic damage. The activation of oxygen-mediated reactions, leading to enhanced formation of products such as lipid peroxides,[16] may play a role in this process. Levels of the endogenous lipid-soluble antioxidant α-tocopherol are also remarkably decreased during ischemia, and especially after reperfusion.[17]

In addition, sustained generation of oxygenated metabolites of AA occurs during reperfusion, as shown by the rise of the concentrations of all CO products, especially of thromboxane, in the brain cortex of gerbils[11] and rats[13] that, after a period of occlusion of common carotid arteries, were reperfused.

Products of the AA lipoxygenase, such as the hydroxylated fatty acid 12-HETE,[9] were also detected in the brain during ischemia; and various types of hydroxylated fatty acids (5-HETE, 11-HETE, 12-HETE, 15-HETE) are actively produced by brain tissue upon incubation.[18,19] The dynamics of eicosanoid production in *in vitro* systems, however, is very different from that in the *in vivo* situation. Elevation of LTC_4 and B_4 in the gerbil brain during ischemia, and especially after reperfusion, has been shown by Moskowitz and Levine;[20] but due to analytical difficulties in measuring endogenous levels of these compounds in tissues, further information is not available. Again, production of leukotrienes has been characterized in incubated and stimulated slices of cerebral tissues,[21] and a neuroendocrine role has been attributed to these[22] and other[23] metabolites formed through the AA lipoxygenase.

The formation of such a complex variety of lipid products, and especially the oxygenated derivatives (eicosanoids, lipid peroxides, etc.), which is summarized in TABLE 2, certainly contributes to the onset of cellular lesions, tissue edema, and vasospasm that are initiated during ischemia and enhanced during the reperfusion phase. The amplification of these processes when blood flow and oxygen are supplied to the tissue may explain the aggravation of cell damage during reperfusion following ischemia and/or during incomplete ischemia.

TABLE 2. Lipid Metabolites and/or Mediators Generated from Complex Lipids in the Ischemic and Reperfused Brain

Ischemic	Reperfused
Free fatty acids and free arachidonate	CO products
Lysophospholipids	LO products (leukotrienes, hydroxy fatty acids)
Products of phosphoinositide breakdown (e.g., diacylglycerol, phosphatidic acid)	Lipoperoxides
Platelet-activating factor (PAF)	

PHARMACOLOGICAL CONTROL OF BRAIN EICOSANOIDS IN ISCHEMIA/RECOVERY

The participation of several endogenous mediators or factors in the onset of the functional and metabolic alterations occurring during ischemia, and especially in the reperfusion phase, has guided pharmacological approaches to the control of ischemic damage at the experimental and clinical levels.

The involvement of several eicosanoids, especially TxA_2 and PGI_2, in the modulation of cerebrovascular tone and cerebral blood flow (CBF) is supported by considerable evidence. The effects of various prostaglandins on isolated cerebral arteries have been studied and have been shown to be influenced by various factors. The role of endogenous eicosanoids has also been interpreted on the basis of the effects of drugs affecting eicosanoid synthesis on brain circulatory parameters, such as cerebral blood flow. Indomethacin, for example, has been consistently reported to reduce CBF in experimental animals and humans and to reduce considerably the response to hypercapnia (see Refs. 24 and 25 for reviews). These data suggest that vasodilating eicosanoids, such as prostacyclin, are the major CO products generated in the brain vascular compartment under basal conditions. The above effects, however, are not shared with other CO inhibitors and may be mediated by mechanisms different from the inhibition of prostaglandin synthesis. In addition there are also some species differences in the response of CBF to indomethacin.

Since elevation of vasocostricting CO products, such as TxA_2 and $PGF_{2\alpha}$, is a major alteration of eicosanoid metabolism in incomplete ischemia[12,13] and during reperfusion,[11] the use of indomethacin or other CO inhibitors has been tested by several investigators. Inhibition of TxB_2 accumulation during incomplete ischemia followed by reperfusion in the rat[13] or during reperfusion in a gerbil brain ischemia model[12] was associated with improved recovery. Indomethacin treatments were shown also to improve recovery in various other ischemic conditions. In addition, indomethacin does not inhibit the formation of prostacyclin in the brain during reperfusion, and this may be relevant to the recovery process. The use of indomethacin and other nonsteroidal antiinflammatory agents has been shown also to reduce vasospasm, which may be a contributing factor in the induction of ischemia.[26] The pharmacological effects of inhibitors of AA CO on indices of tissue damage during brain ischemia and/or reperfusion may not, however, be attributed completely to their action on eicosanoid synthesis, since data on this parameter are very limited. In addition, two distinct forms of CO are present in the brain,[27] and these may be differentially affected by various drugs.

Various inhibitors of thromboxane synthetase have also been tested and shown to be effective, for instance in reducing ischemic damage,[28] especially in models based on AA-induced platelet aggregation.[29] On the other hand, no pharmacological treatment is actually available to control the formation of LO products in brain ischemia.

Corticosteroid treatments have also been tested in situations of neural traumatic injury, and improvement of blood flow and carbohydrate metabolism[30] in cat spinal cord and of glucose utilization in rat brain[31] have been described. The relationship between corticosteroid treatment and prostaglandin synthesis in brain ischemia, however, has not been elucidated, since these drugs do not prevent the accumulation of various CO products in the brain after ischemia.[12,32] Corticosteroids, however, have a complicated range of actions in addition to the effects on phospholipases and AA metabolism.

Treatments of impaired cerebral circulation due to thrombotic or spastic events are also based on infusions of vasodilating and antithrombotic agents, such as prostacyclin or its analogues. PGI_2, alone or in combination with indomethacin, has been shown, in fact, to reduce ischemic damage or to improve recovery from ischemia.[33-37]

In general, the pharmacological treatments (schematically represented in FIG. 1) aimed at controlling eicosanoid levels in the ischemic brain, and especially during the recovery phase, are essentially based on the concept of maintaining a low ratio of constricting to dilating endogenous compounds—for example, thromboxane vs. prostacyclin—at the cerebrovascular level. This is actually obtained by the use of CO inhibitors—such as indomethacin—which appear to reduce TxB_2 levels in the reperfused brain more than those of prostacyclin; or by infusing PGI_2.

The effects of vasoactive drugs on eicosanoid production in tissues during ischemia and recovery have not been widely studied. It may be of interest, in this respect, that a derivative of carbochromene, the compound AD_6—which induces sustained dilation of coronary vessels,[38] inhibits platelet aggregation in the dog stenosed coronary artery,[39] reduces the *ex vivo* production of TxB_2 in stimulated platelets without affecting the conversion of exogenous AA,[40] and inhibits the release of AA by thrombin-stimulated human platelets[41]—has also been shown to enhance prostacyclin release in different conditions.[42,43] We have evaluated the effects of pretreatment with AD_6 (4 mg/kg ip 2 h before) on the levels of TxB_2 and 6-keto-$PGF_{1\alpha}$ in the rat brain after hypoxia and recovery, and also on the ability of stimulated cerebral cortical slices to produce leukotrienes. The results are summarized in TABLE 3.[44] Pretreatment with AD_6

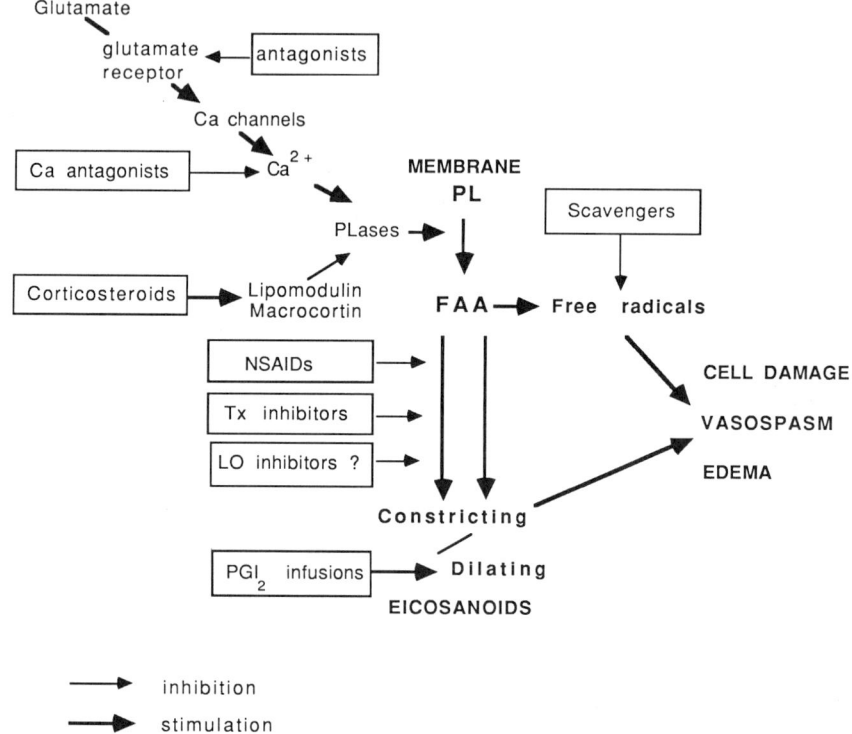

FIGURE 1. Pharmacological control of eicosanoids in brain ischemia and recovery. PL = phospholipid; FAA = free arachidonate; NSAIDs = nonsteroidal antiinflammatory drugs; Tx = thromboxane; LO = lipoxygenase.

TABLE 3. Levels of TxB_2 and 6-Keto-$PGF_{1\alpha}$ in the Brain Cortex of Control and AD_6-pretreated Rats after Hypoxia and Recovery

	Nonhypoxia		Hypoxia		Recovery	
	Control	AD_6	Control	AD_6	Control	AD_6
TxB_2 (ng/g fw)	3.7 ± 0.4	3.6 ± 0.5	3.5 ± 0.4	2.5 ± 0.3	6.2[a] ± 0.4	3.4[b] ± 0.5
6-Keto-$PGF_{1\alpha}$ (ng/g fw)	11.0 ± 2.0	33.0[c] ± 4.0	9.8 ± 1.7	9.1 ± 1.6	12.1 ± 2.7	8.1 ± 2.4

NOTE: Values are the average ± SEM of measurements carried out in 10 animals/group in each condition. Hypoxia was obtained by respiration of 5% O_2 in N_2 in a metabolic cage for 30 min, and recovery was carried out for 5 min by respiration of air. Animals were sacrificed by focused microwave radiation. Products were measured after extraction and purification by specific solid-phase enzyme immunoassay according to Pradelles, Grassi, and Maclouf.[68] AD_6 (8 monochloro-3-β-diethylaminoethyl-4-methyl-7-ethoxy carboxyl methoxy coumarin) was administered ip at a dose of 4 mg/kg 24 h before the beginning of hypoxia. Tx = thromboxane.
[a] $p < 0.01$ vs. nonhypoxic and hypoxic conditions (Dunnett test).
[b] $p < 0.05$ vs. controls (Dunnett test).
[c] $p < 0.01$ vs. controls (Dunnett test).

induced a selected elevation of 6-keto-PGF$_{1\alpha}$ in the brain of normoxic animals, a reduction of TxB$_2$ levels at the end of the hypoxic phase, and prevention of the accumulation of TxB$_2$ during recovery, in comparison to nontreated animals. In addition, generation of leukotrienes by incubated cerebral slices upon stimulation with the calcium ionophore A23187 and AA was reduced in samples obtained from pretreated animals as compared to controls (TABLE 4). Although the effects of the drug on other parameters were not studied, the reduction of the TxB$_2$/6-keto-PGF$_{1\alpha}$ ratio in the brain induced in normoxic, hypoxic, and recovering animals may exert protecting effects on brain cells in the experimental conditions used. However, the detailed effects of this type of drug on the eicosanoid balance in the nervous system in conditions of hypoxia/ischemia and recovery, in relation also to biochemical, functional, and morphologic indices of the brain status need further evaluation.

An indirect effect on eicosanoid generation in the brain could be exerted also by drugs affecting some of the early steps involved in the activation of lipolytic enzymes. The intracellular calcium increase associated with ischemic depolarization of cell membranes[45] is a major factor in the activation of phospholipases. Calcium inhibitors

TABLE 4. Levels of LTB$_4$ and C$_4$ in Brain Slices from Control and AD$_6$-pretreated Rats in Nonstimulated and Stimulated Conditions

	Control		Treated	
	Nonstimulated	Stimulated	Nonstimulated	Stimulated
LTB$_4$ (ng/g fw)	0.9 ± 0.3	15.8 ± 1.9	0.8 ± 0.2	10.6^a ± 1.7
LTC$_4$ (ng/g fw)	2.4 ± 0.3	30.4 ± 1.8	2.3 ± 0.3	17.4^b ± 1.7

NOTE: Data are average ± SEM of triplicate analyses of samples from a pool (8–10) of sliced brains, obtained from controls and AD$_6$-pretreated rats. Samples were incubated at 37 °C in phosphate buffer for 60 min in the presence of arachidonic acid (75 μM) and calcium ionophore A23187 (5 μM) after 10 min of preincubation. Products were measured after extraction with chloroform/methanol/water (6:3:2), phase separation, purification on Sep-pack C$_{18}$ cartridges, and RIA. AD$_6$ = 8 monochloro-3-β-diethylaminoethyl-4-methyl-7-ethoxy carboxyl methoxy coumarin; LT = leukotriene.
$^a p < 0.05$ vs. controls.
$^b p < 0.02$ vs. controls.

have been shown to exert cerebroprotective actions in ischemia.[46–48] Improved recovery of EEG activity after recirculation following ischemia was observed in rats pretreated with nimodipine, but the accumulation of free fatty acids (FFA) in the brain during ischemia was not prevented.[49] FFA were not measured during reperfusion. Apparently, the effects of calcium antagonists on eicosanoid production in brain ischemia and reperfusion have not yet been studied.

We have tested the effects of pretreatment with nimodipine of rats subjected to reversible ischemia by ligation of common carotid arteries followed by reperfusion on levels of free arachidonate (FAA) and TxB$_2$ in the cerebral cortex. In the nontreated animals (TABLE 5) levels of FAA increased at the end of ischemia, in comparison to values in the nonischemic animals, and tended to return to basal values at 5 min of reperfusion. Levels of TxB$_2$ were increased moderately at the end of ischemia and markedly at 5 min of reperfusion. In the treated animals, levels of FAA were lower than in controls in the nonischemic and reperfused situations, but no difference in the levels of TxB$_2$ in the various conditions was observed between treated and control animals. It appears from these data that the calcium antagonist used, although it affected levels of FAA in basal conditions and during reperfusion in the brain, did not

TABLE 5. Levels of Free Arachidonate and TxB_2 in the Rat Brain Cortex after Ischemia and Reperfusion in Control and Nimodipine-pretreated Rats

	Nonischemia		Ischemia		Reperfusion	
	Controls ($n = 6$)	Treated ($n = 6$)	Controls ($n = 8$)	Treated ($n = 8$)	Controls ($n = 8$)	Treated ($n = 8$)
Free arachidonate (ng/mg protein)	112 ± 8	$60^a \pm 13$	$268^b \pm 40$	$220^c \pm 8$	$202^b \pm 34$	$65^d \pm 19$
TxB_2	2.4 ± 0.7	2.3 ± 0.8	$5.4^b \pm 1.0$	$4.5^b \pm 1.0$	$43.1^c \pm 5.6$	$44.1^c \pm 11.9$

NOTE: Groups of male rats were subjected to transient ischemia by ligation of both common carotid arteries (total of 20 min, including the last 5 min of hypoxia by respiration of 5% O_2 in N_2) and were subsequently reperfused for 5 min. Nonischemic (sham operated), ischemic, and reperfused animals were sacrificed by focused microwave radiation. Free arachidonate was measured by quantitative GLC of methyl esters prepared after chromatographic separation of free fatty acids; TxB_2 (thromboxane B_2) was measured by RIA after extraction and purification. Nimodipine treatment: 1 mg/kg ip 1 h before surgery. Values are the average ± SEM.
[a] $p < 0.02$ vs. control animals (Dunnett test).
[b] $p < 0.05$ vs. nonischemic animals (Dunnett test).
[c] $p < 0.001$ vs. nonischemic animals (Dunnett test).
[d] $p < 0.05$ vs. control animals (Dunnett test).

influence the activation of lipolytic processes during ischemia, as already described.[49] This possibly explains the lack of changes of the CO product TxB_2 also in the reperfusion phase, at least in the experimental conditions tested.

MEMBRANE PROTECTING AGENTS AND BRAIN ISCHEMIA

One of the key phenomena in the onset of irreversible damage during and after an ischemic event is the lesion to the plasma membrane, resulting from a wide spectrum of metabolic derangements. In this process, the generation of metabolic products—including eicosanoids and lipoperoxides, products with biological or cytotoxic activities, and products derived from complex lipids within membranes—can be considered both an index of cell damage and also a major factor for the progression of the lesions.

The complex glycosphingolipids containing sialic acid—the gangliosides—are components of cellular membranes that are localized in the outer leaflet of the lipid bilayer; they are particularly abundant in nerve tissue. The possible functional roles of gangliosides concern neuronal development, synaptogenesis, and synaptic transmission.[50-52] The administration of gangliosides has also been shown to facilitate the regeneration of damaged peripheral nerves[53] or the central nervous system.[54] GM1, one of the major gangliosides in the mammalian brain, when administered exogenously, penetrates the blood-brain barrier[55] and is also actively incorporated into neuronal membranes.[56] The interaction of gangliosides with brain membranes is accompanied by various metabolic effects, such as increased activity of adenylate cyclase[57] and phosphodiesterase,[58] enhanced release of dopamine,[59] and modifications of Na, K-ATPase activity.[60] Exogenous gangliosides were shown to reduce edema[61] and the loss of enzymatic activities[62] in the brains of rats that had sustained open head injuries. Administration of GM1 after occlusion of the middle cerebral artery in cats resulted in greater local CBF, reduced local cerebral glucose metabolism, and reduced histological damage.[63] In another study of a gerbil model of ischemia, GM1 and its inner ester AGF_2 (which has a longer half life in serum than GM1), when administered soon after surgery, reduced cerebral edema, protected from loss of ATPase activity, and decreased mortality.[64] GM1 and AGF_2 were also able to reduce Ca^{++} overload in the brain and K^+ efflux from cells, in addition to improving CBF and reducing the extent of cell damage, in the postischemic period following transient ischemia in the rat.[65] It has been postulated that gangliosides may play a role as endogenous modulators of the translocation of protein kinase C[66] (PKC) from cytosol to plasma membrane. This process increases the phosphorylation of specific membrane proteins after activation of calcium influx. The translocation of PKC appears to involve glutamate receptor–operated cationic channels,[67] and gangliosides may thus limit the cell damage caused by glutamate-mediated calcium influx. The protective action of gangliosides with respect to alterations induced in the brain by ischemia, and the possible modulation by these compounds of membrane processes that appear to be associated with early stages of cell activation, have prompted us to study the effects of pretreatment with the ganglioside derivative AGF_2 on levels of lactate, FAA, and CO products in the rat brain during ischemia and reperfusion (TABLE 6). In nontreated animals, marked elevations of lactate, FAA, and 6-keto-$PGF_{1\alpha}$, together with a smaller increment of TxB_2, occurred in the brain after ischemia. At 5 min of reperfusion, values of lactate and FAA were reduced with respect to values in the ischemic rats, although they still remained higher than in nonischemic animals. Concentrations of TxB_2 and 6-keto-$PGF_{1\alpha}$, on the other hand, were markedly increased over values both in the nonischemic and in the ischemic animals. In the animals pretreated with AGF_2, the

TABLE 6. Levels of Lactate, Free Arachidonate, TxB$_2$, and 6-Keto-PGF$_{1\alpha}$ in Brain Cortex of Control and AGF$_2$-pretreated Rats Subjected to Cerebral Ischemia and Reperfusion

	Nonischemia		Ischemia		Reperfusion	
	Control	Treated	Control	Treated	Control	Treated
Lactate (μg Moles/g)	1.95 ± 0.46	2.0 ± 0.46	13.5^a ± 2.6	9.9^b ± 1.2	5.2^c ± 1.4	4.3^c ± 0.8
Free arachidonate (ng/mg protein)	40 ± 5	37 ± 5	361^d ± 90	339^d ± 81	70^e ± 10	64^e ± 14
TxB$_2$ (pg/mg protein)	1.4 ± 0.2	1.3 ± 0.2	3.9^f ± 7	2.5 ± 0.7	46.3^g ± 13.5	5.4^c ± 1.1
6-Keto-PGF$_{1\alpha}$ (pg/mg protein)	2.7 ± 0.6	5.5^h ± 1.1	16.1^a ± 1.4	8.6^i ± 1.8	102.1^e ± 23.0	20.4^{c,j} ± 4.4

NOTE: Experimental conditions as described in TABLE 5. Pretreatment with AGF$_2$ as carried out by ip injections of 10 mg/kg for three days twice a day, with a last treatment 2 h before ischemia. Tx = thromboxane. Values are the average ± SEM of 8 animals in each group. Statistical analysis is according to the Dunnett test.

$^a p < 0.01$ vs. nonischemic animals.
$^b p < 0.005$ vs. nonischemic animals.
$^c p < 0.05$ vs. ischemic animals.
$^d p < 0.02$ vs. nonischemic animals.
$^e p < 0.005$ vs. ischemic animals.
$^f p < 0.05$ vs. nonischemic animals.
$^g p < 0.02$ vs. ischemic animals.
$^h p < 0.005$ vs. control animals.
$^i p < 0.025$ vs. control animals.
$^j p < 0.001$ vs. control animals.

modifications of lactate and FAA in the ischemic phase were similar to those occurring in controls, but the eicosanoids were only marginally modified with respect to values in the treated, nonischemic animals. The effects of ganglioside pretreatment on brain eicosanoid levels were very pronounced in the animals that were reperfused for 5 min, since both products were only marginally elevated over values in the nonischemic animals, in contrast with the situation in the nontreated animals. In addition, the TxB_2/6-keto-$PGF_{1\alpha}$ ratio in the brain of pretreated animals at 5 min of reperfusion was quite lower than in controls. These data indicate that gangliosides affect parameters, such as the accumulation of TxB_2 during reperfusion, that are both factors for the progression of cerebrovascular impairments and possible indices of responses to cytotoxic conditions. These effects may be partly responsible for the protecting action of gangliosides in brain ischemia and recovery.

In conclusion, various pharmacological treatments known to affect eicosanoid production—especially TxB_2 generation—in tissues have been shown to improve functional parameters and to reduce cell damage in the brain during the ischemic and the reperfusion phases. On the other hand, control of the eicosanoid changes associated with the ischemic and recovery conditions is obtained also with the use of compounds—such as the gangliosides—that appear to exert a membrane protecting action, possibly as modulators of metabolic processes at the membrane site. In addition, control of the generation of LO products, which may play an important role in the pathophysiology of ischemic lesions, is a pharmacological approach that deserves greater attention in future studies.

REFERENCES

1. ICHIDA, S., H. TOKUNAGA, M. MORIYAMA, Y. ODA, S. TANAKA & T. KIDA. 1982. Effects of neurotransmitter candidates on $^{45}Ca^{++}$ uptake by cortical slices of rat brain: Stimulatory effects of L-glutamic acid. Brain Res. **248**: 305–311.
2. CHEN, S. T., C. Y. HSU, E. L. HOGAN, H. Y. JUAN, N. L. BANIK & J. D. BALENTINE. 1987. Brain calcium content in ischemic infarction. Neurology **37**: 1227–1229.
3. SCHWARCZ, R., A. C. FOSTER, E. D. FRENCH, W. O. WHETSELL & C. KOHLER. 1984. Excitotoxic models for neurogenerative disorders. Life Sci. **35**: 19–32.
4. YASUDA, H., K. KISHIRO, N. IZUMI & M. NAKANISHI. 1983. The presence and physiological significance of dual phases in brain arachidonate acid liberation during ischemia. J. Cereb. Blood Flow Metab. **3** (Suppl. 1): S345–S346.
5. ABE, K., K. KOGURE, H. YAMAMOTO, M. IMAZAWA & K. MIYAMOTO. 1987. Mechanism of arachidonic acid liberation during ischemia in gerbil cerebral cortex. J. Neurochem. **48**: 503–509.
6. ANNABLE, C. R., L. M. MCMANUS, K. D. CAREY & R. N. PINCKARD. 1985. Isolation of platelet-activating factor (PAF) from ischemic baboon myocardium. Fed. Proc. **44**(4): 1271.
7. KOCHANEK, P., A. DUTKA, K. KUMAROO & J. HALLENBECK. 1986. Platelet activating factor receptor blockade enhances early neuronal recovery after multifocal brain ischemia in the dog (abstract). Second International Conference on Platelet Activating Factor and Structurally Related Alkyl Ether Lipids. Gatlinburg, TN.: 118.
8. PANETTA, T., V. L. MARCHESELLI, P. BRAQUET, B. SPINNEWYN & N. G. BAZAN. 1987. Effects of a platelet activating factor antagonist (BN 52021) on free fatty acids, diacylglycerols, polyphosphoinositides and blood flow in the gerbil brain: Inhibition of ischemia-reperfusion induced cerebral injury. Biochem. Biophys. Res. Commun. **149**: 580–587.
9. SPAGNUOLO, C., L. SAUTEBIN, G. GALLI, G. RACAGNI, C. GALLI, S. MAZZARI & M. FINESSO. 1979. PGF_2 Thromboxane B_2 and HETE levels in gerbil brain cortex after ligation of common carotid arteries and decapitation. Prostaglandins **18**: 53–61.

10. GAUDET, R. J. & L. LEVINE. 1979. Transient cerebral ischemia and brain prostaglandins. Biochem. Biophys. Res. Commun. **86:** 893–901.
11. GAUDET, R. J., I. ALAM & L. LEVINE. 1980. Accumulation of cyclooxygenase products of arachidonic acid metabolism in gerbil brain during reperfusion after bilateral common carotid occlusion. J. Neurochem. **35:** 653–658.
12. GAUDET, R. J. & L. LEVINE. 1980. Effects of unilateral common carotid artery occlusion on levels of prostaglandins D_2, $F_{2\alpha}$, 6-keto $PGF_{1\alpha}$ in gerbil brain. Stroke **11:** 648–652.
13. SHOHAMI, E., J. ROSENTHAL & S. LAVY. 1982. The effect of incomplete cerebral ischemia on prostaglandin levels in rat brain. Stroke **13:** 494–499.
14. WOJTCZAK, L. 1976. Effect of long chain fatty acids and Acyl CoA on mitochondrial permeability, transport and energy coupling processes. J. Bioenerg. Biomembr. **8:** 293–311.
15. CHAN, P. H. & R. A. FISHMAN. 1978. Brain edema: Induction in cortical slices by polyunsaturated fatty acids. Science **201:** 358–360.
16. WATSON, B. D., R. BUSTO, W. J. GOLDBERG, M. SANTISO, S. YOSHIDA & M. D. GINSBERG. 1983. Lipid peroxidation *in vitro* induced by diffuse forebrain ischemia in rat brain. J. Cereb. Blood Flow Metab. **3** (Suppl. 1): S325–S326.
17. YOSHIDA, S., K. ABE, R. BUSTO, B. D. WATSON, K. KOGURE & M. D. GINSBERG. 1982. Influence of transient ischemia on lipid-soluble anti-oxidants, free fatty acids and energy metabolites in rat brain. Brain Res. **245:** 307–316.
18. WOLFE, L. S., H. M. PAPPIUS, R. POKRUPA & A. HAKIM. 1985. Involvement of arachidonic acid metabolites in experimental brain injury. Identification of lipoxygenase products in brain. Clinical studies on prostacyclin infusion in acute cerebral ischemia. *In* Advances in Prostaglandin, Thromboxane and Leukotriene Research, Vol. 15. O. Hayaishi & S. Yamamoto, Eds.: 585–588. Raven Press. New York, NY.
19. SHOHAMI, E., T. P. JACOBS, J. M. HALLENBECK & G. FEUERSTEIN. 1987. Increased Thromboxane A_2 and 5-HETE production following spinal cord ischemia in the rabbit. Prostagland. Leuk. Med. **28:** 169–181.
20. MOSKOWITZ, M. A., K. J. KIWAK, K. HEKIMIAN & L. LEVINE. 1984. Synthesis of compounds with properties of leukotrienes C_4 and D_4 in gerbil brains after ischemia and reperfusion. Science **224:** 886–888.
21. LINDGREN, J. A., T. HOKFELT, S. V. DAHLEN, C. PATRONO & B. SAMUELSSON. 1984. Leukotrienes in the rat central nervous system. Proc. Natl. Acad. Sci. USA **81:** 6212–6216.
22. LINDGREN, J. A., A. L. HULTING, T. HOKFELT, S. E. DAHLEN, P. ENEROTH, S. WERNER, C. PATRONO & B. SAMUELSSON. 1985. Occurrence of leukotrienes in rat brain. Evidence for a neuroendocrine role of leukotriene C_4. *In* Advances in Prostaglandin, Thromboxane and Leukotriene Research, Vol. 15. O. Hayaishi & S. Yamamoto, Eds.: 561–564. Raven Press. New York, NY.
23. SNYDER, G. D., J. CAPDEVILA, N. CHACOS, S. MANNA & J. R. FALCK. 1983. Action of luteinizing hormone-releasing hormone: Involvement of novel arachidonic acid metabolites. Proc. Natl. Acad. Sci. USA **80:** 3504–3507.
24. SIESJO, B. K., & B. NILSSON. 1982. Prostaglandins and the Cerebral Circulation. Prostaglandins and the Cardiovascular System. J. A. Oates, Ed.: 367–380. Raven Press. New York, NY.
25. PICKARD, J. D., & V. WALKER. 1984. Current concepts of the role of prostaglandins and other eicosanoids in acute cerebrovascular disease. *In* Neurotransmitters and the Cerebral Circulation, Vol. 2. E. T. Mackenzie, J. Seylar & A. Bes, Eds.: 191–218. Raven Press. New York, NY.
26. WHITE, R. P. & J. T. ROBERTSON. 1983. Comparison of piroxicam, meclofenamate, ibuprofen, aspirin and prostacyclin efficacy in a chronic model of cerebral vasospasm. Neurosurgery **12:** 40–46.
27. LYSZ, T. W. & P. NEEDLEMAN. 1982. Evidence for two distinct forms of fatty acid cyclooxygenase in brain. J. Neurochem. **38:** 1111–1117.
28. TAMURA, A., T. ASANO, K. SANO, T. TSUMAGARI & A. NAKAJIMA. 1979. Protection from cerebral ischemia by a new imidazole derivative (Y-9179) and pentobarbital. A comparative study in chronic middle cerebral artery occlusion in cats. Stroke **10:** 126–134.
29. FREDRICKSSON, K., I. ROSEN, B. JOHANSSON & T. WIELOCH. 1983. The thromboxane

synthetase inhibitor OKY-1581 prevents cerebral ischemia and neural transmission failure induced by sodium arachidonate platelet aggregation. J. Cereb. Blood Flow Metab. 3(Suppl. 1): S293–S294.
30. BRAUGHLER, J. M. & E. D. HALL. 1983. Lactate and pyruvate metabolism in injured cat spinal cord before and after a single large intravenous dose of methylprednisolone. J. Neurosurg. **59:** 256–261.
31. PAPPIUS, H. M. & L. S. WOLFE. 1983. Involvement of serotonin and catecholamines in functional depression of traumatized brain. J. Cereb. Blood Flow Metab. 3 (Suppl. 1): S226–S227.
32. CROCKARD, H. A., K. K. BHAKOO & P. F. LASCELLES. 1982. Regional prostaglandin levels in cerebral ischemia. J. Neurochem. **38:** 1311–1314.
33. PICKARD, J. D., A. TAMURA, M. STEWART, A. MCGEORGE & W. FITCH. 1980. Prostacyclin, indomethacin and the cerebral circulation. Brain Res. **197:** 425–431.
34. HALLENBECK, J. M., & T. W. FURLOW, JR. 1979. Prostaglandin I_2 and indomethacin prevent unpairment of post-ischemic brain reperfusion in the dog. Stroke **10:** 629–637.
35. HALLENBECK, J. M., T. P. JACOBS & A. I. FADEN. 1983. Combined PGI_2, indomethacin and heparin improve neurological recovery after spinal trauma in cats. J. Neurosurg. **58:** 749–754.
36. HALLENBECK, J. M., D. R. LEITCH, A. J. DUTKA, L. J. GREENBAUM & A. E. MCKEE. 1982. Prostanglandin I_2, indomethacin and heparin promote post-ischemic neuronal recovery in dogs. Am. Neurol. **12:** 145–156.
37. GRYGLEWSKI, R. J., S. NOWAK, E. KOSTKA-TRABKA, J. KUSMIDERSKI, A. DEMBINSKA-KIEC, K. BIERON, M. BASISTA & B. BLASZCZYK. 1983. Treatment of ischemic stroke with prostacyclin. Stroke **14:** 197–202.
38. APORTI, F., M. FINESSO & L. GRANATA. 1978. Effects of 8-monochloro-3β-diethylamino-ethyl-4 methyl-7-ethoxy carbonyl methoxy coumarin (AD_6) on the coronary circulation of the dog. Pharmacol. Res. **10:** 469–473.
39. PROSDOCIMI, M., M. FINESSO, F. TESSARI, A. GORIO, L. R. LANGUINO, G. DE GAETANO & E. DAIANA. 1985. Inhibition by AD_6 (8-monochloro-3β-diethylaminoethyl-4 methyl-7-ethoxy carbonyl methoxy courmarin) of platelet aggregation in dog stenosed coronary artery. Thromb. Res. **39:** 399–405.
40. GALLI, C., E. AGRADI, A. PETRONI & A. SOCINI. 1980. Effects of 8-monochloro-3β-diethylaminoethyl-4 methyl-3 ethoxy carbonyl methoxy coumarin (AD_6) on aggregation, arachidonic acid metabolism and thromboxane B_2 formation in human platelet. Pharmacol. Res. Commun. **12:** 329–337.
41. PORCELLATI, S., V. COSTANTINI, M. PROSDOCIMI, R. PISTOLESI, P. PORROVECCHIO, G. G. NENCI & G. GORACCI. 1987. AD_6 (8-monochloro-3β-diethylaminoethyl-4 metnyl-7 ethoxycarboxyl-methoxy coumarin) inhibits the release of arachidonic acid in human platelets stimulated by thrombin. Thromb. Res. **47:** 15–24.
42. PETRONI, A., A. SOCINI, M. BLASEVICH, A. BORGHI & C. GALLI. 1985. Differential effects of various vasoactive drugs on basal and stimulated levels of TxB_2 and 6-keto-$PGF_{1\alpha}$ in rat brain. Prostaglandins **29:** 579–587.
43. DEJANA, E., C. DE CASTELLRNAU, G. BALCONI, D. ROTILIO, A. PIETRA & G. DE GAETANO. 1982. AD_6, a coronary dilating agent, stimulates PGI_2 production in rat aorta ex vivo and in human endothelial cells in culture. Pharmacol. Res. Commun. **14:** 779–724.
44. BERTAZZO, A., A. PETRONI, S. SARTI, C. COLOMBO & C. GALLI. 1988. The carbochromene derivative AD_6 reduces the TxB_2/6-keto-$PGF_{1\alpha}$ ratio in cerebral cortex during hypoxia and recovery and leukotriene synthesis in brain tissue, in the rat. Prostaglandins **35:** 15–29.
45. NAYLER, W. G., P. A. POOLE-WILSON & A. WILLIAMS. 1979. Hypoxia and calcium. J. Mol. Cell. Cardiol. **11:** 683–706.
46. HEFFEZ D. S. & J. V. PASSONNEAU, 1985. Effect of nimodipine on cerebral metabolism during ischemia and recirculation in the Mongolian gerbil. J. Cereb. Blood Flow Metab. **5:** 523–528.
47. FUJISAWA, A., M. MATSUMOTO, T. MATSUYAMA, H. UEDA, A. WANAKA, S. YONETA, K. KIMURA & T. KAMADA. 1986. The effect of the calcium antagonist nimodipine on the gerbil model of experimental cerebral ischemia. Stroke **17:** 748–752.
48. BIELENBERG, G. W., T. BECK, D. SAUER, M. BURNIOL & J. KRIEGLSTEIN. 1987. Effects of

cerebroprotective agents on the cerebral blood flow and post-ischemic energy metabolism in the rat brain. J. Cereb. Blood Flow Metab. **7:** 480–488.
49. MABE, H., H. NAGAI, T. TAKAGI, S. UMEMURA & M. OHNO. 1986. Effect of nimodipine on cerebral functional and metabolic recovery following ischemia in the rat brain. Stroke **17:** 501–505.
50. WILLINGER, M. & M. SCHACHNER. 1980. GM1 ganglioside as a marker for neuronal differentiation in mouse cerebellum. Dev. Biol. **74:** 101–117.
51. ROISEN, F. J., H. BARTFELD, R. NAGELE & G. YORKE. 1981. Ganglioside stimulation of axonal sprouting in vitro. Science **214:** 577–578.
52. RAHMAN, H., W. PROBST & M. MUHLEISEN. 1982. Gangliosides and synaptic transmission. Jpn. J. Exp. Med. **52:** 275–286.
53. SPARROW, J. R. & B. GRAFSTEIN, 1982. Sciatic nerve regeneration in ganglioside treated rats. Exp. Neurol. **77:** 230–235.
54. KARPIAK, S. E. 1983. Ganglioside treatment improves recovery of alternation behavior after unilateral entorhinal cortex lesion. Exp. Neurol. **81:** 330–339.
55. ORLANDO, P., G. COCCIANTE, G. IPPOLITO, P. MOSSARI, S. ROBERTI & G. TETTAMANTI. 1979. The fate of tritium labelled GM1 ganglioside injected in mice. Pharmacol. Res. Commun. **11:** 759–770.
56. TOFFANO, G., D. BENVEGNU, A. C. BONETTI, L. FACCIO, A. LEON, P. ORLANDO, R. GHIDONI & G. TETTAMANTI. 1980. Interactions of GM1 ganglioside with rat brain neuronal membranes. J. Neurochem. **35:** 861–866.
57. PARTINGTON, C. R. & J. W. DALY. 1979. Effect of gangliosides on adenylate cyclase activity in rat cerebral cortical membranes. Mol. Pharmacol. **15:** 484–491.
58. DAVIS, C. W. & J. W. DALY. 1979. Activation of rat cerebral cortical 3', 5' cyclic nucleotide phosphodiesterase activity by gangliosides. Mol. Pharmacol. **17:** 206–211.
59. CUMAR, F. A., B. MAGGIO & R. CAPUTTO. 1978. Dopamine release from nerve endings induced by polysialogangliosides. Biochem. Biophys. Res. Commun. **84:** 65–69.
60. LEON, A., G. TETTAMANTI & G. TOFFANO. 1981. Changes in functional properties of neuron membranes by insertion of exogenus ganglioside. In Gangliosides in Neurological and Neuromuscular Function, Development and Repair. M. M. Rapport & A. Gorio, Eds.: 45–54. Raven Press. New York, NY.
61. KARPIAK, S. E. & S. P. MAHADIK. 1984. Reduction of cerebral edema with GM1 ganglioside. J. Neurosci. Res. **12:** 485–492.
62. KARPIAK, S. E. & S. P. MAHADIK. 1984. GM1 ganglioside limits CNS pathology. In Cellular and Pathological Aspects of Glycoconjugate Metabolism. H. Dreyfus, R. Massarelli, L. Freysz and G. Rebel, Eds.: 585–598. INSERM. Paris.
63. TANAKA, K., E. DORA, R. URBANICS, J. H. GREENBERG, G. TOFFANO & M. REIVICH. 1986. Effect of the ganglioside GM1 on cerebral metabolism, microcirculation, recovery kinetics of ECoG and histology, during the recovery period following focal ischemia in cats. Stroke **17:** 1170–1178.
64. KARPIAK, S. E., Y. S. LI & S. P. MAHADIK. 1987. Gangliosides (GM1 and AGF$_2$) reduce mortality due to ischemia: Protection of membrane function. Stroke **18:** 184–187.
65. CAHN, J., M. G. BORZEIX & G. TOFFANO. 1986. In Gangliosides and Neuronal Plasticity. FIDIA Res. Series, Vol. **6.** G. Tettamanti, R. W. Ledeen, K. Sandhoff, Y. Nagai & G. Toffano, Eds.: 435–443. Liviana Press. Padova.
66. MACDERMOTT, A. B., M. L. MAYER, G. L. WESTBROOK, S. J. SMITH & J. L. BARKER. 1986. NMDA-receptor activation increases cytoplasmatic calcium concentration in cultured spinal cord neurones. Nature (London) **321:** 519–522.
67. VACCARINO, F., A. GUIDOTTI & E. COSTA. 1987. Ganglioside inhibition of glutamate-mediated protein kinase C translocation in primary cultures of cerebellar neurons. Proc. Natl. Acad. Sci. USA **84:** 8707–8711.
68. PRADELLES, P., J. GRASSI & J. MACLOUF. 1985. Anal. Chem. **57:** 1170–1173.

PART VI. ARACHIDONIC ACID AND ITS METABOLITES IN NORMAL AND ABNORMAL BRAIN FUNCTIONS: SLEEP, TEMPERATURE REGULATION, ALCOHOL EFFECTS, AND MENTAL DISORDERS

The Aging Brain

A Normal Phenomenon with Not-So-Normal Arachidonic Acid Metabolism[a]

ALBERTO GAITI

Department of Experimental Medicine and Biochemical Sciences
University of Perugia
Perugia, Italy

INTRODUCTION

Aging is a property of any multicellular organism and is characterized by a measurable decline of physiological functions. The brain, which is composed of postmitotic nonrenewable cells, is a particularly strong candidate for an organ that plays a crucial role in biological aging. Even if the causes of this decline are still unknown, several hypotheses have been advanced in the attempt to explain the gradual loss of this organ's ability to adapt to the environment. Among these, the membrane deterioration theory is considered one of the most important factors in explaining the aging phenomena.

Membranes are made up of a bimolecular leaflet of phospholipids and cholesterol interacting with proteins through ionic and hydrophobic forces.[1] Protein-lipid interaction may play an important role in regulating some of the membrane functions, and, in addiction, the acyl groups of membrane phospholipids are also important to the activity of membrane-bound enzymes. The degree of unsaturation, the cholesterol content, and membrane lipid asymmetry are thought to be important in maintaining membrane fluidity in highly functional membranes; and any modification of these parameters leads to a variation of the membrane functions. Modifications of membrane functions related to the alterations of these parameters in aged animal models have been described.[2-5]

Among other parameters, a high degree of unsaturation is important in order to maintain a liquid crystalline state of the membrane, while the presence of polyunsaturated fatty acids in the membrane is undesiderable due to the liability of these molecules to oxidation and free radical attack,[6] which may facilitate the aging process. The "free radical theory of aging" was proposed by Harman in 1956[7]; it states that a major contributor to the aging processes is the continuous production of oxygen radicals. One of the most evident consequences of lipid peroxidation started by radicals is the accumulation of lipofuscin with age.[8]

The above findings lead one to expect that age induces a modification of the phospholipid polyunsaturated fatty acid profile. The first report on this field was that of O'Brien and Sampson, who in 1965 determined the fatty acid composition of lipids

---

[a]This work was supported in part by Consiglio Nazionale delle Richerche, Progetto Finalizzato, Medicina Preventiva e Riabilitativa, SP "Meccanismi di invecchiamento," Grant 115.07444.87.00299.56.

from gray and white matter and myelin from four human brains of widely different ages.[9] Later, Svennerholm and coworkers published more extensive studies on the acyl group profile of the human brain phospholipids related to age.[10] These results, subsequently more-or-less confirmed for other animal species as well (see Reference 11 for review), indicate that the major modifications of the fatty acid profile occur during development and maturation, while only slight modifications are present in the elderly. On the other hand, a quite relevant modification of the fatty acyl composition of the microsomal diacylglycerols (as phospholipid precursors) was found in the whole brain of adult and aged rats[12] (TABLE 1).

More precisely, the percent of the content of monoenoic and dienoic species increases noticeably with a corresponding decrease of that of arachidonate. However, little information was present in the literature regarding the metabolism of fatty acids in the brain lipids during aging.

A source of much of the fatty acid in brain phospholipid is its uptake from the circulation,[13,14] in the steady state the amount of free fatty acid transported into the brain is balanced by fatty acid released from brain lipids.[15] The lipids cross the endothelium cells of brain microvessels that constitute the major component of the so-called blood-brain barrier[16] and mix with endogenous pools. This passage through

TABLE 1. Fatty Acyl Composition of Microsomal Diacylglycerols of 24-Month-Old (Aged) Rats as Compared with That of 4-Month-Old (Adult) Rats[a]

	4-Month-Old Rats	24-Month-Old Rats
Diacylglycerols (μg/mg protein)	10.4 ± 3.2	8.4 ± 1.2[b]
Difference in fatty acid composition		
16:1		+67%
18:1		+21%
18:2		+88%
20:4		−20%

[a]Modified from Brunetti et al.[12]
[b]$p < 0.05$.

endothelium cells of brain microvessels is not a passive process. Both fatty acid oxidation[17] and arachidonoyl-CoA synthesis[18] are present in this very specific structure and might play a role in the uptake of serum lipids.

The fatty acids are then utilized by the brain structure and, if labeled acids are injected intraperitoneally, labeling takes place in mitochondrial, synaptosomal, microsomal, and myelin membranes.[19] Fatty acid may be elongated and desaturated,[15] while oxidation seems of little importance for energy production in the adult brain, since acetyl-CoA from beta-oxidation is reincorporated into other fatty acids.[20]

When labeled fatty acids are injected intracerebrally or, better, in the lateral ventricle of the brain of experimental animals, long-chain fatty acids are readily taken up by the brain tissue and incorporated into membrane lipids, the rate of arachidonate uptake being usually more rapid than that of saturated fatty acids.[21]

The initial step for fatty acid utilization is the enzymatic formation of acyl-CoA (EC 6.2.1.3). This is a nearly obligatory step prior to fatty acid oxidation and esterification into polar and neutral lipids. In the brain, this enzymatic activity depends both on the length and the degree of unsaturation of the acyl chain.[22,23] In particular, Reddy and Bazan[24] demonstrated that a specific arachidonoyl-CoA synthetase is present in the brain microsomes and hypothesized that this activity might be involved in limiting eicosanoid formation as well as other metabolic fates and also participate in the retention of essential fatty acids in the central nervous system (CNS).

Arachidonic acid is preferentially incorporated into diacylglycerophosphoinositides (IPG) and diacylglycerophocholines (choline phosphoglycerides: CPG).[15,21] In general, arachidonoyl-IPG turnover in the brain membranes was more rapid than that of other phosphoglycerides, so that the existence of two different metabolic pools of archidonate has been suggested: a small pool with a rapid turnover rate (half-life in hours) and a larger one with a longer half-life (days).[21]

A relatively high specific radioactivity is also found in triacylglycerols (TG), which are trace components of the brain.[15] This has led to the suggestion that TG may regulate the fatty and metabolism, functioning as a reservoir between free fatty acids and glycerolipids.[20,25,26]

In spite of the rapid accumulation of polyunsaturated fatty acid in the IPG and CPG, these two lipids contain a relatively low number of polyunsaturated fatty acids, which, on the contrary, are present in high proportions in ethanolamine and serine phosphoglycerides (EPG and GPS) (see Reference 10 as a review).

These results indicate that brain phospholipid acyl groups undergo active turnover, IPG are rapidly converted into diacylglycerols (DG) by the IPG-dependent phospholipase C,[27] which may be utilized in the phospholipid biosynthesis *ex novo* pathway as wall as retransformed into free fatty acids. The remodeling of the phospholipid molecule may be also determined by a combined action of phospholipase A activity with subsequent reacylation, Land's cycle.[28]

EFFECTS OF AGE ON FATTY ACID METABOLISM IN THE BRAIN

When labeled arachidonic acid is injected into the lateral ventricle of the brain of 4-month- and 24-mont-old rats, its utilization differs according to the brain area examined and the age of the animal. The rate of fatty acid incorporation into lipids is always lower from aged than from adult rat brain areas.[26] In the cortex the differences between adult and aged animals are dramatic (FIG. 1).

Only a slight failure of arachidonic acid incorporation takes place in the hippocampus of the aged rat brain. The same difference is also evident in the lipidic precursors DG and phosphatidic acid (PA) (FIG. 2).

Interestingly, the specific activity of arachidonic acid in all the areas examined in both adult and aged animals draw together to the same value at about 24 hours after the injection of the labeled precursor.

These first results indicate that in the aged, as compared to the adult, rat brain, there are: (1) different arachidonic acid metabolisms according to the brain area examined; (2) failure of fatty acid utilization, at least in the fast pool (see above); and (3) a tendency to lose fewer fatty acids (as demonstrated by the specific activity slopes of lipids from aged animals).

The last finding seems to indicate a decrease of the arachidonic acid turnover rate in the lipids that may act as storage sites, thus partly counteracting the decline of its incorporation. To verify this hypothesis we tested *in vitro* the phospholipase A activities. The activity of these enzymes has been postulated to play such different roles in the cells as the regulation of the biosynthesis of phospholipid molecular species and phospholipid breakdown and turnover.[29]

The effect of age on phospholipase activity differs greatly according to the substrate used (CPG and EPG) and the cerebral area tested.[30] Although there is a decrease or slight stimulation of phospholipase A_2 activity when arachidonic acid containing EPG is used as substrate, a stimulation of about 200% is seen in some areas

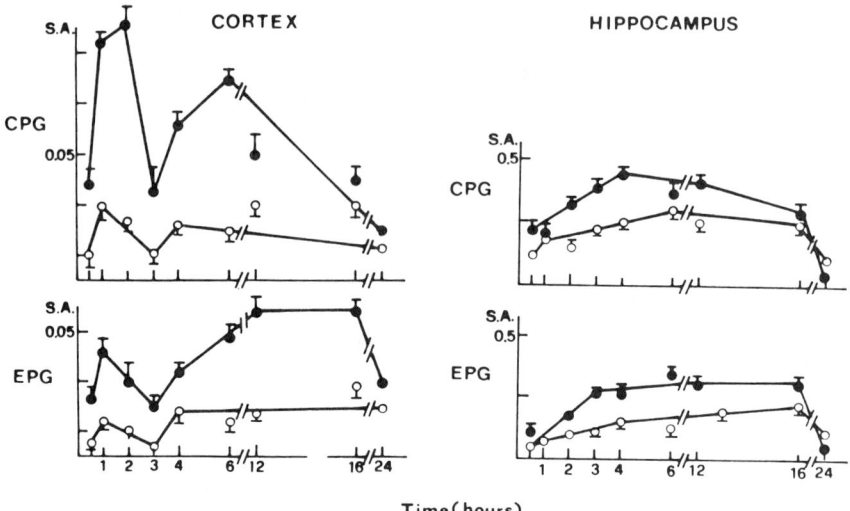

FIGURE 1. Arachidonic acid incorporation *in vivo*. Time–specific activity slopes of different lipids from the cortex and hippocampus. S.A. = specific activity (nCi/μg phospholipid P); *open circles* = 4-month-old (adult) rats; *solid circles* = 24-month-old (aged) rats. Two μCi of 1-^{14}C arachidonic acid (together with palmitic acids differently labeled) were injected into the lateral ventricle of the rat brain with the aid of stereotaxis apparatus in a total volume of 10 μl of sucrose 0.32 M in Tris-HCl 50 mM pH 7.4 containing BSA 1 mg/ml. The animals were sacrificed at various times after the injection. (Adapted from Gatti *et al.*[26])

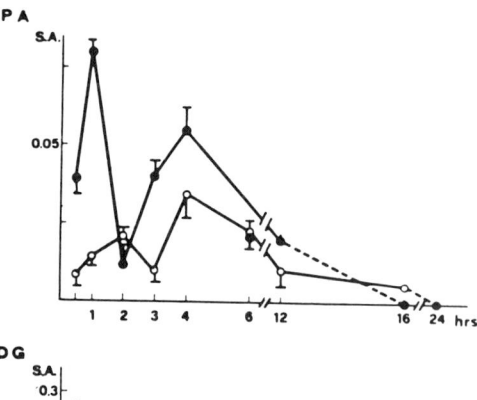

FIGURE 2. Time–specific activity slopes of phosphatidic acid (PA) and diacylglycerols (DG) from the cortex. S.A. = specific activity (nCi/μg phospholipid P); *open circles* = 4-month-old adult rats; *solid circles* = 24-month-old (aged) rats. For details see legend to FIG. 1. (Adapted from Gatti *et al.*[26])

of the brain of aged rats when the activity is tested with arachidonic acid containing CPG. Interestingly, when phospholipase A_2 activity decreases as an effect of age, its affinity for the substrates increases. On the contrary, age has no effect on enzyme K_m in an area such as the hippocampus, where the activity rate remains either not affected or poorly affected.[30,31]

These results point to a more efficient reutilization of arachidonic acid in brain areas of aged animals. This hypothesis was confirmed by testing arachidonic acid incorporation into 2-lyso phosphoglycerides *in vitro,* where either no variation or stimulation of the acylation process was observed[32] (FIG. 3). Interestingly, both the phospholipase activities and the reacylation system are increased in aged rat brain areas when choline lipids are used as substrates. As CPG is one of the lipids involved in the arachidonic acid fast turnover pool, we have further support for our previous hypothesis.

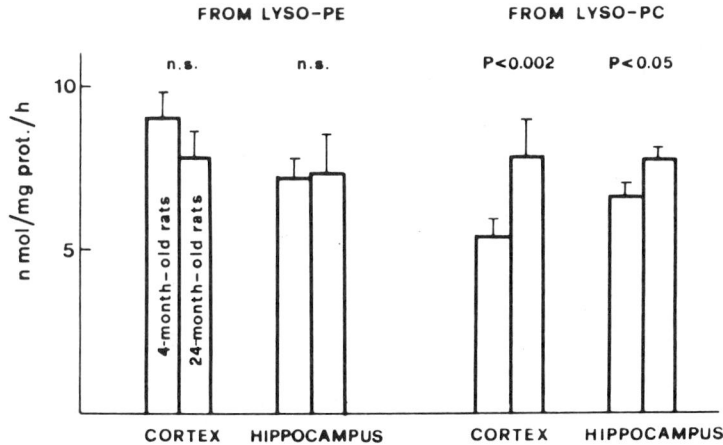

FIGURE 3. Arachidonic acid incorporation into lysophosphoglycerides *in vitro.* Lyso-PC = 2-lyso-1-acylglycerophosphocholine; Lyso-PE = 2-lyso-1-acylglycerophosphoethanolamine; n.s. = not significant. For each pair of columns, the left represents 4-month-old (adult) rats, the right 24-month-old (aged) rats. Tubes were incubated 20 min at 37 °C at pH 7.4 (50 mM tris-HCl, 20 mM $MgCl_2$, in the presence of ATP 5 mM, CoA 1 mM, DTT 0.1 mM, BSA 5 mg/ml and 1-^{14}C arachidonic acid 80 μM (specific activity 1.25 Ci/mol).[31,32,36]

If the above results clearly indicate that the aged rat brain structure is able to utilize arachidonic acid more efficiently than the adult rat brain, we still have to explain the reasons for the reduced incorporation of this acid into the phospholipids during the first hours from the labeled precursor injection (see FIG. 1). One of the possible causes may be found in the age-dependent decrease of the *de novo* glycerophospholipid biosynthesis as demonstrated by using water-soluble precursors.[33] However, this is not sufficient to explain such a high decrease of arachidonic acid incorporation (about 70%; see FIG. 1).

To gain more information about the phenomenon, we are testing the arachidonic acid uptake and successive metabolic transformations in slices from the cortex and hippocampus of adult and aged rat brain.

The slopes of time-dependent content of free labeled arachidonic acid in cells from cortex slices are shown in FIG. 4A. At all times, a higher content of the free labeled acid is evident in the cortex of aged rats than in that of adults. This higher content leads, in the aged animal, to a higher amount of arachidonoyl-CoA (FIG. 4B); however, the slope of the CoA derivative labeling becomes about constant after 10 min of incubation, indicating a probable failure of the transformation mechanism. In our opinion, this saturation of the system is confirmed by the highest value of free arachidonic acid labeling found in the aged cortex after 60 min of incubation.

The labeling of the DG is still slightly higher in the cortex of aged rats than in that of adults (FIG. 5A), even if the differences are less significant, while the labeling in the polar lipid fraction of aged rat cortex is lower than that of adults (FIG. 5B).

CONCLUSIONS

These preliminary results offer us the possibility of understanding better the effect of age on arachidonic acid metabolism in the brain. Leaving aside the problem of the blood-brain barrier, which is under investigation, arachidonic acid enters the cerebral cells of aged animals at a rate that is either comparable to (hippocampus, data not shown) or higher than that for adults. The subsequent free acid metabolic transformations are modified by age, probably due to reduced energy availability.[34,35] This is evident by examining the time-dependent slopes of labeling of both the arachidonoyl-CoA and, better, the polar lipid extracted from the cortex. The reduced content of labeling of polar lipids from the aged as compared to the adult cortex in spite of the higher content of arachidonoyl-CoA may be a result of the combined failure of both the enzymatic assembling of DG with the hydrophilic head of the phospholipid[33] and the reduced availability of activated bases (cytidine diphospho bases), for the synthesis of which an energy supply is required.

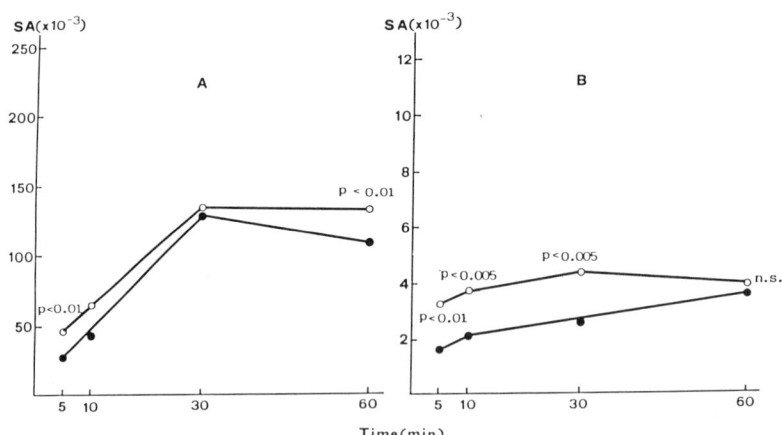

FIGURE 4. Content of free labeled arachidonic acid (**A**) and arachidonoyl-CoA (**B**) as nCi/mg wet weight $\times 10^{-3}$ at different incubation times. SA = specific activity; *open circles* = 4-month-old (adult) rats; *solid circles* = 24-month-old (aged) rats. Slices 400 μm thick were incubated at 37 °C in oxygenated Krebs solution in the presence of 250 nCi (+1 μmole of cold acid) of 5,6,8,9,11,12,14,15-^{3}H arachidonic acid (specific activity 80 Ci/mmol). *p:* ANOVA test of statistical significance.

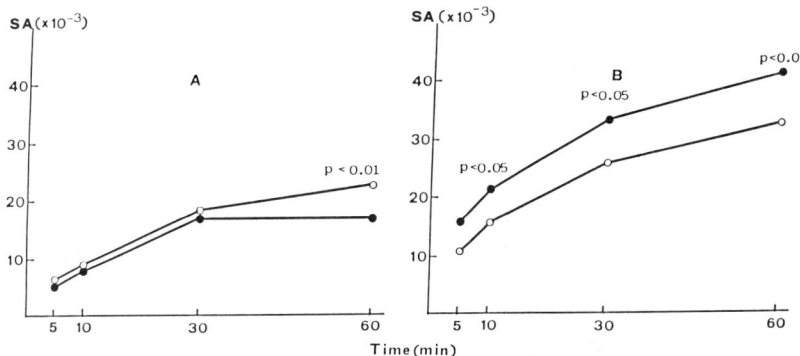

FIGURE 5. Content of labeled diacylglycerols (DG) (**A**) and total polar lipids (LP) (**B**) as nCi/mg wet weight $\times\ 10^{-3}$ at different incubation times. SA = specific activity; *open cirles* = 4-month-old (adult) rats; *solid circles* = 24-month-old (aged) rats. Incubation as in legend to FIG. 4.

In this way, the reduction of polyunsaturated fatty acid incorporation into the lipidic fast pools in the aged brain has several concomitant causes. These pools are the main pathway to storage and distribution of fatty acids to membrane lipids, in spite of their unaffected uptake into the cells. The decrease of arachidonic acid incorporation into the fast pools may also explain the reduced content of this acid in the endogenous DG (see TABLE 1). The altered fatty acid profile of these precursors contributes to the failure of phospholipid *ex novo* biosynthesis, as we previously clearly demonstrated by almost completely restoring the CPG and EPG biosynthesis *in vitro* when DG prepared from the adult rat brain were incubated with enzyme preparation from the aged rat brain.[12]

On the other hand, the brain structure of the aged animal tries to counteract the failure of *de novo* biosynthesis with a more efficient reutilization of arachidonic acid and, presumably, of other polyunsaturated fatty acids. However, such a decline of incorporation may have a dangerous effect on membrane integrity as it becomes more difficult for the cell to renew all its lipidic molecules damaged by such causes as lipid peroxidation.[6] As a consequence, changes in membrane composition induce variations in its functions. In particular, if it is true that age has a negative effect on the uptake of phospholipid water-soluble precursors,[36] the modification in membrane composition may reduce the uptake even more, hence further affecting phospholipid metabolism and membrane composition.

In conclusion, the balance between negative effects and compensative mechanisms becomes unable to counteract the effects of increasing age, and a failure of membrane functions becomes more and more evident, as is indirectly confirmed by such pathological situations as senile dementia, in which a profound modification of physiological functions are connected with a noticeable modification of membrane composition.[37]

REFERENCES

1. SINGER, S. J. 1974. The molecular organization of membranes. Annu. Rev. Biochem. **43:** 805–815.
2. SUN, A. Y. & G. Y. SUN. 1979. Neurochemical aspects of the membrane hypothesis of aging. Interdiscip. Top. Gerontol. **15:** 34–53.

3. BONETTI, A. C., A. BATTISTELLA, G. CALDERINI, S. TEOLATO, F. T. CREWS, A. GAITI, S. ALGERI & G. TOFFANO. 1983. Biochemical alterations in the mechanism of synaptic transmission in aging brain. In Aging of the Brain. D. Samuel, S. Algeri, S. Gershon, V. E. Grimm & G. Toffano, Eds.: 171–181. Raven Press. New York, NY.
4. CALDERINI, G., A. C. BONETTI, A. BATTISTELLA, F. T. CREWS & G. TOFFANO. 1983. Biochemical changes of rat brain membranes with aging. Neurochem. Res. **8:** 483–492.
5. SCHROEDER, F. 1984. Role of membrane lipid asymmetry in aging. Neurobiol. Aging **5:** 323–333.
6. CUTLER, G. R. 1984. Free radicals and aging. In Molecular Basis of Aging. A. K. Roy & B. Chatterjee, Eds.: 263–354. Academic Press. New York, NY.
7. HARMAN, D. 1956. Aging: A theory based on free radical and radiation chemistry. J. Gerontol. **11:** 298–301.
8. ALOJ TOTARO, E., P. GLEES, F. A. PISANTI, Eds. 1985. Advances in Age Pigments Research. Pergamon Press. Oxford.
9. O'BRIEN, J. S. & E. L. SAMPSON. 1965. Fatty acid and aldehyde composition of the major brain lipids in normal human gray matter, white matter and myelin. J. Lipid Res. **6:** 545–551.
10. SVENNERHOLM, L. 1968. Distribution and fatty acid composition of phosphoglycerides in normal human brain. J. Lipid Res. **9:** 570–679.
11. SUN, G. Y. & L. L. FOUDIN. 1985. Phospholipid composition and metabolism in the developing and aging nervous system. In Phospholipids in the Nervous System. J. Eichberg, Ed.: 79–129. John Wiley & Sons. New York, NY.
12. BRUNETTI, M., A. GAITI & G. PORCELLATI. 1979. Synthesis of phosphatidylcholine and phosphatidylethanolamine at different ages in rat brain in vitro. Lipids **14:** 925–931.
13. DHOPESHWARKAR, G. A. & J. F. MEAD. 1973. Uptake and transport of fatty acids into the brain and role of the blood-brain barrier system. Adv. Lipid Res. **11:** 109–142.
14. MORAND, O., M. MASSON, N. BAUMANN & J. M. BOURRE. 1981. Exogenous 1-14C lignoceric acid uptake by neurons, astrocytes and myelin, as compared to incorporation of 1-14C palmitic and stearic acids. Neurochem. Int. **3:** 329–334.
15. HORROCKS, L. A. 1985. Metabolism and function of fatty acids in brain. In Phospholipids in the Nervous System. J. Eichberg, Ed.: 173–195. John Wiley & Sons. New York, NY.
16. OLDENDORF, W. H. 1977. The blood-brain barrier, a review. Exp. Eye Res. **25** (Suppl): 177–190.
17. MORISAKI, N., Y. SAITO & A. KUMAGAI. 1982. Fatty acid oxidation of rat brain microvessels in hypertension, aging and experimental diabetes. Atherosclerosis **42:** 221–227.
18. MORAND, O., J. B. CARRÉ, P. HOMAYOUN, E. NIEL, N. BAUMANN & J. M. BOURRE. 1987. Arachidonoyl-CoA synthetase and nonspecific acyl-CoA synthetase activities in purified rat brain microvessels. J. Neurochem. **48:** 1150–1156.
19. SUN, G. Y. & L. A. HORROCKS. 1973. Metabolism of palmitic acid in the subcellular fractions of mouse brain. J. Lipid Res. **14:** 206–214.
20. COOK, H. W. 1982. Chain elongation in the formation of polyunsaturated fatty acids by brain: Some properties of the microsomal system. Arch. Biochem. Biophys. **214:** 695–704.
21. SUN, G. Y. 1982. Metabolic turnover of arachidonoyl groups in brain membrane phosphoglycerides. In Phospholipids in the Nervous System, Vol. 1: Metabolism. L. A. Horrocks, G. B. Ansell & G. Porcellati, Eds.: 75–89. Raven Press. New York, NY.
22. MURPHY, M. G. & M. W. SPENCE. 1980. Long-chain fatty acid: CoA ligase in rat brain in vitro: A comparison of activities with oleic and cis-vaccenic acids. J. Neurochem. **34:** 367–373.
23. MURPHY, M. G. & M. W. SPENCE. 1982. Acid-Coenzyme A ligase in brain: Fatty acid specificity in cellular and subcellular fractions. J. Neurochem. **38:** 675–679.
24. REDDY, T. S. & N. G. BAZAN. 1983. Kinetic properties of archidonoyl-CoA synthetase in rat brain microsomes. Arch. Biochem. Biophys. **226:** 125–133.
25. MIZOBUCHI, M., N. MORISAKI, N. MATSUOKA, Y. SAITO & A. KUMAGAI. 1982. Incorporation of 1-^{14}C Palmitic acid into neutral lipids and phospholipids of rat cerebral cortex in vitro. J. Neurochem. **38:** 1365–1371.
26. GATTI, C., K. NOREMBERG, M. BRUNETTI, S. TEOLATO, G. CALDERINI & A. GAITI. 1986.

Turnover of palmitic and arachidonic acids in the phospholipids from different brain areas of adult and aged rats. Neurochem. Res. **11:** 241–252.
27. DAWSON, R. M. C. 1985. Enzymic pathways of phospholipid metabolism in the nervous system. *In* Phospholipids in the Nervous System. J. Eichberg, Ed.: 45–73. John Wiley & Sons. New York, NY.
28. LAND, W. E. M. 1960. Metabolism of glycerolípids II. The enzymatic acylation of lysolecithin. J. Biol. Chem. **235:** 2233–2237.
29. VAN DEN BOSCH, H. 1980. Intracellular phospholipase. A. Biochim. Biophys. Acta **604:** 191–246.
30. GAITI, A., C. GATTI, M. BRUNETTI, S. TEOLATO, G. CALDERINI & G. PORCELLATI. 1985. Phospholipase activities in rat brain areas during aging. *In* Phospholipid in the Nervous System, Vol. 2. Physiological Roles. L. A., Horrocks, J. N. Kanfer & G. Porcellati, Eds.: 155–162. Raven Press. New York, NY.
31. GAITI, A., M. PULITI, M. BRUNETTI, C. GATTI & G. CALDERINI. 1986. Importance of alternative pathways for phospholipid biosynthesis in aged rat brain. *In* Neuroendocrine System and Aging. P. Vezzadini, A. Facchini & G. Labò, Eds.: 205–210. EURAGE. Rijswijk. The Netherlands.
32. GAITI, A., C. GATTI, M. PULITI & M. BRUNETTI. 1986. Phospholipid metabolism in aging brain. *In* Phospholipid Research and the Nervous System: Biochemical and Molecular Pharmacology. L. A. Horrocks, L. Freysz & G. Toffano, Eds.: 225–231. Liviana Press/Springer Verlag. Padova & Berlin.
33. GAITI, A., M. BRUNETTI, G. L. PICCININ, L. WOELK & G. PORCELLATI. 1982. The synthesis in vivo of choline and ethanolamine phosphoglycerides in different brain areas during aging. Lipids **17:** 291–296.
34. HOYER, S. 1985. The effect of age on glucose and energy metabolism in brain cortex of rats. Arch. Gerontol. Geriatr. **4:** 193–203.
35. LEONG, S. F., J. C. K. LAI, L. LIM & J. B. CLARK. 1981. Energy metabolising enzymes in brain regions of adult and aging rats. J. Neurochem. **37:** 1548–1556.
36. GAITI, A. & C. GATTI. 1988. Phospholipid interconversion reactions in different brain areas and their possible importance in brain aging. *In* Phospholipid in the Nervous System: Biochemical and Molecular Pathology. N. Bazan, L. A. Horrocks & G. Toffano, Eds. Liviana Press/Springer Verlag. Padova & Berlin. In press.
37. GOTTFRIES, C. G., I. KARLSSON & L. SVENNERHOLM. 1985. Senile dementia: A white matter disease? *In* Normal Aging, Alzheimer's Disease and Senile Dementia. C. G. Gottfries, Ed.: 111–118. Editions de l'Université de Bruxelles. Bruxelles.

Prostaglandin D$_2$ and Sleep

OSAMU HAYAISHI

*Hayaishi Bioinformation Transfer Project
Research Development Corporation of Japan
Osaka 569, Japan*

Until recently, prostaglandin D$_2$ had long been considered a minor and biologically inactive prostanoid or even a nonenzymic decomposition product of prostaglandin H$_2$. In the late 1970s, the presence of a relatively large amount of PGD$_2$ was reported in the central nervous system (CNS) of the rat and other mammals, including humans, indicating that prostaglandin D$_2$ is unique among the prostaglandins in having a high concentration in the mammalian brain. We therefore investigated the metabolism and enzymes involved in the biosynthesis and degradation of prostaglandin D$_2$ in the CNS. Our results indicated that prostaglandin D$_2$ is actively synthesized and metabolized by specific enzymes in neurons and glial cells. We then decided to investigate the neural functions of prostaglandin D$_2$ in the brain.

In order to approach this problem, we isolated, partially purified, and characterized binding proteins, or the putative receptors, of prostaglandins in the CNS. We also studied the intracerebral distribution of these binding proteins by radioautography combined with computer-assisted image processing with color coding. The results indicate that the binding protein for prostaglandin D$_2$ is localized in the gray matter—namely, the neuron-rich areas—and is highly concentrated in certain specific areas, such as the olfactory bulb, cerebral cortex, occipital cortex, hippocampus, hypothalamus, and preoptic area. This in turn indicates that PGD$_2$ may be involved in certain specific neural functions.[1] Much less binding is seen in the cerebellum, brain stem, and midbrain.

The preoptic area has long been known as a center of regulation of sleep. For example, when the preoptic area of a rat is destroyed, slow-wave sleep is no longer observed.[2] On the other hand, slow-wave sleep can be induced by electric stimulation of the preoptic area.[3] However, the chemical mechanisms involved in the induction of sleep were not elucidated until now. When saline was injected into the preoptic area of the control rats under conditions of sleep deprivation, the rats were awake most of the time. However, when several nanomoles of PGD$_2$ were microinjected into the preoptic area, the awake period was decreased by almost 50%, and the amount of sleep was increased more than fivefold.[4] The site of action was specific for the preoptic area. The effect was dose-dependent and quite specific for PGD$_2$.

Sleep is a very complex phenomenon; the synopsis presented in FIGURE 1 is obviously oversimplified. Wakefulness and two major types of sleep—namely, slow-wave sleep (SWS) and rapid eye movement (REM) sleep—can be judged by the animal's behavior. However, precise qualitative and quantitative analyses of the sleep-wake pattern are carried out by recordings of brain wave, or EEG (the electroencephalogram); eye movement, or EOG (the electrooculogram); and muscle tension, or EMG (the electromyogram). During slow-wave sleep, EEG recordings show characteristic slow waves, and eye movement is practically absent. On the other hand, the EEG and EOG patterns during REM sleep resemble those of wakefulness, whereas muscle is almost completely relaxed, as indicated by the flat EMG recordings.

In order to obtain more quantitative data and to critically evaluate the effect of

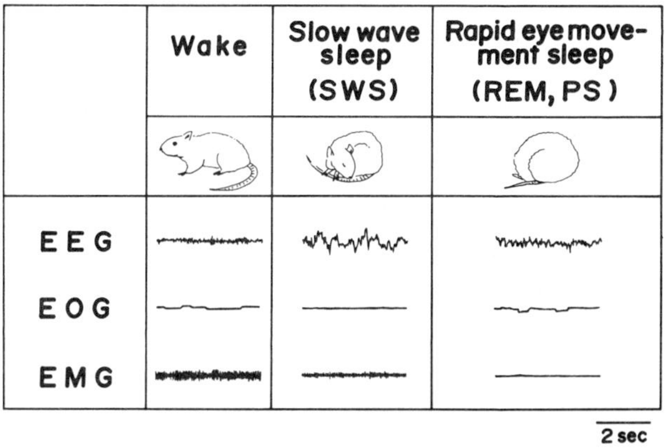

	Wake	Slow wave sleep (SWS)	Rapid eye movement sleep (REM, PS)
	🐀	🐀	🐀
EEG	~~~	~~~	~~~
EOG	___	___	___
EMG	~~~	~~~	___

2 sec

FIGURE 1. Parameters of wakefulness and sleep. EEG = electroencephalogram; EOG = electrooculogram; EMG = electromyogram.

PGD_2 on sleep, we employed the more sophisticated continuous-infusion sleep bioassay system that was originally developed by Professor Inoué of Tokyo Medical and Dental University (FIG. 2). Male Sprague-Dawley rats weighing about 300 g were used for most of these experiments. Various electrodes and a cannula were implanted into the rats at least 7 days before the experiments. PGD_2 was infused through the cannula continuously for 10 h into the third ventricle of the brain. The sleep stages were determined on the bases of the polygraphic recordings of EEG, EMG, and locomotion, and the sleep scores were computed by and stored in a central processing unit. The behavior of the rat was monitored by a video-recording system. FIGURE 3 shows the

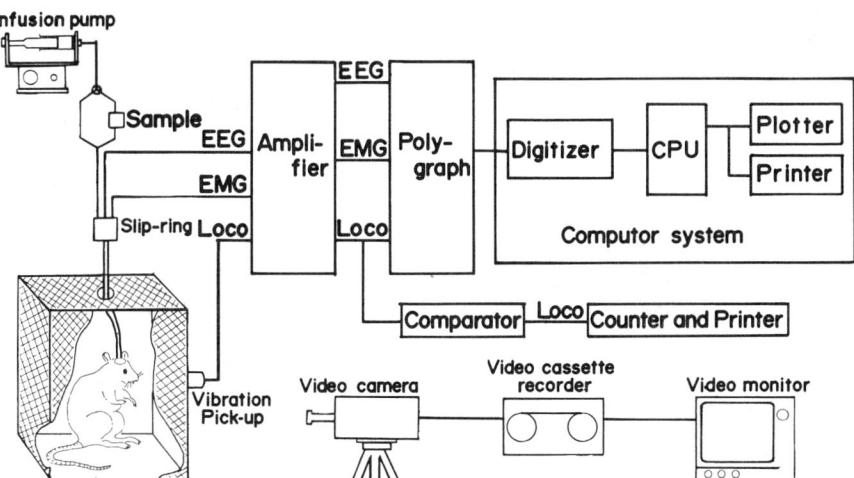

FIGURE 2. Bioassay system for sleep analysis. EEG = electroencephalogram; EMG = electromyogram; Loco = locomotion.

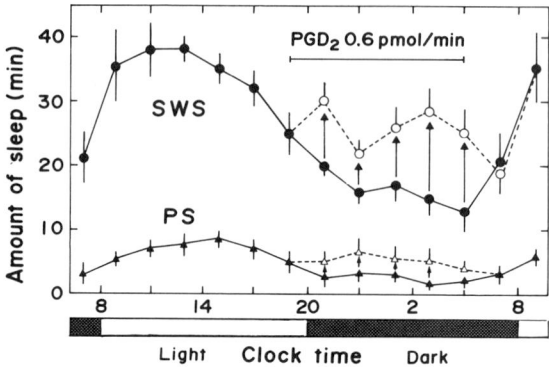

FIGURE 3. Effect of PGD$_2$ on sleep patterns. Vertical axis indicates minutes of sleep in each hour. Horizontal axis indicates time schedule. The period of infusion of PGD$_2$ is indicated by the *horizontal line* on the upper right. *Solid circles and triangles* = control; *open circles and triangles* = treated animals; SWS = slow-wave sleep; PS = paradoxical (= rapid eye movement, REM) sleep.

effect of PGD$_2$ on sleep patterns, when a small amount of the PG was slowly and continuously infused into the third ventricle. Rats are nocturnal animals—they sleep during the day but are awake most of the time during the night. When PGD$_2$ was infused at a rate of 0.6 pmol per minute during the night, both slow-wave sleep and REM sleep increased as shown here. The effect was dose-dependent and specific for PGD$_2$. As little as one femtomole (10^{-15} mol) per second was effective in inducing excess sleep. Sleep induced by PGD$_2$ was indistinguishable from physiological sleep as judged by EEG, EMG, locomotor activities, body temperature, heart rate, and general behavior of the rat.[5] In order to prove that the effect of PGD$_2$ is not pharmacological, but physiological, we did the following experiments.

PGD synthetase activity exhibits a circadian fluctuation in parallel with the sleep/wake cycle (FIG. 4). In the light period, when rats mainly sleep, PGD$_2$ is more actively synthesized than in the dark period. However, the specific activity of PGD$_2$ dehydrogenase remains almost the same. Furthermore, the administration of inhibitors of prostaglandin synthesis, such as indomethacin and diclofenac sodium, results in a decrease in the amount of diurnal sleep.

When diclofenac sodium was infused intravenously into rats during the day, the amount of sleep decreased dose-dependently (FIG. 5). After the termination of infusion, there was a rebound, and nocturnal sleep was increased to a significant

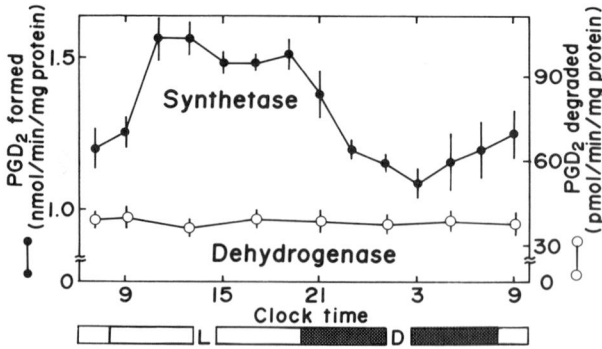

FIGURE 4. Circadian changes in PGD$_2$ synthetase and PGD$_2$ dehydrogenase in the rat brain. L = light; D = dark.

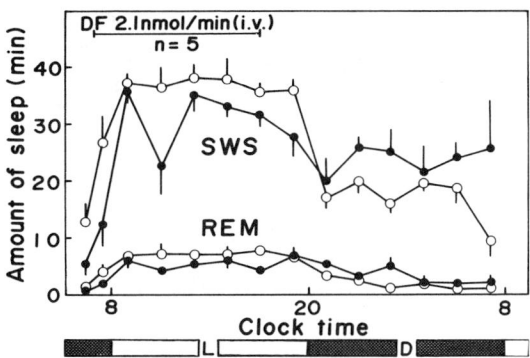

FIGURE 5. Effect of diclofenac sodium (DF) on the diurnal sleep of the rat. Vertical axis indicates minutes of sleep in each hour. The period of infusion of DF is indicated by the *horizontal line* on the upper left. *Open circles* = control; *solid circles* = treated animals: SWS = slow-wave sleep; REM = rapid eye movement sleep; L = light; D = dark.

extent. These results are consistent with the interpretation that PGD$_2$ is involved physiologically in sleep induction in the brain of rats.

More recently, we found that intraventricular infusion of PGE$_2$ reduces the amount of diurnal sleep of rats (FIG. 6). Here prostaglandin E$_2$ was infused at a rate of 10 pmole/min into the third ventricle of a rat during the day. The amount of slow-wave sleep was reduced to about 70% of the control, the amount of REM sleep to about 40%.[6] After the termination of infusion, there was a rebound, and nocturnal sleep was increased to a significant extent; but the sleep pattern returned to normal during the next day. Whether or not this effect of PGE$_2$ on sleep is a primary effect of this particular PG is currently under investigation in my laboratory.

Because the sleep pattern of rats is somewhat different from that of primates, we further extended these studies to the rhesus monkey (*Macaca mulatta*).[7] Adult male monkeys weighing about 5-8 kg were used for the experiments. Various electrodes and a cannula were implanted into the monkeys at least one month before the experiments. The samples were dissolved in an artificial cerebrospinal fluid (CSF), which was then infused into the lateral or third ventricle through a cannula for 6 hours from 11:00 A.M. to 5:00 P.M. Sleep stages were monitored and determined by essentially the same method as that employed for the rat experiments, except that the EOG was also recorded simultaneously. FIGURE 7 shows the sleep patterns of a rhesus monkey before, during, and after PGD$_2$ infusion. The sleep diagrams of artificial CSF–infused and untreated control monkeys were very similar, if not exactly identical. Like some human

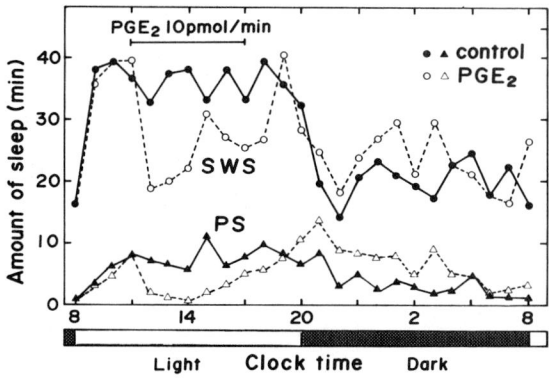

FIGURE 6. Effect of PGE$_2$ on the diurnal sleep of the rat. Vertical axis indicates minutes of sleep in each hour. The period of infusion of PGE$_2$ is indicated by the *horizontal line* on the upper left. SWS = slow-wave sleep; PS = paradoxical (= rapid eye movement, REM) sleep.

beings, this particular monkey takes a nap in the early afternoon. However, when about 500 pmoles/minute of PGD_2 were infused into the lateral ventricle from 11 A.M. until 5 P.M., sleep was induced almost immediately, followed by the occasional appearance of deep SWS and REM sleep. Such a sleep pattern is almost identical to that of physiological sleep during the night. Through the video recording system, one can watch the monkey during these sleep stages, which are shown in FIGURE 8.

In FIGURE 8A the monkey is wide awake, as is indicated by the characteristic low-amplitude and high-frequency fast-wave EEG and a continuous high-amplitude EMG. Eye movement is evident from the EOG. When a picomolar amount of PGD_2 is infused, the monkey almost immediately goes into sleep (FIG. 8B). During slow-wave sleep, high-amplitude and low-frequency EEG tracings are observed. On the other hand, the EMG is reduced, and eye movement has completely ceased. During REM sleep (FIG. 8C), the EEG is similar to that observed during the awake period; but the EMG is completely flat, and rapid eye movement is observed by EOG recording and through the video recording system. These results indicate that the sleep patterns of

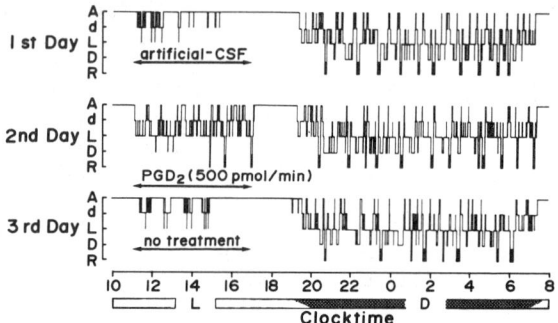

FIGURE 7. Sleep patterns of a rhesus monkey before, during, and after PGD_2 infusion. The period of infusion of artificial cerebrospinal fluid (CSF) and PGD_2 and the corresponding time for untreated monkeys are indicated by *horizontal lines with arrows*. A = awake; d = drowsy; L = light slow-wave sleep; D = deep slow-wave sleep; R = rapid eye movement sleep. On horizontal axis: L = light; D = dark.

man and monkey are similar and that PGD_2 induces sleep that is indistinguishable from natural sleep. The effect of PGD_2 infusion is dose-dependent and relatively specific. Among the other PGs tested, only D_3 is somewhat active, whereas $F_{2\alpha}$, D_1, 9β-D_2, and D_2 methyl ester are much less effective or inactive, and PGE_2 is inhibitory. This specificity coincides well with that of PGD_2 receptors in the monkey brain *in vitro*, suggesting that the process is probably receptor mediated.

In order to provide further evidence to show that PGD_2 induces physiological sleep, we compared EEG recordings and power spectral data of a rhesus monkey infused with artificial CSF, PGD_2, or a benzodiazepine derivative during the day with those obtained during the night (FIG. 9). The power spectral analysis permits dissection of an EEG signal into its frequency components at a certain time during the EEG recordings and provides more qualitative and quantitative information about the nature of sleep. The power spectral data and EEG recordings obtained by the infusion of PGD_2 during the day were essentially identical to those observed during the infusion of a vehicle during the day when the monkey takes a nap and also to those during the night,

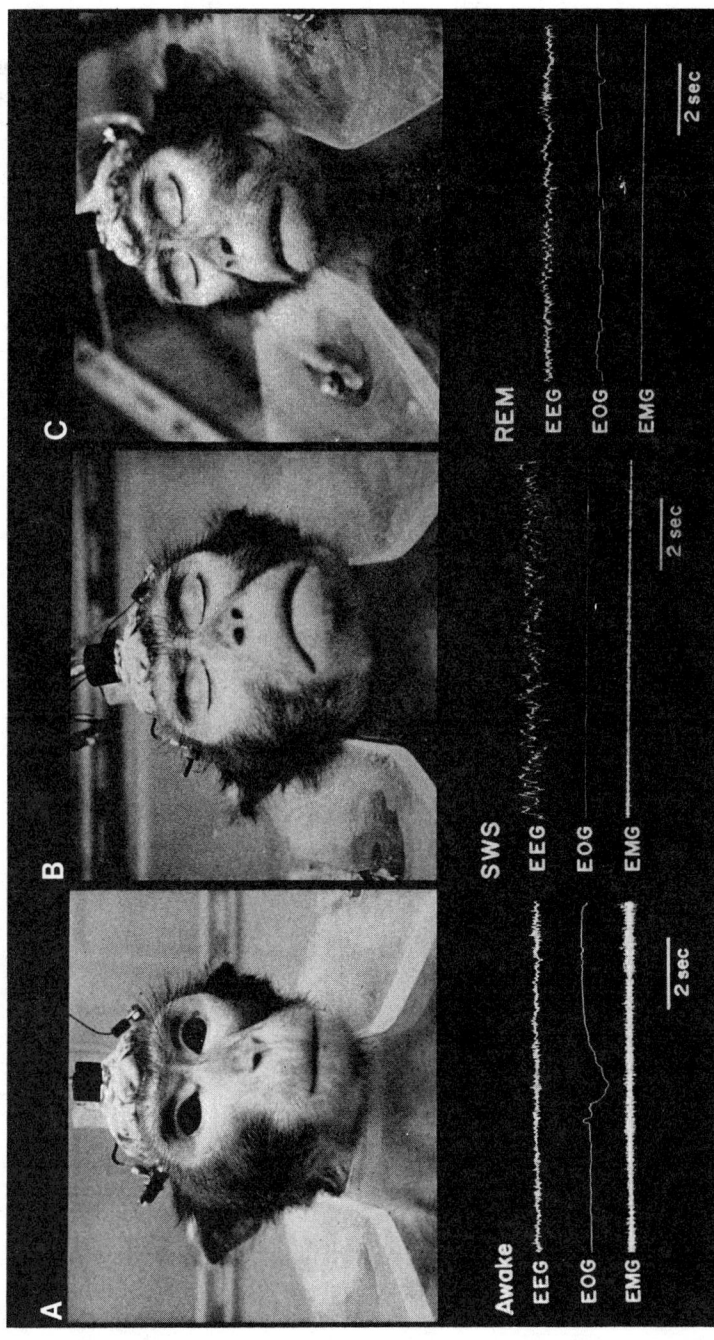

FIGURE 8. Video, electroencephalographic (EEG), electrooculographic (EOG), and electromyographic (EMG) recordings of three phases of sleep of a rhesus monkey: (**A**) awake, (**B**) slow-wave sleep (SWS), and (**C**) rapid eye movement (REM) sleep. Sleep was induced by infusion of PGD_2.

indicating that the sleep induced by PGD_2 during the day is indistinguishable from natural sleep based on these criteria.

On the other hand, when nitrazepam, a popular benzodiazepine derivative, was administered, the EEG tracings and power spectral arrays were clearly different in that there was a sharp peak in the δ wave region of 0.5 to 3 Herz, whereas the θ band of around 4 to 7 Herz was almost nonexistent. Instead, the so-called benzodiazepine fast-wave peak around 20 Herz was clearly evident. These data demonstrate that sleep induced by a sleep-inducing drug is easily distinguishable from natural or PGD_2-induced sleep on the basis of EEG analysis.

In summary:

1. PGD_2 is a major PG in the CNS of the rat and other mammals, including humans.
2. PGD_2 receptors are highly concentrated in the preoptic area, which is considered to be a center of sleep regulation.

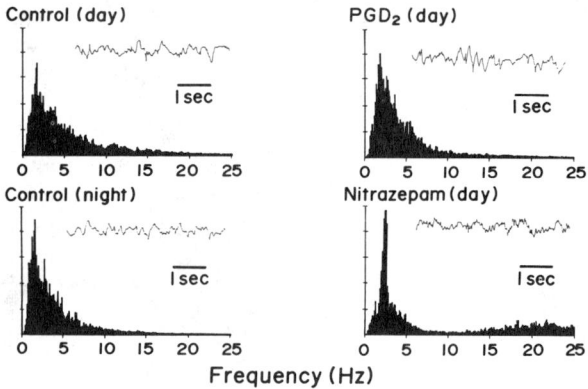

FIGURE 9. Power spectra and EEG tracings (*insets*) of the sleep of a rhesus monkey.

3. Microinjection of PGD_2 into the preoptic area or intracerebroventricular infusion of as little as femtomolar amounts of PGD_2 into rats and monkeys induces sleep that is indistinguishable from natural sleep on the basis of EEG, EMG, EOG, behavior, and other criteria.
4. The effect is dose-dependent and specific for PGD_2. Other PGs are much less effective or totally inactive.
5. Inhibitors of PG synthesis decrease the amount of rats' diurnal sleep, as does PGE_2.

On the basis of these various lines of evidence, we conclude that prostaglandin D_2 induces sleep that is indistinguishable from physiological sleep and that PGD_2 and E_2 are the endogenous sleep-regulating substances that have been looked for by a number of investigators for many years. This is obviously not the final answer to the mystery of this complex phenomenon. However, it does provide clues that should lead to our ultimate understanding of the biological significance and biochemical mechanism of this interesting process.

ACKNOWLEDGMENTS

This work has been carried out with the collaboration of the following coworkers: H. Onoe, H. Osama, K. Kin, H. Matsumura, and R. Ueno, Research Development Corporation of Japan, Takatsuki; Y. Ishikawa, and T. Nakayama, Osaka University, Osaka; K. Naitoh, K. Honda, and S. Inoué, Tokyo Medical and Dental University, Tokyo; and I. Fujita, H. Nishino, and Y. Oomura, National Institute for Physiological Sciences, Okazaki.

REFERENCES

1. YAMASHITA, A., Y. WATANABE & O. HAYAISHI. 1983. Autoradiographic localization of a binding protein(s) specific for prostaglandin D_2 in rat brain. Proc. Natl. Acad. Sci. USA **80:** 6114–6118.
2. NAUTA, W. J. H. 1946. Hypothalamic regulation of sleep in rats. An experimental study. J. Neurophysiol. **9:** 285–316.
3. STERMAN, M. B. & C. D. CLEMENTE. 1962. Forebrain inhibitory mechanisms: Sleep patterns induced by basal forebrain stimulation in the behaving cat. Exp. Neurol. **6:** 103–117.
4. UENO, R., Y. ISHIKAWA, T. NAKAYAMA & O. HAYAISHI. 1982. Prostaglandin D_2 induces sleep when microinjected into the preoptic area of conscious rats. Biochem. Biophys. Res. Commun. **109**(2): 576–582.
5. UENO, R., K. HONDA, S. INOUÉ & O. HAYAISHI. 1983. Prostaglandin D_2, a cerebral sleep-inducing substance in rats. Proc. Natl. Acad. Sci. USA **80:** 1735–1737.
6. MATSUMURA, H., K. HONDA, Y. GOH, R. UENO, T. SAKAI, S. INOUÉ & O. HAYAISHI. 1989. Awaking effect of prostaglandin E_2 in freely moving rats. Brain Res. **481:** 242–249.
7. ONOE, H., R. UENO, I. FUJITA, H. NISHINO, Y. OOMURA & O. HAYAISHI. 1988. Prostaglandin D_2, a cerebral sleep-inducing substance in monkeys. Proc. Natl. Acad. Sci. USA. **85:** 4082–4086.

The Role of Arachidonic Acid Metabolites in Mediating Ethanol Self-Administration and Intoxication[a,b]

FRANK R. GEORGE[c]

Behavior Genetics Laboratory, Preclinical Pharmacology Branch
National Institute on Drug Abuse, Addiction Research Center
Alcohol, Drug Abuse, and Mental Health Administration
United States Public Health Service
United States Department of Health and Human Services
Baltimore, Maryland 22124
and
Department of Pharmacology and Toxicology
School of Pharmacy
University of Maryland
Baltimore, Maryland 21201

INTRODUCTION

The sequence of biochemical events by which ethanol produces its central intoxicating and reinforcing effects remains unknown. However, over the past ten years a consistent body of literature has developed concerning the role of membrane phospholipid composition and metabolism related to prostaglandin (PG) synthesis and the involvement of PGs in mediating the central, and possibly some of the peripheral, effects of alcohols. The first evidence that PGs might mediate ethanol's behavioral effects appeared several years ago, when it was shown that pretreatment with inhibitors of PG synthesis (PGSI) decreased central nervous system (CNS) sensitivity to ethanol, propanol, and t-butanol, but did not affect sensitivity to pentobarbital or chloral hydrate.[1] In addition, the potency of each PGSI was found to be perfectly rank-order correlated with its potency in inhibiting PG synthesis, and the antagonism seen was shown to be due to a decrease in neural sensitivity to ethanol and not due to metabolic changes.

Several reports have since appeared replicating, substantiating, and systematically expanding these original findings. PGSIs have been shown to antagonize ethanol-induced activation, hypothermia, and mortality.[2-9] PGSI treatment during gestation prevents some of the morphological anomalies seen with fetal exposure to ethanol.[10] Biochemically, ethanol affects peripheral PG metabolism[11] and enhances PGE_1-stimulated cAMP accumulation in rat brain cortical slices.[12] Administration of PGE_1

---

[a]This research was supported in part by NIMH grant 1T1MH10679, and by New Investigator Research Award AA-06104 and AA-06924 from the National Institute on Alcohol Abuse and Alcoholism.

[b]The animals used in this study were maintained in facilities fully accredited by the American Association for the Accreditation of Laboratory Animal Care (AAALAC).

[c]Address for correspondence: Dr. Frank R. George, NIDA Addiction Research Center, Box 5810, Baltimore, Maryland 21224.

FIGURE 1. Potency correlation for a series of cyclooxygenase inhibitors. Y axis represents dose of PGSI required to reduce duration of loss of righting reflex, i.e., sleep time, by 50% in response to a 4.0-g/kg ip dose of ethanol in HS/Ibg male mice. X axis represents μm concentration of PGSI for 50% inhibition of cyclooxygenase. IND = indomethacin, ASP = aspirin, FLU = flufenamate, MEF = mefenamate, ACE = acetaminophen. Data from Reference 1.

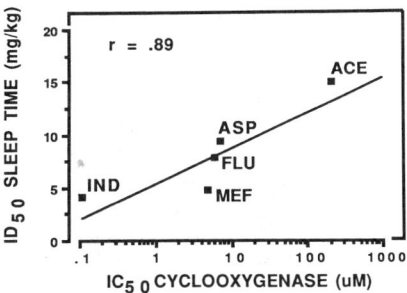

and prostanoid precursors enhance ethanol's sedative effects, and PGE_1 reduces ethanol withdrawal severity.[9,12] In addition, ethanol increases *in vivo* brain PG levels in a dose-dependent manner, and these changes covary with changes in blood ethanol levels over time.[13-16] Ethanol has also recently been shown to increase PGE levels in mouse uterine/embryonic tissue, an effect blocked by aspirin.[17]

Two important criteria for establishing a biochemical mechanism of action for a behavioral response to a drug are a potency correlation and a genetic correlation. To obtain a significant potency correlation, a series of antagonists must bind to a specific molecular site with biochemical affinities that form a high rank-order correlation with their potencies as antagonists at the behavioral level. FIGURE 1 shows that a highly significant potency correlation exists between the IC_{50} doses of indomethacin (INDO) for sleep time and cyclooxygenase inhibition, suggesting that the CNS depressant effects of ethanol are mediated through a cyclooxygenase mechanism.

To obtain a high genetic correlation, there must exist a significant qualitative and quantitative rank-order relationship for two variables—for instance, a behavioral response to a drug and a biochemical effect of the drug—across a number of genetically specified populations, such as inbred mouse strains. In this regard, animals that are more sensitive to ethanol require larger amounts of PGSI to antagonize ethanol-induced sleep time and behavioral activation, as shown in FIGURE 2.

Further genetic evidence to substantiate the PG hypothesis regarding the acute intoxicating effects of ethanol has been obtained through the use of the LS/Ibg (LS) and SS/Ibg (SS) mice. The LS and SS mice were produced through selective breeding for differential sensitivity to the depressant effects of ethanol;[18] thus any biological factors also differing between these lines may contribute to the casual basis of response to ethanol. It has been shown that there exists a strong inverse correlation between baseline PG levels, ethanol-induced changes in PG levels, and neural sensitivity to

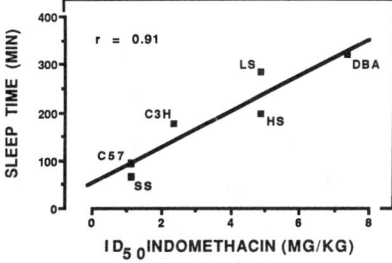

FIGURE 2. Genetic correlation for a number of inbred mouse strains. Y axis represents duration of loss of righting reflex, i.e., sleep time, in response to a 4.0-g/kg ip dose of ethanol. X axis represents dose of INDO required for 50% inhibition of sleep time. C57 = C57Bl/6J, SS = SS/Igb, C3H = C3H/HeJ, LS = LS/Ibg, HS = HS/Ibg, DBA = DBA/2J. Data from References 1, 2, 4, 5, 7.

ethanol across line and sex within the LS and SS mice, providing yet another line of evidence implicating PGs as primary mediators of ethanol's effects.

Another important aspect of ethanol is that this drug can serve as a powerful reinforcer. That is, animals will perform work contingent upon obtaining ethanol as a reward. In the 1960s a line of research developed that differed from the traditional two-bottle choice studies in both techniques and conceptual basis. Procedures were devised so that laboratory animals could intravenously inject drugs into themselves, and it has been demonstrated that drugs from a number of pharmacological classes can serve as reinforcers for animals.[19-21] Findings in this area have been consistent; and in general, results obtained in one laboratory have been duplicated in other laboratories.[22]

Ethanol, self-administered orally, has been shown to serve as a powerful reinforcer in mice, rats, rhesus monkeys, and baboons.[23-25] Since PGs have repeatedly been shown to play an important role in acute response to ethanol, one hypothesis would be that PGs would also play a role in determining the reinforcing effects of ethanol. If PGSI treatment reduces CNS sensitivity to ethanol, then a partial antagonism could result in a reduced but still present CNS response to ethanol. This could produce increased consumption of ethanol solutions. A greater antagonism could reduce the effects of ethanol to the point where there is no interoceptive effect—that is, the organism is unable to discriminate between drug and water, resulting in a decrease in ethanol drinking. An additional possibility addresses the hypothesis that animals consume ethanol for its caloric content and not its CNS effects. If calories are important determinants of animals' ethanol drinking, then PGSI antagonism of ethanol's CNS effects should have little or no effect on ethanol consumption, especially in situations where animals are maintained at reduced body weights.

In the studies that follow, the purpose was to establish the extent to which a group of rats would orally self-administer ethanol over a range of conditions, and then to determine if the PGSI antagonism of acute ethanol-related behaviors can be extended to include antagonism of the reinforcing effects of ethanol. If a PGSI effect was found, an additional purpose was to examine the specificity of this effect by testing the ability of PGSI treatment to decrease responding to a nonalcohol reinforcer.

METHODS

Animals

Five experimentally naive male Sprague-Dawley rats (BioLab), 16 weeks old and weighing 280–320 g at the start of the experiment, were housed individually in a temperature-controlled room (26 °C) with a 12-hr light-dark cycle (0700–1900 lights on) and given free access to Purina rat chow and tap water prior to initiation of the experiments.

Apparatus

Ten sound-attentuated operant conditioning chambers (LVE 1414, Lehigh Valley Equipment) equipped with two levers and a solenoid-driven liquid dipper (LVE 1351) were used. Three colored lights above each level were used to provide visual stimuli. The dipper cup (0.11 ml) was available unless driven by a lever press, at which time it dropped for 1 s into a liquid-filled reservoir to refill. A 2000-Hz tone was also presented during the 1-s interval. Programming and data recording were controlled by equipment located in an adjacent room.

Data Analysis

Since the rats had identical treatment histories, a group design was used, incorporating within subjects repeated-measures analysis of variance (ANOVA), analyzed using BMDP2V statistical software.[26] The Dunnett test for multiple comparisons was used for post-hoc analyses.[27] Stable responding was defined as five consecutive days with no significant deviation in responses as determined by visual analysis of the data. The mean for N minus the first two days was determined for each animal under each condition. The mean values were used as the animal's scores for analysis. Self-administration of ethanol was measured in several ways, including number of level presses, number of ethanol deliveries, volume of liquid consumed, and blood ethanol levels.

Blood Ethanol Assay

On the last day of the 8% retest, replicate 10-μl blood samples were obtained from the tail of each rat at the end of the experimental session. Since most ethanol drinking occurred at the beinning of the one-hour sessions, these tail blood samples provided a conservative estimate of circulating ethanol levels. In addition, unpublished data from our laboratory indicate that blood alcohol levels determined from tail blood provides a correlated but low estimate of brain alcohol levels. The blood samples were placed in 190 μl of cold 0.55-M perchlorate, shaken, then centrifuged at 700 × g for five min. One hundred seventy μl of supernatant was removed and placed in a separate test tube, to which 30 μl of deionized water and 200 μl of 0.222-M K_2CO_3 were added. The tubes were vortexted and centrifuged for two min. Aliquots of 80 μl were removed in replicate and added to 640 μl of cold 0.50-M Tris buffer at pH 8.8, 40 μl of 50-mM NAD^+, and 40 μl alcohol dehydrogenase (ADH) (Sigma, 500 units/ml). The samples were vortexted, incubated at room temperature for one hour, then analyzed for the formation of NADH by measuring spectrophotometric absorbance at 340 nm. Samples were compared to concurrently prepared standards.

Procedure

Ethanol solutions were prepared using 95% EtOH mixed in room-temperature tap water. Fresh solutions were prepared immediately prior to the beginning of each experimental session. Ethanol was established as a reinforcer using procedures similar to those previously described.[28] Initially, the rats were reduced to, and maintained at, 80% of their 16-week free-feeding weights. They were then water deprived and received their daily food allowance before the experimental session. The rats were next trained to lever-press to receive a water delivery. Once responding was stable for all animals, ethanol solutions of 2, 4 and 8% (w/v) were available during the sessions for 3, 4, and 6 days, respectively.

After this initial exposure to ethanol, the rats were subsequently fed 15 min after the end of each experimental session, and had free 23-hour access to water in their home cages for the remainder of the experiments. All animals were then exposed to 8, 16, and 32% (w/v) ethanol. Each concentration was given until all rates showed stable responses over at least 5 consecutive sessions. Retests at 8% and 0% were then given under identical conditions.

Under a continuous reinforcement schedule (fixed ratio [FR] 1), these rats responded the highest, and consumed the greatest amounts of liquid at 8%. The values for 8%, 16%, and 8% retest were significantly greater than 0% (repeated-measures

ANOVA: $p < 0.005$; Dunnett's t: 8% vs. 0% = 4.07, $p < 0.01$; 16% vs. 0% = 3.00, $p < 0.05$; 32% vs. 0% = 1.14, not significant). At 8% w/v ethanol, the volume consumed averaged 6.4 ml, ethanol intake averaged 2.1 g/kg for each one-hour session, and the rats exhibited postsession blood ethanol levels (BEL) of 98 ± 8 mg/dl. Volume of liquid consumed was linearly related to number of deliveries, $r = .98$. Importantly, most responding occurred at the beginning of the session. Observation of the animals revealed frequent postsession episodes of ataxia at 8 and 16%. Since 8% w/v ethanol maintained the greatest amount of responding, this concentration was chosen for the INDO studies.

EXPERIMENT 1: EFFECTS OF INDOMETHACIN TREATMENT ON ORAL SELF-ADMINISTRATION OF ETHANOL

After determining the pattern and extent of ethanol self-administration, as described above, the effect of INDO pretreatment on ethanol-reinforced responding was determined.

Method

All sessions were run on an FR 1 schedule using 8% (w/v) ethanol, as described above, but now with the addition of injections administered 20 min prior to the start of the sessions. Drug solutions were prepared as follows. INDO (Sigma, St. Louis, Missouri, USA) was dissolved in a 1% ethanol, 1% polysorbate 80, 0.9% saline solution at a concentration of 10.0 mg/ml and administered at a volume of 2.0 ml/kg body weight. Additional concentrations were made from dilutions of this stock solution. The rats were pretreated daily via intraperitoneal (ip) injection with one of several doses of INDO or vehicle control. For each day of testing, injections were given contralateral to the injection side of the previous day. Several doses and conditions, including sham injection, 0 (vehicle), 1.25, 1.9, 2.5 and 5.0 mg/kg INDO were tested in nonconsecutive order. Vehicle retests were performed after each drug condition. Rats were given daily injections with each dose for five consecutive days, then given two days' recovery time. This was repeated once for each condition, and provided an additional control for possible cumulative effects of INDO. In this way, each PGSI dose was compared to pre- and postcondition vehicle groups—that is, an $AB_1AB_2A \ldots B_nA$ design. Plasma levels of INDO were not obtained; however, other reports[29,30] suggest that the INDO would be metabolized within a 24-hr period. Blood ethanol levels were measured as described in EXPERIMENT 1 on the final day of the 5.0 mg/kg and vehicle retest conditions.

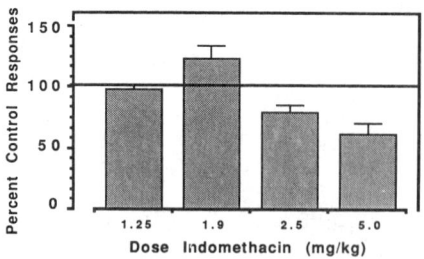

FIGURE 3. Number of deliveries (X ± SEM) of 8% ethanol under a FR 1 schedule as a function of INDO dose. Amount of ethanol consumed was linearly related to number of deliveries, $r = .99$. Repeated-measures ANOVA: Dose $p < 0.01$. Dunnett's test: vehicle (V) vs. 1.25, not significant; V vs. 1.9, $p < 0.05$; V vs. 2.5, $p < 0.05$; V vs. 5.0, $p < 0.1$.

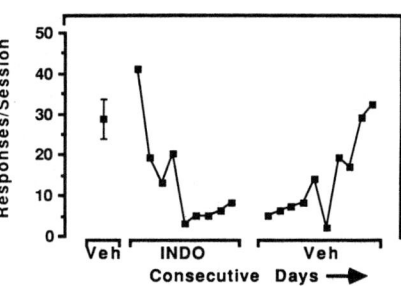

FIGURE 4. Daily response record for Rat P1. Note typical extinction pattern of ethanol self-administration as a function of indomethacin (INDO) treatment, and spontaneous recovery as a function of termination of daily INDO treatment. Veh = vehicle.

Results

The handling and injection stress introduced by the sham injection condition produced a temporary decrease in responding that lasted no more than two days for any animal. All animals returned to preinjection levels of responding. There were no significant differences found between any of the vehicle retest conditions, and these data were therefore pooled within each rat to obtain a mean control value for each animal, which was used in subsequent analyses.

FIGURE 3 shows that INDO produced dose-related changes in ethanol intake. A statistically significant increase in responding was found at 1.9 mg/kg, while significant decreases were seen at 2.5 and 5.0 mg/kg. At these latter two doses of INDO, some rats completely extinguished responding, while others were marginally affected. The patterns of responding seen in FIGURE 4 for one rat show that while INDO produced an extinction of ethanol self-administration, cessation of INDO treatment produced no long-lasting effects on responding, as indicated by the return to baseline levels of responding following termination of INDO treatment. In addition, the fact that the vehicle retests between each INDO dose did not differ also suggests that there were no long term effects of INDO pretreatment. Blood ethanol levels were 58 ± 6 and 87 ± 7 mg/dl for the 5.0 mg/kg and vehicle conditions, respectively, suggesting that INDO did not affect ethanol intake by interfering with ethanol metabolism or distribution. This is consistent with previous reports.[1]

EXPERIMENT 2: EFFECTS OF INDOMETHACIN TREATMENT ON ORAL SELF-ADMINISTRATION OF SACCHARIN

This experiment was designed to provide initial information concering the specificity of the INDO effect on ethanol self-administration. An important question is whether the effects of INDO on ethanol self-administration are due to a specific PGSI antagonism of CNS responses to ethanol or result from a nonspecific effect on motivation or baseline level of operant activity. In addition, it was important to substantiate the results of Experiment 1, which suggested that the reduction by INDO of responding for ethanol was not due to taste-aversion conditioning.

Method

A second group of Sprague-Dawley rats were trained to self-administer a saccharin solution. Drug solutions were prepared as described above. A saccharin concentration of 0.0625% was prepared by diluting 0.25 g saccharin in 4.0 l tap water. This concentration was used because it produced a level of responding at FR 1 similar to the FR1 level of responding for 8% w/v ethanol.

INDO, 5.0 mg/kg, was administered as described above. Once responding for saccharin was stable and the effects of vehicle injection on saccharin responding were measured for five sessions, experimental conditions were presented in the following order: 0, 5.0, 0, 5.0 mg/kg INDO. Each condition was presented until five consecutive stable sessions were obtained for all rats. Blood samples were not taken in this experiment.

Results

The results of INDO treatment on saccharin-reinforced responding are summarized in Table 1. INDO had no effect on oral self-administration of saccharin. This suggests that INDO antagonism of responding for ethanol may be specific. In addition, it substantiates the conclusion that the effects of INDO on responding for ethanol are not due to the development of taste aversions, since INDO should also have produced an aversion to saccharin.

TABLE 1. Effect of 5.0 mg/kg Indomethacin (INDO) on Saccharin Self-Administration in Male Sprague-Dawley Rats ($n = 7$) under a Fixed Ratio (FR) 1 Schedule

Condition	Mean Responses ± SEM
Saline	36.3 ± 8.4
INDO	39.3 ± 6.5
Saline	38.0 ± 8.0
INDO	30.4 ± 4.1

NOTE: Repeated-measures ANOVA: $F(3,18) = 0.99$; not significant.

DISCUSSION

These studies demonstrate that PGSI treatment significantly alters responding for ethanol in a dose-dependent manner in rats for which ethanol was serving as a positive reinforcer. The results are consistent with the hypothesis that INDO served significantly but partially to antagonize the reinforcing effects of ethanol. PGSIs have repeatedly been shown to decrease CNS sensitivity to ethanol.[1-10] However, the antagonism seen is usually a partial effect, typically in the range of 40–80%. Therefore, at marginally active PGSI doses ethanol consumption should increase in relation to the slightly shifted CNS sensitivity of the animal to ethanol. At maximally effective PGSI doses, CNS sensitivity to ethanol could be decreased to the extent that ethanol is no longer able to function as a reinforcer. In the studies presented here, at 1.9 mg/kg, INDO produced an increase in responding for 8% ethanol, while at 2.5 and 5.0 mg/kg INDO produced a significant decrease in responding. The similar levels of baseline responding seen during the saline retests between each INDO dose indicate that the changes in ethanol intake were not due to an INDO-induced taste aversion to ethanol. In addition, the shifts in responding produced by INDO treatment provide another area of evidence indicating that animals are not working for ethanol solely for the caloric content of this drug. Subsequent testing of INDO pretreatment on saccharin-maintained responding produced no effect, suggesting that the INDO effect on ethanol responding was not due to a generalized effect on self-administration behavior or to the development of taste-aversion conditioning.

The results of this study are consistent with the findings of acute studies, in which INDO has been shown specifically to antagonize ethanol depression and not to affect behavioral responses to other substances.[1] However, since only a single substitute reinforcer—namely, saccharin—was tested, this result should be accepted with caution. It remains to be shown conclusively that the INDO antagonism of oral ethanol self-administration seen in this study is a PG-mediated event, specific to ethanol. However, the results are consistent with a significant data base indicating that prostaglandins are involved in mediating many ethanol-related behaviors.

While the results of the present studies are consistent with previous studies suggesting that ethanol acts by enhancing the formation of PGs, it is not clear from the currently available data whether differences within each PG type in the brain exist in response to ethanol and whether regional differences in ethanol-PG interactions might be found. For example, it has been shown that differences exist between the LS and SS mice with regards to cerebellar Purkinje cell depression in response to ethanol, but no differences exist between these lines in hippocampal cell response to ethanol.[31] Since Purkinje cell activity is known to have a norepinephrine-PGE component,[32] it would be useful to examine the relationships between ethanol, PGE, norepinephrine release and cellular activity within this cell type and brain region. It is possible that the ataxic effects of ethanol could result from an increase in cerebellar PGE, causing a decrease in NE release onto Purkinje postsynaptic terminals.

Other recent studies have shown that PGs are involved in the mediation of dopaminergic activity.[33,34] The antagonism of ethanol's reinforcing effects could be due to an INDO antagonism of PG-mediated dopaminergic activity within the nucleus accumbens. Ethanol could also have important effects on other PGs, on other components of the arachidonate cascade, and on other related pathways such as leukotriene synthesis.[1,14,35-37] Clearly, elucidation of the specific roles played in the CNS by the numerous metabolites of arachidonic acid will greatly increase our ability to understand the interactions between these compounds and ethanol. This should, in turn, increase the probability of developing novel therapeutic agents for the treatment of ethanol-related problems.

SUMMARY

Prostaglandin synthesis inhibitors antagonize the effects of alcohols, indicating that some aspect of cyclooxygenase activity and arachidonic acid metabolism is involved in the mechanism of action of alcohols. In addition, ethanol increases *in vivo* brain PGE and PGF levels in a manner correlated across dose and time with the absorption phase of ethanol. These results have provided systematic evidence in support of the hypothesis that ethanol produces its intoxicating effects to a significant degree through a prostaglandin-mediated mechanism. This report has presented an overview of this work, as well as additional results from a series of recent studies that examined the effects of pretreatment with INDO, a potent PGSI, on ethanol self-administration. The results of these self-administration studies indicate that INDO can decrease responding for ethanol in a dose-related manner. The pattern of changes suggests that INDO decreases ethanol self-administration by decreasing the reinforcing effects of ethanol and not by producing a conditioned aversion to ethanol. In a subsequent study, INDO did not affect saccharin self-administration. These results suggest that there exists a common prostaglandin-related mechanism that is important in the mediation of both acute sensitivity to ethanol and the reinforcing properties of this drug. These findings may provide for the development of novel pharmaceutical treatments for acute alcohol overdose as well as for chronic alcohol abuse.

ACKNOWLEDGMENTS

The author wishes to thank Theresa Crimmins and Joseph Raphael for technical assistance, and Dr. Richard A. Meisch for helpful suggestions with this research.

REFERENCES

1. GEORGE, F. R. & A. C. COLLINS. 1979. Pharmacol. Biochem. Behav. **10**: 865–869.
2. GEORGE, F. R., S. J. JACKSON & A. C. COLLINS. 1981. Psychopharmacology **74**: 241–244.
3. RITZ, M. C., F. R. GEORGE & A. C. COLLINS. 1981. Subst. Alcohol Actions/Misuse **2**: 289–299.
4. GEORGE, F. R., G. I. ELMER & A. C. COLLINS. 1982. Subst. Alcohol Actions/Misuse **3**: 267–274.
5. GEORGE, F. R., T. C. HOWERTON, G. I. ELMER & A. C. COLLINS. 1983. Pharmacol. Biochem. Behav. **19**: 131–136.
6. GREIZERSTEIN, H. B. 1984. Psychopharmacology **84**: 101–104.
7. GEORGE, F. R., M. C. RITZ & A. C. COLLINS. 1985. Psychopharmacology **85**: 151–153.
8. GRUPP, L. A., J. ELIAS, E. PERLANSKI & R. B. STEWART. 1985. Psychopharmacology **87**: 20–24.
9. SEGARNICK, D. J., D. M. CORDASCO & J. ROTROSEN. 1985. Pharmacol. Biochem. Behav. **23**: 71–75.
10. RANDALL, C. L. & R. F. ANTON. 1984. Alcoholism Clin. Exp. Res. **8**: 513–515.
11. PENNINGTON, S. N. & C. P. SMITH. 1979. Prostaglandins Med. **2**: 43–50.
12. ROTROSEN, J., D. MANDIO, D. SEGARNICK, L. J. TRAFICANTE & S. GERSHON. 1980. Life Sci. **26**: 1867–1876.
13. ANTON, R. F., C. J. WALLIS & C. L. RANDALL. 1984. Alcoholism Clin. Exp. Res. **8**: 80.
14. GEORGE, F. R. & A. C. COLLINS. 1985. Alcoholism Clin. Exp. Res. **9**: 143–146.
15. GEORGE, F. R., M. C. RITZ, G. I. ELMER & A. C. COLLINS. 1986. Life Sci. **39**: 1069–1075.
16. GEORGE, F. R. 1986. Alc. Alcoholism Suppl. **1**: 675–678.
17. RANDALL, C. L., R. F. ANTON, H. C. BECKER & N. M. WHITE. 1988. Alcoholism Clin. Exp. Res. **12**: 340.
18. MCCLEARN, G. E. & R. KAKIHANA. 1973. Behav. Genet. **3**: 409–410.
19. DENEAU, G., T. YANAGITA & M. H. SEEVERS. 1969. Psychopharmacologia **16**: 30–48.
20. THOMPSON, T. & C. R. SCHUSTER. 1964. Psychopharmacologia **5**: 87–94.
21. WEEKS, J. R. 1962. Science **138**: 143–144.
22. GRIFFITHS, R. R., G. E. BIGELOW & J. E. HENNINGFIELD. 1980. Similarities in animal and human drug-taking behavior. *In* Advances in Substance Abuse. N. K. Mello, Ed. Vol. 1: 1–90. JAI Press. Greenwich. CT.
23. ELMER, G. I., R. A. MEISCH & F. R. GEORGE. 1986. Pharmacol. Biochem. Behav. **24**: 1417–1421.
24. HENNINGFIELD, J. E. & R. A. MEISCH. 1981. J. Stud. Alcohol **42**: 192.
25. MEISCH, R. A. 1977. Ethanol self-administration: Infrahuman studies. *In* Advances in Behavioral Pharmacology. T. Thompson & P. B. Dews, Eds. Vol. 1: 35–84. Academic Press. New York, NY.
26. DIXON, W. J. 1983. BMDP Statistical Software. University of California Press, Berkely, CA.
27. ROSCOE, J. T. 1975. Fundamental Research Statistics for the Behavioral Sciences. 2nd ed.: Holt, Rhinehart & Winston. New York, NY.

28. MEISCH, R. A. 1975. Pharmacological Rev. **27:** 465–473.
29. GEORGE, F. R., T. C. HOWERTON, G. I. ELMER & A. C. COLLINS. 1983. Pharmacol. Biochem. Behav. **19:** 131–136.
30. HUCKER, H. B., S. C. STAUFFER, S. D. WHITE, R. E. RHODES, B. H. ARISON, E. R. UMBENHAUER, R. J. BOWER & F. G. MCMAHON. 1973. Drug MEtab. Dispos. **1:** 721–736.
31. SORENSEN, S., T. DUNWIDDIE, G. MCCLEARN, R. FREEDMAN & B. HOFFER. 1981. Pharmacol. Biochem. Bheav. **14:** 227–234.
32. COOPER, J. R., F. E. BLOOM & R. H. ROTH. 1982. The Biochemical Basis of Neuropharmacology. 4th edit. Oxford Press. New York, NY.
33. SCHWARZ, R. D., N. J. URETSKY & J. R. BIANCHINE. 1982. Pharmacol. Biochem. Behav. **17:** 1233–1237.
34. MILLIA, C., F. NICOLETTI, A. A. GRASSO, F. PATTI, D. F. CONDORELLI, E. RAPISARDA, L. RAMPELLO, G. COSTA & U. SCAPAGNINI. 1983. J. Neurochem. **41:** 1190–1191.
35. WESTCOTT, J. Y. & R. C. MURPHY. 1983. Prostaglandins **26:** 223–240.
36. SEGARNICK, D. J., H. RYER & J. ROTROSEN. 1985. Biochem. Pharmacol. **34:** 1343–1346.
37. NOE, M., D. OLIVA, A. CORSINI, M. SOMA, R. FUMAGALLI & S. NICOSIA. 1985. J. Cyclic Nucleotide Protein Phosphor. Res. **10:** 293–308.

Thermoregulatory Actions of Eicosanoids in the Central Nervous System with Particular Regard to the Pathogenesis of Fever

A. S. MILTON

Department of Pharmacology
University of Aberdeen
Marischal College
Aberdeen, Scotland

If a definition of life were required, it might be most clearly established on that capacity, by which the animal preserves its proper heat under the various degrees of temperature of the medium in which it lives. The most perfect animals possess this power in a superior degree, and to the exercise of their vital functions this is necessary. The inferior animals have it in a lower degree, in a degree however suited to their functions. In vegetables it seems to exist, but in a degree still lower, according to their more limited powers, and humbler destination...

There is reason to believe, that while the actual temperature of the human body remains unchanged, its health is not permanently interrupted by the variation in the temperature of the medium that surrounds it; but that a few degrees of increase or diminution of the heat of the system, produces disease and death. A knowledge therefore of the laws which regulate the vital heat, seems to be the most important branch of physiology.

—JAMES CURRIE, 1808

So wrote James Currie in his book entitled "Medical Reports on the Effects of Water as a Remedy in Fever and Other Diseases."[1]

Of all the symptoms of disease, fever is the one most easily recognized as being of pathological significance. The first action that every physician takes on examining sick patients is to record their temperature; in hospitals patients' temperatures are recorded at least once a day.

The symptoms of fever—shivering, cold and clammy extremities, the burning forehead, profuse sweating, and the subjective feeling of heat and cold—have been recorded throughout history. The very words we use stem from the classical languages: fever from the Latin *febris,* and pyrexia and pyretic from the Greek *pyretos.*

Modern studies on pyretics and antipyretics and our understanding of fever stem from two important developments. The first was the introduction of the clinical thermometer. The first thermometer is properly attributed to Galileo, who is said to have invented it sometime between the years 1593 and 1597. The first clinical thermometer was described by Sanctorius in 1625, but it was not until the second decade of the eighteenth century that the measuring thermometer was described by Fahrenheit. The second important development occurred in 1763, when the Reverend Edward Stone of Chipping Norton in Oxfordshire, England presented to the Royal Society in London the results of his observations on the use of the bark of the willow tree in the treatment of ague.[2] From that time until 1970 we had no idea how infection raised body temperature or how antipyretics reduced fever. The modern era commenced in 1970, when Milton and Wendlandt injected various prostaglandins

(PGs) into the cerebroventricular system of the conscious cat.[3] (A full account of the history of the experiments that led to this discovery is fully documented in the review chapter written in 1982 by the author of the present paper.[4])

THE ROLE OF PROSTAGLANDINS IN FEVER AND THE MODE OF ACTION OF ANTIPYRETIC DRUGS

The first experiments showed that PGE_1 in microgram quantities produced a marked rise in deep body temperature accompanied by shivering and vasoconstriction

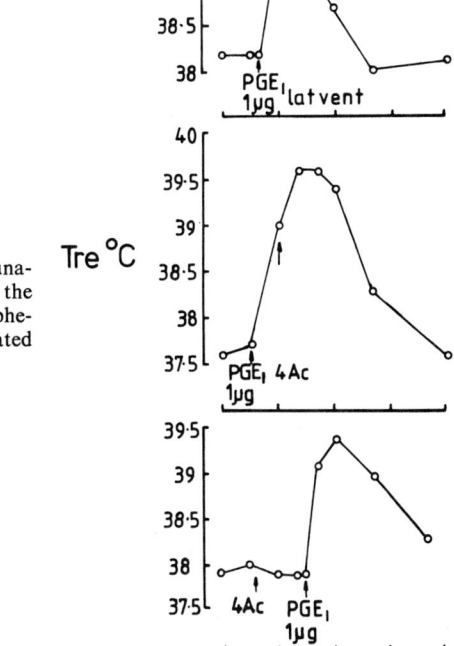

FIGURE 1. Rectal temperature (Tre) of an unanesthetized rat. $PGE_{1\alpha}$ (1 µg) was injected into the right lateral cerebral ventricle. 4-Acetamidophenol (4-AC) was injected 50 mg/kg ip, as indicated by the *arrows*.

and with the animal adopting a "curled up" position, symptoms very similar to those observed following the central administration of bacterial endotoxins. A report of this first observation was published by Milton and Wendlandt in 1970.[3] One of the most exciting findings of this early work was the observation that the antipyretic drug 4-acetamidophenol (4-Ac) (paracetamol, acetaminophen) had no effect on the febrile response to PGE_1 (Fig. 1), in contrast to its action in suppressing fever produced by the central administration of endotoxin, which Milton and Wendlandt had previously reported in 1968.[5] From their observations with PGE_1 and 4-Ac, Milton and Wendlandt put forward the proposal that "PGE_1 may be acting as a modulator in temperature regulation and that the action of antipyretics may be to interfere with the release of PGE_1 by pyrogen." At that time there was no experimental evidence to indicate how antipyretic drugs might affect the release of prostaglandins; however, the answer was to come a few months later when in 1971 Vane showed that the nonsteroidal, antiinflammatory drugs including aspirin inhibited the synthesis of prostaglandins from arachidonic acid by lung homogenate.[6] Vane suggested that since fever could be mimicked by prostaglandins, and because of the proposed involvement of prostaglandins in inflammation and pain, the prostaglandins were mediators in all three of these pathological conditions, and the nonsteroidal, antiinflammatory drugs produced their antipyretic, antiinflammatory, and analgesic actions by inhibiting the synthesis of the prostaglandins. This proposal of Vane provided an answer to the question of why aspirinlike drugs should have these three apparently dissimilar therapeutic actions.

In their paper in 1970 on the effects of the prostaglandins Milton and Wendlandt found that prostaglandin A_1, F_{1a} and F_{2a} were inactive at the same dose levels as PGE_1 with respect to thermoregulatory effects. In a more detailed investigation published in 1971 Milton and Wendlandt showed that prostaglandin E_2 produced exactly the same thermoregulatory response in the cat as PGE_1 and also that PGE_1 and PGE_2 were equally potent.[7] They also showed that PGE_1 was hyperthermic in the rabbit. In another publication in 1971 Milton and Wendlandt reported on the hyperthermic effects of PGE_1 in the rat.[8] By 1971 Feldberg and Saxena had confirmed the original observations of Milton and Wendlandt on the hyperthermic effects of PGE_1 in the cat and had also shown that this substance was hyperthermic in the rabbit and rat.[9] In addition they made two important discoveries: first, that when PGE_1 was infused into the cerebroventricular system of the cat, the hyperthermia produced was sustained for only as long as the infusion lasted; thereafter, deep body temperature returned to the preinfusion level. Secondly, they located the site of action of PGE_1 as the preoptic area of the anterior hypothalamus (PO/AH). The observations of Milton and Wendlandt and of Feldberg and Saxena indicated that prostaglandins would be an ideal endogenous substance for modulating increases in body temperature, including fever, since it was active in very small amounts, its duration of action was short, it acted in the area of the brain considered to be the center of thermoregulation, and it was hyperthermic in all the species in which it had at that time been administered.

In 1970 Milton and Wendlandt reported that a prostaglandin-like substance had been found in cat cerebrospinal fluid (CSF) during pyrogen fever;[3] and in 1973 Feldberg and Gupta obtained CSF from the third cerebral ventricle in the conscious cat[10] and assayed it for contractile activity, using the rat fundus strip preparation of Vane.[11] They found that in afebrile animals activity was very low or absent; whereas during fever produced by injecting pyrogen directly into the third cerebral ventricle, the activity was considerably greater. On administration of the antipyretic 4-Ac, the fever abated, and the contractile activity of the CSF was again low. In 1973 Feldberg, Gupta, Milton, and Wendlandt collected CSF from the cisterna magna in the conscious cat and assayed it for PG-like activity.[12] They found that the O-somatic antigen of *Shigella dysenteriae* produced a fever when administered both into the third ventricle and into the cisterna magna, and also when given intravenously. In all cases during the febrile response, the PG-like activity of the CSF increased, and the three antipyretic drugs acetylsalicylic acid (aspirin), 4-Ac, and indomethacin all abolished fever; and at the same time the PG-like content of the CSF fell (see FIG. 2). Thin-layer chromatography of the CSF samples followed by bioassay and radioimmunuoassay indicated that the prostaglandin presence in the CSF of the cat during fever was prostaglandin E_2. As previously reported by Milton and Wendlandt in 1971 in the cat, PGE_2 is of equal potentcy to PGE_1 in producing hyperthermia.[7] It was therefore concluded by Feldberg et al. in 1973 that the prostaglandin released during pyrogen fever and responsible for the hyperpyrexia was PGE_2.[12]

Bacterial endotoxins, tissue damage, and other stimuli that produce fever are thought to do so by stimulating the synthesis and release of a low-molecular-weight protein that was originally called either leucocyte pyrogen or endogenous pyrogen (EP) but is now referred to as interleukin 1 (IL1). Harvey and Milton in 1975 prepared EP from cat peritoneal exudate cells and injected it either intravenously in a single dose or infused it intravenously into conscious cats; the CSF was collected and assayed for PGE_2.[13] Doses of EP prepared from 5×10^6 cells produced a mean rise in temperature of 1.5 °C, and PGE_2 increased from less than 1 ng/ml to a mean of 3.2 ng/ml at the

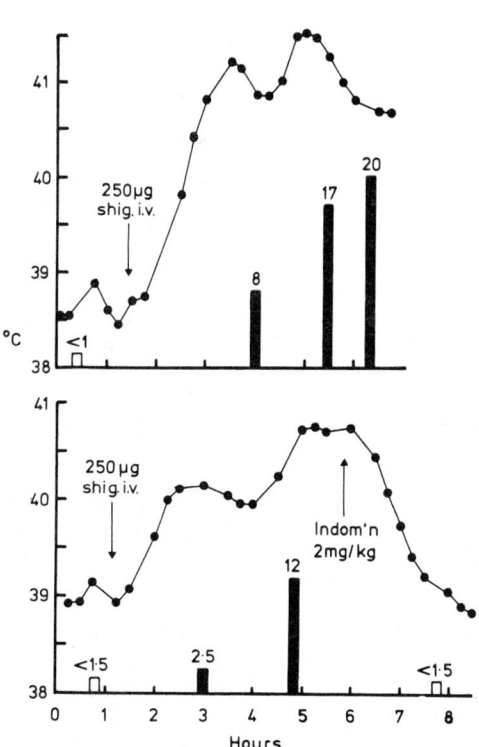

FIGURE 2. Records of rectal temperature from two unanesthetized cats. The height of the columns and the values above them refer to PGE_1-like activity in ng/ml of cisternal cerebrospinal fluid; the position of the columns refers to the time (but not the duration) of the CSF collection. The *arrow* on the left in *both panels* indicates an iv injection of 250 μg of pyrogen (the O-somatic antigen of *Shigella dysenteriae,* shig.). The second *arrow* in the *bottom panel* indicates an ip injection of indomethacin (indom'n), 2 mg/kg. (From Feldberg, Gupta, Milton, and Wendlandt.[13] Reprinted by permission from *Journal of Physiology*.)

height of the febrile response. If the EP (4×10^6 cell exudate per ml) was infused at a rate of 0.5 ml/min for 5 minutes followed by 0.05 ml/min, a rapid rise in deep body temperature was produced and was sustained for as long as the infusion was continued; and PGE_2 levels rose from less than 1 ng/ml to between 2.7 and 5 ng/ml and remained elevated until the infusion was stopped. Harvey and Milton also obtained plasma from cats during fever produced by the administration of the O-somatic antigen of *S. dysenteriae* injected either intravenously or into the cerebroventricular system. The plasma was infused into the jugular vein of conscious cats previously made tolerant to *S. dysenteriae*. This was to prevent any possibility of a febrile response to *S. dysenteriae* endotoxin that might have still been circulating in the donor animal, though this was unlikely as endotoxin is very rapidly removed from the circulation by body tissue.

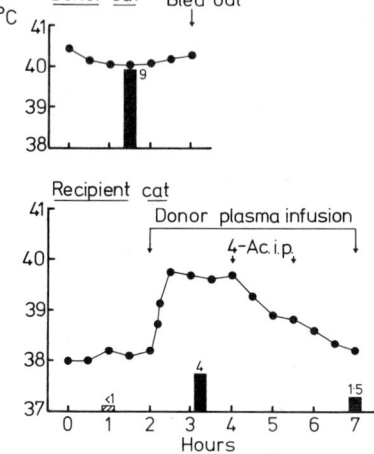

FIGURE 3. Rectal temperature records from two unanesthetized cats. The length of the columns and the values above them refer to PGE$_2$-like activity in cisternal cerebrospinal fluid, expressed as ng/ml. The *top panel* shows a cat with a postoperative fever. The *lower panel* shows an endotoxin-resistant cat. Between the *large arrows*, the plasma from the febrile cat was injected iv (5 ml/kg), followed by an infusion of 0.1 ml/min. At the *small arrows*, 4-acetamidophenol (4-Ac), 50 mg/kg, was injected ip.[13] (From Milton.[4] Reprinted by permission from Springer-Verlag.)

When the plasma was taken from cats receiving endotoxin intravenously and infused into the recipient cats, an increase in deep body temperature was observed, and this was associated with an increase in the CSF PGE$_2$ levels. Plasma obtained from the donor that had received no endotoxin, but 0.9% sodium chloride instead, was found to be nonpyrogenic when infused into recipient cats; and no increase in CSF PGE$_2$ levels were found. In a cat that developed a postoperative fever, the deep body temperature was found to be 40.5 °C. A sample of CSF was taken and found to contain 7.8 ng/ml PGE$_2$. Plasma taken from this animal was infused into a recipient cat and produced a sustained fever, the temperature rising by 1.5 °C; and the PGE content of the CSF of the recipient increased from less than 1 ng to 3.8 ng.

In experiments in which Harvey and Milton injected EP into the conscious cat, they found that the antipyretic 4-Ac not only reduced the fever and lowered the elevated prostaglandin levels following central administration of EP, but also did so during intravenous infusion of EP. When the antipyretic agent was given while the EP infusion was maintained, antipyresis occurred in the presence of circulating EP. Similar results were obtained when plasma from a febrile cat was infused into an afebrile recipient animal. Again 4-Ac reduced the fever. (FIG 3)

Saxena, Begg, Singhal, and Ahmad in 1979 measured the prostaglandin-like activity of human CSF obtained from pyrexic patients with bacterial or viral infections.[14] The CSF was obtained by lumbar puncture and tested for biological activity on the rat fundus strip preparation. Biological activity was assayed against a known solution of prostaglandin E$_1$. PGE-like activity was found in the CSF of patients suffering from high fever (39 °C) of short duration (less than 3 days). From their experimental records it would appear that a 1-ml sample of CSF obtained from a patient with tubercular meningitis contained approximately 1 ng PGE, and a sample from another patient with typhoid fever contained 3 ng PGE/ml. Prostaglandin-like activity was found in patients suffering from viral encephalitis or pyrogenic meningitis, and also in cases of undiagnosed fever. Prostaglandin-like activity was only occasionally detectable when the fever was of a lower magnitude (less than 39 °C) or of longer duration (5 days or more). No activity was present in the CSF of afebrile patients. The authors suggest that prostaglandins may play some role in the initial stages of pyrexia in man.

THERMOREGULATORY MECHANISMS BY WHICH PROSTAGLANDINS INCREASE BODY TEMPERATURE

In order to study the way in which prostaglandins raise deep body temperature Bligh and Milton in 1973 observed the effects of infusing PGE_1 into the cerebroventricular system of the conscious Welsh Mountain sheep.[15] The sheep was chosen as the experimental animal for this study because of its ability to maintain a constant deep body temperature when exposed to a wide range of ambient air temperatures, varying from below freezing to above deep body temperature. It does this by regulating both heat loss and heat gain mechanisms. The responses can be regularly monitored. Bligh and Milton used three ambient temperatures, namely 10, 18, and 45 °C and recorded deep body temperature, ear-skin temperature, respiratory rate, and the presence or absence of shivering. The results of their experiments on one particular sheep are shown in Table 1. PGE_1 was infused at a rate of 2.5 μg/min. When the ambient air temperature was cold (10 °C), respiratory rate was low (minimizing evaporative heat loss), and the ear-skin temperature was the same as the air temperature, indicating vasoconstriction. Occasional bursts of electrical activity recorded from a thigh muscle indicating shivering. These measurements showed that the animal was maintaining its deep body temperature by minimizing heat loss and occasionally increasing heat production. When PGE_1 was infused, there was no change in ear-skin temperature, the respiratory rate dropped slightly, and violent shivering was recorded. This resulted in an immediate rise in deep body temperature. The elevated temperature was maintained so long as the infusion of PGE_1 lasted. However, as soon as the infusion was stopped, the animals began to pant and continued to do so until all the heat gained during the infusion of the PGE_1 had been lost and body temperature had returned to normal. In contrast, when the animals were exposed to an ambient temperature of 45 °C—that is, when the ambient temperature was above deep body temperature—the ear blood vessels were fully dilated, and vigorous panting was observed, with no sign of shivering. The animals were therefore actively preventing deep body temperature rise by evaporative heat loss. Under these conditions, when the PGE_1 infusion was started,

TABLE 1. PGE_1 Infusion into the Lateral Ventricle of Sheep

	Control	Effects of PGE_1 Infusion	Measurements 1 Hour after PGE_1 Infusion
Ambient temperature 10 °C			
T. rec. (°C)	39.3	40.8	40.2
T. ear. (°C)	10.8	9.9	11.0
Resp. rate/min	35	30	105
EMG	0/+	+++	0
Ambient temperature 45 °C			
T. rec. (°C)	39.0	42.5	41.0
T. ear. (°C)	44.0	44.7	44.6
Resp. rate/min	220	30	324
EMG	0	0	0
Ambient temperature 18 °C			
T. rec. (°C)	39.5	41.2	40.5
T. ear. (°C)	28.0	23.5	28.2
Resp. rate/min	150	30	270
EMG	0	++	0

NOTE: T. rec. = rectal temperature; t. ear = ear temperature; EMG = electromyographic recording from thigh muscle.

the respiratory rate dropped dramatically; but there was no vasoconstriction, and no shivering was observed. Deep body temperature rose rapidly due to the depression of evaporative heat loss with the animals being unable to lose heat. Immediately the PGE_1 infusion was stopped, panting recommenced, and the respiratory rate rose well above the preinfusion level. This was maintained until deep body temperature had returned to normal. When the sheep were maintained at 18 °C the ear-skin temperature lay between air temperature and deep body temperature, indicating controlled vasomotor tone. There was no shivering, but a relatively rapid respiratory rate was recorded, indicating some measure of evaporative heat loss. It should be remembered that though the animals were at room temperature, a temperature of 18 °C is considerably greater

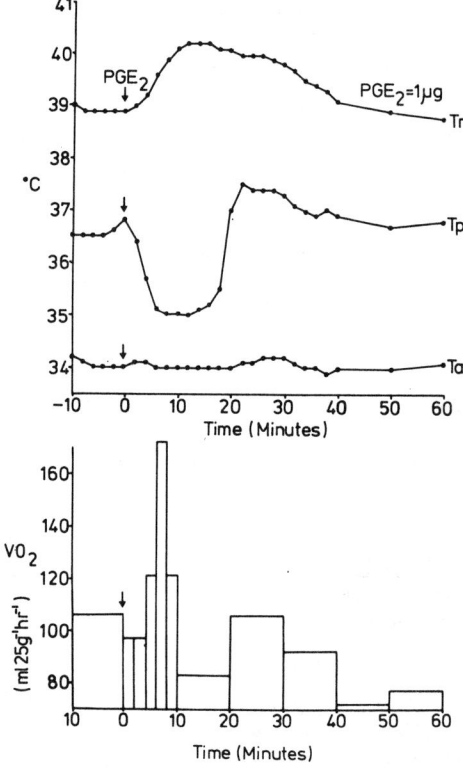

FIGURE 4. Effect of PGE_2 (icv) on body temperature of MF1 mouse. *Upper panel, top curve:* rectal temperature, showing increase in deep body temperature following the administration of 1 μg PGE_2 at *arrow: middle curve:* paw temperature, showing decrease in temperature indicating vasoconstriction and diminution of heat loss; *bottom curve:* ambient temperature. *Lower panel:* oxygen consumption, expressed as ml/25 g body weight/hour, showing an increase in oxygen consumption during the rise in deep body temperature, indicating heat production.

than that normally experienced during a summer day in the mountains. The PGE_1 infusion produced a fall in respiratory rate, a decrease in ear-skin temperature—indicating vasoconstriction—and an occasional burst of shivering. Deep body temperature rose rapidly. When the PGE_1 infusion was stopped, shivering ceased, ear-skin temperature rose—indicating vasodilation—and the respiratory rate rose, indicating evaporative heat loss. The deep body temperature soon returned to normal.

These experiments on the Welsh Mountain sheep provide considerable insight into our understanding of the thermoregulatory effects of the prostaglandins. They show that PGE_1 increases deep body temperature by inhibiting the heat loss mechanisms through inhibition of evaporative heat loss by panting, and by inhibiting surface heat loss through vasoconstriction. The prostaglandins stimulate heat grain mechanisms by increasing metabolic heat production through shivering.

Using the 1971 model of Bligh, Cottle, and Maskrey,[16] these results can be interpreted as indicating an action for PGE_1 somewhere on the pathway between cold sensors and heat production in the effectors before the origin of a crossed-inhibitory influences on the pathways between warm sensors and heat loss effect. The predominant pattern of thermoeffector activity depended upon ambient air temperature and therefore on the thermoregulatory pathways being driven at that time. During the infusion of the PGE_1, the maintained elevated temperature reflects a new equilibrium between heat gain and heat loss. There is no need to postulate the archaic view that the prostaglandins and therefore fever produce a resetting of the body thermostat to a higher temperature. Of particular interest were the observations that as soon as the PGE infusion was stopped, the animals rapidly lost the heat they had gained, and deep body temperature was rapidly restored to normal. This is reminiscent of the effects of antipyretic drugs in reducing fever. Again it is unnecessary to postulate that antipyretic drugs act by resetting the thermostat back to normal.

Milton, Pertwee, and Todd in 1982[17] and 1983[18] showed that in the endotoxin-resistant MF1 mouse injection of PGE_2 icv produced a coordinated increase in oxygen consumption, vasoconstriction, and rise in deep body temperature (see FIG. 4).

PROSTAGLANDINS AND BODY TEMPERATURE REGULATION

Though there can be no doubt that prostaglandins are involved in fever, the evidence would point to their not being involved in the control of normal body temperature. Cammock, Dascombe, and Milton in 1976 subjected conscious cats to both heat (45 °C) and cold (0 °C), collected CSF from the cisterna magna, and measured the PGE content by radioimmunoassay.[19] They found that during cold stress lasting for approximately two hours, the animals assumed a crouched position to conserve body heat and exhibited vigorous and continuous shivering, vasoconstriction, and piloerection. The animals' deep body temperature was maintained during the cold stress. However, the PGE levels of the CSF were unchanged from those measured when the animals were maintained at an ambient temperature of 25 °C. In contrast, when the animals were exposed to heat stress, they stretched out to maximize heat loss, panted, and sweated from the paw pads. However, they were unable to maintain their deep body temperature, which rose steadily. No changes in the PGE levels of the CSF were observed, however. Subsequently Bernheim, Gilbert, and Stitt in 1980 subjected rabbits to cold and heat exposure and also to cooling and heating of the hypothalamus.[20] They collected CSF from the third ventricle and assayed it for PGE activity by radioimmunoassay. Neither exposure to heat or cold nor changes in hypothalamic temperature produced any changes in the PGE levels of the CSF, whereas administration of endogenous pyrogen to the same animals produced marked increases in PGE.

In contrast to their antipyretic action, the cyclooxygenase inhibitors do not impair normal thermoregulation, giving support to the view that prostaglandins are not involved.[21-23] Occasionally the cyclooxygenase inhibitors have been observed to lower resting deep body temperature, but only minimally.[24] Recent experiments by Abul, Davidson, Milton, and Rotondo in 1987 have shown that at rest there are detectable levels of PGE_2 circulating in the blood, and these are reduced to undetectable levels by the cyclooxygenase inhibitor ketoprofen.[25] At the same time they observed a slight fall in deep body temperature (see FIG. 5a). Interestingly, they found that heat stress, producing increases in deep body temperature, was without effect on circulating PGE_2 levels (see FIG. 5b).

PYROGENS AND CIRCULATING PROSTAGLANDIN LEVELS

In 1987 Abul, Davidson, Milton, and Rotondo reported that not only bacterial endotoxin but also the interferon-inducer Poly I:C and endogenous pyrogen/interleu-

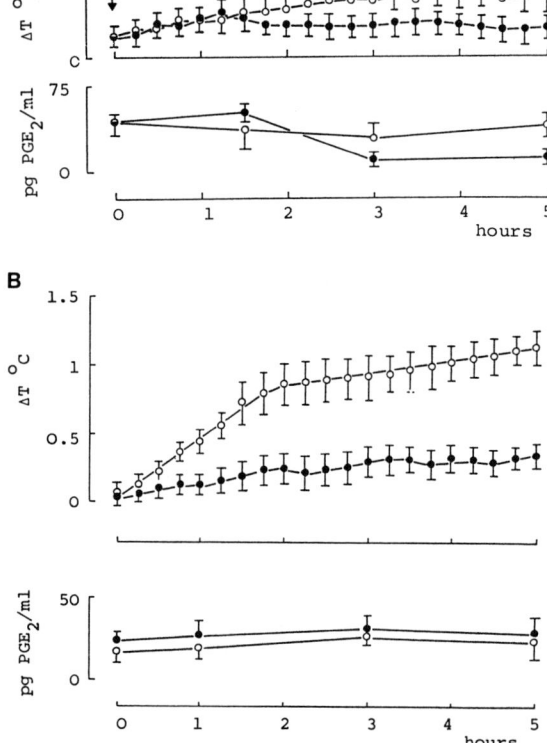

FIGURE 5. (A) Effect of ketoprofen on body temperature (*upper panel*) and blood PGE_2 levels (*lower panel*). At the *arrow* on the left iv saline was introduced; at the *arrow* on the right ketoprofen (3 mg/kg) (*solid circles*) and saline (control, *open circles*) were introduced. (B) Effect of high ambient temperature (45 °C, *open circles*) and room temperature (20 °C, *solid circles*) on changes in deep body temperature (ΔT °C, *upper panel*) and blood PGE_2 levels (pg/ml, *lower panel*).

kin 1 all increase circulating blood levels of PGE_2.[25] The increase was parallel to the increase in body temperature, increasing as fever developed and falling as the fever abated. Prior administration of the nonsteroidal antiinflammatory drug ketoprofen completely abolished the rise in body temperature and the rises in PGE_2 levels, whereas dexamethasone given one hour before the pyrogens only attenuated these parameters. Ketoprofen given during the peak of fever produced rapid and complete defervescence; blood PGE_2 levels decreased to undetectable levels.

In a subsequent study in 1989, Milton, Abul, Davidson, and Rotondo measured the levels of PGE_2 in CSF in rabbits in which a cannula had previously been implanted into the third cerebral ventricle, using push-pull perfusion.[26] During the febrile response to Poly I:C, they found a marked increase in PGE_2 released from brain tissue into the perfusate. Dexamethasone administered 1 hour before the pyrogen attenuated the PGE_2 release. Separate experiments carried out on PGE_2 release from monocytes showed that all three pyrogens stimulated PGE_2 release and that dexamethasone attenuated this release. The protein synthesis inhibitor anisomycin antagonized the inhibitory actions of dexamethasone.

These studies clearly demonstrate that the antipyretic action of dexamethasone occurs simultaneously with decreases in the pyrogen-stimulated elevation of both blood and CSF PGE_2 levels. Monocytes were used as a model for pyrogen-stimulated PGE_2 release, as they could contribute to the elevation of blood PGE_2 levels *in vivo* in the presence of pyrogens. The requirement for a one-hour pretreatment with dexamethasone *in vivo* is consistent with the view that glucocorticoids exert their action via the induction of protein synthesis. As will be mentioned in a subsequent section, it is thought that the antiinflammatory actions of glucocorticoids are mediated through the induction of lipocortin, an anti–phospholipase A_2 protein. This would account not only for the necessity of having to administer dexamethasone one hour prior to the pyrogens, but also for the observation that the protein synthesis inhibitor anisomycin antagonized the inhibitory effects of dexamethasone on the PGE_2 release from monocytes. This antagonism indicates that the dexamethasone-induced reduction of PGE_2 release involves a protein synthesis step—possibly the induction of lipocortin.

EFFECTS OF PROSTAGLANDINS ON NEURONAL ACTIVITY IN THE PREOPTIC ANTERIOR HYPOTHALAMIC AREA

Conflicting and confusing results have been obtained from studies comparing the effects of prostaglandin, pyrogens, and antipyretic drugs on neuronal activity in the PO/AH. The results that have been obtained appear to depend upon the techniques used and on whether the animals were anesthetized or conscious.[29-31] More recently Watanabe, Morimoto, and Murakami in 1987[32] and also Ono, Morimoto, Watanabe, and Murakami, also in 1987,[33] have investigated the effects of endogenous pyrogen and prostaglandin E_2 on hypothalamic neurons in guinea pig brain slices and found that both endogenous pyrogen and prostaglandin E_2 appear to have the same effects.

One caveat that is important when discussing all experiments on brain cellular recordings, particularly from isolated cells, is that any damage done to the cells during their preparation will almost certainly trigger the synthesis of prostaglandins; and therefore the cells will already be under prostaglandin influence when they are examined. In addition it should be remembered that the increase in body temperature produced by the prostaglandins is possibly an efferent effect on heat gain and heat loss mechanisms; and therefore prostaglandin E_2 may be stimulating efferent neuronal pathways that themselves are not thermosensitive. That being so, one would not expect prostaglandins to affect thermosensitive neurons.

ARACHIDONIC ACID

Splawinski, Reichenberg, Vetulani, Marchaj, and Kaluza in 1974;[34] Clark and Cumby in 1976;[35] and Laburn, Mitchell, and Rosendorff in 1977[36] all reported that arachidonic acid given intracerebroventricularly (icv) produced a rise in deep body temperature. Splawinski *et al.* showed that intragastric administration of aspirin to rats significantly reduced the hyperthermic response to arachidonic acid. However, Clark and Cumby in their paper indicate that this dose of salicylate should have been hypothermic in the rat. These two authors showed that sodium salicylate antagonized the hyperthermia due to sodium arachidonate, but only after 3 to 4 hours' latent period—as did paracetamol. However, this substance was much more active in reducing the fever due to icv bacterial endotoxin. Indomethacin was ineffective, in contrast to its ability to block both lipopolysaccharide (LPS) and EP fever. Clark and Cumby conclude from their results that if prostaglandins do mediate pyrogen-induced fever, the primary action of these antipyretics is an indirect decrease of prostaglandin synthesis by inhibition of an early step, such as combining with the pyrogen receptor or reducing the availability of prostaglandin precursors. Laburn, Mitchell, and Rosendorff injected both sodium arachidonate and PGE_1 into the lateral cerebral ventricle of the rabbit and showed that the response to PGE_1 could be antagonized by the prostaglandin antagonist SC99220 and attenuated by the antagonist HR446, whereas these blocking drugs only attenuated the hyperthermia produced by sodium arachidonate. They also showed that the hyperthermia due to arachidonate could be blocked by indomethacin. They therefore concluded from their results that the hyperthermic actions of arachidonate are due to its derivatives and not to the parent compound. Since the response was not blocked by the prostaglandin antagonists, whereas prostaglandin E_1 was, these researchers suggested that a derivative of arachidonic acid such as either an endoperoxide or a thromboxane was responsible for fever, not prostaglandin itself. The main criticism of this paper is that extraordinarily high doses of inhibitors were given, 15 μmol SC19220 and 440 nmol HR446, against a dose of only 4 nmol PGE_1. Another criticism is, of course, that PGE_2 and not PGE_1 is the E prostaglandin formed from arachidonic acid. In addition, during fever, PGE_2 will be produced in the brain; and the concentration of PGE_2 at the necessary receptors may differ quite fundamentally from that occurring by the addition by PGE_2 icv. Similarly, the PGE antagonists, when given icv, will reach similar receptors to those reached by icv PGE_1 but may not reach all the receptors reached by endogenously formed PGE_2.

Recently Milton and Sawhney (1987) have shown that the hyperthermic response to arachidonic acid is completely inhibited by the protein synthesis inhibitor anisomycin.[37] Since there is no evidence that arachidonic acid itself is hyperthermogenic, the complete inhibition of the hyperthermic response to arachidonic acid by anisomycin suggests that protein synthesis is necessary for the development of fever. Possibly prostaglandin synthesis itself is dependent upon new protein synthesis (e.g., one of the enzymes in the eicosanoid cascade).

When considering experiments in which arachidonic acid is added icv, it is important to remember that prostaglandin synthesis would normally appear to be triggered by pathological events that in a controlled manner make available arachidonic acid, which is converted intracellularly to prostaglandins. This situation may differ considerably to that where large amounts of arachidonic acid are administered extracellularly. In addition, arachidonic acid itself is most unstable and undergoes spontaneous degradation. This may occur during infusion of arachidonic acid solutions.

PROSTACYCLIN

Prostacyclin (PGI_2), a cyclic derivative of arachidonic acid, was discovered by Moncada, Gryglewski, Bunting, and Vane in 1976;[38] it is a major metabolite of arachidonic acid in certain arterial walls and is present in other tissues, including the CNS. Its immediate precursors are the endoperoxides: mainly PGH_2, and to some extent PGG_2. PGI_2 is extremely labile at physiological pH and is rapidly degraded to the stable metabolite 6-oxo-$PGF_{1\alpha}$. In 1980 Milton, Cremades-Campos, Sawhney, and Bichard injected PGI_2 and its metabolite into the third cerebral ventricle of conscious cats and rabbits and compared their actions on body temperatures with that of PGE_2.[39] In cats, the injection of 100 and 200 μg PGI_2 into the third cerebral ventricle produced a rise in deep body temperature within a few minutes, associated with vigorous shivering, ear-skin vasoconstriction, and piloerection. Some shivering was also observed after a lower dose of 50 μg, although no effect on body temperature was observed. Sedation was a consistent feature of all three doses. No significant differences were observed between the responses to 100 and 200 μg PGI_2, both producing less hyperthermia than 1 μg PGE_2. The hyperthermic response to PGI_2 lasted several hours—considerably longer than that produced by PGE_2. 6-Oxo-$PGF_{1\alpha}$ (50, 100, and 200 μg) was also injected into the third cerebral ventricle of cats. The lower dose had no effect on body temperature or on the behavior of the animal. Both the 100- and 200-μg doses produced temperature responses very similar to those

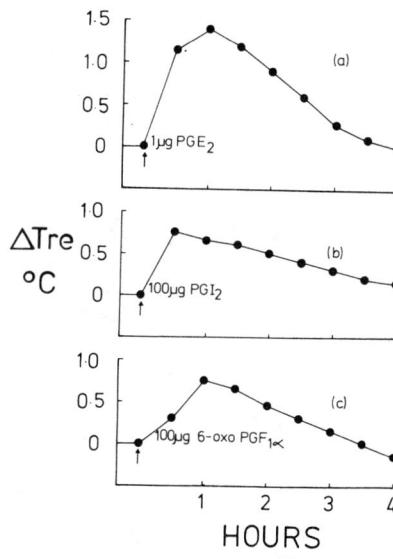

FIGURE 6. Febrile responses of unanesthetized cats to intraventricular injections of (a) 1 μg PGE_2; (b) 100 μg PGI_2; (c) 100 μg 6-oxo-$PGF_{1\alpha}$. ΔTre = change in temperature. (From Milton, Cremades-Campos, Sawhney, and Bichard.[39] Reprinted by permission from S. Karger, Basel).

produced by PGI_2, but the behavioral effects were different: restlessness and an increase in the frequency of respiration often accompanied the rise in deep body temperature, but vigorous shivering and vasoconstriction did not appear to be associated with the rise in temperature (see FIG. 6). PGI_2, when injected in doses of 10, 50, and 100 μg into the third cerebral ventricle of rabbits produced a dose-related hyperthermia. The maximum increase in temperature following 100 μg PGI_2 was similar to that occurring after 5 μg PGE_2; however, the duration of the response to PGI_2 was greater than that of PGE_2. The behavioral effects produced by PGI_2 in the rabbit also differed from those produced by PGE_2 in that the animals became very active immediately after the injection of PGI_2, whereas PGE_2 produced sedation. 6-Oxo-$PGF_{1\alpha}$ (100 μg) produced effects on temperature and behavior in rabbits very similar to those observed after the same dose of PGI_2. The differences in the responses of PGI_2 and 6-oxy-$PGF_{1\alpha}$ compared with PGE_2 and their very low potency compared with PGE_2 would suggest that prostacyclin is not involved in the pathogenesis of fever.

THROMBOXANES

There is little evidence to suggest that thromboxanes are involved in fever; in fact, all the evidence is against such an idea. In 1980 Cremades-Campos and Milton[40] and Milton, Cremades-Campos, Sawhney, and Bichard (1979)[39] investigated the thermoregulatory effects of two prostaglandin endoperoxidase derivatives—namely, (15s)-hydroxyl-11, 9a (epoxymethano) prosta-5Z, 13E-dienoic acid (Upjohn-46619), and (15s)-hydroxy-11, 9a (methanoepoxy) prosta-5Z, 13E-dienoic acid (Upjohn-44069). U46619 is known to be a potent thromboxane A_2 mimetic. They found that in the conscious cat icv injection of U46619, which they refer to as 9_α PGM_2, produced a marked fall in deep body temperature (see FIG. 7). In contrast, the other endoperoxide derivative, 11_α PGM_2, which is thought to resemble more closely the stable prostaglandins, had a hyperthermic action. In the rabbit U46619 was without effect in low doses, whereas larger doses were toxic; the animals died rapidly after icv injection of the substance. They also found that imidazole, a selective inhibitor of thromboxane synthesis, did not reduce the hyperthermic response to arachidonic acid.

LEUKOTRIENES

From a hypothetical or logical point of view one would not expect leukotrienes to be involved in fever. They are produced from arachidonic acid via the lipoxygenase pathway, and the enzymes involved are not inhibited by the antipyretic cyclooxygenase inhibitors. In 1974 O'Rourke and Rudy injected leukotrienes B4, D4, and E4 both

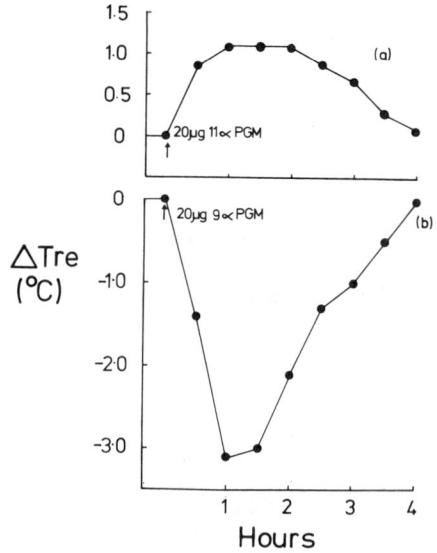

FIGURE 7. Febrile responses of unanesthetized cats to intraventricular injections of (*upper panel*) 20 μg 11α-PGM_2 (U44069); (*lower panel*) 20 μg 9α-PGM_2 (U46619). ΔTre = change of temperature. (From Milton, Cremades-Campos, Sawhney, and Bichard.[39] Reprinted by permission from S. Karger, Basel.)

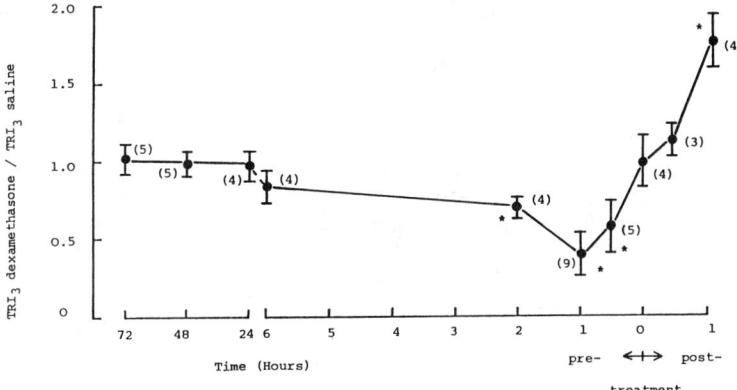

FIGURE 8. Time course of the effects of dexamethasone on the febrile response of rabbits to Poly I:C. Dexamethasone was injected iv at various times before (pretreatment) or after (posttreatment) the injection of Poly I:C (5 μg/kg iv). Results for the zero time-point were obtained by injecting both dexamethasone and Poly I:C simultaneously. Results are expressed as the means ± S.E. of the ratios of TRI_3 for dexamethasone treatment to that of TRI_3 for saline (control) for each rabbit. TRI_3 was calculated from the injection of Poly I:C. Numbers in brackets indicate number of different rabbits used for each time-point. * denotes $p < 0.05$ versus mean for 72 hours. (From Abul, Davidson, Milton, and Rotondo.[42] Reprinted by permission from Springer-Verlag.)

intracerebroventricularly and into the preoptic area of the rat and found that none of them had any effect on deep body temperature.[4]

The observations of Abul, Davidson, Milton, and Rotondo[25] that dexamethasone, thought to exert its effect through lipocortin, which inhibits all eicosanoid synthesis including the leukotrienes, has no effect on normal body temperature would mitigate any argument in favor of the leukotrienes' being involved in normal body temperature regulation.

ANTIPYRETIC ACTION OF STEROIDS

It has recently been proposed that the antiinflammatory actions of glucocorticoids are mediated through the induction of a protein known as lipocortin, which inhibits the enzyme phospholipase A_2 (PLA_2). Inhibition of PLA_2 should prevent mobilization of arachidonic acid from membrane phosphatides and so reduce the synthesis of the eicosanoids. This is thought to account for the antiinflammatory action of the steroids. Since, as previously discussed, PGE_2 is the central mediator of fever, the antiinflammatory steroids should also be antipyretic.

Abul, Davidson, Milton, and Rotondo in 1987 studied the antipyretic action of dexamethasone in great detail.[42] Dexamethasone is a synthetic glucocorticoid with an antiinflammatory potency some 25-fold greater than hydrocortisone.[43] Abul *et al.* found that dexamethasone significantly reduced the febrile response to three different pyrogens—namely, bacterial lipopolysaccharide (LPS), Poly I:C, and endogenous pyrogen. However, the time course of the inhibitory action of dexamethesone was of particular interest. A maximum effect was seen when the dexamethasone was administered 1 hour before Poly I:C, with a smaller effect seen at either 2 hours or 30 minutes before the pyrogen administration. No effect was observed when the steroid was given 6–72 hours before the pyrogen (see FIG. 8). When the steroid and the pyrogen were administered together, there was no reduction in the febrile response; when given one hour after the pyrogen, the steroid potentiated the febrile response. Also of interest was the dose response curve. A maximum effect was observed with 3 mg/kg; however, 6 mg/kg resulted in a lesser effect.

With all three pyrogens studied, the maximum effect of the dexamethasone was to reduce the febrile response by approximately 50% (FIG. 9). Complete inhibition was not observed as with the cyclooxygenase inhibitors and also in contrast to the cyclooxygenase inhibitors, which are true antipyretics and bring down the febrile response once it has been initiated. Dexamethasone was unable to bring down a febrile response and, as mentioned previously, actually potentiated it.

LIPOCORTIN

As previously mentioned, it is now thought that the antiinflammatory steroids exert their action by stimulating the synthesis of the phospholipase A_2 inhibitor lipocortin. Since dexamethasone can reduce the development of fever, it would therefore be expected that lipocortin should be involved in this action. Recent experiments by Flower, Davidson, Milton, and Peers (unpublished) have provided evidence that lipocortin given iv can indeed reduce the development of fever to the interferon-inducer Poly I:C. Since lipocortin is a protein and would not be expected to cross the blood-brain barrier, the results obtained so far would indicate a peripheral site of

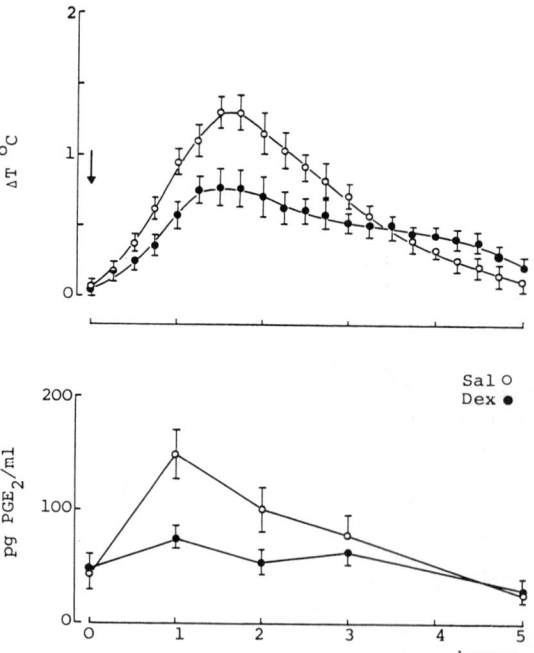

FIGURE 9. Effect of dexamethasone (3 mg/kg) on febrile response to interleukin 1 in the conscious rabbit. *Open circles:* interleukin 1 (75 units) iv plus saline control. *Filled circles:* interleukin 1 plus dexamethasone. *Upper panel:* trace changes in deep body temperature (ΔT °C); *lower panel:* blood PGE_2 levels (pg/ml). Dexamethasone was given 1 hour before time zero, IL1 at time zero.

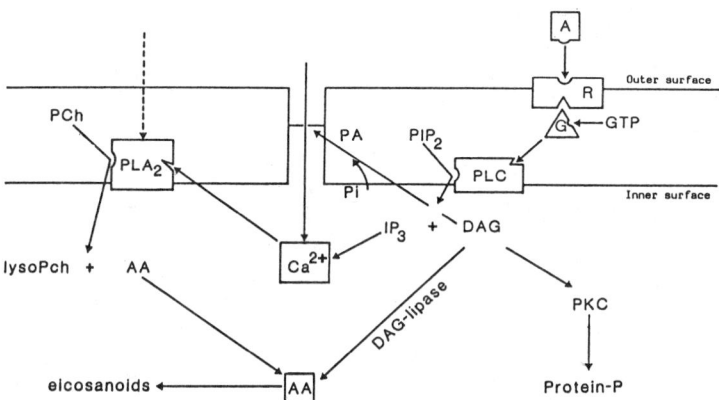

FIGURE 10. Schematic representation of involvement of phospholipases in production of arachidonic acid. PLA_2 = phospholipase A_2; PLC = phospholipase C; A = agonist; R = receptor; G = GTP-binding protein; PA = phosphatidic acid; DAG = diacyglycerol; PIP_2 = phosphatidyl-inositol-bis-phosphate; IP_3 = inositol-trisphosphate; AA = arachidonic acid; lyso Pch = lysophosphatidyl-choline; PKC = protein kinase C; DAG lipase = diacyglycerol-lipase; PCh = phosphatidyl-choline.

action, producing further evidence that the source of the prostaglandins responsible for fever may be peripheral and not central.

ACTIONS OF PYROGENS ON PHOSPHOLIPASE A_2 ACTIVITY

The primary event in the synthesis of the prostaglandins and other eicosanoids is the availability of arachidonic acid. Arachidonic acid does not exist in the free form but only as a constituent of endogenous cell phospholipids. There are two separate pathways involved in making arachidonic acid available from cell constituents—one involving phospholipase A_2 and the other a diacylglycerol-lipase (see FIG. 10).

Phospholipase A_2 catalyzes the hydrolysis of arachidonic acid from the 2-position of phosphatidyl-choline and other phosphatides present in cell membranes. Diacylglycerol-lipase hydrolyzes diacylglycerol (DAG), this substrate having been made available by the action of phospholipase C on phosphatidylinositol.

In 1987 Milton and Rotondo investigated the effects of rabbit endogenous pyrogen, recombinant human interleukin 1 (rhIL1), and tumor necrosis factor (TNF) on PLA_2 activity in purified synaptic plasma membranes and mononuclear leucocyte subcellular fractions from rabbit and purified PLA_2 from snake venom.[44] In addition they studied the effects of bacterial lipopolysaccharide, Poly I:C, and PGE_2 on the purified PLA_2. PLA_2 activity was estimated by measuring the production of [^{14}C]-arachidonic acid from [^{14}C]-arachidonyl phosphatidyl-choline after incubation with calcium ions and calmodulin.

They found that rabbit EP increased the PLA_2 activity of both the mononuclear leucocyte fractions and the purified PLA_2 in the order of threefold; rhIL1 also signifcantly increased the activity of both preparations, though only 1.3-fold. Preincubation of both EP and rhIL1 at 80 °C abolished their stimulating activity. In contrast, TNF inhibited the PLA_2 activity of both preparations, LPS inhibited the purified PLA_2 preparation, and Poly I:C and PGE_2 were without effect. The PLA_2 activity of the synaptic membrane was much less than that of the mononuclear leucocyte fractions. None of the pyrogens had any effect.

Milton and Rotondo conclude from their results that endogenous pyrogen and interleukin 1 stimulate PLA_2 activity in mononuclear leucocytes but not in neuronal membranes and that this may be a direct effect on the enzyme itself.

PHOSPHOLIPASE C: ACTION OF PYROGENS ON INOSITOL-PHOSPHATE ACCUMULATION IN CELLS

Much attention has been paid recently to the role of phosphatidlyinositol (PI) metabolism in the transduction of extracellular signals into intracellular events. It has been shown that the hydrolysis of membrane phosphatidyl-inositol 4-5 bis-phosphate is an important early event in cell activation in a variety of systems.[45] Hydrolysis of phosphatidyl-inositol 4-5 bis-phosphate catalyzed by phospholipase C produces two prospective intracellular messengers: inositol 1-4-5 tris-phosphate (IP_3) and diacylglycerol. IP_3 functions to mobilize calcium ions from intracellular stores, whereas DAG activates protein-kinase C and in addition may be broken down to arachidonic acid by the enzyme DAG lipase. Thus indirectly phospholipase C increases the intracellular availability of arachidonic acid and hence increases eicosanoid biosynthesis (see FIG. 9). The ability of IP_3 to mobilize the intracellular calcium necessary for phospholipase A_2 activity in a variety of tissues raises the possibility that bacterial lipopolysaccharide and other pyrogenic immunomodulators may stimulate phosphatidyl-inositol turnover in leucocytes. Kozak, Milton, and Rotondo reported in 1988 on the results of the experiments that they had carried out on the effects of lipopolysaccharide, muramyl-dipeptide (MDP), and Poly I:C on the accumulation of inositol-phosphates (IP) in leucocytes.[46] They found that all three pyrogens increase the IP level in monocytes, with the maximum increase occurring when the cells were incubated with the pyrogens for 2 hours. If incubations were carried out for less than 1 hour, no accumulation occurred. In a separate series of experiments they found that the protein synthesis inhibitor anisomycin reduced the LPS-stimulated IP increase. In contrast to the effects of LPS, Poly I:C, and MDP, interleukin 1 increased the IP levels in the monocytes within ten minutes, the maximum being reached after 30 minutes. The action of IL1 was not inhibited by anisomycin. They conclude that in view of the longer period required by the exogenous immunomodulators before a significant increase in IP level was observed and the inhibition by anisomycin, it would appear that the increase in IP levels in response to LPS in particular requires a protein mediator. A likely candidate for this protein mediator is IL1, as a rapid increase in the IP levels were observed when this immunomodulator was used. These results suggest that the increase in IP levels in response to the exogenous immunomodulators does not occur directly and that this is not a likely mechanism by which the exogenous immunomodulators trigger the biosynthesis of interleukin 1. It would appear more likely that interleukin 1 exerts its vast array of actions, including possibly prostanoid production, by this signal transduction mechanism.

CALCIUM CHANNEL BLOCKING DRUGS

Since phospholipase A_2, the enzyme responsible for making available arachidonic acid, is stimulated directly by interleukin 1 in the presence of calcium ions and calmodulin,[44] and indeed *in vivo* depends upon intracellular calcium ions, it could be predicted that calcium ion channel blocking drugs are antipyretic. Abul, Davidson, Milton, and Rotondo in 1987 therefore investigated the effects of the calcium channel blocking drug verapamil on the febrile response to the interferon inducer Poly I:C, to bacterial lipopolysaccharide, and to interleukin 1, given iv; and to the direct injection of PGE_2 into the third cerebral ventricle.[47] Poly I:C in the dose of 5 μg/kg iv produced the well-documented biphasic febrile response with a thermal response index (TRI_5) of 4.57. When verapamil was administered iv 30 minutes prior to the Poly I:C in a dose of 1 mg/kg, the resulting fever was significantly reduced with a TRI_5 of 2.23 ($p > 0.01$). Verapamil also attenuated the pyrogenic responses to bacterial pyrogen and IL1. In contrast the monophasic hyperthermic response to icv PGE_2 (0.5 μg) was completely unaffected by the prior administration of verapamil.

The results obtained were as predicted, with the calcium channel blocking agent showing antipyretic activity. The observation that verapamil had no effect on the PGE_2 hyperthermia indicates that the antipyretic action could not be accounted for by interference with the efferent control of body temperature. It is most likely that the effect of verapamil is either an effect on the production of interleukin 1 or a direct effect on the biosynthesis of prostanoids.

CONCLUSION

The results described in this paper indicate that prostaglandin E_2, but not any other eicosanoid derivative, is responsible for the rise in deep body temperature that occurs in fever. The evidence for this is that minute amounts of PGE_2 applied to the thermoregulatory center activate heat-gain and inhibit heat-loss mechanisms to elevate body temperature. During fever produced either by bacterial pyrogens or interleukin 1, the PGE_2 level of the cerebrospinal fluid is increased, and the increase parallels the rise in deep body temperature. The nonsteroidal, antiinflammatory, antipyretic drugs that act by inhibiting the fatty acid cyclooxygenase enzyme responsible for the synthesis of the prostaglandins not only produces antipyresis, but at the same time reduces the levels of PGE_2 in the CSF found during fever. Dexamethasone (a steroidal antiinflammatory) the mode of action of which is thought to involve lipocortin (a phospholipase A_2 inhibitor), reduces the febrile response and also reduces the central and peripheral levels of circulating PGE_2. IL1, the common mediator for fever, stimulates the activity of the enzyme PLA_2, which is responsible for making available arachidonic acid for eicosanoid synthesis. IL1 and other pyrogens stimulate the accumulation of inositolphosphates, suggesting that the alternative pathway of prostaglandin synthesis through diacylglycerol may also be activated by pyrogens. The antipyretic action of the calcium channel blockers indicate the importance of calcium ions in eicosanoid synthesis.

Finally, no evidence can be found to indicate that arachidonic acid metabolites are involved in normal body temperature regulation.

REFERENCES

1. CURRIE, J. 1808. Medical Reports on the Effects of Water as a Remedy in Fever and other Diseases, 4th London, Edit. Philadelphia, PA.
2. STONE, E. 1763. Philos. Trans. **53:** 195–200.
3. MILTON, A. S. & S. WENDLANDT. 1970. J. Physiol. (London) **207:** 76–77P.
4. MILTON, A. S. 1982. Pyretics and Anti-pyretics, A. S. Milton, Ed.: 257–303. Springer-Verlag. Berlin.

5. MILTON, A. S. & S. WENDLANDT. 1968. Br. J. Pharmacol. **34:** 215–216P.
6. VANE, J. R. 1971. Nature (London) New Biol. **213:** 232–235.
7. MILTON, A. S. & S. WENDLANDT. 1971. J. Physiol. (London) **218:** 325–336.
8. MILTON, A. S. & S. WENDLANDT. 1971. J. Physiol. (London) **217:** 33–34P.
9. FELDBERG, W. & P. N. SAXENA. 1971. J. Physiol. (London) **217:** 547–556.
10. FELDBERG, W. & K. P. GUPTA. 1973. J Physiol (London) **228:** 41–53.
11. VANE, J. R. 1957. Br. J. Pharmacol. **12:** 344–349.
12. FELDBERG, W., K. P. GUPTA, A. S. MILTON & S. WENDLANDT. 1973. J. Physiol. (London) **234:** 279–293.
13. HARVEY, C. A. & A. S. MILTON. 1975. J. Physiol. (London) **250:** 18–20P.
14. SAXENA, P. N., M. M. A. BEGG, K. C. SINGHAL & M. AHMAD. 1979. Indian J. Med. Res. **70:** 495–498.
15. BLIGH, J. & A. S. MILTON. 1973. J. Physiol. (London) **229:** 30–31P.
16. BLIGH, J., W. H. COTTLE & M. MASKREY. 1971. J. Physiol. (London) **212:** 377–392.
17. MILTON, A. S., R. G. PERTWEE & D. A. TODD. 1982. J. Physiol. (London) **322:** 59P.
18. MILTON, A. S., R. G. PERTWEE & D. A. TODD. 1983. Environment, Drugs and Thermoregulation. P. Lomax & E. Schönbaum, Eds.: 150–152. S. Karger. Basel.
19. CAMMOCK, S., M. J. DASCOMBE & A. S. MILTON. 1976. Adv. Prostaglandin Thromboxane Res. **1:** 375–380.
20. BERNHEIM, H. A., T. M. GILBERT & J. T. STITT. 1980. J. Physiol. (London) **301:** 69–78.
21. ROSENDORFF, C. & W. I. CRANSTON. 1968. Clin. Sci. **35:** 81–91.
22. CLARK, W. G. 1970. J. Pharmacol. Exp. Ther. **175:** 469–475.
23. CLARK, W. G. & H. R. CUMBY. 1975. J. Physiol. (London) **248:** 625–638.
24. MILTON, A. S. 1973. Adv. Biosci. **9:** 495–500.
25. ABUL, H., J. DAVIDSON, A. S. MILTON & D. ROTONDO. 1987. J. Physiol. (London) **391:** 94P.
26. MILTON, A. S., H. ABUL, J. DAVIDSON & D. ROTONDO. 1989. Thermoregulation Research in Clinical Applications. P. Lomax & E. Schönbaum, Eds.:74–77. S. Karger. Basel.
27. FORD, D. M. 1974. J. Physiol. (London) **242:** 142–143P.
28. STITT, J. T. & J. D. HARDY. 1975. Am. J. Physiol. **229:** 240–245.
29. GELL, R. M. & P. SWEETMAN. 1977. Can. J. Physiol. Pharmacol. **55:** 560–567.
30. SCHOENER, W. P. & S. C. WANG. 1976. Brain Res. **117:** 157–162.
31. GORDON, C. J. & J. E. HEATH. 1980. Brain Res. **183:** 113–121.
32. WATANABE, T., A. MORIMOTO & N. MURAKAMI. 1987. J. Appl. Physiol. **63:** 918–922.
33. ONO, T., A. MORIMOTO, T. WATANABE & N. MURAKAMI. 1987. J. Appl. Physiol. **63:** 175–180.
34. SPLAWINSKI, J. A., K. REICHENBERG, J. VETULANI, J. MARCHAJ & J. KALUTZA. 1974. Pol. J. Pharmacol. Pharm. **26:** 101–107.
35. CLARK, W. G. & H. R. CUMBY. 1976. J. Physiol. (London) **257:** 581–595.
36. LABURN, H., D. MITCHELL & C. ROSENDORFF. 1977. J. Physiol. (London) **267:** 559–570.
37. MILTON, A. S. & V. SAWHNEY. 1977. Naunyn-Schmiedeberg's Arch. Pharmacol. **336:** 332–341.
38. MONCADA, S., R. J. GRYGLEWSKI, S. BUNTING & J. R. VANE. 1976. Nature (London) **263:** 663–665.
39. MILTON, A. S., A. CREMADES-CAMPOS, V. K. SAWHNEY & A. BICHARD. 1979. Pharmacology Thermoregulation. B. Cox, P. Lomax, A. S. Milton & E. Schönbaum, Eds.: 87–92. S. Karger. Basel.
40. CREMADES-CAMPOS, A. & A. S. MILTON. 1982. J. Physiol. (London) **325:** 39P.
41. O'ROURKE, S. E. & T. A. RUDY. 1984. Brain Res. **295:** 283–288.
42. ABUL, H., J. DAVIDSON, A. S. MILTON & D. ROTONDO. 1987. Naunyn-Schmiedeberg's Arch. Pharmacol. **335:** 305–309.
43. MOORE, P. K. & J. R. S. HOULT. 1980. Nature (London) **228:** 269–270.
44. MILTON, A. S. & D. ROTONDO. 1987. J. Physiol. (London) **391:** 95P.
45. BERRIDGE, M. J. 1984. Biochem. J. **220:** 345–360.
46. KOZAK, W., A. S. MILTON & D. ROTONDO. 1988. Br. J. Pharmacol. **94:** 337P.
47. ABUL, H., J. DAVIDSON, A. S. MILTON & D. ROTONDO. 1987. J. Physiol. (London) **394:** 133P.

Polyunsaturated Fatty Acids, Prostaglandins, and Schizophrenia

DANIEL P. VAN KAMMEN, [a]JEFFREY K. YAO, AND
KENNETH GOETZ

Highland Drive Veterans Administration Hospital
Pittsburgh, Pennsylvania 15206
and
Department of Psychiatry
Western Psychiatric Institute and Clinic
Pittsburgh University School of Medicine
Pittsburgh, Pennsylvania 15213

INTRODUCTION

A number of phenomena in schizophrenia may be explained by an excess or deficiency of certain prostaglandins (PGs) or by abnormalities in arachidonic acid (AA) metabolism.[1-5] Studies of polyunsaturated fatty acids (PUFA), prostaglandin (PG) synthesis, PGE_1 receptor activity and cAMP production in platelets, and platelet aggregation have revealed significant differences between schizophrenic patients and controls. Moreover, clinical trials of the antipsychotic efficacy of PG precursor supplementation, PGs, or PG antagonists link these compounds to the pathophysiology of schizophrenia.

Prostaglandins are synthesized mainly from two series of essential fatty acids (EFA), the cis,cis-9,12-octodecadienoic acid [18:2(n-6)] and the cis,cis-9,12,15-octodecatrienoic acid [18:3(n-3)] series. Fatty acids of both series are important in maintaining the structure and function of neural and other cellular membranes. Previous studies using chemical labels, phospholipases, and phospholipid exchange proteins have demonstrated that the phospholipid constituents are asymmetrically distributed over both sides of the membrane.[6] In human red blood cells (RBCs), the outer monolayer contains predominantly the choline-containing phospholipids—phosphatidyl-choline and sphingomyelin—while the inner monolayer contains predominantly the aminophospholipids—phosphatidylethanolamine and phosphatidylserine. Despite the highly asymmetric location of phospholipids in the membrane, the lipid bilayer exhibits a remarkably high degree of stability.[7] Selective modification of the molecular species of phosphatidylcholine in the outer monolayer may destabilize the structural matrix of the RBC membrane.[8] It is also apparent that small changes in fatty acid turnover may accompany changes in membrane function and morphology.[9] In normal subjects, the desaturase enzymes that metabolize essential fatty acids have a higher affinity for the linolenic series.[10-12] It is hypothesized that the desaturase enzymes present in schizophrenic patients have a greater affinity for the linoleic series.[13] Thus a low level of linoleate and a high level of AA and linolenate are expected to be found in schizophrenic patients. The changes in membrane PUFA composition may have a profound impact on lipid fluidity.

---

[a]Address for correspondence: Dr. Daniel P. van Kammen, Chief of Staff, Professor of Psychiatry, Highland Drive VA Medical Center, Pittsburgh, Pennsylvania 15206.

In this paper we shall review the recent findings implicating abnormalities of PUFAs and PGs in schizophrenia. We shall also discuss the hypotheses relating PG synthesis to turnover of dopamine and norepinephrine in schizophrenia.

POLYUNSATURATED FATTY ACIDS

Blood Fatty Acid Composition

Although fatty acid abnormalities in schizophrenic patients are thought to be unequivocally present,[13] there are very few published reports regarding fatty acid composition in plasma or RBCs of psychotic patients. Ellis and Sanders[14] first noted an increase of 20:5(n-3) and 22:6(n-3, but not of 20:4(n-6), in plasma phosphatidylcholine of patients with endogenous depression.[14] Obi and Nwanze later reported a significant increase in linolenic acid, 18:3(n-3), in both plasma and RBCs of schizophrenic patients.[15] Hitzeman and Garver also showed a decrease in linoleic acid, 18:2(n-6), in RBCs of schizophrenic patients.[16] Concomitantly, there was a marked increase in AA, 20:4(n-6). Their results may explain a reduced synthesis of PGE_1 in platelets[17] and high levels of PGE_2 in the cerebrospinal fluid (CSF) of schizophrenics.[18] However, Vadadi et al. have recently shown that schizophrenics had significantly lower levels of 18:2(n-6) and 20:4(n-6), with higher levels of 18:3(n-6) than controls.[19] On the other hand, Rudin hypothesized that schizophrenia may be related to a deficiency of the metabolites of the linolenic acid (n-3) series.[20] Thus, whether a PUFA deficiency is a basis for decreased PG activity in schizophrenia awaits further investigation. The above studies were carried out some time ago, using methods with insufficient resolution of fatty acid separation. Given today's advancements in gas chromatography—that is, capillary column—and high pressure liquid chromatography, there is obviously a need for reevalution of fatty acid composition in psychotic disorders under rigid experimental conditions, including diet control.

Arachidonic Acid Metabolism in Platelets

Demisch et al. have recently studied the incorporation of [^{14}C]arachidonic acid into platelets from 56 psychiatric (33 unmedicated and 23 medicated) patients and 31 normal controls.[21] Incorporation of [^{14}C]arachidonic acid into platelet phospholipids was 50% less in unmedicated patients with schizophreniform ($n = 11$) and schizoaffective ($n = 6$) disorder than in controls. The decrease in AA incorporation was not affected by sex or age. However, the mean incorporation rate in patients treated with haloperidol was slightly higher than that of untreated patients. This suggests that haloperidol increases the incorporation of AA into platelet phospholipids.[21] On the other hand, there was no significant difference between unmedicated schizophrenic patients ($n = 10$) and controls. Thus, it is likely that the altered incorporation of AA into platelets is related to subtype and the course of the psychiatric disorder without showing any specificity towards a specific group of symptoms or their intensity.[21]

Platelet phospholipids are enriched with AA, which is of particular importance in platelet funciton. The main source of AA for PG and thromboxane synthesis appears to derive from phospholipase A_2 activity.[22,23] This enzyme has been found to be increased in the plasma of drug-free schizophrenic patients.[24] Membrane-bound phospholipase A_2 could be responsible for some of the reported changes in membrane phospholipids as well as for subsequent PG biosynthesis in schizophrenia (see below). It is uncertain, however, whether in plasma such increase reflects the enzyme activity or an artifact.

CEREBROSPINAL FLUID AND PLASMA PROSTAGLANDIN LEVELS

In spite of methodological difficulties, several reports indicate changes in PG levels in schizophrenic patients compared to normal or other psychiatric control groups (TABLE 1). Mathé et al. first reported an increase in total PGEs, but not of thromboxane, in the CSF of 8 drug-free schizophrenic patients.[18] Recently, Kaiya et al. have added data that the mean value of plasma PGE_2 was significantly higher in 40 schizophrenic patients than in 23 normal controls.[25] Elevated PGE_2 levels were also demonstrated in the CSF[26] and plasma of depressed patients.[27,28] On the other hand, Linnoila et al. noted that CSF PGE_2 was undetectable in drug-free bipolar depressed and schizophrenic patients;[26] while Gerner and Merill did not find any differences in total CSF PGE levels among 18 drug-free schizophrenics, 20 affective disorder patients, and 18 normal subjects.[29] Recently, Mathé et al. have shown decreased plasma levels of a major PGE_2 metabolite in twins with a schizophrenic disorder.[30]

TABLE 1. Prostaglandin Measurements in Schizophrenic Patients

	Subjects	Compound	Assay	Results
Cerebrospinal fluid				
Mathé et al. (1980)	8 DF schiz	PGE_2	RIA	PGE_2 ↑
	9 NC	Tbx		Tbx =
Linnoila et al. (1983)	11 DF schiz	PGE_2, PGF_1	RIA	PGF ND (S)
	12 AD	6-keto-PGF_2		PGF ↑↑ (AD)
Gerner & Merrill (1983)	18 schiz	PGE	RIA	=
	18 NC			
Plasma				
Mathé et al. (1986)	10 DF schiz	PGE_2 metab	RIA	↓ schiz
	14 NC			= dep
	5 DF dep			
Kaiya et al. (in press)	3 DF schiz	PGE_2	RIA	↑ DF schiz
	37 med schiz			↑ NL schiz
	15 psychotics			
	23 NC			

NOTE: DF = drug free; schiz, S = schizophrenic patient; RIA = radioimmunoassay; NC = normal controls; Tbx = thromboxane; AD = affective disorder; dep = depressed patient; NL = neuroleptic treated; ND = not detectable.

PROSTAGLANDIN BIOSYNTHESIS, PROSTAGLANDIN E_1 RECEPTOR ACTIVITY, AND cAMP

In one of the first studies of PG biosynthesis in schizophrenic patients, Abdulla and Hamadi reported that in vitro high doses of adenosine-di-phosphate (ADP) greatly increased [^{14}C]PGE_1 synthesis in platelets of normal controls and affective disorder subjects, but not of schizophrenics.[17] However, the synthesis of PGE_1 from [^{14}C]dihomo-gamma-linolenic acid (DHLA) alone did not differ among schizophrenic, manic, depressed, and normal control subjects.

Subsequently, several groups have studied PGE_1 stimulation of cAMP synthesis in schizophrenia (TABLE 2). The cAMP response may reflect PGE_1 receptor sensitivity, adenylcyclase activity, or the coupling between the receptor and its adenylcyclase. Rotrosen et al.[31] and Kafka et al.[32] reported independently on a decreased cAMP response to PGE_1 stimulation in platelets of schizophrenic patients. Similar findings

TABLE 2. ^{3}H-cAMP Accumulation Following Prostaglandin E_1 Stimulation of Platelets of Schizophrenic Patients

Authors	Subjects	Tissue	PGE_1	PGE_1 + NE	Comments
Pandey et al. (1975)	9 schiz 10 NC	plat	AS ↑ (=4) CS = (=5)		small numbers
Rotrosen et al. (1979)	20 S 21 NC	PRP	AS ↓ CS		
Kafka et al. (1979)	20 schiz 39 NC	plat	→		M < F NaF ↓
Rotrosen et al. (1980)	11 DF schiz 20 med schiz 29 N	PRP	→		M = F
Garver et al. (1982)	20 schiz 11 NC	plat	→		M = F NaF =
Kafka & van Kammen (1983)	20 schiz 23 dep 31 NC	plat	→	→*	NaF ↓ GTP reverses ↓
Kafka et al. (1985)	83 S 38 dep 51 NC	plat	→	*	adenylcyclase forskolin stim.
Kanof et al. (1986)	99 S 38 dep 33 NC	plat leuc	→ =		leucocytes cAMP synthesis =

NOTE: plat = platelet; AS = acute schizophrenic patient; CS = chronic schizophrenic patient; M = male; F = female; leuk = leukocyte; PRP = platelet-rich plasma; GTP = guanidine-tri-phosphate. Other abbreviations as in TABLE 1.

were also demonstrated in their follow-up studies,[33-35] and in reports by Garver et al.[36] and Kanof et al.[37] Pandey et al., who published the first report on PGE$_1$ stimulation of cAMP synthesis in platelets of schizophrenic patients, found an increased cAMP response to PGE$_1$ in acute patients ($n = 4$), compared to both chronic patients ($n = 5$) and normal controls ($n = 10$).[38] The small number of subjects may explain the inconsistent findings of this early report.

Because the level of PGE$_1$-induced cAMP did not correlate with psychosis ratings and did not vary significantly over time, Kafka et al. raised the possibility that this decrease in cAMP production was a trait or vulnerability marker.[32,34] However, Kanof et al. found a relationship between PGE$_1$-induced cAMP levels and symptom intensity in schizophrenic patients (Brief Psychiatric Rating Scale, BPRS), although not in depressed patients (Hamilton Depression Scale).[37] Van Kammen and Kafka (unpublished data, 1983) found a significant relationship following suppression of stimulated cAMP with NE ($r = -0.34$, $n = 40$, $p = 0.03$). However, the relationship between global psychosis and cAMP levels following PGE$_1$ stimulation with and without NE suppression was significant only in the 19 female patients ($r = -0.57$, $p = 0.01$; $r = 0.47$, $p = -0.04$, respectively) and not in the 21 males ($r = 0.04$, $p = NS$; $r = 0.02$, $p = NS$, respectively).

In addition, Kafka et al. reported a decreased cAMP response to NaF in schizophrenic patients,[32] which Garver et al. could not replicate.[36] Subsequent studies on the adenylcyclase enzyme complex have shown that adenylcyclase stimulation of forskolin was decreased in platelet membranes of schizophrenic patients.[35] This finding further suggests that there is an alteration in the adenylcyclase catalytic unit, either in changes in the number of units or in the unit's structure or conformation.[35]

The PGE$_1$-stimulated cAMP synthesis in platelets was not altered by addition of psychotropic drugs *in vitro*.[33] Chronic treatment with neuroleptic drugs or lithium carbonate did not change the cAMP response either, while high doses of propranolol increased the cAMP production without affecting the number of alpha$_2$ receptors.[34] Unfortunately, treatment response for individual patients was not provided.

A similar reduction in PGE$_1$-stimulated cAMP production was also observed in depressed patients, compared to normal controls.[32,34,35,37] There were, however, some differences between the schizophrenics and depressives. Kafka et al. found normal suppression (54%) by NE of the PGE$_1$-stimulated cAMP production in schizophrenics, but a significantly lower suppression (16%, $p < 0.05$) in depressives.[35] This suggests a defect in schizophrenic patients in the adenylcyclase complex or the coupling of the alpha$_2$ receptor to that complex, rather than a reduction in the absolute magnitude of the inhibitory action of NE, as was observed in the depressed patients.[39] Although in depressed patients psychosis levels were not assessed, the data seem to suggest that this decrease may be associated with regulation of psychosis in both schizophrenia and mood disorders. According to Kafka et al., the decrease can also be observed in some hypo- and hypertensive disorders, indicating an association with the autonomic nervous system in the psychotic disorders.[35] Recently, Mooney et al. showed that activities of PGD$_2$ and NAF-stimulated adenylcyclase were linearly related in depressed patients who responded to the benzodiazepine alprazolam, but not in non-responding patients.[40] The PGD series have not been well studied in schizophrenia.

PLATELET AGGREGATION RESPONSE TO PROSTAGLANDIN E$_1$

Kaiya et al. reported that the platelet aggregation response to epinephrine was diminished in 18 unmedicated, but not in 13 medicated, schizophrenic patients.[41] Clinical improvement was observed in 7 patients after neuroleptic treatment, which increased the aggregation response to AA, epinephrine, dopamine, and serotonin. The inhibitory effect of PGE_1 on ADP-induced aggregation was significantly decreased in all unmedicated schizophrenic patients. Neuroleptic treatment tended to normalize the response to PGE_1, although acute treatment increased the inhibitory response (TABLE 3).

Whalley et al. found that the platelet aggregation-disaggregation response to ADP was significantly lower in 8 subchronic, neuroleptic treated patients than in controls.[42] The difference between the maximum aggregation response to AA and ADP was significantly greater in these patients as well as in 6 drug-free schizophrenic patients (TABLE 3). These authors suggest defective release of AA from membrane phosphatidylcholine by phospholipase A_2 reaction.

Since the platelet aggregation response is not mediated by PGE_1, these studies do not evaluate the PGE_1 deficiency or subsensitivity hypothesis, but raise the possibility of a change in phospholipase A_2 activity in schizophrenia.

TREATMENT EVALUATION

Based upon a hypothesized altered biosynthesis of PGE_1 in schizophrenia, several groups have attempted to correct such a defect with different therapeutic approaches (TABLE 4).

TABLE 3. Platelet Aggregation Studies in Schizophrenic Patients

Authors	Subjects	Stimulus	Response
Kaiya et al. (1983)	18 DF schiz	ADP	no difference
	13 med schiz	epinephrine	↑ DF schiz
	13 NC	AA	↓ following NLs
		ADP + PGE_1	PGE_1 effect ↓ in DF schiz
Whalley et al. (1984)	6 DF schiz	ADP	ADP aggregation in 8 NL and 6 DF schiz
	8 med schiz		
	38 NC	AA	difference between maximum AA and ADP aggregation response: schiz > NC

NOTE: ADP = adenosine-di-phosphate; AA = arachidonic acid. Other abbreviations as in TABLE 1.

Precursor Deficiency

The main sources of the 1- and 2-series PGs are derived from DHLA (20:3(n-6)) and AA, respectively. Linoleic acid (LA, 18:2(n-6)), the main EFA in food, is the precursor for both DHLA and AA. Prior to the formation of DHLA and AA, LA is first converted to gamma-linolenic acid (GLA) by delta-6 desaturase. If this step is blocked, supplementation with GLA, DHLA, or AA is needed for the subsequent PG biosynthesis. Human milk and evening primrose oil (EPO) or onager oil are major sources of GLA. Whether these will lead to increase in PGE_1 or PGE_2 is still controversial.

Vaddadi replaced chronic neuroleptic treatment in 6 chronic schizophrenic patients with phenoxymethyl penicillin and EPO (100 mg/day GLA and 700mg/day cLA).[43] Two patients improved in this open study. He reported on another study with

TABLE 4. Treatment Evaluation

Author	Drug	Subjects	Design	Response
PGE_1 supplementation				
Kaiya et al. (1984)	40–100 mg iv	4 DF schiz	open	3 NL nonresponders no effects; 3 responded
Kaiya et al. (1985)	PGE_1 100–250 mg iv PGE_1	2 Med schiz 7 schiz	open	2 patients: 50% ↑ BPRS (PGE_1 − IR ↑)
PG inhibition				
Falloon et al. (1978)	acetominophen	10 DF schiz	placebo crossover	no ↓ psychosis ↓ in temp
PG precursor or synthesis enhancement				
Chouinard et al. (1978)	phenoxy-methyl-penicillin	10 schiz (CPZ)	open	CPZ dose ↓.4
Vaddadi (1979)	GLA (100 mg/day) cLA (700 mg/day) phenoxy-methyl-penicillin	6 schiz DF	open replacement of NL	psychosis ↓.2
Vaddadi (1981)	GLA (100 mg/day) cLA (700 mg/day)	3 schiz, NL resistant	open	patients became worse: TLE?
Holman & Bell (1983)	GLA (100 mg/day) cLA (700 mg/day)	13 schiz NL	crossover	no effect, 2 patients on active treatment: seizures
Vaddadi et al. (1986)	DHLA (1 g/day)	21 schiz NL resistant	random placebo crossover	no antipsychotic effects, dyskinetic movements ↓
Soulairac et al. (1983)	Onager oil (0.4–2.4 g/day)	14 schiz	open	most SS improved
Bourguignon et al. (1984)	Onager oil (2–4 g/day)	10 schiz	open	3, 6 or 12 months, no effect
Wolkin et al. unpublished (1983) (In Rotrosen & Wolkin, 1987)	GLA (300 mg/day) placebo	14 schiz NL treated	double blind	6 weeks, no effects

NOTE: BPRS = Brief Psychiatric Rating Scale; GLA = gamma-linolenic acid; DHLA = di-homo-gamma-linolenic acid; IR = immunoreactivity; CPZ = chlorpromazine; cLA = linoleic acid; TLE = temporal lobe epilepsy; SS = subjects. Other abbreviations as in TABLE 1.

EPO without penicillin in 3 neuroleptic-resistant patients. They worsened and showed clinical signs consistent with temperal lobe epilepsy (TLE).[44] Vaddadi suggested that EPO could help to differentiate between TLE and schizophrenia. Holman and Bell reported that 2 patients on EPO developed seizures as well, and suggested that EPO could enhance the epileptogenic effects of neuroleptics.[45] On the other hand, no improvements in positive or negative symptoms were reported in schizophrenic patients after treatment with 300 mg/day (Wolkin et al., unpublished data, see Ref. 1) or 600 mg/day[46] of GLA. In France, Soulairac et al. reported successful treatment of 14 schizophrenic patients with onager oil,[47] which contains over 70% of GLA, although Bourguignon et al. were unable to replicate this finding in 10 schizophrenic patients.[48] If there are no pretreatment abnormalities in EFA precursors of PGE, presumably no treatment effects of precursor treatment are to be expected.

Vaddadi et al. reported on a negative but controlled trial of 1 g/day DHLA, another precursor of PGE_1, in 21 neuroleptic-resistant chronic schizophrenic patients.[19] Two groups received DHLA, one with a placebo injection and one with depot neuroleptic. Another group was treated with a DHLA placebo and depot neuroleptic. In spite of overall improvement in all three groups, the DHLA-alone group showed the most symptomatic improvement. Improvement in dyskinetic movements was also observed.

Direct Supplementation of Prostaglandin E_1

Kaiya et al. administered 40–100 μg PGE_1 intravenously to 4 drug-free and 2 medicated schizophrenic patients in an open study.[49] PGE_1 and prolactin levels were monitored along with behavioral changes. The two patients with elevated pretreatment PGE_1 levels improved markedly. Neuroleptic-nonresponsive patients did not improve ($n = 3$). Prolactin levels did not change. Following PGE_1 treatment discontinuation and behavioral worsening, PGE_1 levels decreased. Subsequent neuroleptic treatment led to behavioral improvement and an increase in PGE_1 levels. Later, Kaiya et al. published a second report with higher doses of PGE_1 (100–250 mg/day) in 7 drug-free schizophrenic patients.[50] Two patients showed a decrease of 50% in BPRS ratings. These same patients showed the highest PGE_1-immunoreactivity in plasma prior to treatment (TABLE 4).

Effects of Drugs on Prostaglandin Biosynthesis

If schizophrenic symptoms are related to a PGE_1 deficiency, then drugs that enhance PGE_1 synthesis, such as penicillin, should improve psychotic symptoms, while drugs such as aspirin, acetaminophen, or indomethacin should worsen schizophrenia. Indeed, Greer et al. reported that hallucinations and agitation may be induced by chronic intoxication with aspirin.[51] Aspirin does not easily cross the blood-brain barrier. It is uncertain whether this effect of aspirin resembles an organic brain syndrome or a genuine schizophrenia-like psychosis. Furthermore, the dose of aspirin did not correlate with the inhibition of PGE_1 synthesis.[52] Similarly, increasing the synthesis of PGE_1 should lead to improvement. On the other hand, if an excess is present, improvement should follow synthesis inhibition.

Falloon et al.[53] tested the Feldberg[2] hypothesis of increased PGE activity in schizophrenia. They reported on a double-blind treatment evaluation of acetaminophen, which is known to decrease PGE levels in the hypothalamus. Ten schizophrenic patients were given 1 g of acetaminophen QID. Except for a decrease in the diurnal variations in temperature at 10 A.M. and 10 P.M., no significant differences in behavior were observed between acetominophen or placebo after one week of treatment. The one-week evaluation may have been too short to assess either a PG excess or deficiency hypothesis.

Chouinard et al. were able to reduce the dose of chlorpromazine in four of ten schizophrenic patients by concomitant administration of phenoxymethyl penicillin, which is thought to enhance PGE_1 synthesis.[54]

Most of the reported studies have less-than-optimal designs and poor patient sampling—for instance, neuroleptic-treated or neuroleptic-nonresponsive patients. Neuroleptic replacement or withdrawal studies may lead to the wrong conclusions, as it may take some time before relapse occurs. Additionally, some stable patients may improve following drug withdrawal.[55,56] In spite of these mostly negative findings, the reported studies should lead to better study designs.

The antidyskinetic effects resulting from the presumed increase in PGE_1 synthesis warrant further exploration in man. In experimental animals, dyskinetic movements induced by intrastriatal injections of dopamine (DA), could be greatly reduced by

TABLE 5. Prostaglandin Hypotheses of Schizophrenia

A. PG Excess Hypothesis (Feldberg, 1975)
   a. $PGE_1 \rightarrow$ cataleptic effects
   b. Endotoxine-induced cataleptic states $\rightarrow \uparrow PGE_1$
   c. Psychotic and catatonic episodes $\rightarrow$ febrile symptoms

B. PGE_1 Deficiency Hypothesis (Horrobin, 1977, 1978, 1979)
   a. $\downarrow$ flare and wheel with histamine skin test
   b. $\downarrow$ flushing with niacin
   c. Pain tolerance
   d. Inflammation resistant
   e. Prolactin $\uparrow$ PG synthesis
   f. PG antagonists: induce psychotic states
   g. PGE_1 synthesis unresponsive to ADP
   h. PGE_1 receptor subsensitivity

supplementation of either DHLA[57] or PGs.[58] This decrease was reversed in the presence of the PG inhibitor aspirin.

PROSTAGLANDIN HYPOTHESES OF SCHIZOPHRENIA

A PG hypothesis pertinent to the etiology of schizophrenia was first formulated by Feldberg in 1976, who proposed that schizophrenia may be associated with an excess in prostaglandins (TABLE 5a).[2] He based his hypothesis on the PGE-induced cataleptogenic effects in animals, and on reports that brain and CSF levels of PGs are elevated in endotoxin-induced cataleptic states. In addition to PGE and endotoxins, neuroleptics in high doses can induce cataleptic states in animals and neuroleptic malignant syndrome in man. Feldberg pointed out that febrile episodes may occur with catatonic episodes or during activation of psychosis, particularly early in the illness. In such instances worsening of psychosis could be due to increased PG synthesis. Consistent with this hypothesis is the report by Mathé et al., who found increased PGE levels in the CSF of schizophrenic patients.[18] Unfortunately, PGE_1 and PGE_2 were not separately reported. On the other hand, fever is not always associated with increased

PG synthesis[59] or psychosis. Furthermore, PG antagonists have not been found to have therapeutic effects in schizophrenia.[53]

Horrobin subsequently suggested that schizophrenia was related to a PGE_1 deficiency (TABLE 5b).[3-5] His hypothesis was based primarily on the following anecdotal and circumstantial clinical evidence of decreased PGE_1 activity in schizophrenia: (1) schizophrenic patients have been reported to have a lesser response to a histamine skin test (flare and wheel). (2) Niacin-induced flushing, which resembles flushing induced by PGE_1 administration,[60,61] is absent in 80% of schizophrenics. This reduced flushing response, however, could not be confirmed by Fiedler et al.[62] (3) Schizophrenic patients are known to be pain tolerant[63] and resistant to inflammation. Rheumatoid arthritis is rarely observed in schizophrenic patients.[64] (4) Prolactin, which stimulates PG synthesis, is elevated by antipsychotic drugs.[3,4,65] However, increased prolactin levels per se do not lead to decreases in psychosis. (5) PG antagonists like chloroquin, quinine, and quinacrine can induce "schizophrenia"-like episodes or an organic brain syndrome in healthy subjects.[3,43,54] The PG deficiency hypothesis is further supported by the report that PGE_1 synthesis in schizophrenic patients is unresponsive to ADP stimulation,[17] and that PGE_1 receptors are subsensitive (TABLE 2).

COMMENTS

There are several other reasons to explore AA metabolism and PGs in the psychotic disorders than the anecdotal and indirect observations proposed above. First, there is the interaction of PGs with the monoamines, which are believed to play a role in schizophrenia. Second, the role of leukotrienes in the immune system could lead to a bridge with the autoimmune hypothesis of schizophrenia.[66] Third, membrane abnormalities seem to be present in schizophrenia, which could relate to the variability in so many biochemical findings. Finally, PGE elevation may underly the neuroleptic malignant syndrome.

Decreased PGE_1 function is consistent with the DA hypothesis of schizophrenia, because such a decrease could enhance release of DA. It would also affect other neurotransmitter systems believed to be involved in schizophrenia such as NE[67] and serotonin.[68] Additionally, there is evidence that during certain states of the illness a hypodopaminergic[69] or hypoadrenergic[67] condition may be present. PGs may play an important role in monoamine receptor activity, as they can affect the affinity between neurotransmitter receptors and adenylcyclase. This is particularly relevant, since increased affinity of the D_1 receptor for its adenylcyclase has been reported in schizophrenic autopsy brains.[70]

Conceivably, platelet PGE_1 receptors reflect neuronal PGE_1 receptors associated with DA, NE, or 5HT. Platelets are considered a peripheral model of brain neurons,[71,72] because platelets originate from the same embryonal tissue as the brain. Kanof et al. did not observe decreased cAMP stimulation with PGE_1 when leukocytes were used instead of platelets, suggesting tissue specificity of this response.[37] We also do not know whether PGE^1 receptors in the brain are linked to DA- or NE-associated adenylcyclase. Most experiments on PG modulation of the DA system involve the nigrostriatal pathway rather than the mesolimbic or mesocortical systems. PGs increase NE turnover in the cortex and have physiological effects at many different systems in the brain. At this time it is unclear whether these effects would be specifically related to the synapses of DA and NE, which are presumed to mediate psychotic symptoms and their intensity.[76] Kanof et al. linked PGE_1 synthesis to the DA system,[37] while Kafka and van Kammen stressed the role of NE in schizophrenia.[34]

Interestingly, we have recently found that CSF NE levels in schizophrenia are state dependent, being higher in patients who have relapsed—who show an increase in psychosis—than in patients who remain clinically stable.[73]

There is general agreement that PGE_1-stimulated cAMP production is reduced in platelets of schizophrenic patients. Significant correlations between symptom intensity and these cAMP levels, with and without NE suppression, have been observed. However, there is considerable overlap with normal values, while repeat measures seem to indicate that the cAMP levels in response to PGE_1 do not change substantially. Conceivably, the PGE_1 response sets the limit as to how disturbed the patient can become, while the NE levels determine the symptomatology at a given time. Clearly, the clinical condition of the patient at the time of the blood drawing will determine whether significant relationships will be observed, since behavioral states may reflect different biochemical states. In this light, drug response or relapse prediction studies may provide a better understanding of the role of these disturbances. As Kafka and van Kammen pointed out, this adenylcyclase-related observation may be caused by a down regulation of the PG receptors through increased circulating PGs of the E series or a defect in the coupling of adenylcyclase to the PGE_1 receptor.[34]

Most of the studies so far support some kind of a disturbance of AA metabolism or prostaglandin activity in schizophrenia, even though treatment studies are not very promising so far. The hypotheses of PGE_2 excess and PGE_1 deficiency are not incompatible,[4] as PGE_1 inhibits PGE_2 synthesis. Most findings support one hypothesis or the other. Systematic studies are needed to clear up the confusion about disturbances at different levels of the metabolic cascade. Neuroleptic treatment either has no effect or tends to normalize the reported abnormalities. Duration of illness may be more important than total chronic neuroleptic exposure. Studies of PUFAs, AA metabolism, and activity of phospholipase A_2 and PGEs may help to clarify the variability in course, symptoms, and drug response in schizophrenia,[73] including the neuroleptic malignant syndrome and response to lithium, as well as to help to explore the autoimmune hypothesis. Other areas of interest to the study of psychotic disorders relevant to AA metabolism and PGs include studies of cerebral blood flow and brain metabolism (positron emmision tomography). In conclusion, PGE and PUFA metabolism could play a role in the pathophysiology of schizophrenia. Their potential role in the etiology is still uncertain at most.

SUMMARY

Psychotic disorders, particularly schizophrenia, are associated with clinical phenomena that can be explained by disturbances in polyunsaturated fatty acid and prostaglandin metabolism. Previous studies of PUFA, PG synthesis, PGE_1 receptor activity and aggregation responses in platelets, and clinical treatment trials suggest a role for PGE in the pathophysiology of schizophrenia. Since a decrease in PGE_1 activity can be associated with an increase of dopamine release, a deficiency of PGE_1 is consistent with the dopamine hypothesis of schizophrenia. State-of-the-art assay and clinical trial methodology should clarify the role of PUFA metabolism in schizophrenia.

REFERENCES

1. ROTROSEN, J. & A. WOLKIN. 1987. Phospholipid and prostaglandin hypotheses of schizophrenia. *In* Psychopharmacology: The Third Generation of Progress. H. Y. Meltzer, Ed.: 759–764. Raven Press. New York, NY.

2. FELDBERG, W. 1976. Psychol. Med. **6:** 359–369.
3. HORROBIN, D. F. 1977. Lancet **1:** 936–937.
4. HORROBIN, D. F., A. I. ALLY, R. A. KARMALI, M. KARMAZYN, M. S. MANKU & R. O. MORGAN. 1978. Psychol. Med. **8:** 43–48.
5. HORROBIN, D. F. 1979. Lancet **1:** 529–531.
6. OP DEN KAMP, J. A. F. 1979. Am. Rev. Biochem. **48:** 47.
7. VAN MEER, G., B. DE KRUIJFF, J. A. F. OP DEN KAMP & L. L. M. VAN DEENEN. 1980. Biochem. Biophys. Acta **596:** 1.
8. ROELOFSEN, B., G. VAN MEER & J. A. F. OP DEN KAMP. 1981. Scand. J. Clin. Lab. Invest. **41** (Supp. 156): 111–115.
9. DISE, C. A., D. B. P. GOODMAN & H. FASMUSSEN. 1980. J. Lipid Res. **21:** 292–300.
10. HOLMAN, R. T. 1966. Essential fatty acid deficiency. *In* Progress in the Chemistry of Fats and Other Lipids. R. T. Holman, Ed.: 275–348. Pergamon Press, New York, NY.
11. BRENNER, R. R. 1974. Mol. Cell Biochem. **3:** 41–52.
12. MEAD, J. F. & A. J. FULCO. 1976. Unsaturated and Polyunsaturated Fatty Acids in Health and Disease. C. C. Thomas. Springfield, IL.
13. HORROBIN, D. F. & Y. S. HUANG. 1983. Med. Hypothesis **10:** 329–336.
14. ELLIS, F. R. & T. A. B. SANDERS. 1977. J. Neurol. Neurosurg. Psychiatry **40:** 168–169.
15. OBI, F. O. & E. A. C. NWANZE. 1979. J. Neurol. Sci. **43:** 447–454.
16. HITZEMANN, R. & D. GARVER. 1982. Psychopharmacol. Bull. **18:** 190–193.
17. ABDULLA, Y. H. & K. HAMADAH. 1975. Br. J. Psychiatry **127:** 591–595.
18. MATHÉ, A. A., G. SEDWALL, F. A. WIESEL & H. NYBACK. 1980. Lancet **1:** 16–17.
19. VADDADI, K. S., C. J. GILLEARD, R. H. MINDHAM & R. BUTLER. 1986. Psychopharmacology **88**(3): 362–367.
20. RUDIN, R. O. 1981. Biol. Psychiatry **16:** 837–850.
21. DEMISCH, L., H. GERBALDO, P. GEBHART, K. GEORGI & H. J. BOCHNIK. 1987. Psychiatry Res. **22:** 275–282.
22. IMAI, A., K. YANO, Y. KAMEYAMA & Y. NOZAWA. 1982. Jpn. J. Exp. Med. **52:** 99–105.
23. SIESS, W., P. CUATRECASAS & E. G. LAPETINA. 1983. J. Biol. Chem. **258:** 4683–4686.
24. GATTAZ, W. F., M. KOLLISCH, T. THUREN, J. A. VIRTANEN & P. K. J. KINNUNEN. 1987. Biol. Psychiatry **22:** 421–426.
25. KAIYA, H., M. UEMATSU, M. OFUJI, K. TAKEUCHI, M. NOZAKI & E. IDAKA. In press. J. Neural Transm.
26. LINNOILA, M., A. R. WHORTON, D. R. RUBINOW, R. W. COWDRY, P. T. NINAN & R. N. WATERS. 1983. Arch. Gen. Psychiatry **40:** 405–406.
27. LIEB, J., R. KARMALI & D. HORROBIN. 1983. Prostagland. Leuk. Med. **10:** 361–367.
28. CALABRESE, J. R., R. G. SKWERER, B. BARNA, A. D. GULLEDGE, R. VALENZUELA, A. BUTKUS, S. SUBICHIN & N. E. KRUPP. 1986. Psychiatry Res. **17:** 41–47.
29. GERNER, R. H. & J. E. MERRILL. 1983. Biol. Psychiatry **18**(5): 565–569.
30. MATHÉ, A. A., G. EBERHARD, J. SAAF & L. WETTERBERG. 1986. Biol. Psychiatry **21:** 1024–1030.
31. ROTROSEN, J., A. D. MILLER, D. MANDIO, L. J. TRAFICANTE & S. GERSHON. 1978. Life Sci. **23:** 1989–1996.
32. KAFKA, M. S., D. P. VAN KAMMEN & W. E. BUNNEY. 1979. Am. J. Psychiatry **136**(5): 685–687.
33. ROTROSEN, J., A. D. MILLER, D. MANDIO, L. J. TRAFICANTE & S. GERSHON. 1980. Arch. Gen. Psychiatry **37:** 1047–1054.
34. KAFKA, M. S. & D. P. VAN KAMMEN. 1983. Arch. Gen. Psychiatry **40:** 264–270.
35. KAFKA, M. S., L. J. SIEVER, J. I. NURNBERGER, T. W. UHDE, S. TARGUM, D. M. M. COOPER, D. P. VAN KAMMEN & N. S. TOKOLA. 1985. Psychopharmacol. Bull. **21**(3): 599–602.
36. GARVER, D. L., C. JOHNSON & D. R. KANTER. 1982. Life Sci. **31:** 1987–1992.
37. KANOF, P. D., C. JOHNS, M. DAVIDSON, L. J. SIEVER, E. F. COCCARO & K. L. DAVIS. 1986. Arch. Gen. Psychiatry **43:** 987–993.
38. PANDEY, G. N., D. L. GARVER, C. TAMMINGA, S. ERICKSON, S. I. ALI & J. M. DAVIS. 1977. Am. J. Psychiatry **134**(5): 518–522.
39. SIEVER, L. J., M. S. KAFKA, S. TARGUM & C. R. LAKE. 1984. Psychiatry Res. **11:** 287–302.

40. MOONEY, J. J., A. F. SCHATZBERG, J. O. COLE, P. P. KIZUKA, M. SALOMON, J. LERBINGER, K. M. PAPPALARDO, B. GERSON & J. J. SCHILDKRAUT. 1988. Biol. Psychiatry 23: 543–559.
41. KAIYA, H., H. IMAI, Y. MURAMATSU, M. NOZAKI, H. FUJIMURA, S. ADACHI & M. NAMBA. 1983. Psychiatry Res. 9: 309–318.
42. WHALLEY, L. J., H. W. READING & R. ROSIE. 1984. Psychol Med. 14: 207–211.
43. VADDADI, K. S. 1979. Prostaglandins Med. 2: 77–80.
44. VADDADI, K. S., C. J. GILLEARD, R. H. S. MINDHAM & R. BUTLER. 1986. Psychopharmacol. 88: 362–367.
45. HOLMAN, C. P. & A. F. J. BELL. 1983. Orthomol. Psychiatry 12:302–304.
46. WOLKIN, A., B. JORDAN, E. PESELOW, M. RUBINSTEIN & J. ROTROSEN. 1986. Am. J. Psychiatry 143: 912–914.
47. SOULAIRAC, A., H. LAMBINET & J. C. NEUMAN. 1983. Ann. Med. Psychol. 141(8): 883–891.
48. BOURGUIGNON, A., B. JACOTOT, P. LACROIX, M. MAILLE & A. MANUS. 1984. Encéphale 10(5): 241–244.
49. KAIYA, H. 1984. Biol. Psychiatry 19(3): 457–463,
50. KAIYA, H., A. TAKAI & MORITA. 1985. In Clinical and Pharmacological Studies in Psychiatric Disorders. G. D. Burrows & T. R. Norman, Eds. John Libbey. London.
51. GREER, H. D. P. WARD & K. B. CORBIN. 1965. J. Am. Med. Assoc. 193: 555–558.
52. COLLIER, J. G. & R. J. FLOWER. 1971. Lancet II: 852–853.
53. FALLOON, I., D. C. WATT, K. LUBBE, A. MACDONALD & M, SHEPHERD. 1978. Psychol. Med. 8: 495–499.
54. CHOUINARD, G., L. ANNABLE & D. F. HORROBIN. 1987. IRCS J. Med. Sci. 6: 187–188.
55. MARDER, S. R., D. P. VAN KAMMEN & W. E. BUNNEY, JR. 1979. Arch. Gen. Psychiatry 36: 1080–1085.
56. VAN KAMMEN, D. P., S. R. MARDER, D. L. MURPHY & W. E. BUNNEY, JR. 1978. Am. J. Psychiatry 135: 567–569.
57. COSTALL, B., E. KELLY & R. J. NAYLOR. 1984. Br. J. Pharmacol. 83: 733–740.
58. COSTALL, B., S. W. HOLMES & M. E. KELLY. 1985. Br. J. Pharmacol. 85: 943–949.
59. CRANSTON, W. I., R. F. HELLON & D. J. MITCHELL. 1975. J. Physiol. 248: 28.
60. EKLUND, B., L. KAYSER, J. NOWACK & A. WENMALM. 1979. Prostaglandins 17: 821–830.
61. HORROBIN, D. F. 1980. Lancet 1: 706–707.
62. FIEDLER, P., A. WOLKIN & J. ROTROSEN. 1986. Biol. Psychiatry 21: 1344–1347.
63. DAVIS, G. C., M. BUCHSBAUM, D. P. VAN KAMMEN & W. E. BUNNEY, JR. 1979. Psychiatry Res. 1:61–69.
64. OSTERBERG, E. 1978. Acta Psychiatr. Scand. 58: 339–359.
65. RUBIN, R. T. 1987. Prolactin and schizophrenia. In Psychopharmacology: The Third Generation of Progress. H. Y. Meltzer, Ed.: 803–808. Raven Press. New York, NY.
66. DELISI, L. E. 1987. Viral and immune hypotheses for schizophrenia. In Psychopharmacology: The Third Generation of Progress. H. Y. Meltzer, Ed.: 765–772. Raven Press. New York, NY.
67. VAN KAMMEN, D. P. & J. GELERNTER. 1987. Biochemical instability in Schizophrenia I: The norepinephrine system, In Psychopharmacology: The Third Generation of Progress. H. Y. Meltzer, Ed.: 745–752. Raven Press. New York, NY.
68. VAN KAMMEN, D. P. & J. GELERNTER. 1987. Biochemical instability in schizophrenia II: The serotonin and gamma-aminobutyric acid systems. In Psychopharmacology: The Third Generation of Progress. H. Y. Meltzer, Ed.: 753–758. Raven Press, New York, NY.
69. FRIEDHOFF, A. J. 1986. Ann. N.Y. Acad. Sci. 463: 47–52.
70. HESS, E. J., H. S. BRACHA, J. E. KLEINMAN & I. CREESE. 1987. Life Sci. 40: 1487–1497.
71. PLETSCHER, A. 1981. Br. J. Pharmacology 72: 349–354.
72. STAHL, S. M. 1977. Arch. Gen. Psychiatry 34:509–516.
73. VAN KAMMEN, D. P., J. PETERS, A. NUGENT, W. B. VAN KAMMEN, K. L. GOETZ, J. YAO & M. LINNOILA. Biol. Psychiatry. In press.
74. VAN DER VELDE, C. D. 1976. Arch. Gen. Psychiatry 33: 489–496.

PART VII. POSTER PAPERS

Regenerative Arachidonic Acid Oxygenation Waves as Back-Propagating Neural Signals

STEPHEN C. BAER[a]

Cambridge, Massachusetts 02238

In neural network models of learning it is widely assumed that knowledge is stored as synaptic strength changes, for each synapse, evoked in part by a signal from its *post*synaptic neuron. In some models, learning vastly improves when these back-propagating signals can pass *through* the synapse and travel (in effect, at least) rapidly up its presynaptic axon into the cell body and out the input synapses, and so on.[1] Signals with this type of propagation could also be useful for searching synaptic memory to find goal-fulfilling plans.[2] But for real axons, unfortunately, fast back-propagating signals have not yet been described.

Certain presynaptic endings in the mammalian brain appear to strengthen in response to a signal from their postsynaptic neuron, initiated at NMDA receptors[3,4] and perhaps involving diffusion of arachidonic acid (AA) oxygenation products in the backward direction across the synaptic cleft.[5] The likely presence of free AA in axons (after spike bursts) and the chain reaction kinetics of the AA oxygenating enzymes cyclooxygenase[6] and lipoxygenase[7] may allow this chain reaction of eicosanoid synthesis to continue up the axon as a regenerative wave. After oxygenase product diffuses across the synaptic cleft, it would bind to substrate-rich but inactive oxygenase, kindling it to make more product eicosanoid, which activates more oxygenase, and so on, sending a propagating signal of interkindled eicosanoids (psike) up the axon (FIG. 1).

Some back-propagation models[2,8] require facilitating backward conduction through channels whose parallel forward channels had recently been active. With psikes as backward signals, spike-dependent Ca^{++} entry, causing AA release, could implement this facilitation.

Reacting cyclooxygenase emits light,[9] and light can stimulate polyunsaturated fatty acid oxygenation,[10] but the extremely low intensity of the emitted light argues against photoexcitation of adjacent oxygenation reactions as a plausible mechanism for wave propagation. However, applying the Hemler-Lands cyclooxygenase model[6] to the start of an enzyme activity burst, when H_2O_2 is the dominant cytoplasmic peroxide, synthesis of a seed eicosanoid molecule requires binding of H_2O_2, which is then converted to bound $HO_2\cdot$. Due to an overlap of emission and absorption bands, singlet oxygen ($^1O_2$) can efficiently excite nearby $HO_2\cdot$ via energy transfer of a 1.27-μm IR photon.[11] Since cyclooxygenase may generate $^1O_2$,[9] a form of the enzyme both blocked in this $HO_2\cdot$ binding state and also triggered by $HO_2\cdot$ electronic excitation might allow rapid transfer of activation between enzyme molecules, for fast wave propagation.

Agents that block NMDA receptors or their associated Ca^{++} channels can block some forms of synaptic plasticity, produce psychotic symptoms, induce general

[a]Address for correspondence: S.C. Baer, Box 1181, Cambridge, Massachusetts 02238.

anesthesia, and protect against seizures and ischemic brain damage.[4] That NMDA receptor activation may lead to local AA oxygenation[5] is consistent with eicosanoid models for these phenomena. The link may also involve propagation of oxygenation waves from the activated receptors. For example, such waves might be the target of

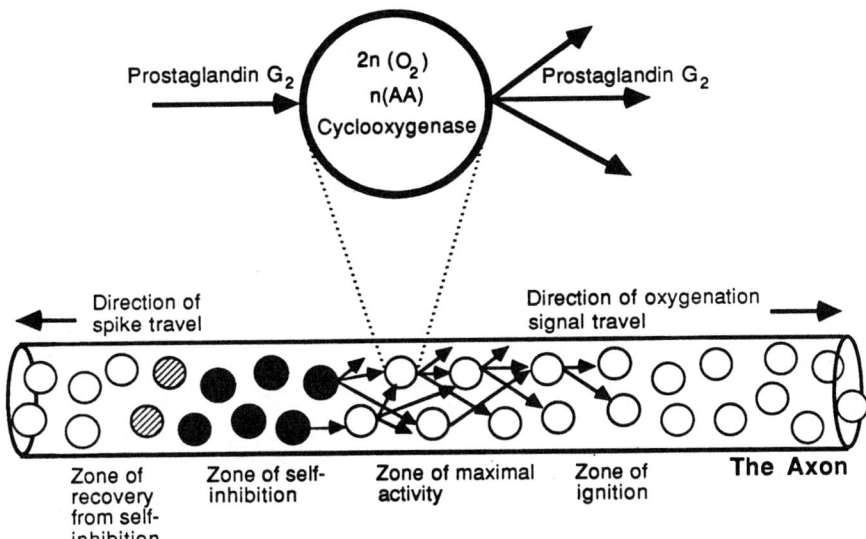

FIGURE 1. The hypothetical AA oxygenation wave propagating up an axon. Each *circle* represents a volume of cytoplasm containing one cyclooxygenase complex and its substrates, arachidonic acid (AA) and oxygen. Since, according to the Hemler-Lands model,[6] under conditions of very low cytoplasmic peroxide concentration, cyclooxygenase requires a molecule of one of its products, prostaglandin G_2, for activation, the cyclooxygenase acts as a replicator for this molecule. A collection of these enzyme complexes in a channel could support, in effect, an "epidemic" of prostaglandin G_2 synthesis. Because cyclooxygenase is self-inhibiting (on a slower time scale than its self-excitation),[6] the wave would experience an automatic turn-off before exhaustion of substrates. Partial recovery of enzyme activity following self-inhibition,[6] in combination with synthesis of new enzyme, could reset the axon for conduction of successive waves. (Note that the product molecules are assumed to diffuse away from the enzyme in every direction, but only those diffusing towards the right in this figure encounter still-unactivated enzyme; for simplicity, these are the only ones shown here by *arrows*.) Lipoxygenase, or possibly a chain oxidizing enzyme dependent on a reducing substrate other than AA or an oxidant other than O_2, might substitute for cyclooxygenase. Free radicals or electronically excited states produced by the enzyme might—via charge transfer or energy transfer, respectively—transmit excitation to an inactive enzyme complex much faster than possible with a diffusing molecule messenger, for potentially very fast wave propagation. The psike might travel in the collection of coupled glial elements surrounding the axon, rather than through the axon itself.

those general anesthetics inhibiting luciferase (an oxygenase) with potencies that, over several homologous series, parallel their anesthetic potency.[12]

The report that cyclooxygenase is many times more abundant in corpus callosum than in the cerebellum,[13] for instance, suggests a possible role in signal conduction along cerebral cortical axons. Whether this or another oxygenase in (or around) axons shows regenerative burst kinetics[6] under physiological conditions, and whether such activity bursts propagate up the axons, might be studied by attempting to trigger the bursts by light pulses delivered by an optical fiber or microscope objective (far UV to make free radicals, or, with axons containing a photosensitizer, visible light to make $^1O_2$). Any ensuing local reaction or propagation of reaction waves from the triggering site might, initially, be detected indirectly as electrical changes in the stimulated axons or corresponding cortical regions, or as transients in optically monitorable parameters (e.g., $[Ca^{++}]$, $[H^+]$) likely to be perturbed by passage of such a wave. Propagation might also be demonstrated by quick-freezing the axons shortly after stimulation, and detecting trapped free radicals by ESR measurement on regions at varying distances from the stimulus site.

REFERENCES

1. RUMELHART, D. E., G. E. HINTON & R. J. WILLIAMS. 1986. Learning internal representations by error propagation. *In* Parallel Distributed Processing, Vol. 1. D. E. Rumelhart & J. L. McClelland, Eds.:318. MIT Press. Cambridge, MA.
2. BAER, S. C. 1986. Problem solving cellular automata. *In* Cellular Automata '86 Conference. C. H. Bennett, T. Toffoli & S. Wolfram, Eds. MIT Lab. Comp. Sci. Tech. Rep. TM-317.
3. COLLINGRIDGE, G. L. & T. V. P. BLISS. 1987. NMDA receptors—their role in long-term potentiation. Trends. Neurosci. **10:** 288.
4. COTMAN, C. W., D. T. MONAGHAN & A. H. GANONG. 1988. Excitatory amino acid neurotransmission: NMDA receptors and Hebb-type synaptic plasticity. Ann. Rev. Neurosci. **11:** 61.
5. BLISS, T. V. P., M. L. ERRINGTON, M. A. LYNCH & J. H. WILLIAMS. 1988. The lipoxygenase inhibitor nordihydroguaiaretic acid (NDGA) blocks the induction of both tetanus-induced and calcium-induced long-term potentiation in rat hippocampus. Pflügers Arch. 411 Suppl. **1:** 229.
6. HEMLER, M. E. & W. E. M. LANDS. 1980. Evidence for a peroxide-initiated free radical mechanism of prostaglandin biosynthesis. J. Biol. Chem. **255:** 6253.
7. SIEGEL, M. I., R. T. MCCONNELL, S. L. ABRAHAMS, N. A. PORTER & P. CUATRECASAS. 1979. Regulation of AA metabolism via lipoxygenase and cyclooxygenase by 12-HPETE. Biochem. Biophys. Res. Commun. **89:** 1273.
8. MILNER, P. M. 1974. A model for visual shape recognition. Psychol. Rev. **81:** 521.
9. CADENAS, E., H. SIES, W. NASTAINE & V. ULLRICH. 1983. Singlet oxygen formation detected by low-level chemiluminescence during enzymatic reduction of prostaglandin G_2 to prostaglandin H_2. Hoppe-Seyler's Z. Physiol. Chem. **364:** 519.
10. MIHELICH, E. D. 1980. Novel endoperoxides isolated from sensitized photooxidation of methyl linoleate. Implications for prostaglandin biosynthesis. J. Am. Chem. Soc. **102:** 7141.
11. BECKER, K. H., E. H. FINK, P. LANGEN & U. SCHURATH. 1974. Near infrared emission bands of the HO_2 radical. J. Chem. Phys. **60:** 4623.
12. FRANKS, N. P. & W. R. LIEB. 1985. Mapping of general anaesthetic target sites provides a molecular basis for cutoff effects. Nature **316:** 349.
13. YOSHIMOTO, T., K. MAGATA, H. EHARA, K. MIZUNO & S. YAMAMOTO. 1986. Regional distribution of prostaglandin endoperoxide synthase studied by enzyme-linked immunoassay using monoclonal antibodies. Biochim. Biophys. Acta. **877:** 141.

Platelet-Activating Factor Receptor Blockade Decreases Early Posttraumatic Cerebral Edema in Rats

D. C. BUCHANAN,[a,b] P. M. KOCHANEK,[a,b]
E. M. NEMOTO,[a] J. A. MELICK,[a]
AND R. J. SCHOETTLE[a,b]

*Departments of [a]Anesthesiology/Critical Care Medicine
and [b]Pediatrics
University of Pittsburgh
Pittsburgh, Pennsylvania 15213*

INTRODUCTION

Platelet-activating factor (PAF), an ether phospholipid, is found in small quantities in the normal brain.[1] It potently increases vascular permeability and exhibits cerebrovascular and cerebrometabolic effects.[2,3] We hypothesized that PAF is involved in the pathogenesis of posttraumatic vasogenic edema and tested the effect of a PAF-receptor blocker in a rat model of concussive cerebral injury.

METHODS

Twenty Wistar rats were anesthetized with 1% halothane, 66% N_2O, and 33% O_2, intubated, mechanically ventilated, and paralyzed with pancuronium. Femoral arterial and venous catheters were inserted to monitor arterial blood pressure, withdraw arterial blood samples, and for iv drug infusion. Rectal temperature was controlled at 38 ± 0.20 °C. The rats were placed in a stereotaxic device, and a craniotomy was made over the right parietal cortex. Inspired halothane was reduced to 0.4%, and equilibration was allowed for 1 h. Rats were randomly assigned to 4 groups. Two groups received an iv bolus of the PAF-receptor blocker BN 52021 (10 mg/kg) and two received vehicle (DMSO) immediately before trauma. The investigator was unaware of the agent used. A metal rod weighing 10 g was then dropped from either 5 or 10 cm through a plastic guide tube. Immediately thereafter, the bone flap was replaced and sealed with plastic cement. After 2 h of mechanical ventilation, the rats were decapitated and the brains removed and divided into hemispheres. The percent brain water of each hemisphere was determined by comparison of wet/dry weights. Right-left hemispheric difference in brain water was calculated for each animal, and the Wilcoxon rank sum test was used to compare the treated and untreated groups.

RESULTS

Controlled physiologic variables were similar in treated and untreated groups before and after trauma. BN 52021 significantly decreased edema formation in rats subjected to a 50 g × cm traumatic insult ($p < 0.014$) (see Fig. 1). In rats subjected to

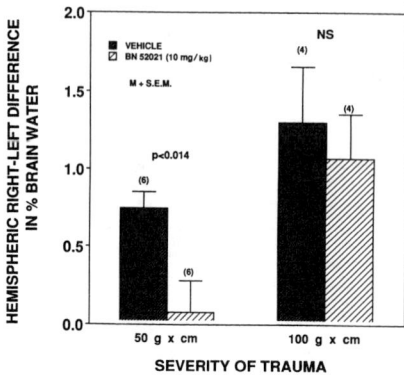

FIGURE 1. Effect of BN 52021 on early posttraumatic cerebral edema in rats.

a 100 g × cm traumatic insult the effect of BN 52021 on water content was not significant ($p > 0.10$). Because of the small number of animals in this group, statistical power was insufficient for conclusive results.

DISCUSSION

This study demonstrates that treatment with the PAF-receptor blocker BN 52021 attenuates the development of early posttraumatic cerebral edema in rats subjected to a mild traumatic insult. We further speculate that PAF may be involved in the pathogenesis of posttraumatic cerebral edema.

REFERENCES

1. TOKUMURA, A., K. KAMIYASU, K. TAKAUCHI & H. TSUKATANI. 1987. Evidence of existence of various homologues and analogues of platelet activating factor in a lipid extract of bovine brain. Biochem. Biophys. Res. Commun. **148:** 415–425.
2. PIPER, P. J. & A. W. B. STANTON. 1986. Intracranial circulatory effects of platelet-activating factor and indomethacin in the anaesthetized pig. Br. J. Pharmacol. **88:** 239.
3. KOCHANEK, P., E. NEMOTO, J. MELICK, R. EVANS & D. BURKE. 1987. Platelet-activating factor alters cerebral blood flow and metabolism in rats. Circulation **75** (Suppl. 4): 53.

Nerve Growth Factor Stimulates PC12 Cell Eicosanoid Synthesis

A Role in Nerve Fiber Growth

J. J. DeGEORGE,[a] R. WALENGA

State University of New York Medical Center
Syracuse, New York 13210

S. T. CARBONETTO

The Neuroscience Unit
Montreal General Hospital Research Institute
Montreal, Quebec H3G-1A4, Canada

Nerve growth factor (NGF) stimulates neuronal growth and differentiation by binding to receptors in the plasma membrane. The intracellular events involved in coupling NGF-receptor binding to its physiological effects, including nerve fiber growth, are not known. Several studies have indicated that NGF stimulates phospholipid metabolism in neuronal cells.[1,2] Since phospholipid metabolism is often associated with the liberation of arachidonic acid[3] (AA), we examined the effect of NGF on the synthesis of AA metabolites, eicosanoids, in PC12 cells. PC12 cells respond to NGF treatment by expressing many neuronal characteristics, including extension of nerve fibers.[4]

TABLE 1. Comparison of the Effects of Nerve Growth Factor and Epidermal Growth Factor on Production of Arachidonic Acid Metabolites in PC12 Cell Homogenates

Metabolite	NGF-Treated	Control	EGF-Treated
PGF2	16 ± 4	3.3 ± 2.1	4.4 ± 1.1
PGE2	22 ± 4	4.9 ± 1.1	5.2 ± 0.5
PGD2	13 ± 3	3.8 ± 0.9	3.8 ± 0.5
HHT	3.3 ± 2.8	2.1 ± 2.7	1.9 ± 1.9
15-HETE	16 ± 4	9.2 ± 3.3	8.9 ± 2.7
Unidentified	3.2 ± 2.7	1.1 ± 0.2	0.8 ± 0.3
AA	33 ± 3	49 ± 14	36 ± 1
Neutral Lipid	112 ± 16	115 ± 5	155 ± 8
Origin	45 ± 5	48 ± 12	54 ± 13

NOTE: Cell homogenates were prepared to reflect equal cell numbers and incubated with $1-^{14}C$ AA (0.25 μCi/assay) for 30 min at 27 °C. Figures are cpm $\times 10^{-3}$/sample. Data are from 3 experiments in duplicate, $n = 6$. Similar results were obtained diluting homogenates to equal protein content. NGF = nerve growth factor; EGF = epidermal growth factor; HHT = hydroxyheptadecatrienoic acid; 15-HETE = 15(s)-hydroxyeicosatetraenoic acid; AA = arachidonic acid.

[a]Current address: Laboratory of Neurosciences, National Institute on Aging, National Institutes of Health, Bethesda, Maryland 20892.

PC12 cells were cultured in suspension with or without βNGF (100 ng/ml) or epidermal growth factor, (EGF; 100 ng/ml) for 7 days. Homogenates were prepared and were incubated with 1-^{14}C AA to examine the production of eicosanoids. Lipids were extracted and eicosanoids were separated by TLC.[5] NGF pretreatment increased the synthesis of both cyclooxygenase and lipoxygenase eicosanoids (TABLE 1). EGF, which has many effects on PC12 cells similar to NGF but does not stimulate nerve fiber growth,[6] did not alter AA metabolism (TABLE 1). The NGF-stimulated eicosanoid synthesis expressed by the cell homogenates was independent of prior cell attachment to the substratum or nerve fiber growth (total eicosanoids synthesized from 1-^{14}C AA: 271 ± 19, 244 ± 11, and 100 ± 12, mean $\pm$ SEM cpm $\times 10^{-2}$, $n = 6$; cultured in suspension plus NGF, cultured attached to the substratum plus NGF, and cultured attached to the substratum without NGF, respectively).

The effect of inhibitors of AA metabolism on nerve fiber growth was also examined (TABLE 2). Inhibitors of AA release from membrane phospholipids (mepacrine and

TABLE 2. Effect of Inhibitors of Arachidonic Acid Metabolism On Nerve Fiber Growth by Primed PC12 Cells

Treatment	Cells with Nerve Fibers (% of Total)
Control	78 ± 4
4-Bromphenacyl bromide (5 μM)	28 ± 7
Mepacrine (100 μM)	6 ± 5
Aspirin (1 mM)	78 ± 2
Indomethacin (20 μM)	93 ± 2
BW755c (100 μM)	10 ± 3
Baicalein (10 μM)	16 ± 4
Eicosatetraynoic acid (25 μM)	22 ± 1

NOTE: PC12 cells incubated in suspension with βNGF for seven days were seeded onto collagen-coated culture dishes. Drugs were added 10 min after seeding, and the cultures were incubated for 3 h. Only cells extending nerve processes longer than one cell diameter were scored as having extended nerve processes. More than 100 cells per culture examined. Data are means $\pm$ SEM, $n = 6$.

4-bromphenacyl bromide) and inhibitors of lipoxygenase metabolism of AA (BW755c, eiscosatetraynoic acid, and baicalein) decreased nerve fiber growth by "NGF-primed"[4] PC12 cells. Inhibitors of cyclooxygenase metabolism of AA (aspirin and indomethacin) did not inhibit growth.

Our data suggest that NGF treatment of PC12 cells increases the capacity of the cells to synthesize eicosanoids, and that synthesis of some eicosanoids, the lipoxygenase metabolites, may be necessary for growth of nerve fibers.

REFERENCES

1. LAKSHMANAN, J. 1979. J. Neurochem. **32**: 1599.
2. TRAYNOR, A. E. 1984. Dev. Brain Res. **14**: 205.
3. IRVINE, R. F. 1982. Biochem. J. **204**: 3.
4. GREENE, L. et al. 1982. Dev. Biol. **91**: 305.
5. DEGEORGE, J. J. et al. 1986. J. Biol. Chem. **261**: 3428.
6. HUFF, K. R. & G. GUROFF. 1979. Biochem. Biophys. Res. Commun. **89**: 175.

Effects of Traumatic Brain Injury on Arachidonic Acid Metabolism and Brain Water Content in the Rat

PAUL DEMEDIUK,[a] ALAN I. FADEN, ROBERT VINK,
ROBERT ROMHANYI, AND TRACY K. McINTOSH

Center for Neural Injury
Department of Neurology
University of California
San Francisco, California 94143
and
Neurology Service
Veterans Administration Medical Center
San Francisco, California 94121

During the past decade, it has become increasingly clear that central nervous system trauma may produce tissue injury through both direct and indirect mechanisms.[1] Direct effects occur acutely as a result of mechanical disruption, with subsequent rapid cell death. Indirect effects are delayed and develop over a period of minutes to hours following the initial trauma. A variety of biochemical and physiological changes have been postulated to contribute to this delayed, secondary injury process, including: alterations in lipid metabolism,[2] disruption of magnesium ion homeostasis,[3] and edema formation.[4] In the present study, preliminary results on changes in tissue lipids, magnesium, and edema following experimental traumatic brain injury to rats[5] are reported. Any statistically significant differences among the control and experimental groups were determined by analysis of variance (ANOVA) with a Dunnett's posthoc test (* = significantly different from controls, $p \leq 0.05$).

Tissue levels of free fatty acids (FFA), total phospholipid, cholesterol, thromboxane B_2, and water content were measured over time in the brains of rats subjected to fluid-percussion traumatic brain injury of moderate severity (2.0–2.2 atmospheres). Brains of injured animals and sham-operated controls were frozen *in situ* with liquid N_2 at 10 min, 4 h, and 24 h postinjury, and the area that has been shown histologically to be the site of maximal injury (left parietal cortex) was dissected out. Trauma resulted in small increases in FFA levels at the site of injury at 10 min and 4 h, and much larger increases at 24 h. Among the FFA, the largest increases were observed in stearate (control = 1.5 ± 0.1, 10 min = 6.9 ± 0.1*, 4 h = 7.4 ± 0.6*, 24 h = 17.3 ± 1.1* μg/mg protein) arachidonate (control = 0.1 ± 0.01, 10 min = 0.6 ± 0.02*, 4 hr = 1.2 ± 0.1*, 24 hr = 2.4 ± 0.2*) and docosahexaenoate (control = 0.1 ± 0.01, 10 min = 0.1 ± 0.01, 4 h = 1.1 ± 0.1*, 24 h = 2.7 ± 0.2*). Total brain phospholipid and cholesterol levels were significantly decreased at all postinjury time points studied. Thromboxane levels were markedly elevated at 10 min postinjury, substantially declined by 4 h, and approached control values at 24 h (control = 8.7 ± 2.8, 10 min = 636.4 ± 33.1, 4 h = 110.8 ± 11.4, 24 hr = 18.1 ± 8.3

---

[a] Address for correspondence: Paul Demediuk, Ph.D., Neurology Service (127), Veterans Administration Medical Center, 4150 Clement Street, San Francisco, California 94121.

pg/mg protein). Surprisingly, no changes in brain water content were observed at any of the postinjury timepoints. Small decreases in tissue potassium occurred at 4 h postinjury (control = 400.1 ± 13.3, 10 min = 409.5 ± 8.8, 4 h = 304.8 ± 12.2*, 24 h = 396.6 ± 7.8 μmol/g dry weight), and tissue sodium levels increased slightly at 24 h postinjury (control = 149.2 ± 1.8, 10 min = 163.1 ± 1.8, 4 h = 155.2 + 5.9, 24 h = 197.6 ± 7.2* μmol/g dry weight). Total tissue magnesium levels were significantly reduced at 4 and 24 h after brain injury (control = 29.9 ± 0.5, 10 min = 29.3 ± 0.7, 4 h = 23.9 ± 0.6*, 24 h = 23.6 ± 0.9*). These results suggest that changes in lipid metabolism and magnesium content in the brain may play a role in the pathophysiology of posttraumatic tissue damage. In contrast, significant edema formation does not occur after moderate fluid-percussion brain injury in rats and therefore does not appear to be a factor in the injury process.

REFERENCES

1. SIESJÖ, B. K. 1981. Cell damage in the brain: A speculative synthesis. J. Cerebral Blood Flow Metab. **1**: 155–186.
2. DEMEDIUK, P. & A. I. FADEN. 1988. Arachidonic acid metabolites and membrane lipid changes in central nervous system injury. *In* Pharmacological Approaches to the Treatment of Brain and Spinal Cord Injury. D. G. Stein & B. A. Sabel, Eds.: 23–42. Plenum. New York, NY.
3. VINK, R., T. K. MCINTOSH, P. DEMEDIUK, M. W. WEINER & A. I. FADEN. 1988. Decline in intracellular free Mg^{2+} is associated with irreversible tissue injury after brain trauma. J. Biol. Chem. **263**: 757–761.
4. CHAN, P. H. & R. A. FISHMAN. 1986. Brain edema. *In* Handbook of Neurochemistry, Vol. 10. A. Lajtha, Ed.: 153–174. Plenum. New York, NY.
5. MCINTOSH, T. K., A. I. FADEN, M. R. BENDALL & R. VINK. 1987. Traumatic brain injury in the rat: Alterations in brain lactate and pH as characterized by ^{1}H and ^{31}P nuclear magnetic resonance. J. Neurochem. **49**: 1530–1540.

Eicosanoid Production after Traumatic Spinal Cord Injury in the Rat

Inhibition by BW755c and Potentiation by Hypomagnesia

PAUL DEMEDIUK[a] AND ALAN I. FADEN

Center for Neural Injury
Department of Neurology
University of California
San Francisco, California 94143
and
Neurology Service
Veterans Administration Medical Center
San Francisco, California 94121

Traumatic mechanical insults to the mammalian spinal cord are followed by delayed, progressive tissue death. There is increasing evidence to indicate that this self-propagating cell death is mediated by the release or production of a variety of pathophysiological chemical factors, including metabolites of membrane glycerophospholipids.[1,2] Of the experimentally observed changes in membrane lipid metabolism, the release of arachidonic acid and its oxidative conversion to physiologically active forms (eicosanoids) is thought to be of particular importance in the injury process.[3] Arachidonic acid is normally metabolized to eicosanoids via two different enzymatic pathways:[4] the cyclooxygenase pathway produces prostaglandins, thromboxanes, and prostacyclin; the lipoxygenase pathway produces leukotrienes, hydroperoxy and hydroxy forms of arachidonic acid. Diverse cyclooxygenase and lipoxygenase products of arachidonic acid can be generated by most mammalian cells. However, the types and amounts of each reaction product may vary considerably among different cell types. Recent results suggest that alterations in magnesium ion homeostasis may also contribute to the progression of secondary injury after spinal cord trauma,[5] possibly through potentiation of eicosanoid production.[6] In the present study a rat model of spinal cord trauma[7] was used to examine the effects on eicosanoid production of injury severity, inhibition of synthesis, and dietary magnesium deficiency.

Spinal cord samples from rats subjected to three different levels of impact trauma (25, 50, 100 g-cm) were examined for immunoreactive thromboxane B_2 and 6-sulfidopeptide–containing leukotrienes. Prostaglandin $E_{2\alpha}$ levels were measured at 1 hr posttrauma in samples subjected to 100 g-cm injury. Trauma resulted in pronounced increases in thromboxane levels as early as 5 min after injury, with maximum values at 1 hour. Although thromboxane values then slowly declined, they remained significantly above control values for up to 7 days. Significantly smaller thromboxane values were found in rats subjected to mild injury (25 g-cm) than in those that received more severe, irreversible impact injury (50 and 100 g-cm). No statistically significant changes were observed in leukotriene levels in any of the experimental

---

[a]Address for correspondence: Paul Demediuk, Ph.D., Neurology Service (127), Veterans Administration Medical Center, 4150 Clement Street, San Francisco, California 94121.

groups. Prostaglandin $E_{2\alpha}$ was greatly increased at 1 hr posttrauma. Treatment with the combined cyclooxygenase/lipoxygenase inhibitor BW755c 1 hour prior to 100 g-cm injury significantly decreased the production of thromboxane B_2 and prostaglandin $E_{2\alpha}$ at 1 hr and 4 hr postinjury. Posttraumatic accumulation of both thromboxane B_2 and prostaglandin $E_{2\alpha}$ in hypomagnesic rats was almost 2-fold higher than in normal rats. These findings are consistent with the hypothesis that cyclooxygenase products of arachidonic acid metabolism may contribute to secondary injury after spinal cord trauma and provides the rationale for the use of cyclooxygenase inhibitors in the treatment of such injury.

REFERENCES

1. DEMEDIUK, P., R. D. SAUDERS, N. R. CLENDENON, E. D. MEANS, D. K. ANDERSON & L. A. HORROCKS. 1985. Changes in lipid metabolism in traumatized spinal cord. Prog. Brain Res. **63**: 211–226.
2. HSU, C. Y., P. V. HALUSHKA, E. L. HOGAN, N. L. BANIK, W. A. LEE & P. L. PEROT. 1985. Alteration of thromboxane and prostacyclin levels in experimental spinal cord injury. Neurology **35**: 1003–1009.
3. DEMEDIUK, P. & A. I. FADEN. 1988. Arachidonic acid metabolites and membrane lipid changes in central nervous system injury. *In* Pharmacological Approaches to the Treatment of Brain and Spinal Cord Injury. D. G. Stein & B. A. Sabel, Eds.: 23–42. Plenum Press, New York, NY.
4. WOLFE, L. S. 1982. Eicosanoids: prostaglandins, thromboxane, leukotrienes, and other derivatives of carbon-20 unsaturated fatty acids. J. Neurochem. **38**: 1–14.
5. LEMKE, M., P. DEMEDIUK, T. K. MCINTOSH, R. VINK & A. I. FADEN. 1987. Alterations in tissue Mg^{2+}, Na^+ and spinal cord edema following impact trauma in rats. Biochem. Biophys. Res. Commun. **147**: 1170–1175.
6. NIGAM, S., R. AVERDUNK & T. GUNTHER. 1986. Alteration of prostanoid metabolism in rats with magnesium deficiency. Prostaglandins Leukotrienes Med. **23**: 1–10.
7. FADEN, A. I., C. J. MOLINEAUX, J. G. ROSENBERG, T. P. JACOBS & B. M. COX. 1985. Endogenous opioid immunoreactivity in rat spinal cord following traumatic injury. Ann. Neurol. **17**: 386–390.

Prostanoids and Ischemic Brain Edema

Human and Animal Study

BOGDAN M. DJURIČIĆ,[a,b] VLADIMIR S. KOSTIĆ,[c] AND
BOGOMIR B. MRŠULJA[b]

[b]Laboratory for Human Neurochemistry
Institute of Biochemistry and
[c]Clinic for Neurology
School of Medicine
11000 Belgrade, Yugoslavia

Ischemia is a pathophysiological substrate of stroke. Reflecting the chemistry of brain extracellular space, cerebrospinal fluid (CSF) provides the tool to study the human correlates of biochemical events known to occur in animal models of ischemia.

FIGURE 1 illustrates changes in CSF prostacyclin (measured as 6-keto-$PGF_{1\alpha}$) and thromboxane A_2 (measured as TXB_2) during the first 24 h of stroke (occlusion of a major supply vessel, verified by computerized axial tomography and/or angiography). Both prostanoids (PIs) appeared in considerable amounts within the first 4 h after stroke onset, whereas they were undetectable in nonneurologic patients' CSF samples (control group, $n = 12$). At the same time $PGF_{2\alpha}$ increased from 54.2 ± 18.1 pg/ml CSF in the controls to 1122 ± 122 pg/ml in patient group I (not shown). During the next 20 h, $PGF_{2\alpha}$ decreased to the levels 500–600 pg/ml, this value being still a 10-fold increase over the controls. PGI_2 and TXA_2 declined slightly, the former more; however, comparison to the nil concentration in controls indicates an abnormal situation. The inset in FIGURE 1 shows the prostanoid tissue pattern in Mongolian gerbils during 15-min ischemia and 1 and 2 h of reflow. Similarity to the CSF pattern (FIG. 1) is remarkable, allowing for the difference in time scale, a probable consequence of the distance between the sites of CSF formation (lateral ventricles) and sampling (lumbar sac).

Brain edema (accumulation of water within cerebral tissue) accompanies ischemia.[1] The first two hours of reflow after 15-min ischemia in gerbils are characterized by considerable brain swelling (FIG. 2, inset), up to 3%. This water accumulation coincides with disturbances in the function of (Na,K)ATPase rather than with the ionic disbalance itself.[2]

Several drugs that influence postischemic prostanoid production were tested in respect to their ability to reduce edema (FIG. 2). Dexamethasone acts as a membrane stabilizer in short-term pretreatment; it reduces brain swelling and postischemic burst in $PGF_{2\alpha}$, but does not change ionic tissue composition. Nimodipine, a calcium channel blocker, reduces both brain edema and $PGF_{2\alpha}$; the latter effect is probably related to

---

[a]Address for correspondence: Dr. Bogdan Djuričić, Institute of Biochemistry, School of Medicine, Višegradska 26, 11000 Belgrade, Yugoslavia.

the preempting of the Ca^{2+}-induced increase of phospholipase A_2 known to occur in ischemia.[3] Propentophyline also prevents Ca^{2+} activation of phospholipase A_2 and acts as a serotonin antagonist; this compound has the most profound effect on the extent of brain swelling. Again, there is a reduction in $PGF_{2\alpha}$ postischemic overproduction (FIG. 2). Finally, inhibition of PI synthesis by indomethacin (FIG. 2) also reduced the extent of postischemic brain swelling. Neither drug affected Na^+ or K^+ contents during reflow (FIG. 2). When a thromboxane synthase inhibitor (UK 38,485) was used, no effect was found on brain swelling or ionic composition (not shown).

Although there is no correlation between the degree of $PGF_{2\alpha}$ increase in CSF and neurological deficit in stroke patients,[4] a role of PIs cannot be ruled out in respect to specific consequences of ischemia—for instance, brain edema. The results shown (FIG. 2) relate reduction in PIs to (partial) prevention of brain edema. The mechanism of PI involvement remains to be elucidated, but large amounts of endoperoxides (PGG_2 and PGH_2) formed during PG brain synthesis burst may damage the cell membrane, as do other free radicals.[5] Also, high and persistent PGI_2 and TXA_2 levels indicate damage in the brain vascular compartment and may be partly responsible for the late, vasogenic, component of ischemic brain edema. Thus, it seems that PIs may be therapeutic targets in stroke therapy.

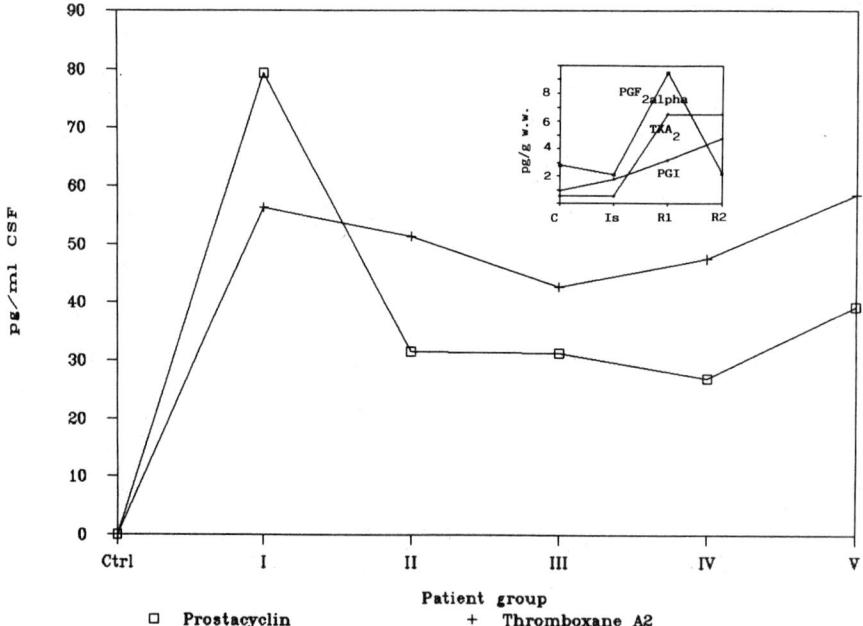

FIGURE 1. Prostacyclin and thromboxane A_2 in stroke patients. Ctrl = controls; I = 0–4 h; II = 5–8 h; III = 9–12 h; IV = 13–16 h; V = 17–24 h after stroke onset; CSF = cerebrospinal fluid. *Inset:* Prostanoids in Mongolian gerbil brain tissue during and after ischemia. C = controls; Is = 15-min ischemia; R1, R2 = one- and two-hour reflow, respectively; Tx = thromboxane. Prostanoids were assayed after extraction by organic solvents using commercially available RIA kits (Amersham, U.K.).

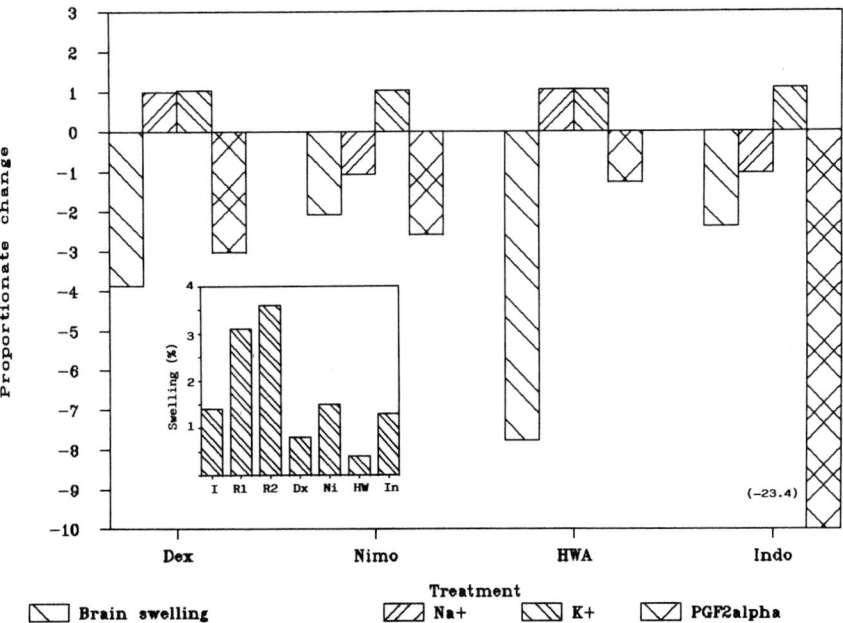

FIGURE 2. Effects of drugs on brain swelling and on sodium, potassium, and $PGF_{2\alpha}$ content in the Mongolian gerbil at one-hour reflow following 15-min ischemia. One-hour reflow values were taken as referent and changes induced by drugs expressed as proportionate changes; these values indicate the magnitude of change in respect to the reference value (value 1 indicates no change). Drugs were administered ip prior to ischemia as follows (mg/kg body weight, min): dexamethasone (Dex, Dx), 2.5, 60; nimodipine (Nimo, Ni), 0.1, 15; propentophyline (HWA, HW), 25, 1; indomethacine (Indo, In), 3, 30. *Inset:* Brain swelling during 15-min ischemia (I), at one (R1) and two (R2) hours of reflow, and at one hour of reflow after drug treatment. Swelling was calculated on the wet/dry weight difference and electrolyte contents measured by flame photometry.

REFERENCES

1. HOSSMANN, K. A. & F. J. SCHUIER. 1979. *In* Brain and Heart Infarcts II. K. J. Zulch, W. Kaufmann, K. A. Hossmann & V. Hossmann, Eds.: 119–129. Springer. Berlin.
2. DJURIČIĆ, B. M., D. V. MIĆIĆ & B. B. MRŠULJA. 1984. *In* Brain Edema. K. G. Go & A. Baethmann, Eds.: 491–498. Plenum. New York, NY.
3. NEMOTO, E. M., G. SHIU & H. ALEXANDER. 1980. Fed. Proc. **39:** 407–409.
4. KOSTIĆ, V. S., B. M. DJURIČIĆ & B. B. MRŠULJA. 1984. Eur. Neurol. **23:** 291–295.
5. YAMAMOTO, M., T. SHIMA, T. UOZOMI, T. SOGABE, K. YAMADA & T. KAWASAKI. 1983. Stroke **14:** 977–982.

The Role of Arachidonic Acid and Prostaglandins in Neurotransmitter Release from Isolated Cerebellar Glomeruli[a]

ROBERT V. DORMAN

Department of Biological Sciences
Kent State University
Kent, Ohio 44242

DAVID M. TERRIAN

Neurosciences Function
United States Air Force School of Aerospace Medicine
San Antonio, Texas 78235

Stimulus-secretion coupling has been correlated with the accumulation of unesterified arachidonate and eicosanoid production in a variety of tissues. The involvement of arachidonate and its metabolites in the evoked release of neurotransmitters was investigated using isolated cerebellar glomeruli, which include the mossy fiber terminals. The glomeruli are able to take up and release D-[^{3}H]aspartate. The release is evoked by membrane depolarization, Ca^{2+} ionophores, arachidonate, and prostaglandin $F_{2\alpha}$. The arachidonate-evoked release is Ca^{2+}-independent and is blocked by cyclooxygenase inhibitors.[1]

Cerebellar glomeruli were radiolabeled *in vitro* with [^{3}H]arachidonate, in order to assess the metabolism of arachidonic acid in this nerve terminal preparation (FIG. 1). Membrane depolarization (45 and 90 mM K^+) stimulated arachidonate accumulation, and EGTA inhibited this response, but only in depolarized terminals. The accumulation observed in nondepolarized glomeruli may be related to internal Ca^{2+} stores. The Ca^{2+} channel blocker verapamil also inhibited arachidonate accumulation. In contrast, the Ca^{2+} ionophore A23187 was able to stimulate arachidonate accumulation. It appears that the evoked accumulation of arachidonate is dependent on external Ca^{2+}. The lipase inhibitors mepacrine and dibucaine reduced [^{3}H]arachidonate accumulation in control and depolarized glomeruli.

Verapamil, mepacrine, and dibucaine were also used to assess the phospholipid source(s) of the free arachidonate. It appeared that inositol glycerophospholipids (IGP) were the primary phospholipid sources of unesterified arachidonate, since membrane depolarization stimulated [^{3}H]arachidonate release from IGP. Also, verapamil, mepacrine, and dibucaine inhibited the depolarization-induced loss of radioactivity from IGP, but did not inhibit choline (CGP) or ethanolamine (EGP) glycerophospholipid catabolism. In fact, EGP and CGP labeling were reduced in the presence of these compounds, suggesting that at least some of the [^{3}H]arachidonate released from IGP was reacylated into EGP and CGP.

---

[a]This work was supported by AFOSR Grants 86-0045 (R.V.D.) and 2312W3 (D.M.T.).

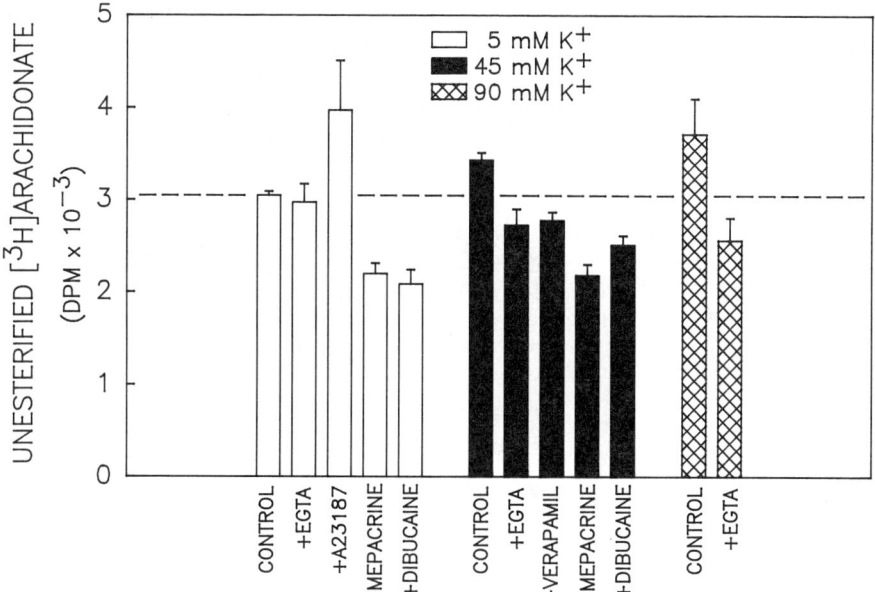

FIGURE 1. Effects of membrane depolarization, Ca^{2+} influx, and lipase inhibitors on arachidonate accumulation in isolated cerebellar glomeruli. Cerebellar glomeruli, including large mossy fiber terminals, were prepared and radiolabeled *in vitro* with [^{3}H]arachidonic acid as described in Reference 1. The glomeruli were then incubated for 0 and 15 min in Krebs-Ringer buffers containing either 5, 45, or 90 mM K^+. Treatments included 1 mM EGTA, 5 μM A23187, 1 mM mepacrine, 1 mM dibucaine, or 100 μM verapamil. Total lipids were extracted and free fatty acids separated by thin-layer chromatography prior to scraping and counting. The results are expressed as changes in labeling (dpm ± SEM) observed during 15-min incubations.

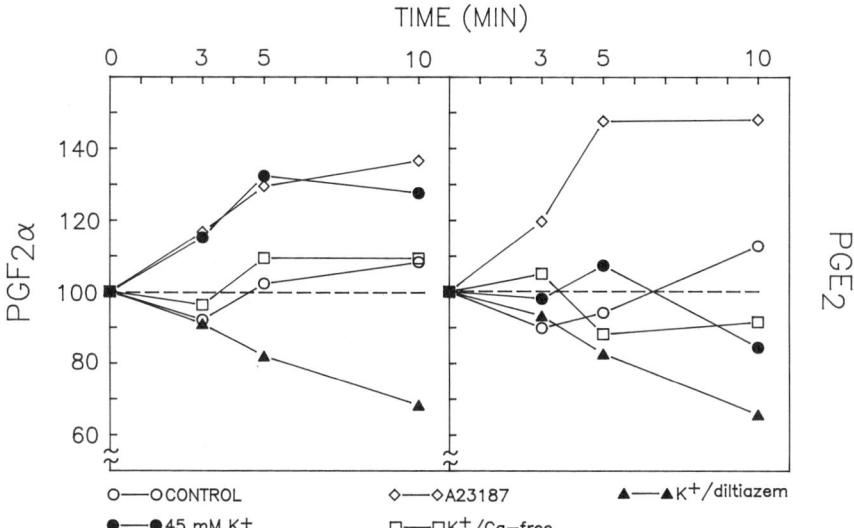

FIGURE 2. Effects of membrane depolarization and Ca^{2+} influx on $PGF_{2\alpha}$ and PGE_2 concentrations. Cerebellar glomeruli were isolated as described in Reference 1. They were incubated for 0, 3, 5, and 10 min in Krebs-Ringer buffer. Treatments included 5 μM A23187, 45 mM K^+, 45 mM K^+ without Ca^{2+}, 45 mM K^+ plus 25 μM diltiazem. The prostaglandins were extracted and quantitated by radioimmunoassay. The results are expressed as % of matched 0 time values.

Two major central nervous system eicosanoids, $PGF_{2\alpha}$ and PGE_2, were examined, since they were shown to affect D-[^{3}H]aspartate release. The effects of depolarization and external Ca^{2+} on the concentrations of these prostaglandins are shown in FIGURE 2. The presence of 45 mM K^+ evoked increased accumulation of $PGF_{2\alpha}$ but had little effect on PGE_2 levels. Exposure of depolarized glomeruli to Ca^{2+}-free conditions reduced the evoked accumulation of $PGF_{2\alpha}$ but had little effect on PGE_2. It appears that depolarization-induced Ca^{2+} influx affected only $PGF_{2\alpha}$ production. The Ca^{2+} channel blocker diltiazem inhibited the accumulation of both prostanoids, while the Ca^{2+} ionophore A23187 stimulated the accumulation of both. We suggest that the evoked release of excitatory amino acid neurotransmitters from cerebellar mossy fiber terminals depends on the Ca^{2+}-dependent accumulation of arachidonate and the subsequent production of $PGF_{2\alpha}$.

REFERENCE

1. DORMAN, R. V., M. A. SCHWARTZ & D. M. TERRIAN. 1986. Brain Res. Bull. **17**: 243–248.

Indomethacin Posttreatment Antagonizes Ethanol-induced Sleep Time

GREGORY I. ELMER AND FRANK R. GEORGE

School of Pharmacy
University of Maryland at Baltimore
Baltimore, Maryland 21201
and
National Institute on Drug Abuse
Addiction Research Center
Baltimore, Maryland 21224

INTRODUCTION

Previous studies in our laboratory have implicated the arachidonic acid cascade as an important system in ethanol's central effects. Pretreatment with prostaglandin synthetase inhibitors (PGSI) antagonize lethal,[1] depressant,[2] activating,[3] and hypothermic[4] responses to ethanol. The dose of inhibitor required to block ethanol's effects is directly proportional to the ethanol sensitivity of the organism.[2] In addition, ethanol increases *in vivo* brain prostaglandin levels in a dose-, sex-, and genotype-dependent manner.[5] The present study investigated the efficacy of indomethacin, a potent PGSI, in antagonizing ethanol-induced hypnosis when given after ethanol.

METHOD

Indomethacin (0, 10.0 mg/kg) was administered ip 15 min pre- and 15, 30, and 60 minutes post-contralateral ip injection of 4.0 g/kg ethanol. Seven male DBA/2J mice were used at each time point for each dose. Following administration of ethanol, animals were placed on their backs in a V-shaped trough. The duration of loss of the righting reflex (sleep time) was used as the measurement for ethanol effect. Animals were judged to be awake when they could right themselves three times within 30 seconds. Waking blood alcohol (WBA) levels were determined at this time via duplicate 10-μl retroorbital blood samples.

RESULTS

Indomethacin decreased ethanol-induced loss of the righting reflex in a time-dependent manner. For example, indomethacin (10 mg/kg) decreased the duration of the loss of the righting reflex by 54% when given 15 minutes after ethanol (FIG. 1). Indomethacin was less effective 30 and 60 minutes postethanol than 15 minutes postethanol. Indomethacin did not significantly alter the rate of ethanol clearance

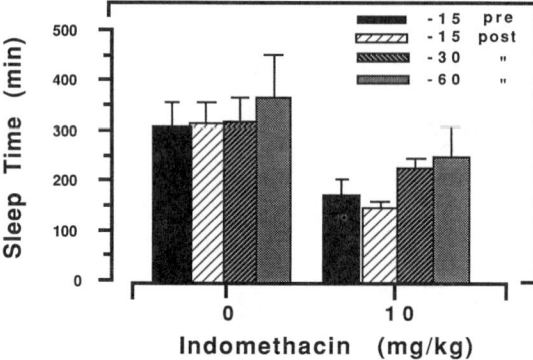

FIGURE 1. Effect of indomethacin on ethanol-induced sleep time. Saline and indomethacin treatments were administered 15 min before and 15, 30, and 60 min after ip injection of 4.0 g/kg ethanol.

from blood. Thus, indomethacin-posttreated animals regained the righting response at significantly higher blood ethanol concentrations than did saline-treated animals (FIG. 2).

DISCUSSION

The present study investigated the efficacy of indomethacin, a potent PGSI, in antagonizing ethanol-induced hypnosis when given after ethanol treatment. The efficacy of indomethacin given 15 min after ethanol is similar to that observed when given 15 min before ethanol. Importantly, WBA levels were consistent with a central nervous system (CNS) effect. It has been shown that ethanol increases the fluidization of biological membranes.[6] Since the arachidonate cascade is a membrane-bound system activated by disruptions in the cell membrane, it is possible that ethanol-induced fluidization increases the activity of the arachidonic acid cascade. These data provide further evidence that ethanol's CNS effects are mediated to a significant extent by the arachidonic acid cascade. In addition, the ability of posttreatment indomethacin to antagonize ethanol-induced sleep time extends the range of conditions under which PGSIs antagonize the behavioral effects of ethanol.

FIGURE 2. Effect of indomethacin on waking blood alcohol level. Saline and indomethacin treatments were administered 15 min before and 15, 30, and 60 min after ip injection of 4.0 g/kg ethanol.

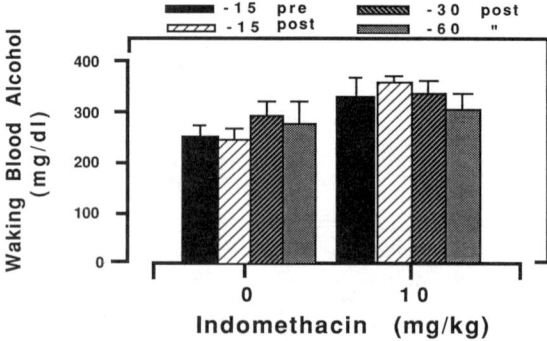

REFERENCES

1. GEORGE, F. R., G. I. ELMER & A. C. COLLINS. 1982. Subst Alcohol Actions/Misuse. **3:** 267–274.
2. GEORGE, F. R., T. C. HOWERTON, G. I. ELMER & A. C. COLLINS. 1983. Pharmacol. Biochem. Behav. **19:** 131–136.
3. RITZ, M. C., F. R. GEORGE & A. C. COLLINS. 1981. Subst. Alcohol Actions/Misuse. **2:** 289–299.
4. GEORGE, F. R., S. J. JAKCSON & A. C. COLLINS. 1981. Psychopharmacology **74:** 241–244.
5. GEORGE, F. R., M. C. RITZ, G. I. ELMER & A. C. COLLINS. 1986. Life Sci. 1069–1075.
6. CHIN, J. H. & D. B. GOLDSTEIN. 1977. Mol. Pharmacol. **13:** 435–441.

Release of Arachidonic Acid Metabolites after Experimental Subarachnoid Hemorrhage

PAOLO GAETANI,[a,b] FULVIO MARZATICO,[c] DANIELA LOMBARDI,[b] ILARIA FULLE,[b] VITTORIO SILVANI,[b] AND RICCARDO RODRIGUEZ Y BAENA[b]

[b]*Department of Surgery, Neurosurgical Section and*
[c]*Institute of Pharmacology*
University of Pavia
I-27100 Pavia, Italy

INTRODUCTION

The activation of lipid peroxidation, the liberation of free radicals, and the enhancement of arachidonic acid (AA) metabolism belong to the neurochemical pattern of brain damage after subarachnoid hemorrhage (SAH). AA metabolites may be involved in different pathogenetic aspects of SAH, because they have specific roles in the regulation of cerebral blood flow (CBF),[1,2] modulation of vascular permeability, and modulation of excitatory and inhibitory neurotransmitter release.[3-6] The accumulation of fatty acids, mainly arachidonate, due to the breakdown of structural membrane lipids, leads to significant variations of prostaglandin (PG) levels in brain tissue.

An active AA metabolism via both the lipoxygenase and the cyclooxygenase pathways has been hypothesized after aneurysmal SAH, as suggested from human cisternal cerebrospinal fluid (CSF) findings.[7,8] Experimental studies regarding the relationship between AA metabolism and SAH have placed special attention on vascular effects of these compounds, with special consideration of the pathogenesis of cerebral vasospasm.[9-10] An important question indirectly arises from available data: do the elevated concentrations of AA metabolites in CSF relate to a temporary accumulation of arachidonate or an *in vivo* enhanced synthesis of the compounds?

In the present study we have investigated the *ex vivo* production of PGD_2, 6-keto-$PGF_{1\alpha}$ (the stable metabolite of prostacyclin), and LTC_4 (metabolite via the lipoxygenase pathway) after experimental induction of SAH in rats in order to verify: (a) the involvement of both metabolic pathways of AA after SAH; and (b) any possible correlation with time-dependent aspects of the disease, such as CBF impairment, vasospasm, and hypoxic neuronal damage.

MATERIALS AND METHODS

The experiments were conducted on male Sprague-Dawley rats (Charles River strain, Calco, Como, Itay) weighing 375–425 g. SAH was induced according to

---

[a]Address for correspondence: Dr. Paolo Gaetani, Department of Surgery, Neurosurgical Section, University of Pavia, Policlinico S. Matteo, I-27100 Pavia, Italy.

Solomon et al.[11] with few modifications.[12] When the rats were in a steady respiratory state (arterial pO_2 and pCO_2, 90 mm Hg and 35–40 mm Hg, respectively) autologous arterial blood was collected (0.35 ml) from the femoral artery, and an aliquot of 0.30 ml was injected into the cisterna magna via a catheter within about 2 minutes.

Animals were divided into the following experimental groups, with 6–8 animals each: (a) sham-operated rats (submitted to surgical procedure and injected with 0.30 ml of saline solution at 37 °C); and (b) the SAH group (rats subjected to SAH procedure with injection of 0.30 ml of autologous arterial blood). Biochemical evaluations were performed at 30 minutes and at 1, 6, and 48 hours after the experimental SAH procedure. Rats were sacrificed by decapitation, and brains were immediately frozen in dry ice and maintained in a prerefrigerated glove box at -22 °C. The cortex slices, weighing approximately 10–15 mg, were bound-cut, weighed, and placed immediately in 1 ml of oxygenated (95% O_2–5% CO_2) Krebs solution, pH 7.4 containing: NaCl 118 mM, KCl 4.7 mM, $MgSO_4$ $7H_2O$ 1.2 mM, KH_2PO_4 1.2 mM, $NaHCO_3$ 25 mM, and glucose 1 g/L. The tubes containing medium with slices were tightly closed. The interval between decapitation and the beginning of incubation was about 3 minutes. Slices were incubated at 37 °C in a shaking water bath for up to 1 hour. At the end of the incubation period the medium was decanted and centrifuged in a refrigerated centrifuge at 3000 rpm at 0 °C. Three aliquots of the supernatant were kept at -80 °C until analysis. Levels of AA metabolites were determined with the radioimmunoassay technique (RIA), as previously described in detail.[7,8,13] Results are expressed in pg/mg of protein. Protein content was determined according to Lowry's method.[29] The assay sensitivity was 6 pg/mg of protein. Statistical analysis was performed using analysis of variance (ANOVA) and the Tukey Test for the multiple comparisons. Statistical significance was accepted for $p < .05$.

RESULTS

TABLE 1 reports the mean *ex vivo* release of PGD_2, 6-keto-$PGF_{1\alpha}$, and LTC_4 in sham-operated rats and in animals subjected to hemorrhage induction at different times. The release of PGD_2 is significantly enhanced at 1 hour and 2 days ($p < .001$) after the SAH procedure; the stable metabolite of prostacyclin is released in a significantly higher amount ($p < .001$) at 2 days after SAH. The metabolite via lipoxygenase pathway shows an increasing trend of *ex vivo* release in the early phases following SAH, after which it remains elevated at 6 hours and 2 days.

DISCUSSION

The *ex vivo* evaluation allows one to study the in-time modifications of metabolic patterns after a pathological event and, as in the case of AA metabolism, to evaluate the variations of each eicosanoid on the basis of its properties. Therefore, with this method the results assume a significance that is quite different from that of data available from measurements of tissue levels. Prostaglandin D_2 is a major prostanoid that is synthesized mainly in the neuronal compartment and is involved in the modulation of excitatory and inhibitory neurotransmitters such as glutamate and γ-aminobutyric acid (GABA);[4] that hyperpolarizes plasma membrane of Purkinje cells *in vitro*;[4] and that has a significant vasoconstrictor effect on cerebral arteries.[10] Since the enhanced release of glutamate has been suggested as a possible mediator of

TABLE 1. *Ex Vivo* Release of Arachidonate Metabolites in Experimental Subarachnoid Hemorrhage (SAH)

Time	PGD_2 (pg/mg protein)		6-keto-$PGF_{1\alpha}$ (pg/mg protein)		LTC_4 (pg/mg protein)	
	Sham-Operated	SAH	Sham-Operated	SAH	Sham-Operated	SAH
	207.53 ± 15.44^a		158.98 ± 14.22^a		24.12 ± 2.55^a	
30 min	226.16 ± 39.6	173.14 ± 21.4	123.15 ± 10.4	117.87 ± 19.7	19.57 ± 2.1	25.91 ± 4.4
1 h	182.40 ± 15.7	256.51 ± 33.1^b	100.95 ± 17.7	113.92 ± 11.5	17.44 ± 0.8	37.98 ± 9.2^c
6 h	223.97 ± 24.0	276.93 ± 88.9	207.64 ± 11.1	198.57 ± 31.8	27.57 ± 4.1	34.02 ± 5.2^b
2 days	257.7 ± 31.2	480.33 ± 42.6^d	158.65 ± 18.3	340.93 ± 65.7^a	25.07 ± 6.8	37.51 ± 7.9^c

[a] Untreated controls.
[b] $p < .02$ vs. sham-operated animals.
[c] $p < .01$ vs. sham-operated animals.
[d] $p < .001$ vs. sham-operated animals.

anoxic-ischemic neuronal damage,[15] we could speculate that the increasing trend of PGD_2 release after experimental SAH is part of an intrinsic defensive mechanism of the brain in the late phase of SAH. Moreover, the increased release of PGD_2 may enhance a vasoconstrictor effect on major cerebral arteries. These findings correlate well with the observed relationship between the perianeurysmal cisternal level of PGD_2 in human CSF and the risk for delayed vasospasm,[7,13] and suggest that the role played by PGD_2 in SAH is very complex.

Recent reports indicate the presence of specific binding sites for LTC_4 in the rat brain and suggest that leukotriene (LT) formation may be regulated by other AA metabolites. The role of LT in cerebral edema formation has been proposed in different experimental conditions and studied in cases of human brain tumors.[16,17] LT have been reported to increase vascular permeability, enhance leukocyte adhesion, promote characteristic changes in subarachnoidal space, and have an *in vitro* vasoconstrictor effect on human basilar arteries. Moreover, increased LTC_4 activity has been found in the cisternal CSF of patients operated on for aneurysmal SAH.[8,13] All these data suggest a possible role for LT in the pathogenesis of cerebral edema and as a vasoactive spasmogen. The results of the present study show that the synthesis capacity for LTC_4 does not significantly change in the early phases after induction of the hemorrhage, while at 1, 6, and 48 hours the brain preserves an elevated capacity for the synthesis of LTC_4. Moreover, there are no significant variations between 1 hour and 2 days after SAH induction; this fact suggests a self-maintaining activation of the lipoxygenase pathway as a consequence of the hemorrhagic insult.

Leukocytes and platelets, together with gray matter, are very rich in lipoxygenase enzyme, and leukocyte adhesion in the subarachnoidal space is a typical morphological aspect of SAH. This would be a significant source for LT, leading to increased permeability of the blood-brain barrier and the formation of brain edema. We could speculate that the release of leukotrienes is a characteristic part of the brain's response to the accumulation of AA after the hemorrhagic insult.

Changes of 6-keto-$PGF_{1\alpha}$ have been studied only in experimental cerebral ischemia, and the variation of metabolite synthesis has been reported as region-specific (in the hippocampus) and closely time-dependent (elevated at 30 minutes after reflow; decreased to 60% of control values at 24 hours). Prostacyclin is involved in microcirculatory regulation, is synthesized by endothelial cells, has a marked vasodilating effect, and prevents blood-brain barrier derangements and the impairment of postischemic brain reperfusion. Moreover, the synthesis of PGI_2 is inhibited by LTC_4. In our experience, *ex vivo* synthesis is lower at 30 minutes and 1 hour after SAH induction when compared to sham-operated animals (although there is no statistical significance). Moreover, 2 days after the hemorrhage, when PGD_2 *ex vivo* release is enhanced and LTC_4 levels are in a steady state, 6-keto-$PGF_{1\alpha}$ levels show a significant increase ($p < .001$). This would be related to a "defensive" response of the brain against the late phase of SAH and CBF variations.

In conclusion, the results of the present study show that: (A) AA metabolism is enhanced after experimental SAH, both via the cyclooxygenase and the lipoxygenase pathways; the activation of the two distinct pathways and the release of AA metabolites are quite different from what is observed in experimental cerebral ischemia, and are strictly time-dependent. (B) The release of AA metabolites after experimental SAH is related more to an enhanced synthesis capacity of brain tissue after the pathological event than it is to the accumulation of arachidonic acid. (C) The activation of the lipoxygenase pathway seems to play a pivotal role in local brain response after the hemorrhage, and this activation also persists in the late phase. The patterns of cyclooxygenase enhancement consist of an early release of factors potentiating edema and local vasoconstriction and a late phase of defensive mechanism activation, such as the release of PGD_2 and prostacyclin.

REFERENCES

1. WALKER, V. & J. D. PICKARD. 1985. Prostaglandins, thromboxane, leukotrienes and the cerebral circulation in health and disease. In Advances and Technical Standards in Neurosurgery. **12:** 3–90.
2. LESLIE, J. B. & W. D. WATKINS. 1985. Eicosanoids in the central nervous system. J. Neurosurg. **63:** 659–668.
3. PICKARD, J. D. 1981. Role of Prostaglandins and arachidonic acid derivatives in the coupling of cerebral blood flow to cerebral metabolism. J. Cerebral Blood Flow Metab. **1:** 361–384.
4. KIMURA, H., K. OKAMOTO & Y. SAKAI. 1985. Modulatory effects of prostaglandin D_2, E_2, F_{2a} on the postsynaptic actions of inhibitory and excitatory amino acids in cerebellar Purkinje cell dendrites "in vitro." Brain Res. **330:** 235–244.
5. KEMPSKY, O., E. SHOAMI, D. VON LUBITZ, J. M. HALLENBECK & G. FEUERSTEIN. 1987. Postischemic production of eicosanoids in gerbil brain. Stroke **18:** 111–119.
6. BHAKOO, K. K., H. A. CROCKARD, P. C. LASCELLES & S. F. AVERY. 1984. Prostaglandin synthesis and edema formation during reperfusion following experimental brain ischemia. Stroke **15:** 891–895.
7. RODRIGUEZ Y BAENA, R., P. GAETANI, G. GRIGNANI, L. PACCHIARINI, T. VIGANÒ, D. ROTA SCALABRINI, V. SILVANI, G. FOLCO & P. PAOLETTI. 1987. Role of arachidonate metabolites in the genesis of cerebral vasospasm. In Advances in Prostaglandins, Thromboxane, and Leukotriene Research, Vol. 17. B. Samuelsson, R. Paoletti & P. W. Ramwell, Eds.: 938–942. Raven Press. New York, NY.
8. PAOLETTI, P., P. GAETANI, G. GRIGNANI, L. PACCHIARINI, V. SILVANI & R. RODRIGUEZ Y BAENA. 1988. CSF leukotriene C_4 following subarachnoid hemorrhage. J. Neurosurg. **69:** 488–493.
9. BOULLIN, D. J., S. BUNTING, W. P. BLASO, T. M. HUNT & S. MONCADA. 1979. Responses of human and baboon arteries to prostaglandin endoperoxides and biologically generated and synthetic prostacyclin—their relevance to cerebral arterial spasm in man. Br. J. Clin. Pharmacol. **7:** 139–147.
10. WHITE, R. P. 1983. Vasospasm I. Experimental findings. In Intracranial aneurysms. J. L. Fox, Ed.: 218–249. Springer. Heidelberg.
11. SOLOMON, R. A., J. LOBO ANTUNES, R. Y. Z. CHEN, L. BLAND & S. CHIEN. 1985. Decrease in cerebral blood flow in rats after experimental subarachnoid hemorrhage. A new model. Stroke **16:** 58–64.
12. MARZATICO, F., P. GAETANI, R. RODRIGUEZ Y BAENA, V. SILVANI, P. PAOLETTI & G. BENZI. 1988. Bioenergetics of different brain areas after experimental subarachnoid hemorrhage in rats. Stroke **19:** 378–384.
13. RODRIGUEZ Y BAENA, R., P. GAETANI & P. PAOLETTI. 1988. A study on cisternal CSF levels of arachidonic acid metabolites after aneurysmal subarachnoid hemorrhage. J. Neurol. Sci. **84:** 329–335.
14. LOWRY, O. H., B. J. ROSEBROUGH, A. L. FARR & R. J. RANDALL. 1951. Protein measurement with the folin phenol reagent. J. Biol. Chem. **193:** 265–275.
15. BENVINISTE, H., J. DREJER, A. SCHOUSBOE & N. H. DIEMER. 1984. Elevation of the extracellular concentrations of glutamate and aspartate in rat hippocampus during transient cerebral ischemia monitored by intracerebral microdialysis. J. Neurochem. **43:** 1369–1374.
16. MOSKOVITZ, M., K. J. KIWAK, K. HEKIMIAN & L. LEVINE. 1984. Synthesis of compounds with properties of Leukotrienes C4 and D4 in gerbil brain after ischemia and reperfusion. Science **224:** 886–889.
17. BLACK, K. L., J. T. HOFF & J. E. MCGILLICUDDY. 1986. Increased leukotriene C4 and vasogenic edema surrounding brain tumors in humans. Ann. Neurol. **19:** 592–595.

Prostaglandin Synthetase Inhibitors Specifically Modulate Ethanol Self-Administration

FRANK R. GEORGE

National Institute on Drug Abuse
Addiction Research Center
Baltimore, Maryland 21224

Pretreatment with prostaglandin synthetase inhibitors (PGSIs) antagonizes acute responses to ethanol.[1-5] This study was designed to examine parametrically the effects of pretreatment with indomethacin (INDO), a potent PGSI, on ethanol self-administration.[6,7] Rats were pretreated daily via ip injection with one of several doses of INDO or vehicle control. Rats were given daily injections with each dose for five consecutive days, then given two days' recovery time. This was repeated once for each condition, providing a control for possible cumulative effects of INDO. Blood ethanol levels were measured on the final day of certain INDO conditions, and on the final vehicle retest day.

There were no significant differences found between any of the vehicle retest conditions. INDO produced significant dose-related changes in ethanol intake. At 1.9 mg/kg, some rats showed a large increase in responding; however, others were not affected. Between 2.5 and 7.5 mg/kg INDO, significant decreases were found in responding for ethanol and intake. Patterns of responding indicate that while INDO produced an extinction of ethanol self-administration, cessation of INDO treatment produced no long-lasting effects on responding, as determined by the return to baseline levels of operant behavior and stability of baseline retests. The pattern of changes in ethanol self-administration suggests that INDO altered responding by decreasing the reinforcing effects of ethanol and not by producing a conditioned aversion to ethanol.[6,7] Blood ethanol levels were reduced by a percentage similar to the reductions seen in responding, suggesting that INDO did not affect ethanol intake by interfering with ethanol metabolism or distribution. In a subsequent experiment, rats were trained to self-administer a saccharin solution. INDO was administered as described above. INDO had no effect on oral self-administration of saccharin, suggesting that INDO did not reduce ethanol drinking via some nonspecific effect on performance or motivation.

These results suggest that there exists a common prostaglandin-related mechanism that is important in the mediation of both acute sensitivity to ethanol and the reinforcing properties of this drug.

REFERENCES

1. GEORGE, F. R. & A. C. COLLINS. 1979. Pharmacol. Biochem. Behav. **10:** 865–869.
2. GEORGE, F. R., T. C. HOWERTON, G. I. ELMER & A. C. COLLINS. 1983. Pharmacol. Biochem. Behav. **19:** 131–136.
3. GRUPP, L. A., J. ELIAS, E. PERLANSKI & R. B. STEWART. 1985. Psychopharmacology **87:** 20–24.

4. RITZ, M. C., F. R. GEORGE & A. C. COLLINS. 1981. Subst. Alcohol Actions/Misuse **2:** 289–299.
5. SEGARNICK, D. J., D. M. CORDASCO & J. ROTROSEN. 1985. Pharmacol. Biochem. Behav. **23:** 71–75.
6. GEORGE, F. R. 1987. Pharmacol. Biochem. Behav. **27:** 379–384.
7. MEISCH, R. A. 1975. Pharmacol. Rev. **27:** 465–473.

Prostaglandin E_2 Administered Intravenously Crosses the Blood-Brain Barrier and Induces Hyperthermia as a Central Action

HIDEYA HAYASHI,[a] NAOMI EGUCHI,[a]
YOSHIHIRO URADE,[b] SEIJI ITO,[a,b] AND
OSAMU HAYAISHI[a,b]

[a]*Hayaishi Bioinformation Transfer Project
Research Development Corporation of Japan
Kyoto 601, Japan*

[b]*Osaka Bioscience Institute
Osaka, Japan*

Prostaglandin (PG) E_2 is well known to be an endogenous mediator of the febrile responses.[1] However, the origin of the PGE_2 that causes the fever is still unclear. Furthermore, the mode of action of pyrogens is a moot point, due to the apparent inability of exogenous and endogenous pyrogens to cross the blood-brain barrier.[2] In the present study, we found that PGE_2 administered systemically induced a potent and dose-dependent hyperthermia in urethane-anesthetized rats.

The intravenous (iv) injection of PGE_2 (0.01–0.1 mg/kg) resulted in remarkable hyperthermia similar to that observed by its intracerebroventricular (icv) administration. As shown in FIGURE 1A, a significant increase in rectal temperature could be seen at doses of 0.05 mg/kg and higher. The maximum change in rectal temperature (ΔT_r max) ranged from 0.50 ± 0.12 °C at 0.05 mg/kg to 1.38 ± 0.16 °C at 1.0 mg/kg.

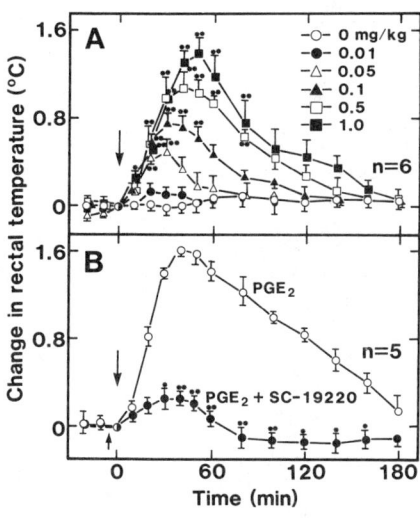

FIGURE 1. (A) Changes in rectal temperature induced by iv injection (at *arrow*) of PGE_2; (B) inhibitory effect of icv preinjection of SC-19220 (2.5 μmol) on hyperthermia caused by iv injection of PGE_2 (0.5 mg/kg). SC-19220 dissolved in dimethyl sulfoxide was administered icv (*small arrow*) 1 min prior to the injection of PGE_2 at 0 min (*large arrow*). $* = p < 0.05$, $** = p < 0.01$ as compared with the control group.

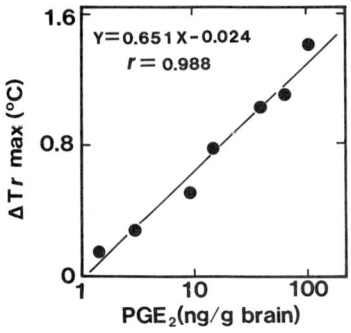

FIGURE 2. Relationship between PGE$_2$ concentration in the brain at 15 s and ΔT_r max value after iv injection of PGE$_2$.

Duration of hyperthermia (80 to 180 min) was also dependent on the dosage. To demonstrate that the PGE$_2$-induced hyperthermia is due to a central action, we examined the inhibitory effect of SC-19220, an antagonist of fever centrally induced by PGE,[3] on the hyperthermic response (FIG. 1B). Pretreatment with icv injection of SC-19220 (2.25 μmol) completely abolished the hyperthermic response with ΔT_r max of 1.5 °C induced by the iv injection of PGE$_2$ (0.5 mg/kg), indicating that hyperthermia casued by the iv injection of PGE$_2$ is mediated by central action(s).

To study the correlation between hyperthermia and the amount of PGE$_2$ that penetrated into the brain, we determined brain uptake of PGE$_2$ by using the tritiated compound and a specific radioimmunoassay for PGE$_2$.[4] In the brain 15 s after PGE$_2$ injection, the PGE$_2$ concentration linearly increased until 102.6 ng/g brain at the highest dose of 1.0 mg/kg. FIGURE 2 shows the relationship between PGE$_2$ content in the brain at 15 s and the ΔT_r max value. In semilogarithmic plots of the PGE$_2$ content in the brain, a linear regression line was seen with a high coefficient ($r = 0.988$). The threshold dose of hyperthermia (0.4 °C) was calculated to be 11 ng of PGE$_2$ in the whole brain, which is almost the same amount as that (3 ng) obtained by icv injection of PGE$_2$. Furthermore, PGE$_2$ showed an uneven regional uptake in the brain, the highest amounts being in the olfactory bulb, basal forebrain, and hypothalamus. These findings indicate that a sizable portion of PGE$_2$ passes through the blood-brain barrier and acts upon the thermoregulatory center to induce fever.

REFERENCES

1. STITT, J. T. 1986. Prostaglandin E as the neural mediator of the febrile response. Yale J. Biol. Med. **59:** 137–149.
2. COCEANI, F., I. BISHAI, J. LEES & S. SIRKO. 1986. Prostaglandin E$_2$ and fever: A continuing debate. Yale J. Biol. Med. **59:** 169–174.
3. CRANSTON, W. I., G. W. DUFF, R. F. HELLON, D. MITCHELL & Y. TOWONSEND. 1976. Evidence that brain prostaglandin synthesis is not essential in fever. J. Physiol. **259:** 239–249.
4. TANAKA, T., S. ITO, O. HIROSHIMA, H. HAYASHI & O. HAYAISHI. 1985. Rat monoclonal antibody specific for prostaglandin E structure. Biochim. Biophys. Acta **836:** 125–133.

The Role and New Action Mechanism of Prostaglandin E_2 in Neurotransmission

SEIJI ITO,[a,b] MANABU NEGISHI,[a] HIDEYA HAYASHI,[b] AND OSAMU HAYAISHI[b]

[a]Department of Cell Biology
Osaka Bioscience Institute
Suita 565, Japan

[b]Hayaishi Bioinformation Transfer Project
Research Development Corporation of Japan
Takatsuki 569, Japan

Prostaglandin E_2 (PGE_2) is known to inhibit the release of norepinephrine from sympathetic nerve terminals in response to acetylcholine. Since acetylcholine stimulates the formation of PGs, Hedqvist proposed that PGE_2 could act as a negative feedback inhibitor of adrenergic transmission.[1] A survey of the distribution of [^{3}H]PGE_2 binding activity in various tissues from several species revealed a highly specific activity in the bovine adrenal medulla.[2] Chromaffin cells of the adrenal medulla synthesize, store, and secrete catecholamines, and the secretory response is elicited via nicotinic cholinergic receptors. Therefore, chromaffin cells are considered as a model system of sympathetic nerve cells, and they have offered insights into the workings of neurotransmission. In this study, we examined the effect of PGE_2 on catecholamine release from cultured bovine chromaffin cells.

FIGURE 1 shows the time course of catecholamine release induced by various stimuli. Neither 1 μM PGE_2 nor 100 μM ouabain, an inhibitor of Na^+, K^+-ATPase, has hardly any effect by itself on catecholamine release over the basal level. However, PGE_2 and ouabain together enhanced the release drastically. The time course of catecholamine release was slow at the onset, and progressive at least until 30 min. Incubation of chromaffin cells with 10 μM nicotine induced a rapid and transient secretion of catecholamines, 11% of the total being released from the cells during a 10-min period. The difference in the rate and magnitude of the secretory response to PGE_2 plus ouabain and nicotine indicates that these two stimuli are acting by different mechanisms.

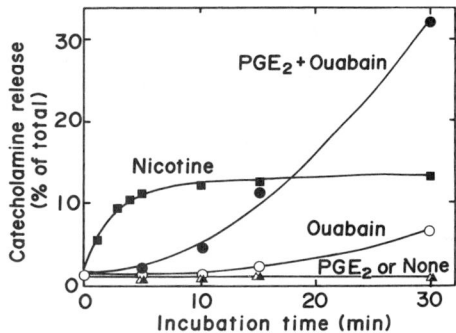

FIGURE 1. Time course of catecholamine release from cultured bovine chromaffin cells. Chromaffin cells (2.5×10^5 cells/assay) were incubated with test agents at 37 °C. At the indicated time, secretion was determined by measuring the percentage of total cellular catecholamines released into the medium. The basal release was 1–2% of the total for 30 min.

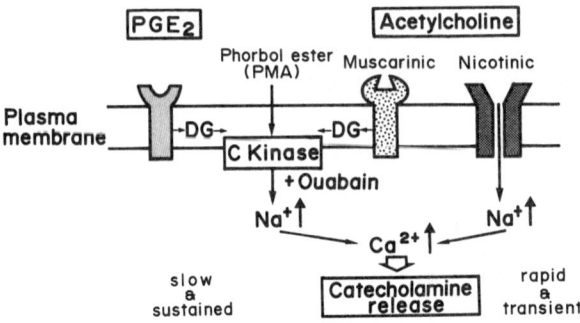

FIGURE 2. Possible mechanism of catecholamine release by PGE_2 from chromaffin cells. DG = diacylglycerol; PMA = phorbol, 12-myristate, 13-acetate.

The synergism of ouabain was also observed with muscarine. PGE_2, like muscarine, induced a time- and concentration-dependent formation of inositol phosphates.[3] This effect on phosphoinositide metabolism was accompanied by an increase in cytosolic free Ca^{2+}. The potency of PGs ($PGE_2 > PGF_{2\alpha} > PGD_2$) to stimulate catecholamine release was well correlated with that to affect phosphoinositide metabolism and that to increase the level of intracellular Ca^{2+}. PGE_2 did not stimulate cAMP formation in chromaffin cells. The synergism of phorbol ester and the Ca^{2+} ionophore A23187 could substitute for the effect of PGE_2 on catecholamine release, demonstrating that protein kinase C activation and Ca^{2+} mobilization are both essential to elicit a full cellular response. FIGURE 2 depicts a possible mechanism of PGE_2-induced catecholamine release in addition to and distinct from the well-known nicotinic pathway.

REFERENCES

1. HEDQVIST, P. 1977. Basic mechanisms of prostaglandin action of autonomic neurotransmission. Annu. Rev. Pharmacol. Toxicol. **17:** 259–279.
2. NEGISHI, M., S. ITO, T. TANAKA, H. YOKOHAMA, H. HAYASHI, T. KATADA, M. UI & O. HAYAISHI. 1987. Covalent cross-linking of prostaglandin E receptor from bovine adrenal medulla with a pertussis toxin–insensitive guanine nucleotide-binding protein. J. Biol. Chem. **262:** 12077–12084.
3. YOKOHAMA, H., T. TANAKA, S. ITO, M. NEGISHI, H. HAYASHI & O. HAYAISHI. 1988. Prostaglandin E receptor enhancement of catecholamine release may be mediated by phosphoinositide metabolism in bovine adrenal chromaffin cells. J. Biol. Chem. **263:** 1119–1122.

Endothelium-derived Relaxing Factor Release from Cultured Endothelial Cells Does Not Require Phospholipase Activation or Arachidonate Mobilization

ROGER A. JOHNS,[a] PETER J. MILNER,[b]
NICHOLAS J. IZZO,[b] JoANNE SAYE,[b]
ALEX L. LOEB,[b] AND MICHAEL J. PEACH[b]

*Departments of [a]Anesthesiology and [b]Pharmacology
University of Virginia Medical Center
Charlottesville, Virginia 22908*

A large body of literature supports the hypothesis that endothelium-derived relaxing factor (EDRF) is a nonprostanoid metabolite of arachidonic acid. These studies have largely involved correlation of inhibition of lipoxygenase or cytochrome P450 pathways for arachidonate metabolism and inhibition of phospholipase activation with decreased endothelium-dependent relaxation of vascular rings. This hypothesis has been questioned because of the nonspecificity of the inhibitors employed, and their uncertain site of action.[1,2]

We used mixed and cocultures of endothelial and vascular smooth muscle cells to investigate the role of phospholipase activation and arachidonate release in the production of EDRF. Bovine aortic or pulmonary artery endothelial cells and rat vascular smooth muscle cells were prepared as previously described.[2] The ability of the phospholipase A_2 inhibitors parabromophenacyl bromide (PBPB; 1×10^{-6} M), dexamethasone (DEX; 1×10^{-6} M), and quinacrine (QUIN; 1×10^{-5} M) as well as the diacylglycerol lipase inhibitor RHC 80267 (4×10^{-5} M) to inhibit melittin-stimulated arachidonate release from cultured endothelial cells and melittin-stimulated EDRF release from cocultures was determined. Arachidonate release was assessed by measuring the amount of ^{3}H-arachidonate or 6-keto-prostaglandin $F_{1\alpha}$ released into fresh medium in response to melittin stimulation (2 μg/ml) in the presence or absence of one or more of the lipase inhibitors and was quantified as percent of control. EDRF release was quantified by determining the amount of cyclic GMP accumulation in co- or mixed cultures in response to melittin stimulation (2 μg/ml) in the presence or absence of one or more lipase inhibitors (HCl extraction followed by radioimmunoassay for cyclic GMP).

As shown in TABLE 1, inhibition of phospholipase A_2 with PBPB, DEX, or QUIN, alone or in combination, blocked arachidonate release by 50–60% but had no effect on EDRF production, as assessed by cyclic GMP accumulation in mixed or cocultures of endothelial and vascular smooth muscle cells. Inhibition of the phospholipase C-diacylglycerol (DAG) lipase pathway of arachidonate release by the DAG lipase inhibitor RHC-80267 also caused partial inhibition of arachidonate release and had no effect on EDRF production. When both phospholipase A_2 and phospholipase C pathways for arachidonate mobilization were inhibited (DEX + RHC 80267), arachidonate release was >90% inhibited, while EDRF release remained intact. We conclude

TABLE 1. Effect of Phospholipase Inhibitors on Arachidonate Release and Endothelium-derived Relaxing Factor Production

	% Inhibition of Melittin-stimulated Arachidonate Release	Melittin-stimulated Cyclic GMP Accumulation (% above Control)
Melittin alone	1	301.8 ± 31.1
+ parabromophenacyl bromide	41.62 ± 4.08*	466.7 ± 123.8
+ dexamethasone	44.09 ± 4.49*	323.3 ± 33.4
+ quinacrine	57.48 ± 5.68*	334.1 ± 41.3
+ dexamethasone and quinacrine	62.99 ± 8.25*	424.1 ± 39.4
+ RHC 80267	49.60 ± 7.86*	401.8 ± 67.1
+ dexamethasone and RHC 80267	90.55 ± 7.82*	351.8 ± 42.4

NOTE: Data expressed as mean ± SEM; $n = 6$ for each group. * = significantly different from melittin control ($p < 0.05$).

that neither phospholipase activation nor arachidonate mobilization is required for EDRF release from cultured bovine endothelial cells.

REFERENCES

1. PEACH, M. J., A. L. LOEB, H. A. SINGER, & J. A. SAYE. 1985. Endothelium-derived relaxing factor. Hypertension 7(Suppl.): I94–I100.
2. JOHNS, R. A. & M. J. PEACH. 1988. Para-bromophenacyl bromide inhibits endothelium-dependent arterial relaxation and cyclic GMP accumulation by effects produced exclusively in the smooth muscle. J. Pharmacol. Exp. Ther. **244:** 2443–2449.

Smooth Muscle Pharmacology of Hydroxylated Docosanoids

JOHN W. KARANIAN, HEE-YONG KIM, TADASHI SHINGU, JAMES YERGEY, AND NORMAN SALEM, JR.

Laboratory of Clinical Studies
National Institute on Alcohol Abuse and Alcoholism
Alcohol, Drug Abuse, and Mental Health Administration
Bethesda, Maryland 20892

It has been suggested that subjects whose diets are high in fish oils have a low risk of cardiovascular disease. Fish oils are rich in eicosapentaenoic acid, as well as docosahexaenoic acid (DHA). We have investigated the proposition that metabolites of DHA may be biologically active and be one of the active components of fish fat. Metabolism of DHA to hydroxy derivatives has been observed in many mammalian tissues, including basophils, the macrophage, platelets, the retina, and the brain, *in vitro*. In this work we have biosynthesized and purified various hydroxylated derivatives of DHA and characterized their structures as well as their smooth muscle pharmacology. Platelets are known to produce 12-lipoxygenase products of DHA. Fresh platelets (10^8 cells/ml × 1 ml from human, monkey, dog, rabbit, guinea pig, or rat) were washed twice and incubated for 20 min at 37 °C with 0.25 μCi of 1-^{14}C-DHA and 1-100 μM unlabelled DHA. Samples were extracted twice with dichloromethane, evaporated, and dissolved in methanol for HPLC analysis. A 5-micron Axxichrom ODS column (4.6 mm × 25 cm) was used with a mobile phase of acetonitrile and 0.1 M ammonium acetate, pH 7.0, using both UV and radioactivity detectors. The two major metabolites of DHA formed by platelets were collected by monitoring their UV absorbance at 235 nm, and then they were extracted, evaporated, and dissolved in Krebs Ringer bicarbonate for subsequent determination of their biological activities. Simultaneously, a portion of these collected fractions were subjected to GC/MS analysis after methylation and trimethylsilylation, and the structures were confirmed to be 11- and 14-hydroxydocosahexaenoic acid (HDHE). Both 5,8,11,14-eicosatetraynoic acid

TABLE 1. Contractile Effect of Hydroxylated Docosanoids in Comparison to That of Some Eicosanoids on Isolated Smooth Muscle

	Tension (mg)[a]	
	Airway[b]	Vascular[c]
11(S) HDHE (2.5 μM)	26 ± 11	ns
14(S) HDHE (2.5 μM)	52 ± 27	ns
17(S) HDHE (2.5 μM)	19 ± 9	ns
12(S) HETE (2.5 μM)	ns	nd
12(S) HPETE (2.5 μM)	ns	nd
TXA$_2$ agonist (2.5 μM) (U46619)	480 ± 96	1,080 ± 70

[a]Expressed as mean ± SE, $n \geq 5$; ns = not significant; nd = not determined.
[b]Guinea pig lung parenchymal strip.
[c]Rat aorta.

TABLE 2. Antagonistic Effect of Hydroxylated Docosanoids in Comparison to That of Some Eicosanoids on U46619-induced Smooth Muscle Contraction

	% Inhibition[a]	
	Airway[b]	Vascular[c]
11(S) HDHE (10 µM)	12 ± 4	35 ± 9[d]
14(S) HDHE (10 µM)	31 ± 8[d]	66 ± 13[d]
17(S) HDHE (10 µM)	27 ± 7[d]	54 ± 16[d]
12(S) HETE (10 µM)	ns	44 ± 11
12(S) HPETE (10 µM)	ns	ns

[a]Mean ± SE inhibition (%) of U46619-induced (2.5 µM) contraction, $n \geq 5$; ns = not significant.
[b]Guinea pig lung parenchymal strip.
[c]Rat aorta.
[d]Significant effect at 1 µM.

(ETYA, 1.0 µM) and the lipoxygenase inhibitor nordihydroguaiaretic acid (NDGA, 40 µM) inhibited the production of HDHE, whereas indomethacin had no effect. Interestingly, ethanol exposure both *in vitro* and *in vivo* by inhalation significantly stimulated rat platelet production of HDHE.

Airway (guinea pig lung parenchymal strip) and vascular (rat aorta) smooth muscle preparations were mounted in 40-ml baths in order to investigate the effects of HDHE on baseline smooth muscle tone and contractility as measured isotonically. The metabolites formed are biologically active, as they are capable of inducing airway smooth muscle contraction; an equimolar concentration of a thromboxane-agonist, U46619, was at least 10–20-fold more efficacious than the HDHE in the lung parenchymal strips (TABLE 1). HDHE may act in part through stimulation of leukotriene production, as increased peptidyl-leukotriene levels were associated with the HDHE-induced contraction in this preparation, and NDGA was capable of a partial blockade of this response. In addition, HDHE antagonizes the contractile effects of the thromboxane agonist but not those of norepinephrine in the preparations studied (TABLE 2). An antithromboxane activity of some specificity may therefore be one property of HDHE. Furthermore, our studies indicate that the 15-lipoxygenase derivative of DHA—that is, 17-HDHE—is also active on these preparations, whereas eicosanoids (12-HETE, 12-HPETE) are not. Our findings suggest that an antithromboxane activity of HDHE may contribute in part to the previously reported inhibitory effect of both ethanol and DHA on thromboxane-induced vascular contractility and platelet aggregation.

Structural Analysis of Oxygenated Metabolites of Polyunsaturated Fatty Acids Using Thermospray Liquid Chromatography/Mass Spectroscopy and Gas Chromatography/Mass Spectroscopy

HEE-YONG KIM, J. W. KARANIAN, AND N. SALEM, JR.

Laboratory of Clinical Studies
National Institute on Alcohol Abuse and Alcoholism
Alcohol, Drug Abuse, and Mental Health Administration
Bethesda, Maryland 20892

Polyunsaturated fatty acids can be oxygenated by either cycloxygenase or lipoxygenase, and the metabolites formed often possess potent biological activity. Structural analysis of these compounds is quite difficult, since complex mixtures of many enzymatic and nonenzymatic products are often formed in biological reactions. Reversed-phase liquid chromatography (LC) in conjunction with on-line thermospray mass spectrometric and UV detection provides a simple and efficient method of qualitative analyses of eicosanoids and related compounds. In this way, complex mixtures are simultaneously separated, and structural information is obtained. In addition to the molecular weight, the number and type of functional groups can often be deduced from the simple fragmentation patterns observed from thermospray spectra of oxygenated metabolites. An example is shown for human platelet docosahexaenoic acid (22:6w3) metabolites. Two major metabolites were observed when

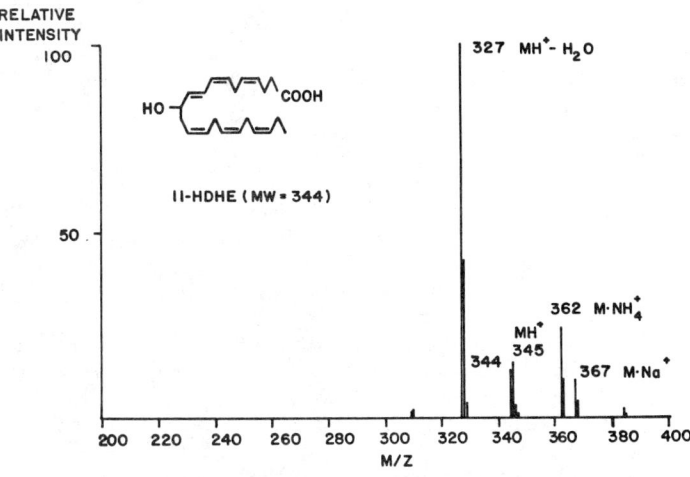

FIGURE 1. Thermospray mass spectrum of 11-hydroxy 22:6w3 produced by human platelets.

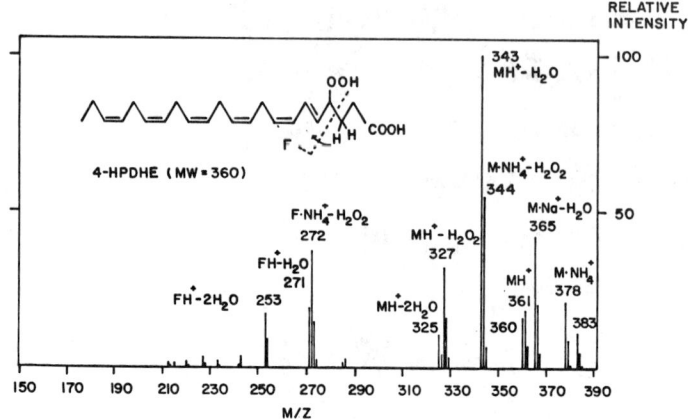

FIGURE 2. Thermospray mass spectrum of 4-hydroperoxy 22:6w3 obtained by autooxidation of 22:6w3.

human platelets were incubated with 22:6w3 in the presence of indomethacin. Both were monohydroxy derivatives, as they gave similar thermospray spectra with the following peaks: $M \cdot NH_4^+ - H_2O$ at m/z 344, MH^+ at m/z 345, $MH^+ - H_2O$ at m/z 327, $M \cdot NH_4^+$ at m/z 362, and $M\,Na^+$ at m/z 367 (11-hydroxy 22:6w3 is shown in FIG. 1). The loss of only one water molecule observed in the spectrum indicates that these are monohydroxy compounds. Since no other significant fragmentation was observed in the thermospray mass spectra of these metabolites, information concerning the position of the hydroxy functions were needed, and this was determined by gas chromatography/mass spectroscopy (GS/MS) analysis after high-pressure liquid chromatography (HPLC) purification and derivatization, including both methylation and trimethylsilylation. However, for hydroperoxy forms of polyunsaturates, thermospray spectra readily provide information regarding the position of the function group. As an example, the spectrum of 4-hydroperoxy 22:6w3 (4-PHDHE) (obtained by autooxidation of 22:6w3) is shown in FIGURE 2. The spectrum includes the usual molecular ion species: $M \cdot NH_4^+$ (m/z 378), MH^+ (m/z 361), $M \cdot NH_4^+ - H_2O$ (m/z 360), $M \cdot NH_4^+ - H_2O_2$ (m/z 344), $MH^+ - H_2O$ (m/z 343), $MH^+ - H_2O_2$ (m/z 327). In addition, the fragments that resulted from the cleavage of the C-C bond adjacent to the hydroperoxy moiety were observed. These fragments are specific to each positional isomer, thus eliminating the need of GC/MS analysis accompanying lengthy purification and derivatization steps. This approach is particularly useful for analyzing lipoxygenase reaction mixtures where reductase activity is absent, such as in some *in vitro* incubations with pure enzyme preparations. Further characterization of structure by configurational analysis was achieved using chiral phase chromatography after methylation. The system used included a dinitrobenzoylphenylglycin (ionic) column (4.6mm × 25 cm) and hexane:isopropanol:acetonitrile 497.5:2.5:0.5 as the mobile phase. Standards of various monohydroxy derivatives of 22:6w3 were prepared by autooxidation. The enantiomers of all the positional isomers were separated in 60 minutes with the exception of the 7- and 4-hydroxy 22:6w3. The optical isomers of the 7-hydroxy derivative were resolved using the pentafluorobenzyl rather than the methyl derivative. Using these methods, the structures of the major platelet liposygenase metabolites of 22:6w3 were determined to be 14-S- and 11-S-hydroxy 22:6w3.

Formation of Lipoxins by the Brain

Ischemia Enhances Production of Lipoxins[a]

SANG JOO KIM[b] AND TEIJI TOMINAGA[c]

[b]Membrane Research Institute
University City Science Center
Philadelphia, Pennsylvania 19104

[c]Division of Neurosurgery
Institute for Brain Diseases
Tohoku University School of Medicine
Sendai 980, Japan

Lipoxygenase products such as 5-HETE, 12-HETE, and 15-HETE have been identified in the central nervous system.[1,2] Ischemic brain tissue has been reported to produce increased levels of sulfidoleukotrienes[3,4] and elevated levels of 15-HETE.[5]

Lipoxins (LXs) are a new class of trihydroxytetraene derivatives of arachidonic acid, first described by Samuelsson's group.[6,7] This series of novel compounds is formed by incubation of 15-H(P)ETE with human leukocytes.[6–10] Purified 12-lipoxygenase from porcine leukocytes is also capable of producing LXs.[11] Subsequently, LXs have been identified in rat alveolar macrophages,[12,13] human eosinophils,[14] rat RBL-1 cells,[15] canine mastocytoma cells,[16] and rat red blood cells.[17]

LXs contain a conjugated tetraene structure and possess diverse biological properties.[10] LXA_4, for example, triggers superoxide anion generation.[6] It activates leukocytes and promotes chemotaxis.[18] LXA_4, in contrast to leukotrienes, induces glomerular hyperperfusion and hyperfiltration.[19] It also provokes changes in microvascular integrity[20] and contraction of lung parenchymal strips.[9] LXA_4 and LXB_4 inhibit natural killer cell function.[21,22] Moreover, LXA_4 activates protein kinase C (PKC)[23,24] with a potency over 30 times greater than diacylglycerol. Interestingly, some of these biological properties are exerted by mechanisms distinct from those of either prostaglandins or leukotrienes.[10]

The present study reports the occurrence of LXs in the rat brain—in particular, elevated levels of LXs in ischemic regions of the brain.

Male Sprague-Dawley rats (Charles River) were anesthetized with nembutal and perfused with saline solution from the ascending aorta. Whole brains were extracted on an ice-cold plate and used as normal brain samples. Rats from the same batch were used to produce focal ischemic lesions. Under halothane anesthesia, the right middle cerebral artery (MCA) and the common carotid artery (CCA) were ligated with a temporary clipping of the left CCA,[25] resulting in cortical infarction in the territory of the right MCA (FIG. 1A). Three days after the surgery, the brain samples were extracted in the same manner, and the ischemic regions of the cerebral cortices (FIG. 1B, C) were dissected out quickly, and homogenized in 3 volumes of phosphate buffered saline with Ca^{2+} (Gibco) at pH 7.4. Similarly, samples were obtained from the nonischemic contralateral hemisphere. The method used for the detection of LXs was essentially Serhan's, with modifications.[13] In brief, the crude homogenate from

---

[a]This work was supported in part by a grant-in-aid from the Institute for Korean-American Studies.

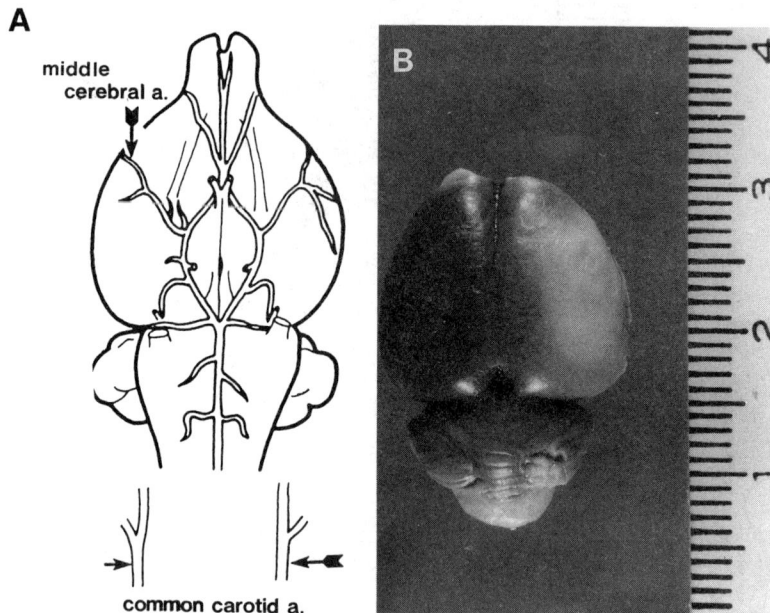
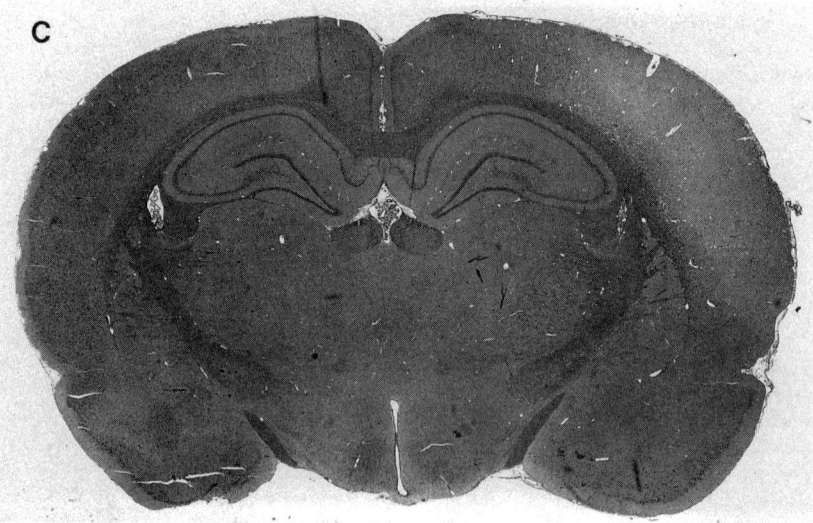

FIGURE 1. (A) A focal cerebral ischemia model. Ischemia was produced by the ligations of the right common carotid artery (CCA) and the middle cerebral artery, combined with temporary occlusion of the left CCA. The sites of vessel occlusion are indicated with *arrows*. (B) Dorsal view of the ischemic rat brain stained with 2,3,5-triphenyl-2H-tetrazolium chloride (TTC) solution. Three days after surgery, the rat was perfused with a saline solution. Then the whole brain was immersed in a 2% TTC solution for 30 min at 37 °C. The ischemic lesion was not stained and appeared white. The nonischemic part was stained dark. The unilateral infarction was well delineated. (C) The coronal section of the ischemic brain (H-E stain). Three days after surgery, the brain was perfused with saline and fixed with 10% buffered formalin. Typical histological changes caused by the ischemic insult were found in the unilateral cerebral cortex, seen as a lighter zone (upper right), compared with the cortex on the opposite side in this picture.

each set of samples was incubated with 15-H(P)ETE (100 μM) and A23187 (5 μM) for 60 min at 37 °C. The reaction mixture was processed[13] and evaluated for RP-HPLC elution profile and UV spectral characteristics compared with those of synthetic standards. The resulting chromatogram (FIG. 2) included several peaks that showed λmax at 301 nm, suggesting the presence of a conjugated tetraene-containing chromophore. Two specific peaks were coeluted with LXA_4 and LXB_4 standards (Cayman Chem. Co.). These two fractions were further examined for their UV spectral characteristics. Both fractions exhibited characteristic UV spectrum with

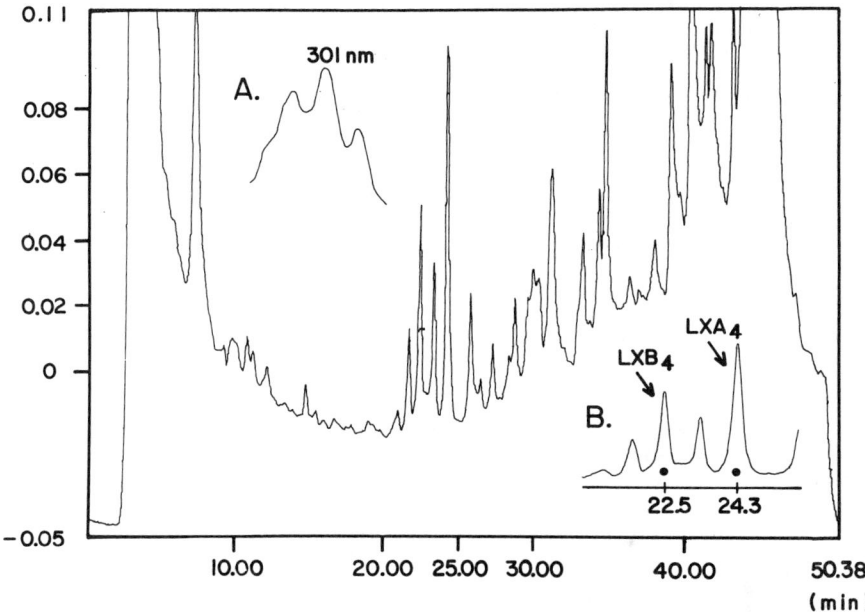

FIGURE 2. A typical RP-HPLC chromatogram of the incubation products of rat brain homogenate with 15-H(P)ETE (100 μM) and A23187 (5 μM) for 60 min at 37 °C. The column was Ultropac TSK-120T(C_{18}-ODS, 5 μm, 4.6 × 250 mm, LKB), and the products were eluted on a linear gradient of methanol/water/glacial acetic acid (50/50/0.05, v/v) to methanol for 40 min at a flow rate of 1 ml/min. The instrument employed was a total LKB HPLC system/IBM PC/Wavescan software package (LKB). *Inset*: A typical UV spectrum (A, λmax 301 nm) of fractions coeluting with standard LXA_4 and LXB_4 (B, retention times; 24.3 min and 22.5 min). The spectrum was recorded in the same solvent using LKB-RSDOU/IBM PC/Wavescan software (LKB).

λmax at 301 nm and shoulders at 289 nm and 316 nm. This spectral feature strongly indicated that the fractions indeed contained a conjugated tetraene chromophore (FIG. 2. inset). These physical properties were similar to those already published. In addition, we observed that the ischemic samples produced consistently higher levels of LXs.

Based on these observations, we conclude that the rat brain has the capacity to form LXA_4, LXB_4, and related isomers; in particular, an ischemically challenged region produces more LXs than the nonischemic region of the brain. It is interesting to note that the brain is one of the highest sources of PKC,[26,27] and that LXs are readily capable of activating this enzyme.[23,24] It is conceivable that activities of PKC-dependent proteins and enzymes could be affected by LXs, thus rendering a molecular basis for a potential novel pathway in this signal transduction system. We propose that the capacity of brain tissue to produce LXs may play an important pathophysiological role, particularly in sequelae associated with brain ischemia.

REFERENCES

1. LINDGREN, J. A., T. HOEKFELT, S. E. DAHLEN, C. PATRONE & B. SAMUELSSON. 1984. Proc. Natl. Acad. Sci. USA **81:** 6212–6216.
2. MIYAMOTO, T., J. A. LINDGREN & B. SAMUELSSON. 1987. Biochim. Biophys. Acta **922:** 372–378.
3. MOSKOWITZ, M. A., K. J. KIWAK, K. HEKIMIAN & L. LEVINE. 1984. Science **224:** 886–889.
4. KIWAK, K. J., M. A. MOSKOWITZ & L. LEVINE. 1985. J. Neurosurg. **62:** 865–869.
5. USUI, M., T. ASANO & K. TAKAKURA. 1987. Stroke **18:** 490–494.
6. SERHAN, C. N., M. HAMBERG & B. SAMUELSSON. 1984. Biochem. Biophys. Res. Commun. **118:** 943–949.
7. SERHAN, C. N., M. HAMBERG & B. SAMUELSSON. 1984. Proc. Natl. Acad. Sci. USA **81:** 5335–5339.
8. FITZSIMMONS, B. J., J. ADAMS, J. F. EVANS, Y. LEBLANC & J. ROKACH. 1985. J. Biol. Chem. **260:** 13008–13012.
9. SERHAN, C. N., K. C. NICOLAOU, S. E. WEBBER, C. A. VEAL, S. E. DAHLEN, T. J. PUUSTINEN & B. SAMUELSSON. 1986. J. Biol. Chem. **261:** 16340–16345.
10. SAMUELSSON, B., S. E. DAHLEN, J. A. LINDGREN, C. A. ROUZER & C. N. SERHAN. 1987. Science **237:** 1171–1176.
11. UEDA, N., C. YOKOYAMA, S. YAMAMOTO, B. J. FITZSIMMONS, J. ROKACH, J. A. OATES & A. BRASH. 1987. Biochem. Biophys. Res. Commun. **149:** 1063–1069.
12. KIM, S. J., B. LAM, H. P. GODFREY, P. Y. K. WONG & Y. KIKKAWA. 1987. (Abstract.) Fed. Proc. **46:** 692.
13. KIM, S. J. 1988. Biochem. Biophys. Res. Commun. **150:** 870–876.
14. SERHAN, C. N., U. HIRSCH, J. PALMBLAD & B. SAMUELSSON. 1987. FEBS Lett. **217:** 242–246.
15. KIM, S. J., A. HAMEED, P. Y. K. WONG & Y. KIKKAWA. 1987. (Abstract.) J. Cell. Biol. **105:** 142.
16. LAZARUS, S. C. & E. ZOCCA. 1988. (Abstract.) FASEB J. **2:** A409.
17. KIM, S. J., A. TAMURA & S. T. OHNISHI. In preparation.
18. PALMBLAD, J., H. GYLLENHAMMAR, B. RINGERTZ, C. N. SERHAN, B. SAMUELSSON & K. C. NICOLAOU. 1987. Biochem. Biophys. Res. Commun. **145:** 168–175.
19. BADR, K. F., C. N. SERHAN, K. C. NICOLAOU & B. SAMUELSSON. 1987. Biochem. Biophys. Res. Commun. **145:** 408–414.
20. DAHLEN, S. E., J. RAUD, C. N. SERHAN, J. BJORK & B. SAMUELSSON. 1987. Acta Physiol. Scand. **130:** 643–647.
21. RAMSTEDT, U., J. NG, H. WIGZELL, C. N. SERHAN & B. SAMUELSSON. 1985. J. Immunol. **135:** 3434–3438.
22. RAMSTEDT, U., C. N. SERHAN, K. C. NICOLAOU, S. E. WEBBER, H. WIGZELL & B. SAMUELSSON. 1987. J. Immunol. **138:** 266–270.
23. HANSSON, A., C. N. SERHAN, J. HAEGGSTROM, M. INGELMAN-SUNDBERG & B. SAMUELSSON. 1986. Biochem. Biophys. Res. Commun. **134:** 1215–1222.
24. KIM, S. J. 1987. Unpublished data.
25. CHEN, S. T., C. Y. HSU, E. L. HOGAN, H. MARICQ & J. D. BALENTINE. 1986. Stroke **17:** 738–743.
26. NISHIZUKA, Y. 1984. Nature (London) **308:** 693–698.
27. NISHIZUKA, Y. 1986. Science **233:** 305–312.

Cerebral Ischemia in Gerbils

Effect of Postischemic Treatment with Oligoprostaglandin B1[a]

D. V. LUBITZ,[b] S. L. COHAN,[b] D. J. REDMOND,[b]
AND M. SHERIDAN[c]

Department of [b]Neurology and
[c]Department of Community and Family Medicine
Georgetown University School of Medicine
Washington, D.C. 20007

Studies by Pollis'[1] and Devlin's[2] groups showed that treatment with a mixture of prostaglandin B1 oligomeres (PGBx) reverses calcium ion overload and restores phosphorylation in mitochondria subjected to anoxia. Also, postischemic administration of PGBx leads to substantially improved survival and better morphological preservation of heart and brain tissue.[3-5] Recently Devlin et al.[6] demonstrated that the biological properties of oligo-PGB (trimer of 16,16' dimethyl-15-dehydroprostaglandin B1) are similar to those of PGBx. We have previously reported[7] that treatment with oligo-PGB1 improves the ability to survive brain ischemia. The results of the continuation of those studies are presented in this paper.

Female gerbils (60-70 g) were subjected to bilateral carotid artery occlusion. In 180 animals the occlusion lasted 15 min, and in 392 gerbils, 20 min. Blood pressure, blood oxygen saturation, body temperature, and cardiac rate were noninvasively monitored during ischemia. After 15-min ischemia, three groups of gerbils ($n = 20$/group) were injected 5 min postischemia at 0.5, 1.0, and 10 mg/kg, respectively, with oligo-PGB dissolved in 4% Na-bicarbonate. Another group ($n = 20$) was injected twice at 10 mg/kg administered 5 min and 24 h postischemia. The controls ($n = 80$) received vehicle injections. Three additional groups of animals ($n = 56$/group) that were exposed to 20 min brain ischemia were given oligo-PGB at 1.0, 5.0, 10.0 mg/kg, respectively. In 56 animals 10 mg/kg of the drug was injected 5 min and 24 hrs postischemia. The controls ($n = 168$) were injected with the vehicle. Behavior and mortality of the animals were monitored for 14 days following ischemia.

There was a dose-dependent improvement in survival of 15 min ischemia after treatment with oligo-PGB (FIG. 1). Sequential injection of the drug (2×10.0 mg/kg, 5 min + 24 h postischemia) resulted in 95% of the animals surviving more than 14 days ($p < 0.001$). In the animals subjected to 20-min occlusion, injections of 10 mg/kg given 5 min and 24 h postischemia resulted in 66% of the gerbils surviving more than 14 days ($p < 0.001$). Lower doses of oligo-PGB administered after 20-min ischemia had no effect; survival was similar to that of the controls (FIG. 2).

The mechanism through which oligo-PGB improves postischemic survival is unknown. It may be related to the already demonstrated physiological properties of the drug—calcium ionophoretic activity or restoration of the postischemic phosphorylation processes. Other possibilities, however, can not be presently discounted.

---

[a]This work was supported by Office of Naval Research Contract N 00014-86-K-0471.

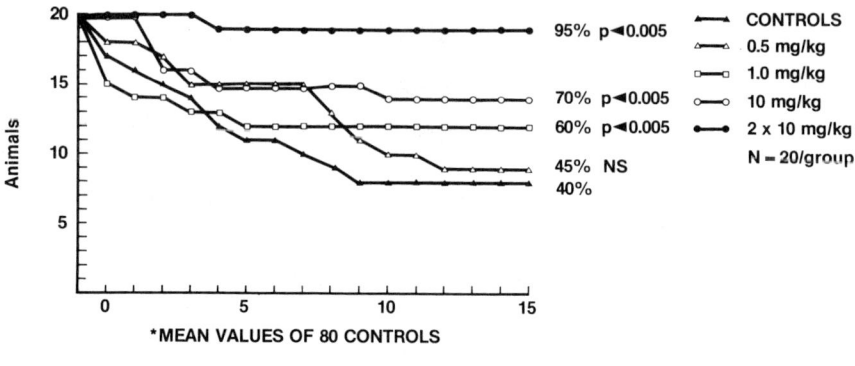

FIGURE 1. Survival of 15-min ischemia after postischemic treatment either with the vehicle (controls) or oligo-PGB.

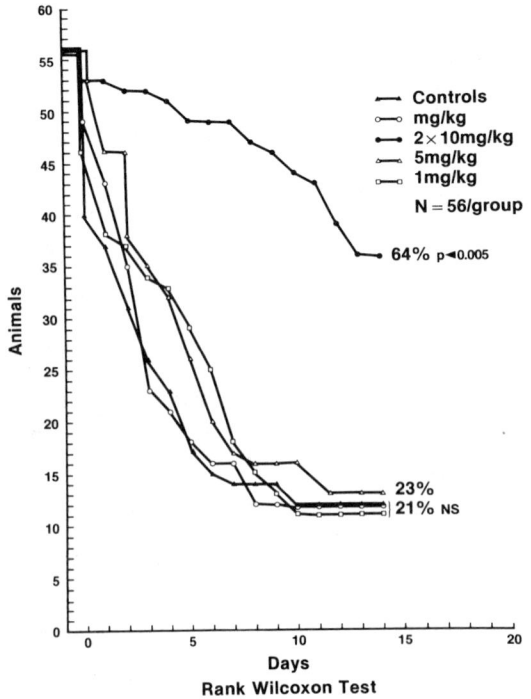

FIGURE 2. Survival of 20-min ischemia after postischemic treatment either with the vehicle (controls) or oligo-PGB.

ACKNOWLEDGMENTS

Dr. G. Nelson, of St. Joseph's University, Philadelphia kindly supplied oligo-PGB.

REFERENCES

1. SHMUKLER, H. W., E. SOFFER, M. G. ZAWRYT, et al. 1982. Physiol. Chem. Phys. **14:** 445–486.
2. OHNISHI, T. S. & T. M. DEVLIN. 1979. Biochem. Biophys. Res. Commun. **89:** 240–245.
3. ANGELAKOS, E. T., R. L. RILEY & D. B. POLIS. 1980. Physiol. Chem. Phys. **12:** 81–96.
4. KOLATA, R. J. & D. B. POLIS. 1980. Physiol. Chem. Phys. **12:** 545–550.
5. MARTINEZ RODRIGUEZ, H. R., R. A. RANGEL GUERRA, B. B. MRSULJA & D. LOWRY. 1986. Rev. Invest. Clin. **38:** 251–260.
6. URIBE, S., R. VILLALOBOS-MOLINA & T. M. DEVLIN. 1987. Biochem. Biophys. Res. Commun. **143:** 1024–1029.
7. COHAN, S. L., D. K. J. E. VON LUBITZ & D. J. REDMOND. 1987. Soc. Neurosci. Abstr. Vol. 13, Part 3.: 1495.

Effects of Platelet-Activating Factor Antagonist BN 52021 on Cerebral Lipid Metabolism following Ischemia Reperfusion in the Gerbil

VICTOR L. MARCHESELLI,[a] THOMAS PANETTA,[a]
PIERRE BRAQUET,[a] KERRY T. THIBODEAUX,[b] AND
NICOLAS G. BAZAN[a]

[a]Louisiana State University School of Medicine
New Orleans, Louisiana 70112

[b]Institut Henri Beaufour
Le Plessis-Robinson, France

Platelet-activating factor (PAF) has been shown to mediate a variety of detrimental effects related to inflammation, bronchoconstriction, platelet aggregation, systemic hypotension, pulmonary hypertension, and increased vascular permeability.[1] Related to the multisystem involvement of PAF in tissue injury, we studied the effects of BN 52021, a potent PAF antagonist,[2] in an ischemia-reperfusion model of cerebral injury.

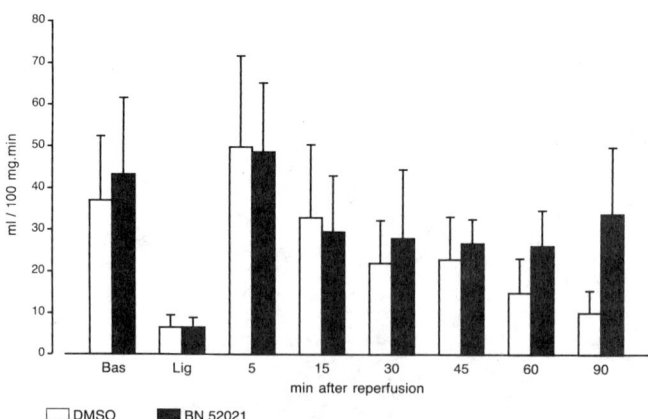

FIGURE 1. Effects of platelet-activating factor antagonist BN 52021 on the cerebral blood flow in the gerbil forebrain following ischemia-reperfusion–induced cerebral injury. Data are expressed as ml/100 gm/min. Values are averages of 7 animals + SEM.

BN 52021, a terpene isolated from *Ginkgo biloba* leaves, has resulted in clinical improvement in animal models of cerebral injury.[1] Cerebral ischemia results in the accumulation of free fatty acids (FFAs) in the brain.[3] During reperfusion, levels of FFA return to normal[4] with increased cyclooxygenase and lipoxygenase[5] reaction products. Bilateral carotid artery ligation and reperfusion results in a significant incidence of death in gerbils.[6] BN 52021 (10 mg/kg) improves survival in gerbils subjected to ischemia-reperfusion injury.[7]

Biochemical and physiological parameters were correlated in a gerbil model of 10 minutes of ischemia followed by 90 minutes of reperfusion. FIGURE 1 depicts the changes in cerebral blood flow during ligation and reperfusion in DMSO vehicle control and BN 52021–treated animals. Control animals had progressive impairment of cerebral blood flow (CBF) after 45 minutes of reperfusion. BN 52021–treated animals recovered, with return of CBF to normal levels. There was an inverse correlation between changes in CBF and release of free fatty acids. Complete forebrain ischemia resulted in a 30-fold increase in FFAs (FIG. 2). Partial midbrain ischemia resulted in only a three-fold increase in FFAs. The patterns of saturated and unsaturated fatty acids released were similar in forebrain and midbrain

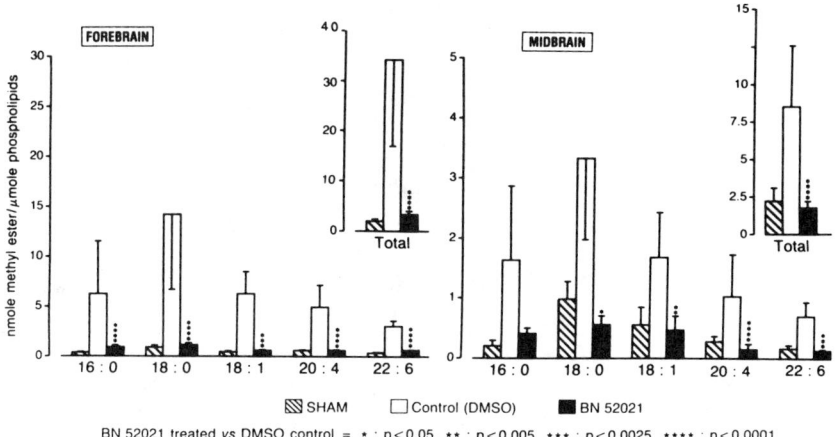

FIGURE 2. Effects of BN 52021 on free fatty acid pools after 90 minutes of reperfusion in the gerbil forebrain and midbrain. Data are expressed as nmole methyl esther/μmole phospholipids. Values are averages of 7 gerbils + SEM.

(18:0 > 16:0 > 18:1 > 20:4 > 22:6). BN 52021 injected at the onset of reperfusion reduced the FFA pool at 90 minutes of reperfusion in the forebrain and midbrain. Inhibition of phospholipase activity may be responsible for the observed effects.

REFERENCES

1. BRAQUET, P., L. TOUQUI, T. Y. SHEN & B. B. VARGAFTIG. 1987. Perspectives in platelet-activating factor research. Pharmacol. Rev. **39**: 97–145.
2. BRAQUET, P., B. SPINNEWYN, M. BRAQUET, R. H. BOURGAIN, J. E. TAYLOR, A. ETIENNE & K. DRIEU. 1985. BN 52021 and related compounds: A new series of highly specific :AF-acether receptor antagonists isolated from Ginkgo biloba. Blood Vessels **16**: 559–572.
3. BAZAN, N. G. 1970. Effects of ischemia and electroconvulsive shock on free fatty acid pool in the brain. Biochim. Biophys. Acta **218**: 1–10.

4. GAUDET, R. J. & L. LEVINE. 1979. Transient cerebral ischemia and brain prostaglandins. Biochem. Biophys. Res. Commun. **86**: 893–901.
5. MOSKOWITZ, M. A., K. J. KIWAK, K. Hekimian & L. LEVINE. 1984. Synthesis of compounds with properties of leukotrienes C_4 and D_4 in gerbil brain after ischemia and reperfusion. Science **244**: 886–889.
6. YOSHIDA, S., S. INOH, T. ASANO, K. SANO, H. SHIMASAKI & N. UETA. 1983. Brain free fatty acids, edema, and mortality in gerbils subjected to transient, bilateral ischemia, and effects of barbiturate anesthesia. J. Neurochem. **40**: 1278–1286.
7. PANETTA, T., V. L. MARCHESELLI, P. BRAQUET, B. SPINNEWYN & N. G. BAZAN. 1987. Effects of a platelet activating factor antagonist (BN 52021) on free fatty acids, diacylglycerols, polyphosphoinositides and blood flow in the gerbil brain. Inhibition of ischemia-reperfusion induced cerebral injury. Biochem. Biophys. Res. Commun. **149**: 580–587.

Eicosanoid Production by Isolated Cerebral Microvessels and Cultured Cerebral Endothelium

STEVEN A. MOORE,[a,b] PAUL H. FIGARD,[c]
ARTHUR A. SPECTOR,[c] AND MICHAEL N. HART[b]

*Departments of [b]Pathology and [c]Biochemistry
The University of Iowa
Iowa City, Iowa 52240*

Many studies indicate that eicosanoids have an important role in normal cerebrovascular physiology and in the cerebrovascular response to brain injury.[1,2] However, little is known about which eicosanoids are contributed by the cells of the cerebral vessels themselves. To examine this contribution more closely, we have been studying the metabolism of arachidonic acid in isolated murine cerebral microvessels and in cultured murine cerebromicrovascular endothelium (CME). Prostaglandins (PG) I_2, E_2, and $F_{2\alpha}$ are produced by cultured CME in response to exogenous arachidonic acid, calcium ionophore A23187, or physiologic agonists including thrombin, bradykinin, serotonin, and acetylcholine. Arachidonic acid and ionophore A23187 stimulated PG production by as much as 30- and 40-fold, respectively, above the background level, while the physiologic agonists increased PG production by 3- to 12-fold above background. Analysis of CME eicosanoids by reverse-phase high-performance liquid chromatography demonstrates production of primarily PGI_2 and E_2 by one line of endothelium (FIG. 1A), while another also produces $PGF_{2\alpha}$, HHT, and a compound with chromatographic properties of 12-hydroxyeicosatetraenoic acid (12-HETE) (FIG. 1B).[3] Two other minor compounds have chromatographic properties of 12-HETE metabolites (FIG. 1B).[3] CME grown on micropore filters and incubated 30 min with 7.5 μM arachidonic acid release PG from both apical and basal surfaces, but primarily from their basal surfaces in a ratio as high as 4:1, basal:apical.[3]

Although PG are the major arachidonic acid metabolites of cultured CME, microvessels isolated from perfused adult mouse brains additionally produce a compound from arachidonic acid with chromatographic properties of a monohydroxyeicosatetraenoic acid (FIG. 1C). Analysis of the trimethylsilyl ether, methyl ester derivative of this metabolite by gas chromatography–mass spectrometry revealed a base peak at m/e 295 and alpha cleavage ions at m/e 215 and 301 from its reduced derivative. Chemical ionization of the reduced derivative in NH_3 revealed a molecular ion at m/e 415. Together these spectra prove that the primary cerebral microvessel metabolite of arachidonic acid is 12-HETE.[4]

While little or no 12-HETE is produced by cultured CME, 12-HETE is rapidly incorporated into CME phospholipids, primarily phosphatidylcholine. 12-HETE is also rapidly metabolized by cultured CME to more polar compounds with chromatographic properties of two of the minor CME arachidonic acid metabolites[3] (FIG. 1). Furthermore, 12-HETE inhibits PG production by cultured CME. When stimulated

---

[a]Address for correspondence: Steven A. Moore, M.D., Ph. D., Department of Pathology, The University of Iowa, Iowa City, Iowa 52242.

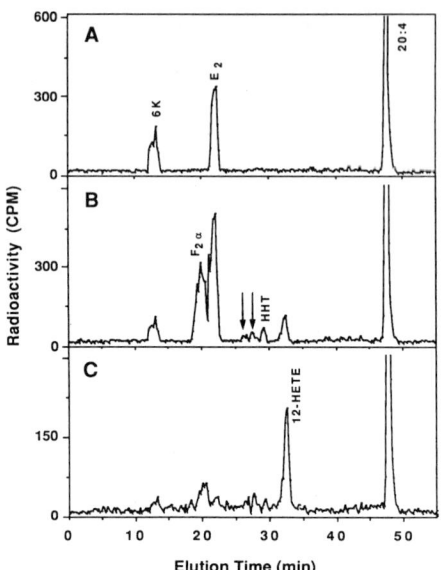

FIGURE 1. Reverse-phase, HPLC chromatograms of radioactive eicosanoids formed by cultured cerebromicrovascular endothelium (CME) and isolated cerebral microvessels. After 1-h incubations of CME with 7.5 μM [^{3}H]-arachidonic acid, one line of CME produces PGI$_2$ (detected as 6-keto-PGF$_{1\alpha}$ [6K]) and PGE$_2$ (**A**), while another also produces PGF$_{2\alpha}$, HHT, and a compound with chromatographic properties of 12-HETE (**B**). Two other minor compounds in (B) have chromatographic properties of CME 12-HETE metabolites[3] (*arrows*). Brain microvessels were isolated from adult mice after transcardiac perfusion with heparinized normal saline. A mixture of arterioles, capillaries, and venules were collected on a 100-μm nylon mesh filter and incubated for 1 h with 7.5 μM [^{3}H]-arachidonic acid, producing primarily 12-HETE (**C**). Protection of the cyclooxygenase enzyme with 10 μM ibuprofen during the isolation procedure resulted in greater PG production by microvessels (as seen here) than when ibuprofen was excluded from the isolation buffer solutions.[3]

TABLE 1. Inhibition of Cerebromicrovascular Endothelial Cell Prostaglandin Production by 12-HETE

	6-Keto PGF$_{1\alpha}$[a]			PGE$_2$[a]		
12-HETE	Control	20:4[b]	A23187[b]	Control	20:4[b]	A23187[b]
0 μM	6.1 ± 0.3	39.7 ± 4.6	38.1 ± 2.5	3.4 ± 0.3	27.2 ± 2.4	32.6 ± 2.9
0.5 μM	5.8 ± 0.2	41.2 ± 3.8	40.3 ± 5.2	3.2 ± 0.2	30.3 ± 3.1	35.1 ± 4.0
1.0 μM	6.2 ± 0.4	19.8 ± 2.0	23.4 ± 2.5	3.8 ± 0.4	12.7 ± 1.8	16.4 ± 2.1
5.0 μM	5.7 ± 0.3	9.1 ± 0.6	13.1 ± 0.9	3.5 ± 0.5	8.7 ± 0.8	12.4 ± 2.3

[a]Data values represent the mean pmole/well ± SE for prostaglandins measured by radioimmunoassay 20 min after stimulation of triplicate wells of cerebromicrovascular endothelium with arachidonic acid or ionophore A23187.

[b]20:4 = 7.5 μM arachidonic acid; A23187 = 2 μM calcium ionophore A23187.

by 7.5 µM arachidonic acid or 2 µM ionophore A23187, PG production is reduced up to 56% by 1 µM and 90% by 5µM 12-HETE; 0.5 µM 12-HETE has no effect on CME PG production (TABLE 1).

These data demonstrate that isolated cerebral microvessels actively metabolize arachidonic acid to a variety of eicosanoids, a property that is maintained in culture by CME. While microvessels convert arachidonic acid primarily to the lipoxygenase derivative 12-HETE, cultured CME produce primarily the cyclooxygenase derivatives PGI_2, E_2, and $F_{2\alpha}$. CME also maintain reactivity to a number of physiologic agonists. PG are released from CME primarily in a basal direction that *in situ* would place them in contact with smooth muscle or neuroglial elements, where they may affect cerebrovascular tone or neuroglial function. These data further suggest that 12-HETE production in the brain (from microvessels or elsewhere) may exert physiologic or pathophysiologic effects by inhibiting CME PG production or by insertion into CME membranes. Eicosanoids derived from cells of the cerebral microcirculation may, therefore, play important roles in both the normal biology of the brain and the pathophysiologic response to brain injuries.

REFERENCES

1. CHAN, P. H. & FISHMAN, P. A. 1984. The role of arachidonic acid in vasogenic brain edema. Fed. Proc. **43**: 210–213.
2. WOLFE, L. S. 1982. Eicosanoids: Prostaglandins, thromboxanes, leukotrienes, and other derivatives of carbon-20 unsaturated fatty acids. J. Neurochem. **38**: 1–14.
3. MOORE, S. A., A. A. SPECTOR & M. N. HART. 1988. Eicosanoid metabolism in cerebromicrovascular endothelium. Am. J. Physiol. **254**: C37–C44.
4. HAMBERG, M. & B. SAMUELSSON. 1974. Prostaglandin endoperoxides. Novel transformations of arachidonic acid in human platelets. Proc. Nat. Acad. Sci. U.S.A. **71**: 3400–3404.

Arachidonic Acid Metabolism in Glutamate Neurotoxicity

TIM MURPHY, ASHISH PARIKH, RONALD SCHNAAR,
AND JOSEPH COYLE

Department of Pharmacology
Johns Hopkins University School of Medicine
Baltimore, Maryland 21205

L-Glutamate (Glu), a putative excitatory neurotransmitter, causes selective neurotoxicity when applied *in vivo* or *in vitro*. Alterations in arachidonic acid (AA) metabolism have been implicated in the neuronal degeneration caused by seizures and ischemia; this degeneration can be prevented by antagonists for certain Glu receptor subtypes. We have examined the role of AA metabolites in Glu cytotoxicity using the N18-RE-105 cell line, which expresses a quisqualate subtype of Glu receptor. Addition of 0.1–1 mM quisqualate or 1–10 mM Glu resulted in up to 85% cell lysis within 24 h; however, 10 mM aspartate, N-methyl-D-aspartate, or kainate were not cytotoxic. Cell lysis was first detected after 6–10 h of Glu exposure, did not involve persistent membrane depolarization by Glu, and was attenuated by reducing calcium in the medium.[1]

PHOSPHOLIPASE AND LIPOXYGENASE INHIBITORS REDUCE L-GLUTAMATE TOXICITY

The phospholipase A2 (PLA2) inhibitors quinacrine and 4-bromophenacyl bromide reduced the toxicity of 10 mM Glu by 92 ± 6 and 67 ± 5%, respectively (TABLE 1). Lipoxygenase inhibitors also reduced 10 mM Glu toxicity, nordihydroguaiaretic acid (NDGA) by 97 ± 1%, and phenidone by 61 ± 8%. However, 5,8,11,14-eicosatetraynoic acid (ETYA) did not reduce Glu toxicity even at 100 μM (TABLE 1). Addition of NDGA (5 μM) after up to 12 h of Glu exposure (well after initiation of cell lysis) completely blocked further Glu toxicity. In contrast, the cyclooxygenase inhibitors acetylsalicylic acid, ibuprofen, and indomethacin at 100 μM had no effect on Glu toxicity (TABLE 1).

ARACHIDONIC ACID RELEASE AND METABOLISM

Release of AA and its metabolites was measured by prelabeling N18-RE-105 cells with [^{3}H]AA for 24 h, washing, and then measuring the amount of radiolabel released into the culture medium over a 10-min period. If Glu was added to cultures of prelabeled cells <10 min prior to collection of medium, no increase in radiolabel release (compared to control cultures) was observed. However if Glu was present for >5 h, a marked increase in release (expressed as % of total [^{3}H]AA incorporated) of radiolabel into the medium was observed 2 h prior to and during Glu-induced cell lysis (6–12 h of Glu exposure) (FIG. 1.) Silica gel thin-layer chromatography, using petroleum ether:ethyl ether:acetic acid (50:50:1) as solvent, of radiolabeled material extracted from the cells indicated that Glu treatment led to an increase in radiolabel with mobilities similar to 15(S)-hydroxy-5-cis-8-cis-11-cis-13-trans-eicosatetraenoic acid (HETE).

ARACHIDONIC ACID TOXICITY

Addition of AA (50–250 μM) to N18-RE-105 cultures was cytotoxic, but the observed toxicity was acute and not completely blocked by NDGA, which differs from the effects observed with Glu treatment. Addition of AA (10–50 μM) to cultures treated with concentrations of Glu that produced submaximal toxicity (1–3 mM) did not result in reproducible potentiation of toxicity.

CALCIUM IONOPHORE TOXICITY AND ARACHIDONIC ACID RELEASE

The calcium ionophore A23187 (10 μM) lysed 81 ± 7% of N18-RE-105 cells, while 1 μM was nontoxic. Unlike Glu toxicity, the cytotoxicity of 10 μM A23187 was

TABLE 1. Effect of Various Proposed Inhibitors of Arachidonic Acid Metabolism on 10 mM L-glutamte (Glu) Toxicity

Compound	μM	% Reduction in 10 mM Glu Toxicity	N
PLA$_2$ inhibitors			
Quinacrine	1	10 ± 5	3
	5	25 ± 7[a]	3
	10	93 ± 6[a]	3
4-Bromo-phenacyl-Br$^-$	10	67 ± 5[a]	3
Lipoxygenase inhibitors			
NDGA	1	47 ± 16[a]	3
	5	97 ± 1[a]	5
Phenidone	10	29 ± 7[a]	3
	25	28 ± 9	4
	50	61 ± 8[a]	3
ETYA	100	NE	2
Cyclooxygenase inhibitors			
Aspirin	100	NE	3
Ibuprofen	100	NE	2
Indomethacin	100	NE	3
Antioxidants			
Vitamin E	1	8 ± 5	3
	10	63 ± 10[a]	3
	100	100 ± 6[a]	3
Ascorbate	50	30	2
Mannitol	10,000	NE	2

NOTE: Indicated compounds were added to N18-RE-105 cell cultures in the presence and absence of Glu, and data expressed as % reduction in 10 mM Glu toxicity. Toxicity was quantified by measurement of cellular and released lactate dehydrogenase. All compounds except mannitol and ascorbate (100× dilution from H20) were diluted from >200× ethanolic stocks (0.5% EtOH alone did not have any effect on Glu cell death or control cell viability). NE = no effect.
[a]$p < 0.05$, two-tailed paired t test.

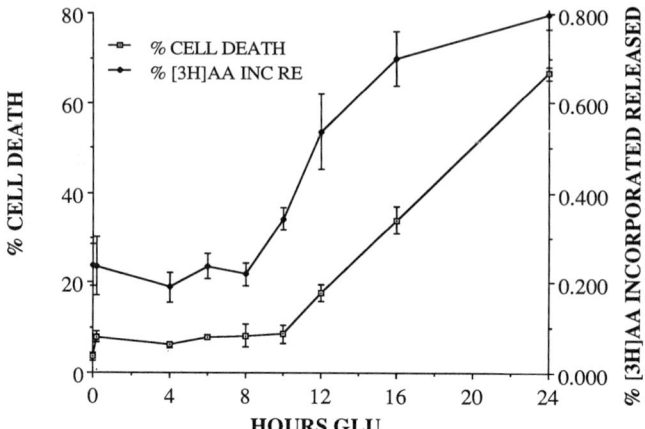

FIGURE 1. Relationship between release of [³H]AA-derived material and Glu-induced cell death in N18-RE-105 cells. Cultures were labeled with [³H]AA for a total of 24 h. Glu (10 mM) was added for the indicated number of hours before measurement of release, such that cells were labeled for the indicated time in the presence of Glu, and for 24 h minus the indicated time in its absence. After washing the cells four times with fresh media, the amount of [³H]AA-derived material released into culture media over 10 min was measured by scintillation counting. Cell death was measured as described in TABLE 1.

minimally reduced by 5 µM NDGA (17% reduction). One µM A23187 increased the release of [³H] product derived from [³H]AA by 97 ± 12% in 10 min, and by 422% in 45–60 min.

PHOSPHATIDYL INOSITOL TURNOVER

Addition of Glu (10 mM) or quisqualate (1 mM) acutely (20 min) or chronically (6–16 h) to N18-RE-105 cells prelabeled with [³H]inositol did not lead to increased levels of cellular inositol phosphates. In contrast, bradykinin (3 µM), which was nontoxic, increased levels of cellular inositol phosphates to 400–500% of control with 20 min of exposure.

PEROXIDE FORMATION

Formation of intracellular peroxides was detected using 2,7 dichlorofluorescin diacetate, which is a nonfluorescent, cell-permeable compound. Upon entering the cell, the compound is deesterified and is subject to oxidation by cellular peroxides to the fluorescent compound 2,7 dichlorofluorescein. When Glu-treated (10 mM Glu, 5–7 h) and control cultures were compared blindly, 14 ± 7% of control cells and 66 ± 10% of Glu-treated cells ($p < .01$) were visible under fluorescence microscopy, and qualitatively Glu-treated cells exhibited greater fluorescence. Consistent with a role for peroxides was the ability of vitamin E completely to block Glu toxicity in a dose-dependent manner.

DISCUSSION

Inhibitors of AA release (PLA_2) and metabolism (lipoxygenase) blocked the cytotoxicity of Glu in N18-RE-105 cells. Increased release of [^{3}H]AA products and formation of its metabolites were detected in Glu-treated cells. However, their relationship to the effects of lipoxygenase and PLA_2 inhibitors remains unclear. In addition, the identity of the [^{3}H] AA metabolite with a mobility similar to 15-HETE remains to be confirmed using better analytical techniques. Nevertheless, Glu-induced formation of peroxides would be consistent with peroxide containing lipoxygenase products. Glu was not able to stimulate acute release of [^{3}H]AA, or increase cellular inositol phosphate production, indicating that N18-RE-105 cells do not possess a Glu receptor–coupled phospholipase C or PLA_2. The time courses of [^{3}H]AA-derived material release, and protection by the lipoxygenase inhibitor NDGA would be consistent with the lack of a Glu receptor coupled to PLA_2 in N18-RE-105 cells, and may indicate that AA metabolism is one of the final events in Glu cytotoxicity in this system. The results from AA addition experiments indicate that AA does not mimic the toxicity associated with Glu. The marked release of [^{3}H]product derived from [^{3}H] AA by nontoxic concentrations of A23187 also suggests that AA release itself is not the primary toxic event in Glu toxicity. Inhibitors and activators of second messenger systems other than AA release and metabolism did not have any effect on Glu toxicity at concentrations reported to be physiologically active; these inhibitors and activators include forskolin, phorbol esters, and calmodulin inhibitors. These data suggest that AA metabolism may be one of several factors contributing to the toxicity of Glu in N18-RE-105 cells.

REFERENCE

1. MURPHY, T. et al. 1988. Brain Res. **444**: 325–332.

Selective Inhibition of Thromboxane Synthase Enhances Reperfusion and Metabolism of the Ischemic Brain[a]

L. C. PETTIGREW,[b,c] L. K. MISRA,[d] J. C. GROTTA,[c]
P. A. NARAYANA,[e] AND K. K. WU[d]

*Departments of [c]Neurology, [d]Internal Medicine
(Division of Hematology), and [e]Radiology
University of Texas Medical School
Houston, Texas 77030*

Selective inhibition of thromboxane (TX) synthase during early reperfusion of the ischemic brain may augment recovery of microcirculatory blood flow leading to preservation of high-energy phosphate metabolism. We tested this hypothesis by studying the effects of 1-benzylimidazole (1-BI), a selective inhibitor of thromboxane synthase, in an animal model of transient forebrain ischemia.

TABLE 1. Cerebral Blood Flow (ml/100 g brain/min)

	Hemisphere		Hippocampus	
Ischemic control ($n = 4$)	42 ± 9	} $p < .01$	51 ± 14	} $p < .04$
1-BI-treated ($n = 3$)	104 ± 13		125 ± 25	
Normal ($n = 6$)	118 ± 9	} $p =$ NS	123 ± 14	} $p =$ NS

NOTE: Figures are ml/100 g brain/min, mean ± standard error of the mean. NS = not significant.

METHODS

Male Wistar rats weighing 250–300 g were subjected to 30 min of transient forebrain ischemia.[1] One group of animals received intravenous infusions of 10 μg/g 1-BI during ischemia and for 30 min afterward. Levels of TXB_2, the stable metabolite of TXA_2, were quantitated by radioimmunoassay in the brain sampled after 60 min of reperfusion.[2]

Hemispheric and hippocampal cerebral blood flow (CBF) were measured by the indicator-fractionation technique[3] and are shown in TABLE 1. A 2-Tesla magnetic resonance spectrometer was used to measure ^{31}P spectra. The integrated areas beneath

---

[a]This work was supported by a grant from the Texas Affiliate of the American Heart Association.
[b]Address for correspondence: L. Creed Pettigrew, M.D., Department of Neurology/UTMSH, P.O. Box 20708, Houston, Texas 77030.

the peaks corresponding to phosphocreatine (PCr) and inorganic phosphorus (Pi) were determined for calculation of the [PCr]/[Pi] ratio. The brain pH was derived from the equation of Petroff and colleagues.[4] Results are shown in TABLE 2.

DISCUSSION

Rats subjected to ischemia for 30 min while receiving 10 μg/g 1-BI ($n = 5$) had a brain TXB_2 level of 11 ± 3 pg/mg protein after 60 min of reperfusion, compared to 101 ± 20 pg/mg protein in ischemic controls ($n = 5$, $p < .002$) and 4 ± 1 pg/mg protein in normals ($n = 10$, $p < .01$). The 1-BI–treated animals showed significant enhancement of CBF (see TABLE 1) and an increase in the [PCr]/[Pi] ratio beyond 45 min of reperfusion. We speculate that TX synthase inhibition augmented perfusion of

TABLE 2. Results of ^{31}P Spectroscopy at Reperfusion Times of 45 and 60 Minutes

	[PCr]/Pi]		pH	
	45 min	60 min	45 min	60 min
Ischemic control ($n = 3$)	4.25 ± 0.56	4.02 ± 0.39	7.20 ± 0	7.12 ± 0.05
1-BI–treated ($n = 3$)	6.33 ± 0.45	6.12 ± 0.82	7.05 ± 0.09	7.05 ± 0.07
Significance	$p < .05$	NS	NS	NS

NOTE: Figures are mean ± standard error of the mean. PCr = phosphocreatine; Pi = inorganic phosphorus; NS = not significant.

ischemic tissue and restored metabolic viability to a large population of threatened cells. There were no significant differences in cerebral pH between the two ischemic groups, indicating that a pH-dependent reduction in PCr within the brains of control animals is probably not the cause of the difference in [PCr]/[Pi] ratios.

REFERENCES

1. PULSINELLI, W. A. & J. B. BRIERLEY. 1979. Stroke 10: 267–272.
2. PETTIGREW, L. C., E. R. HALL, J. C. GROTTA & K. K. WU. 1987. In Cerebral Ischemia and Hemorrheology. A. Hartmann & W. Kuschinsky, Eds.: 272–279. Springer-Verlag. Berlin.
3. VAN UITERT, R. L. & D. E. LEVY. 1978. Stroke 9: 67–72.
4. PETROFF, O. A. C., J. W. PRICHARD, K. L. BEHAR, J. R. ALGER, J. A. DEN HOLLANDER & R. G. SHULMAN. 1985. Neurology 35: 781–788.

Differential Regulation of Two Types of Cation Channel in BC3H-1 Muscle Cells by Arachidonate[a]

R. E. SHERIDAN[b]

Department of Pharmacology
Georgetown University Schools of Medicine and Dentistry
Washington, D.C. 20007

R. McGEE

Department of Pharmacology
Medical College of Ohio
Toledo, Ohio 43699

Significant changes in synaptic responsiveness can result from changes in the number of receptors present on a cell and in the number of ion channels associated with those receptors. The BC3H-1 vascular smooth muscle cell line[1] contains two similar nonselective cation channels. One of these channels is part of the nicotinic receptor (nAChR).[2] The other channel is activated by intracellular calcium[3] and is similar to Ca^{++}-activated cation channels in neuroblastoma[4] and heart.[5] Although these channels have similar electrophysiological properties, they are readily distinguished by their response to exogenous arachidonic acid.

TABLE 1. Arachidonate Suppression of Cation Channels in BC3H-1 Cells

	Culture Conditions	
Channel Type	Control	Arachidonate
Acetylcholine receptor	25/26	3/27
Ca^{++}-activated cation	23/28	13/15

NOTE: Differential suppression of cation channels in arachidonate as measured by physiological responses in patch-clamp recordings. The table shows the fraction of excised membrane patches that contained either the nAChR channel or the Ca^{++}-activated cation channel before and after long-term incubations with 120 μM arachidonic acid at 37 °C. There is a significant reduction ($p < 0.005$) in the number of functional nAChR channels and no change in the number of Ca^{++}-activated cation channels.

Micromolar quantities of arachidonate added to the tissue-culture medium bathing BC3H-1 cells are taken up by the cells and incorporated in the membrane lipids. TABLE 1 shows that this is accompanied by a significant reduction in the number of ion channels associated with the nAChR, with no change in the number of Ca^{++}-activated

---

[a]This work was supported by National Institutes of Health Grant 1 R01 NS22958.
[b]Current address: Neurotoxicology Branch, USAMRICD, Aberdeen Proving Ground, Maryland 21010.

cation channels. This differential loss of ion channels is paralleled by a reduction in the number of receptor sites for acetylcholine.[6] FIGURE 1 shows this loss as a function of the total exogenous arachidonate concentration. These arachidonic acid effects are not rapid. The half-time for disappearance of the nicotinic receptors is approximately one day, comparable to the turnover rate for nicotinic receptors. This time course suggests that arachidonate exerts its effect in this system by preventing synthesis or membrane insertion of new nAChR. The selective loss of nAChRs from the cell surface is limited to treatment with arachidonate. Incubation with similar concentrations of oleic and elaidic acids have no effect on nAChR binding or physiological function. The actions of arachidonic acid on the nAChR are therefore not due to a detergent solubilization of membrane proteins.

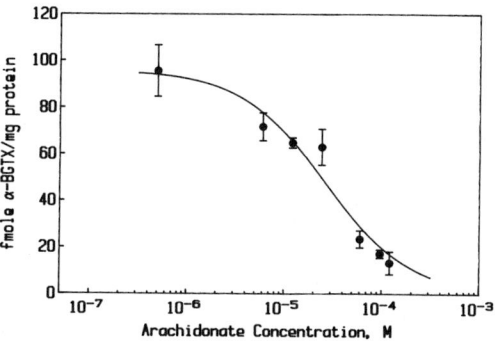

FIGURE 1. Nicotinic receptor changes with arachidonate. The number of nicotinic receptors on the BC3H-1 cell surface is shown as a function of the concentration of arachidonic acid in the culture medium. At 3 days after plating, the culture media was supplemented with 1 mM defatted BSA and the indicated concentration of arachidonate. The cells were maintained in culture for another 6 days, exposed to ^{125}I-*alpha*-bungarotoxin (BGTX), incubated at 37 °C, and washed with ice-cold saline. Nonspecific binding was estimated by residual binding in the presence of 10 mM carbachol. The cells were solubilized in NaOH with aliquots used for determinations of radiolabeled toxin and total protein. The data shown are averages of triplicate measurements ± SEM.

Arachidonic acid can distinguish between two similar cation channels expressed by the BC3H-1 cells and preferentially "down-regulates" nicotinic receptor–coupled channels. In BC3H-1 cells, the Ca^{++}-activated cation channel is probably coupled to an $alpha_1$-adrenergic receptor via an inositol trisphosphate–mediated increase in intracellular calcium.[1] The prolonged presence of circulating arachidonic acid in plasma or cerebrospinal fluid could thus reduce the response to cholinergic input relative to inputs from the adrenergic system.

REFERENCES

1. AMBLER, S. K., R. D. BROWN & P. TAYLOR. 1984. Mol. Pharmacol. **26**: 405–413.
2. SINE, S. M. & J. H. STEINBACH. 1984. Biophys. J. **45**: 175–185.
3. SHERIDAN, R. E. 1986. Neurosci. Abstr. **12**(2): 1200.
4. YELLEN, G. 1982. Nature **296**: 357–359.
5. COLQUHOUN, D., E. NEHER, H. REUTER & C. F. STEVENS. 1981. Nature **294**: 752–754.
6. BOULTER, J. & J. PATRICK. 1977. Biochemistry **16**: 4900–4908.

Increased Peroxidation of Docosahexaenoic Acid in the Rat Brain *in Vitro* and *in Vivo* during Cerebral Ischemia

TADASHI SHINGU, JOHN W. KARANIAN,
HEE-YONG KIM, AND NORMAN SALEM, JR.[a]

Laboratory of Clinical Studies
Division of Intramural Clinical and Biological Research
National Institute on Alcohol Abuse and Alcoholism
Alcohol, Drug Abuse, and Mental Health Administration
Bethesda, Maryland 20892

It is known that free radicals are formed during or after ischemia.[1] We hypothesize that the lipid peroxidation induced by these radicals may lead to brain injury. Polyunsaturated fatty acids such as docosahexaenoate (22:6ω3), which are enriched in the central nervous system,[2] are released from membrane phospholipids during cerebral ischemia and can be rapidly oxidized.[3,4] However, little is known about the factors that contribute to lipid peroxidation during brain trauma. We have studied the peroxidation of docosahexaenoic acid by rat brain homogenate, and we have found that at pH 6.7—a value that commonly occurs during ischemia[5]—there was increased peroxidation.[6] In this report, we discuss the stimulatory effect of oxygen free radicals on lipid peroxidation *in vitro* and on stimulation of lipid peroxidation by cerebral ischemia and reperfusion *in vivo*.

IN VITRO EXPERIMENT

Rat brain was homogenized in 50 mM tris-HCl buffer pH 7.4 or pH 6.5 and incubated with 25 µM [^{14}C]-22:6ω3 free fatty acid for 60 minutes at 37 °C. In our investigations of the effects of free radicals, radical scavengers, and enzyme inhibitors, the following compounds were tested: 100 µM ferrous chloride, 100 µM ferric chloride, 100 µM hydrogen peroxide, 10 µM indomethacin, 40 µM nordihydroguaiaretic acid (NDGA), 50 IU superoxide dismutase (SOD), 100 mM mannitol, and 100 µM alpha-tocopherol. The preparation was acidified to pH 3.5 and extracted twice with equal volumes of dichloromethane. The 22:6ω3 metabolites were then separated by reversed-phase HPLC using an acetonitrile-ammonium acetate (pH 7.0) gradient (20 to 100% acetonitrile in 180 min), and the eluant was monitored using a diode array ultraviolet detector (235 and 280 nm) and a radiodetector. Ferrous iron and Fenton's reagent had a strong stimulatory effect on the formation of 22:6ω3 metabolites. Hydrogen peroxide also stimulated metabolite formation, but to a lesser extent. When boiled homogenate was used in the incubation, the stimulatory effect of Fenton's reagent decreased markedly, and that of hydrogen peroxide disappeared completely. Although neither SOD nor indomethacin had any effect on the stimulation by ferrous

---

[a]Address for correspondence: Norman Salem, Jr., Bldg. 10, Room 3C-218, NIH, 9000 Rockville Pike, Bethesda, Maryland 20892.

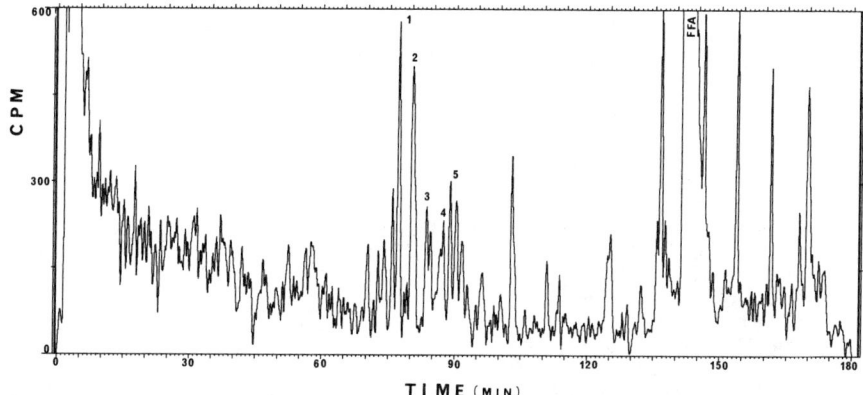

FIGURE 1. Docosahexaenoic acid metabolites produced by ischemic rat brain *in vivo*. The retention times of peaks 1, 2, 3, 4, and 5 corresponded to those of 20-, 17-, 14-, 11-, and 7-hydroxy-docosahexaenoic acids, respectively; the standards were prepared by autooxidation of docosahexaenoic acid and characterized by GC/MS.

iron, Fenton's reagent, or hydrogen peroxide, both NDGA and alpha-tocopherol led to a diminution of the stimulation. On the other hand, mannitol potentiated the hydrogen peroxide–induced stimulation of metabolite formation.

IN VIVO EXPERIMENT

Male spontaneously hypertensive rats (SHR) were lightly anesthetized by chloral hydrate. Both common carotid arteries were occluded by microaneurysm clips, and [^{14}C]-22:6ω3 was injected into the left putamen, using a stereotactic apparatus. Three hours after the occlusion, the rats were decapitated, and the brains were rapidly removed. For the reperfusion study, the clips were removed two hours after the occlusion without anesthesia, and the rats were decapitated one hour after the reperfusion. For the control, rats were sham-operated with respect to the dissection of both common carotid arteries. They were decapitated three hours after the injection of [^{14}C]-22:6ω3 into the left putamen. The brains were homogenized in 100% methanol, and extracts were purified by solid-phase extraction. They were analyzed by reversed-phase HPLC under the same analytical conditions given for the *in vitro* experiment (FIG. 1). Cerebral ischemia stimulated the peroxidation of 22:6ω3 *in vivo* (TABLE 1),

TABLE 1. Effect of Bilateral Carotid Occlusion and Reperfusion on Docosahexaenoic Acid Peroxidation *in Vivo*

Peak No.	3 Hours after Occlusion	1 Hour after Reperfusion
1	142	209
2	241	244
3	188	225
4	222	176
5	131	127

NOTE: Values represent percent change from sham-operated group.

and reperfusion after the ischemia enhanced this stimulatory effect. These results suggest that the peroxidation of 22:6ω3 may have an important role in the pathophysiology of brain injury, since this peroxidation is accompanied by a decrease in tissue pH and iron accumulation.

REFERENCES

1. DEMOPOULOS, H. B. 1973. The basis of free radical pathology. Fed. Proc. **32:** 1859–1861.
2. SALEM, N., JR., H.-Y. KIM & J. A. YERGEY. 1986. Docosahexaenoic acid: Membrane function and metabolism. *In* Health Effects of Polyunsaturated Fatty Acids in Seafoods. A. P. Simopoulos, R. Kifer & R. E. Martin, Eds.: 263–317. Academic Press. New York, NY.
3. SHINGU, T. & N. SALEM, JR. 1987. Role of oxygen radicals in peroxidation of docosahexaenoic acid by rat brain homogenate *in vitro*. *In* Prostaglandin and Lipid Metabolism in Radiation Injury. T. Walden, Jr. & H. N. Hughes, Eds.: 103–108. Plenum. New York, NY.
4. YOSHIDA, S., S. INOH, T. ASANO, K. SANO, M. KUBOTA, H. SHIMAZAKI & N. UETA. 1980. Effect of transient ischemia on free fatty acids and phospholipids in the gerbil brain. Lipid peroxidation as a possible cause of postischemic injury. J. Neurosurg. **53:** 323–331.
5. SIESJÖ, B. K. 1978. Brain Energy Metabolism. John Wiley. New York, NY.
6. SHINGU, T. & N. SALEM, JR. 1986. Mechanism of docosahexaenoic acid oxidation in biological tissue. Trans. Am. Soc. Neurochem. **17:** 193.

Increased 5-HETE Production in the Brain following Head Injury

E. SHOHAMI,[a] Y. SHAPIRA,[b] G. YADID,[a] S. COTEV,[b] AND
G. FEUERSTEIN[c]

Departments of [a]Pharmacology and [b]Anesthesiology
Hebrew University
Hadassah Medical Center
Jerusalem, Israel

[c]Department of Neurology
Uniformed Services University of Health Sciences
Bethesda, Maryland 20814

INTRODUCTION

Edema develops in the brain after various traumatic insults (e.g., ischemia, injury). The chemical mediators of edema formation are not yet identified, and they may differ in the early and late posttraumatic periods. Arachidonate metabolites have been implicated, among other candidates, in the pathological mechanisms leading to increased vascular permeability and edema formation. In a model of closed head injury in rats,[1] edema (measured by microgravimetry) was noted only in the contused hemisphere as early as 15 min after trauma. Edema peaked at 18–24 hours after contusion and gradually returned to normal levels by 7–10 days. The profile of changes in prostaglandin (PG) synthesis was similar—maximal rise in PGE_2 at 18–24 hours and gradual return to normal by 7–10 days.[2] Treatment of traumatized rats with indomethacin or dexamethasone reduced PG synthesis but had no effect on edema development or on the clinical state.[3] Since activation of the 5-lipoxygenase pathway after brain or spinal cord ischemia had been reported previously,[4,5] we attempted to study the activity of several lipoxygenase pathways in the same model of brain contusion in the rat.

MATERIALS AND METHODS

A calibrated weight-drop device was allowed to fall onto the rat skull convexity 1–2 mm lateral (left) from the midline.[1] Edema was determined by measuring tissue specific gravity (SG) in linear gradient columns made of kerosene and bromobenzene and by the dry- to wet-weight ratio. Arachidonic acid metabolism was studied by incubating cortical slices from the injured zone and from the contralateral hemisphere in Krebs-Ringer solution for 1 h at 37 °C. PGs and 5-, 12-, and 15-HETE were determined on aliquots of the incubation medium by radioimmunoassay (RIA) (for PGs, as described,[2] HETES were determined by RIA kits, Seragen).

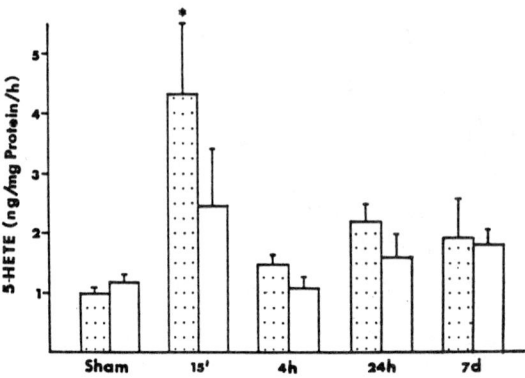

FIGURE 1. The accumulation of 5-HETE during 1-h incubation of cortical slices in oxygenated Krebs-Ringer solution. Slices were taken from the injured (*dotted bars*) and contralateral (*open bars*) hemispheres, at the indicated time after trauma. $* = p < 0.01$ as compared to sham, by ANOVA followed by Student-Newman-Kuel test.

RESULTS AND DISCUSSION

A highly significant increase (400%, $p < 0.01$) of 5-HETE synthesis was found in the injured zone only at 15 min after trauma (FIG. 1). No other HETES were affected, nor did the contralateral hemisphere show any changes in 5-HETE production. By 4 h, 5-HETE synthesis returned to normal, and it remained that way throughout the rest of the experiment.

Some of our earlier findings led us to investigate the lipoxygenase pathway. (1) The *early* (15 min) decrease in SG was not associated with increased PG synthesis (TABLE 1). (2) PG increase occurred in both hemispheres, while edema developed only in the contused one. (3) Inhibition of PG synthesis was not associated with decrease in edema formation.

The present results show that activation of the 5-lipoxygenase pathway after head trauma occurs as early as edema is noticed, and only at the site where SG is reduced. It may therefore have a role in the *early* phase of edema formation after trauma. At the *later* time point, other arachidonate metabolites (PGI_2, PGE_2, and/or leukotrienes) as well as other mediators may be involved in the pathophysiology of edema.

TABLE 1. Specific Gravity, Water Content, and PG Release from Cortical Slices Taken from the Injured Zone of the Contused Hemisphere

	Sham	15 min	1 h	18 h	4 days	10 days
SG	1.04345	1.04258	1.04263	1.03800	1.03985	1.04395
	± 0.00047	± 0.00029^a	± 0.00041^a	± 0.00223^a	± 0.00152^a	± 0.00283
% H_2O	78.52	80.31	79.64	82.27	80.52	78.85
	± 0.12	± 0.45^a	± 0.32^a	± 0.55^a	± 0.64^a	± 0.27
PGE_2[b]	390	365	382	2360	1250	398
	± 45	± 50	± 43	± 450^a	± 215^a	± 45
6-keto-$PGF_{1\alpha}$[b]	215	460	470	400	480	280
	± 32	± 108	± 65^a	± 78	± 160	± 55
TXB_2[b]	260	380	460	280	205	370
	± 50	± 135	± 160	± 75	± 48	± 90

NOTE: Data are means ± SEM; $n = 8$–10 per group. SG = specific gravity.
$^a p < 0.05$ vs. sham.
^{b}Figures are pg/mg protein/h.

REFERENCES

1. SHAPIRA, Y., E. SHOHAMI, A. SIDI, D. SOFFER, S. FREEMAN & S. COTEV. 1988. Crit. Care Med. **16:** 258–265.
2. SHOHAMI, E., Y. SHAPIRA, A. SIDI & S. COTEV. 1987. J. Cereb. Blood Flow Metab. **7:** 58–63.
3. SHAPIRA, Y., E. DAVIDSON, Y. WEIDENFELD, S. COTEV & E. SHOHAMI. 1988. J. Cereb. Blood Flow Metab. **8:**395–402.
4. USUY, M., T. ASANO & K. TAKAKURA. 1987. Stroke **18:** 490–494.
5. SHOHAMI, E., T. P. JACOBS, J. M. HALLENBECK & G. FEUERSTEIN. 1987. Prostaglandins, Leukotrienes and Medicine **28:**169–181.

The Early Effect of Steroidal and Nonsteroidal Antiinflammatory Agents on Neoplastic Epidural Cord Compression

T. SIEGAL,[a,b,c] Tz. SIEGAL,[d] Y. SHAPIRA,[e]
AND E. SHOHAMI[f]

*Departments of [b]Oncology, [c]Neurology, [e]Anaesthesiology,
and [f]Pharmacology
Haddasah University Hospital
and Hebrew University Medical School
Jerusalem, Israel*

*[d]Assuta Hospital
Tel Aviv, Israel*

The purpose of immediate pharmacological intervention in neoplastic spinal cord compression is to halt or delay functional deterioration and allow time for definitive treatment (surgery or radiotherapy) to take place. In paraplegic rats harboring a thoracolumbar epidural tumor we demonstrated a consistent increase in the water content, prostaglandin E2 (PGE2) synthesis, and specific gravity in the compressed cord segments and found them to be targets amenable to pharmacological manipulations.[1,2] The *in vivo* effect of treatment given at the onset of paraplegia with either dexamethasone–sodium phosphate (Dex-p), methylprednisolone–sodium succinate (MP), or indomethacin (INDO) was evaluated after 30 hours of treatment. Tumor-free and tumor-bearing rats were randomized for 3 treatments every 12 hours with 0.4 ml of either sterile saline ($n = 30$), Dex-p (10 mg/kg; $n = 20$), MP (30 mg/kg; $n = 20$), or INDO (10 mg/kg; $n = 20$) and were sacrificed by decapitation 4 hours after the last dose. Following decapitation the cervical (C2-T1) and lumbar (T13-L3) segments were rapidly removed by laminectomy and cut randomly to 3 pieces that were processed for evaluation of water content (by the drying-weighing technique), of specific gravity and of PGE2 synthesis, as previously described.[1] The cervical segments were used as an internal reference control based on previous observations.[1,2] The results of measurements in the cervical and the compressed lumbar areas in each treatment group of normal controls and paraplegic rats are presented in FIGURES 1 and 2. After 30 hours of treatment only INDO reversed all elevated levels (water content, PGE2, and specific gravity) back to normal. Dex-p did correct the elevated specific gravity but failed to affect the increased water content or PGE2 synthesis. MP eliminated the edema and partially reduced PGE2 production but had no effect on the specific gravity.

In keeping with the known role of PGE2 as a mediator of inflammation and edema formation,[3] a rapid antiedematous effect was achieved in this study only when partial or marked reduction of PGE2 production was accomplished by MP or INDO, respectively. Both MP and INDO were equally effective in reducing spinal cord

---

[a]Address for correspondence: Tali Siegal, M.D., Department of Oncology, Haddasah University Hospital, POB 12000, Jerusalem 91120, Israel.

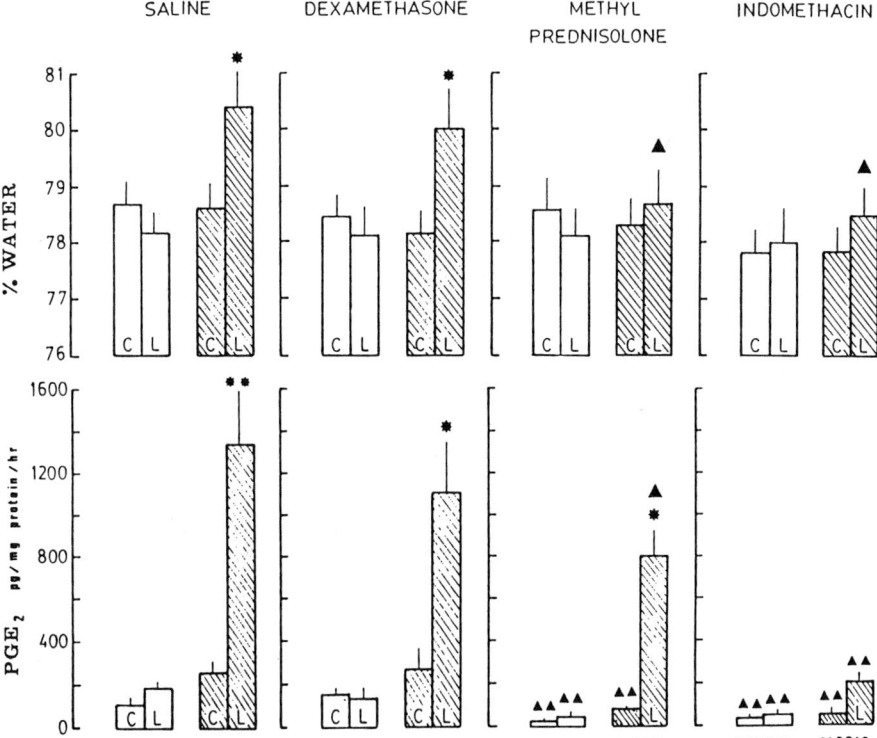

FIGURE 1. Spinal cord water content and prostaglandin E2 (PGE2) production (mean ± SEM) in the cervical (C) and lumbar (L) segments of tumor-free and tumor-bearing paraplegic (plegic) rats evaluated after 30 hours of treatment. Animals were randomized for 3 treatments at 12-hour intervals with 0.4 ml of either sterile saline (controls), dexamethasone–sodium phosphate (10 mg/kg, methylprednisolone–sodium succinate (30 mg/kg), or indomethacin (10 mg/kg). Treatment was started on the day tumor-bearing animals were graded as paraplegic. Saline-treated groups: $n = 30$; treatment groups: $n = 20$. Cervical values served as internal controls. Statistical significance was assessed by a mixed-model ANOVA. *: $p < 0.004$, **: $p < 0.0002$, compared to cervical; ▲: $p < 0.009$, ▲▲: $p < 0.0002$ compared to saline controls.

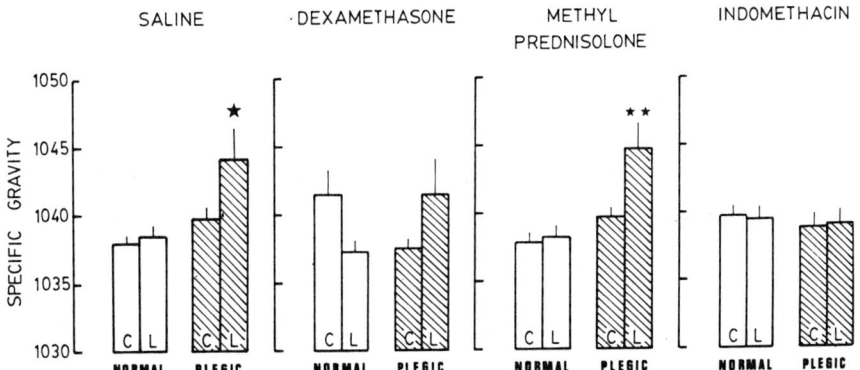

FIGURE 2. Specific gravity (mean ± SEM) of the cervical (C) and lumbar (L) spinal cord segments in tumor-free and tumor-bearing paraplegic rats evaluated after 30 hours of treatment. Animals were randomized for 3 treatments at 12-hour intervals with 0.4 ml of either sterile saline (controls), dexamethasone–sodium phosphate (10 mg/kg), methylprednisolone–sodium succinate (30 mg/kg), or indomethacin (10 mg/kg). Treatment was started on the day tumor-bearing rats were graded as paraplegic. Saline-treated groups: $n = 30$; treatment groups: $n = 20$. Cervical values served as internal controls. Statistical significance was assessed by a mixed-model ANOVA. ★: $p < 0.04$, ★★: $p < 0.01$, compared to cervical.

edema, while Dex-p failed to inhibit PGE2 production after 30 hours of treatment and proved ineffective for early control of spinal cord edema. However, it is the specific gravity that has been shown to be a sensitive measure of complex tissue abnormalities.[1,2] Specific gravity may prove to be a more accurate representation than tissue edema (water content) of a favorable effect of pharmacological intervention.

REFERENCES

1. SIEGAL, T., TZ. SIEGAL, U. SANDBANK, *et al.* 1987. Experimental neoplastic spinal cord compression: Evoked potentials, edema, prostaglandins, and light and electron microscopy. Spine **12:** 440–448.
2. SIEGAL, T., TZ. SIEGAL, Y. SHAPIRA, *et al.* 1988 Indomethacin and dexamethasone treatment in experimental neoplastic spinal cord compression. Part I: Effect on water content and specific gravity. Neurosurgery. **22:** 328-333.
3. JOHNSON, M., F. CAREY & R. M. MCMILLAN. 1983. Alternative pathways of arachidonate metabolism: Prostaglandins, thromboxane and leukotrienes. Essays Biochem. **19:** 41–141.

Primary Structure of Rat Brain Prostaglandin D Synthetase Deduced from the cDNA Sequence

YOSHIHIRO URADE,[a] AKIHISA NAGATA,[b]
YASUHIKO SUZUKI,[b] YUTAKA FUJII,[c]
AND OSAMU HAYAISHI[a]

[a]*Department of Enzymes and Metabolism*
Osaka Bioscience Institute
Suita 565, Japan

[b]*Research Institute for Microbial Diseases*
Osaka University
Suita 565, Japan

[c]*Hayaishi Bioinformation Transfer Project*
Research Development Corporation of Japan
Kyoto 601, Japan

Prostaglandin (PG) D_2 is a major PG produced in the brain of rats and humans. It shows several central actions, such as induction of hypothermia and sleep, and modulation of pain response.

In a previous study, we purified PGD synthetase (prostaglandin H_2 D-isomerase, EC 5.3.99.2) from the rat brain and characterized its molecular and catalytic properties.[1] Furthermore, we found that this enzyme showed unique developmental changes in both its activity[2] and its cellular distribution.[3,4] The PGD synthetase activity is at its highest 1 to 2 weeks after birth, during the period of neural differentiation and early synaptogenesis. At this age, the immunoreactivity of this enzyme is distributed in many neurons. In mature animals, however, the activity decreases to about 50% of that in infant rats, and the immunohistochemical localization of the enzyme shifts mainly to oligodendrocytes.

In this study, we isolated cDNA clones specific for rat brain PGD synthetase from a λgt-11 rat brain cDNA expression library (FIG. 1), and determined the primary structure of this enzyme by a combination of cDNA and protein sequencing (FIG. 2).

Nucleotide sequence analyses of cloned cDNA inserts revealed that this enzyme consisted of a 564-base pair open reading frame coding for a 188-amino acid polypeptide with a M_r of 21,232. About 60% of the deduced amino acid sequence was confirmed by partial amino acid sequencing of tryptic peptides of the purified enzyme.

The recognition sequence for N-glycosylation was seen at two positions of amino acid residues 51–53 and 78–80. Both sites were considered to be N-glycosylated, since two smaller proteins were found during deglycosylation of the purified enzyme with N-glycanase.

The amino acid composition of the purified enzyme indicated that about 20 residues of hydrophobic amino acids of the N-terminus are posttranslationally deleted, probably as a signal peptide.

In Northern blot analysis using an insert from λDS-4 without poly(A) as a probe, a single positive band was seen in the transcripts from the brain and spinal cord at the

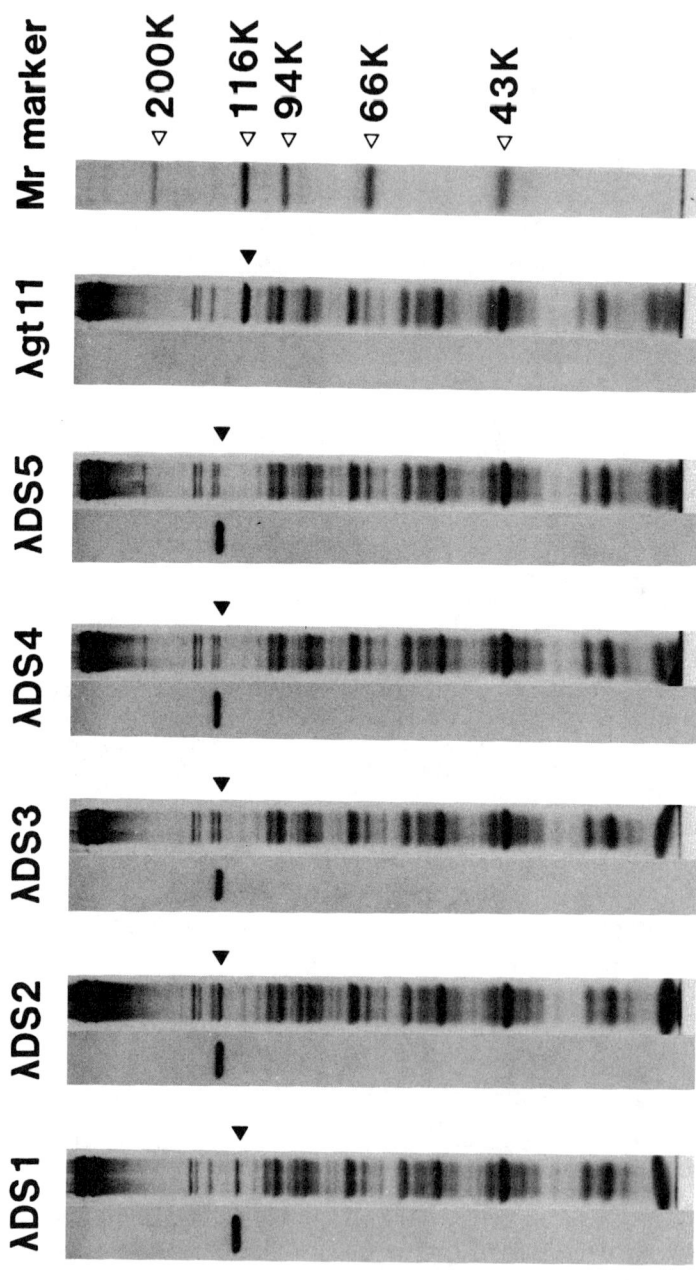

FIGURE 1. Immunoblotting analysis of crude lysates from λgt 11 recombinant lysogens. The lysates from the recombinant lysogens with λDS1-5 and λgt 11 itself were subjected to SDS-PAGE (7.5% gel). After electrophoresis, the protein bands were silver-stained (each *right lane*) or immunostained with antibody (IgG) specific for rat brain PGD synthetase (each *left lane*). The position of each fusion protein is indicated by a *closed arrow head*. The positions of marker proteins (*open arrow heads*) and their Mr values are indicated on the right: myosin (200,000), β-galactosidase (116,000), phosphorylase b (94,000), bovine serum albumin (66,000), ovalbumin (43,000).

```
                                          1                                    34
                               5'--  CCUC AGGCUCAGAC ACCUGCUCUA CUCCAAGCAA

          AUG GCU GCU CUU CCA AUG CUG UGG ACC GGG CUG GUC CUC UUG GGU CUC UUG GGA UUU CCA
          Met Ala Ala Leu Pro Met Leu Trp Thr Gly Leu Val Leu Leu Gly Leu Leu Gly Phe Pro
            1
                      100
          CAG ACC CCA GCC CAG GGC CAU GAC ACA GUG CAG CCC AAC UUU CAA CAA GAC AAG UUC CUG
          Gln Thr Pro Ala Gln Gly His Asp Thr Val Gln Pro Asn Phe Gln Gln Asp Lys Phe Leu
                                                                                 ———  ———
                                                          200
          GGG CGC UGG UAC AGC GCG GGC CUC GCC UCC AAU UCA AGC UGG UUC CGG GAG AAG AAA GAG
          Gly Arg Trp Tyr Ser Ala Gly Leu Ala Ser Asn Ser Ser Trp Phe Arg Glu Lys Lys Glu
              ——— ——— ——— ——— ——— ——— ———      50  ...  ...  ...                     ———

          CUA CUG UUU AUG UGC CAG ACA GUG GUA GCU CCC UCC ACA GAA GGC GGC CUC AAC CUC ACC
          Leu Leu Phe Met Cys Gln Thr Val Val Ala Pro Ser Thr Glu Gly Gly Leu Asn Leu Thr
                      ———                                                     ——— ——— ———
                                 300
          UCU ACC UUC CUA AGG AAA AAC CAG UGU GAG ACC AAG GUG AUG GUA CUG CAG CCG GCA GGG
          Ser Thr Phe Leu Arg Lys Asn Gln Cys Glu Thr Lys Val Met Val Leu Gln Pro Ala Gly
          ——— ——— ——— ——— ———                          ——— ——— ——— ——— ——— ——— ——— ———
                                                                                     100
          GUU CCC GGA CAG UAC ACC UAC AAC AGC CCC CAC UGG CAG CUU CCA CCU CUC AGU GUA
          Val Pro Gly Gln Tyr Thr Tyr Asn Ser Pro His Trp Gln Leu Pro Leu Pro Leu Ser Val
          ——— ——— ——— ——— ——— ———
                      400
          GAA ACC GAC UAC GAU GAG UAC GCG UUC CUG UUC AGC AAG CGG ACC AAG GGC CCA GGC CAG
          Glu Thr Asp Tyr Asp Glu Tyr Ala Phe Leu Phe Ser Lys Arg Thr Lys Gly Pro Gly Gln
                                                                          ——— ——— ——— ———
                                                         500
          GAC UUC CGC AUG GCC ACC CUC UAC AGC AGA GCC CAG CUU CUG AAG GAG GAA CUG AAG GAG
          Asp Phe Arg Met Ala Thr Leu Tyr Ser Arg Ala Gln Leu Leu Lys Glu Glu Leu Lys Glu
          ——— ——— ——— ——— ——— ——— ——— ———
                                              150
          AAA UUC AUC ACC UUU AGC AAG GAC CAG GGC CUC ACA GAG GAG GAC AUU GUU UUC CUG CCC
          Lys Phe Ile Thr Phe Ser Lys Asp Gln Gly Leu Thr Glu Glu Asp Ile Val Phe Leu Pro
          ——— ——— ——— ——— ——— ——— ——— ———
                                               600
          CAA CCG GAU AAG UGC AUU CAA GAG UAA ACACAGGUGA GAGAAGUCAG UCACAGGUAA CACAUGGUGA
          Gln Pro Asp Lys Cys Ile Gln Glu ***
          ——— ——— ——— ———          188
                                                                                       700
          UGUGGCCUCA GGACUCCCGU GCUCUGUCAC UCUUGAGACC CAAGCCCUGG CUCCCCAAAG ACCUUCUCCG

                                              756
          CCCUCCAGCU UUGCCUUGGU GGAGAAAUAA AAUCCAAAGC AAGUC(A)n --3'
```

FIGURE 2. Primary structure of rat brain PGD synthetase mRNA. The nucleotide sequence was deduced from that of the cDNA inserts (λDS-1-5). The predicted amino acid sequence of this enzyme is displayed below the nucleotide sequence. Nucleotide residues are numbered in the 5' to 3' direction, and amino acid residues are in the N to C direction, beginning with the first Met as the initiation site. The site of predicted polyadenylation sequence (AAUAAA) is underlined. The underlined amino acids are confirmed by automated Edman degradation of trypsin-digested peptides. The recognition sequences for N-glycosylation (Asn-X-Ser/Thr) are indicated by a *dotted line*.

same position of ca.850 bases, indicating that most of the nucleotide sequence of mRNA for this enzyme has been determined (the longest sequence is 756 bases plus ca.90-bases of poly(A)).

These results, together with the immunocytochemical localization of this enzyme to rough-surfaced endoplasmic reticulum and outer nuclear membrane of oligodendrocytes,[4] suggest that this enzyme is a membrane-associated protein.

REFERENCES

1. URADE, Y., N. FUJIMOTO & O. HAYAISHI. 1985. J. Biol. Chem. **260:** 12410–12415.
2. UENO, R., H. OSAMA, Y. URADE & O. HAYAISHI. 1985. J. Neurochem. **45:** 483–489.
3. URADE, Y., T. KANEKO, N. FUJIMOTO, Y. WATANABE, N. MIZUNO & O. HAYAISHI. 1985. Adv. Prostaglandin Thromboxane Leukotriene Res. **15:** 549–551.
4. URADE, Y., N. FUJIMOTO, T. KANEKO, A. KONISHI, N. MIZUNO & O. HAYAISHI. 1987. J. Biol. Chem. **262:** 15132–15136.

Functional-Site Study of Prostaglandins in the Monkey Brain Using Quantitative Autoradiography and Positron Emission Tomography

Y. WATANABE,[a,b] B. LÅNGSTRÖM,[c] Y. WATANABE,[a]
K. HAMADA,[a] P-G. GILLBERG,[d] C-G. STÅLNACKE,[e]
M. HATANAKA,[a] H. HAYASHI,[a] AND O. HAYAISHI[a]

[a]*Hayaishi Bioinformation Transfer Project*
Research Development Corporation of Japan
Kyoto 601, Japan

[b]*Department of Neuroscience*
Osaka Bioscience Institute
Osaka 565, Japan

[c]*Department of Organic Chemistry,*
[d]*Academic Hospital, and* [e]*Agricultural Institute*
Uppsala University
Uppsala, Sweden

The functional sites of prostaglandins (PG) in the brain were investigated by quantitative autoradiographic localization of PG receptors and by positron emission tomography (PET) studies.

Monkey brain sections of 10-μm thickness were incubated with 20 nM [^{3}H]PG in the absence or presence of 100 μM PG at 4 °C for 30 min. Autoradiographs were analyzed using a drum-scanning densitometer and image processing system with [^{3}H]microscales as standards. The specific bindings for [^{3}H]PGD$_2$, [^{3}H]PGE$_2$, and [^{3}H]PGF$_{2\alpha}$ were distinctly localized in the nucleus level, and high density was observed in the specific brain regions, as shown in TABLE 1.[1-3] The study in combination with the neurophysiological experiments revealed close relationships between the localization of PG receptors and the known functions of PGs, and also such novel roles as the modulation of PGD$_2$ of the olfactory stimulus-response (TABLE 2).[4]

To extend the study on the localization of PG systems to the higher brain functions or to dynamic aspects, we employed PET technique by using [^{11}C]methyl esters (Me) of PGD$_2$, 9β-PGD$_2$, and total enantiomer of PGD$_2$. The latter two compounds showed little affinity to brain PGD$_2$ binding sites by autoradiography with PGD$_2$-[^{3}H]Me and [^{3}H]stereoisomers and therefore were used as a control for regional blood flow and nonspecific brain uptake. The uptake value of PGD$_2$-[^{11}C]methyl ester into the rhesus brain was about two-fold higher than those of the controls. This difference could be due to the difference in the binding capacities of PGD$_2$-[^{11}C]methyl ester and its stereoisomers, because such a tracer dose of PGD$_2$-Me did not affect any circulatory parameters in the rhesus monkey.

TABLE 1. Summary of Autoradiographic Localization of PGD_2, PGE_2, and $PGF_{2\alpha}$ Binding Sites in *Macaca fuscata* Diencephalon

Brain Region	PGD_2	PGE_2	$PGF_{2\alpha}$
Preoptic area	lat. preop. area	median preop. area med. preop. area	
Hypothalamus	suprachiasmatic n. ant. hypo. n. med. hypo. area dors. hypo. area ventromedial n. mammillaly n. subthalamic n.	med. hypo. area dors. hypo. area lat. hypo. area dorsomedial n. supramammillary n. infundibular n.	supraoptic n. paraventricular n.
Thalamus	anterior n. dorsolateral n. post. lateral n.	anteroventral n. dorsolateral n. centromedian n. paraventricular n. periventricular n. habenular n.	

ABBREVIATIONS: lat., lateral; med., medial; ant., anterior; post., posterior; dors., dorsal; hypo., hypothalamic.

TABLE 2. Correlations between Receptor Localization and Central Action of Prostaglandins

PGs	Localization	Action
PGD_2	mitral cell layer of olfactory bulb	modification of olfactory stimulus-response
	preoptic area	sleep induction
	"	reduction of body temperature
	arcuate nucleus of hypothalamus	inhibition of LHRH release
	suprachiasmatic nucleus of hypothalamus	sleep induction (modification of biorhythm)
	central gray of midbrain	biphasic effects of pain senses
	Purkinje cell layer of cerebellum	modification of GABA, taurine, Glu, Asp action
	substantia gelatinosa of spinal cord	biphasic effects of pain senses
PGE_2	median and medial preoptic area	hyperthermia
	median eminence of hypothalamus	enhancement of LHRH release
	lateral hypothalamic area	anorexia
	substantia gelatinosa of spinal cord	biphasic effects of pain senses
$PGF_{2\alpha}$	paraventricular nucleus & supraoptic nucleus of hypothalamus	enhancement of vasopressin and oxytocin release

REFERENCES

1. WATANABE, Y., Y. WATANABE, T. KANEKO & O. HAYAISHI. 1985. Adv. Prostaglandin, Thromboxane, Leukotriene Res. **15**: 553–554.
2. WATANABE, Y., Y. WATANABE & O. HAYAISHI. 1986. *In* Biomedical Imaging. O. Hayaishi & K. Torizuka, Eds.: 227–238. Academic Press. New York, NY.
3. WATANABE, Y., Y. WATANABE & O. HAYAISHI. 1988. J. Neurosci. **8**(6): 2003–2010.
4. WATANABE, Y., K. MORI, K. IMAMURA, S. F. TAKAGI, & O. HAYAISHI 1986. Brain Res. **378**(1): 216–222.
5. WATANABE, Y., B. LÅNGSTRÖM, C.G. STÅLNACKE, P. GULLBERG, H. SVÄRD, C. HALLDIN & O. HAYAISHI. 1987. Adv. Prostaglandin, Thromboxane, Leukotriene Res. **17**: 939–941.
6. GULLBERG, P., Y. WATANABE, H. SVÄRD, O. HAYAISHI & B. LÅNGSTRÖM. 1987. Appl. Radiat. Isot. **38**(8): 647–649.

Prostaglandins in Human Cerebrospinal Fluid?

JAMES A. YERGEY, NORMAN SALEM, JR.,
JOHN W. KARANIAN, AND MARKKU LINNOILA

*Laboratory of Clinical Studies
Division of Intramural Clinical and Biological Research
National Institute on Alcohol Abuse and Alcoholism
Bethesda, Maryland 20892*

MELVYN P. HEYES

*Laboratory of Neurophysiology
National Institute of Mental Health
Bethesda, Maryland 28092*

INTRODUCTION

The ability of central nervous system tissue to produce prostaglandins (PG) *in vitro* has been known for quite some time, and numerous brain functions have been associated with the PG. It has been assumed that the presence of PG in cerebrospinal fluid (CSF) is indicative of their production in the brain, although there have been disparate results for PG concentrations in the CSF of healthy human volunteers. Values in the literature range from undetectable (e.g., <10 pg/mL CSF) to as much as 1 ng/mL CSF. We have measured PG concentrations in lumbar CSF of healthy human volunteers, in cisternal CSF of rhesus monkeys, and in continuously sampled lumbar CSF of awake rhesus monkeys.

ASSAY

CSF samples were drawn on ice, and exactly 2.0 mL was transferred to a tube containing deuterated internal standards ($^2H_4$-PGE$_2$, $^2H_4$-PGF$_{2\alpha}$, and $^2H_4$-6-keto-PGF$_{1\alpha}$). Samples were then frozen and stored at -70 °C. Indomethacin was found to be unnecessary during sampling. Its contamination of the GC/MS determination was thus eliminated. Thawed samples were treated with 1% MOX-HCL in phosphate buffer at pH 5 overnight to produce the methoxime derivative of the ketone containing PG. Aqueous oximation avoided the use of pyridine and allowed methoximation by-products to be separated from PG during extraction. Solid-phase extraction using C18 cartridges was accomplished by applying the aqueous sample to conditioned columns, rinsing with 80:20 water:methanol, drying the column completely with vacuum, rinsing with dichloromethane, and eluting the sample with methanol. The dried sample was then derivatized sequentially to the pentafluorobenzyl ester (0.1% PFBB, 10% diisopropylethylamine in acetonitrile, 60 °C for 15 min), trimethylsilyl ether (50:50 BSTFA:acetonitrile, 60 °C for 15 min). Using 100-fold less pentafluorobenzyl bromide during esterification greatly reduced electron capturing contaminants. Dried samples were dissolved in 10 μL dodecane, 2 μL were injected on-column for the selected-ion-monitoring, negative chemical ionization GC/MS detection and quantifi-

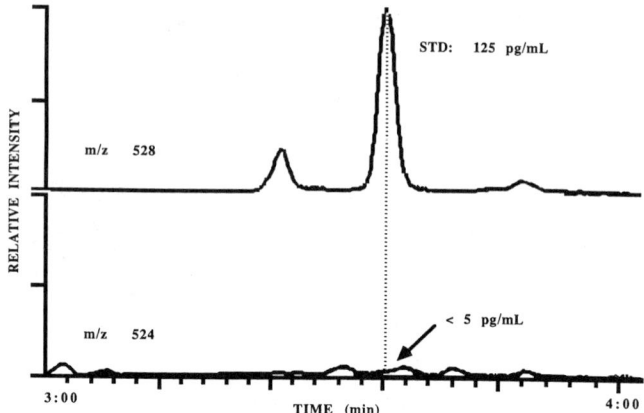

FIGURE 1. GC/MS selected-ion-monitoring trace for prostaglandin E_2 (m/z 524) and its tetradeuterated internal standard (m/z 528) in human CSF.

cation of the MO-PFB-TMS derivative of prostaglandins $E_2, E_1, F_{2\alpha}, F_{1\alpha}$, and 6-keto-$F_{1\alpha}$. Using dodecane as the final solvent reduced the GC/MS cycle time to less than 7 min/sample (RT < 4 min).

DISCUSSION

In contrast to most reports in the literature, our results clearly indicate that CSF from healthy human volunteers contains extremely low concentrations of PG (less than 5 pg/mL). These data have been confirmed by comparisons in our laboratory of human

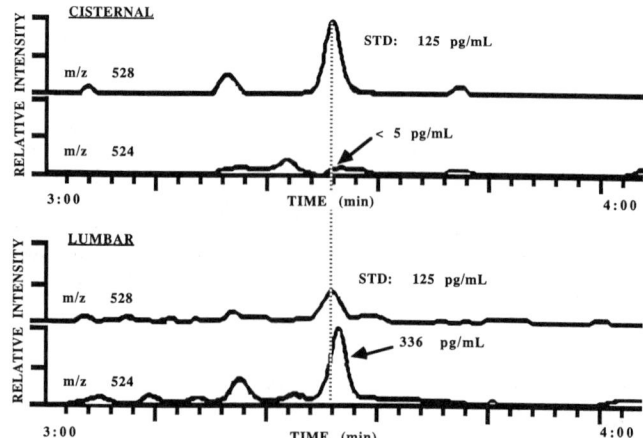

FIGURE 2. GC/MS selected-ion-monitoring trace for prostaglandin E_2 (m/z 524) and its tetradeuterated internal standard (m/z 528) in cisternal and lumbar CSF of rhesus monkeys.

CSF assayed by both GC/MS and radioimmunoassay. Furthermore, continuously sampled monkey CSF contains measurable concentrations of PGE_2, $PGF_{2\alpha}$, and 6-keto-$PGF_{1\alpha}$ (>100 pg/mL), but acutely sampled monkey CSF is similar to human CSF in having immeasurable concentrations of PG. An example of these data for PGE_2 is seen in FIGURES 1 and 2. The very low PG concentrations found in healthy human CSF are conceivably the result of low brain synthesis rates or the result of transport phenomena that limit the bulk CSF concentration.

Inhibition of [1-^{14}C] Arachidonate Incorporation into Synaptosomal Phospholipids by Lipid Peroxides

MALGORZATA M. ZALESKA AND DAVID F. WILSON

Department of Biochemistry and Biophysics
University of Pennsylvania Medical School
Philadelphia, Pennsylvania 19104

It is now well established that the pool of free fatty acids (FA), which are normally present in trace amounts in the brain, increases dramatically through deacylation of phospholipids in various pathological conditions such as ischemia, hypoxia, and hypoglycemia.[1,2] Accumulation of free fatty acids has been implicated in the mechanism(s) generating edema and irreversible funtional damage in ischemic injury.[3,4] It is frequently hypothesized that oxygen contributes to progressive injury occurring in the postischemic reperfusion period, since reoxygenation of the tissues may lead to extensive peroxidation of unsaturated fatty acids and peroxides may both induce further free radical generation and interfere with the repair processes.[3,5,6] The object of this *in vitro* study was to establish whether fatty acid hydroperoxides affect the reacylation of membrane phospholipids in isolated brain nerve ending fraction.

METHODS

Arachidonic (AA) and linoleic acid hydroperoxides (20:4 HPx and 18:2 HPx, respectively) were prepared enzymatically and purified by TLC. Synaptosomes from the rat forebrain were incubated in media adopted from Corbin and Sun:[5] 2.5 mM ATP, 0.1 mM CoA, 0.2 mM DTT, 10 mM MgCl$_2$, 10 mM glucose, 1.27 mM CaCl$_2$, trace amounts of lyso-phospholipids and 0.1 μCi of [1-^{14}C] AA (1.8μM) in Krebs-Henseleit buffer, pH 7.4 for up to 20 min at 37 °C in the presence or absence of hydroperoxides. The reactions were stopped, lipids extracted, the phospholipid fraction separated by TLC, and the radioactivity of appropriate bands counted.

RESULTS AND DISCUSSION

In control incubations there was rapid incorporation of labeled AA into synaptosomal phospholipids with about 20% of the added AA incorporated within 20 min. Addition of either fatty acid hydroperoxide resulted in a concentration-dependent inhibition of AA incorporation (FIG. 1). Approximately 50% inhibition was observed at 20 μM 18:2 HPx and at 30 μM 20:4 HPx. Complete inhibition took place at about 100 μM of either compound. The inhibition was of the noncompetitive type with respect to AA and resulted in a 45% decrease in Vmax, with no effect on the Km value. In the absence of exogenous lyso-phospholipids as acceptors, the incorporation of ^{14}C-AA into synaptosomal phospholipids was significantly lower. However, the degree of inhibition by the fatty acid peroxides remained unaltered.

FIGURE 1. Inhibition of [1-^{14}C]arachidonate incorporation into synaptosomal phospholipids by fatty acid hydroperoxides. Synaptosomes (0.3–0.5 mg protein) were incubated for 20 min at 37 °C in the presence of different concentrations of hydroperoxides. Values are means ± SEM for 3–6 experiments.

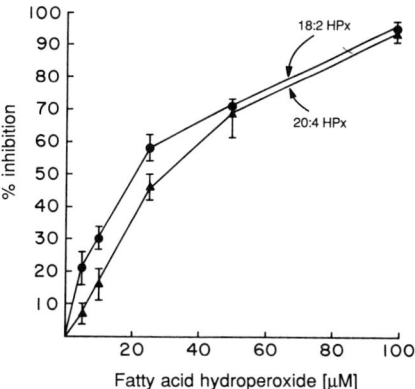

This study demonstrates that low concentrations of fatty acid hydroperoxides directly inhibit the reacylation of synaptosomal phospholipids. This phenomenon may play a significant role in the well-documented decreased ability of postischemic nervous tissue to reacylate membrane phospholipids.[7–9] The decreased capacity for removing free FA and for phospholipid repair may constitute an important mechanism whereby peroxidative events contribute to irreversible brain damage in ischemia.

REFERENCES

1. BAZAN, N. G. 1970. Effect of ischemia and electroconvulsive shock on free fatty acid pool in the rat. Biochem. Biophys. Acta **218**: 1–10.
2. RODRIGUEZ DE TURCO, E. B., G. D. CASCONE, M. F. PEDICONI & N. G. BAZAN. 1977. Phosphatidate, phosphatidylinositol, diacylglycerols and free fatty acids in the brain following electroshock, anoxia or ischemia. Adv. Exp. Med. Biol. **83**: 389–396.
3. CHAN, P. H. & R. A. FISHMAN. 1978. Brain edema: Induction in cortical slices by polyunsaturated fatty acids. Science **201**: 358–360.
4. FISHMAN, R. A. & P. H. CHAN. 1981. Hypothesis: Membrane phospholipid degradation and polyunsaturated fatty acids play a key role in the pathogenesis of brain edema. Ann. Neurol. **10**: 75.
5. CORBIN, D. R. & G. Y. SUN. 1978. Characterization of the enzymatic transfer of arachidonoyl groups to 1-acyl-phosphoglicerides in mouse synaptosome fraction. J. Neurochem. **30**: 77–82.
6. WATSON, B. D., R. BUSTO, W. J. GOLDBERG, M. SANTISO, S. YOSHIDA & M. D. GINSBERG. 1984. Lipid peroxidation in vivo induced by reversible global ischemia in rat brain. J. Neurochem. **42**: 268–274.
7. FOUDIN, L., J. STROSZNAJDER & G. Y. SUN. 1983. Effect of ischemia and severe hypoxia on arachidonic acid uptake by rat brain membranes. Neurochem. Pathol. **1**: 163–170.
8. PEDICONI, M. F., E. B. RODRIGUEZ DE TURCO & N. G. BAZAN. 1983. Effect of postdecapitation ischemia on the metabolism of [^{14}C] arachidonic acid and [^{14}C] palmitic acid in the mouse brain. Neurochem. Res. **8**: 835–845.
9. STROSZNAJDER, J. & G. Y. SUN. 1981. Effect of acute hypoxia on incorporation of [^{14}C] arachidonic acid into glycero-lipids of rat brain. Neurochem. Res. **6**: 767–774.

Index of Contributors

Abe, K., 259–268
Agardh, C.-D., 323–339

Baer, S. C., 424–426
Barkai, A. I., 56–73
Bazan, N. G., 1–16, 296–312, 340–351, 468–470
Beckman, J. S., 282–295
Bengtsson, F., 323–339
Bertazzo, A., 352–364
Bommelaer-Bayet, M. C., 100–111
Braquet, P., 296–312, 340–351, 468–470
Buchanan, D. C., 427–428

Capdevila, J., 192–207
Carbonetto, S. T., 429–430
Chan, P. H., 237–247
Chao, J., 282–295
Chen, S., 237–247
Chu, L., 237–247
Claesson, H.-E., 112–120
Cohan, S. L., 465–467
Cotev, S., 485–487
Coyle, J., 474–477
Crouch, M. F., 153–157

DeGeorge, J. J., 429–430
Demediuk, P., 431–432, 433–434
Demerle, C., 296–312
Djuričić, B. M., 435–437
Dorman, R. V., 438–440
Dray, F., 100–111

Eguchi, N., 451–452
Elmer, G. I., 441–443

Faden, A. I., 431–432, 433–434
Farooqui, A. A., 25–36
Feinmark, S. J., 121–130, 208–218
Feuerstein, G., 313–322, 485–487
Figard, P. H., 471–473
Fishman, R. A., 237–247
Freeman, B. A., 282–295
Fujii, Y., 491–493
Fulle, I., 444–448

Gaetani, P., 444–448
Gaiti, A., 365–373
Galli, C., 352–364
George, F. R., 382–391, 441–443, 449–450
Gerozissis, K., 100–111

Gillberg, P.-G., 494–496
Ginsberg, M. D., 269–281
Goetz, K., 411–423
Goldin, E. 248–258
Grotta, J. C., 478–479
Gustafsson, L. E., 178–191

Hamada, K., 494–496
Harel, S., 248–258
Hart, M. N., 471–473
Hatanaka, M., 494–496
Hayaishi, O., 374–381, 451–452, 453–454, 491–493, 494–496
Hayashi, H., 451–452, 453–454, 494–496
Hertting, G., 84–99
Heyes, M. P., 497–499
Hillered, L., 237–247
Hogan, E. L., 282–295
Horrocks, L. A., 17–24, 25–36
Hosford, D., 296–312
Hsu, C. Y., 282–295

Imaizumi, S., 237–247
Ito, S., 451–452, 453–454
Izzo, N. J., 455–456

Jelsema, C. L., 158–177
Johns, R. A., 455–456
Junier, M. P., 100–111, 192–207

Karanian, J. W., 457–458, 459–461, 482–484, 497–499
Karnushina, I., 112–120
Kim, H.-Y., 457–458, 459–461, 482–484
Kim, S. J., 461–464
Kochanek, P. M., 427–428
Kogure, K., 259–268
Kostić, V. S., 435–437

Långström, B., 494–496
Lapetina, E. G., 153–157
Lindgren, J. Å., 112–120
Linnoila, M., 497–499
Liu, T. H., 282–295
Loeb, A. L., 455–456
Lombardi, D., 444–448
Longar, S., 237–247
Lubitz, D. v., 465–467

MacQuarrie, R. A., 37–55
Magal, E., 248–258

503

Marcheselli, V. L., 296–312, 340–351, 468–470
Marzatico, F., 444–448
McGee, R., 480–481
McIntosh, T. K., 431–432
Melick, J. A., 427–428
Milner, P. J., 455–456
Milton, A. S., 392–410
Misra, L. K., 478–479
Moore, K., 237–247
Moore, S. A., 471–473
Mršulja, B. B., 435–437
Murphy, T., 474–477
Murthy, L. R., 56–73

Nagata, A., 491–493
Narayana, P. A., 478–479
Negishi, M., 453–454
Nemoto, E. M., 427–428

Ojeda, S. R., 192–207

Panetta, T., 340–351, 468–470
Parikh, A., 474–477
Peach, M. J., 455–456
Pellerin, L., 74–83
Pereira, B., 237–247
Petroni, A., 352–364
Pettigrew, L. C., 478–479
Piomelli, D., 121–130, 208–218

Rammohan, K. W., 25–36
Redmond, D. J., 465–467
Rodriguez y Baena, R., 444–448
Romhanyi, R., 431–432
Rossowska, M., 296–312
Rougeot, C., 100–111

Saadi, M., 100–111
Salem, N., Jr., 457–458, 459–461, 482–484, 497–499
Sarti, S., 352–364
Saye, J., 455–456
Schnaar, R., 474–477
Schoettle, R. J., 427–428
Schwartz, J. H., 121–130, 208–218
Seregi, A., 84–99
Shapira, Y., 485–487, 488–490
Shapiro, E., 121–130, 208–218
Sheridan, M., 465–467
Sheridan, R. E., 480–481

Shingu, T., 457–458, 482–484
Shohami, E., 485–487, 488–490
Siegal, T., 488–490
Siegal, Tz., 488–490
Siegelbaum, S. A., 219–236
Siesjö, B. K., 323–339
Silvani, V., 444–448
Smith, M.-L., 323–339
Spector, A. A., 471–473
Spector, R., 146–152
Spinnewyn, B., 296–312
Stålnacke, C.-G., 494–496
Sun, G. Y., 37–55, 282–295
Suzuki, Y., 491–493

Tai, H. H., 282–295
Terrian, D. M., 438–440
Thibodeaux, K. T., 468–470
Tiberghien, C., 100–111
Tomer, A., 248–258
Tominaga, T., 461–464

Urade, Y., 451–452, 491–493
Urbanski, H. F., 192–207

Van Kammen, D. P., 411–423
Vink, R., 431–432
Volterra, A., 219–236

Walenga, R., 429–430
Watanabe, Y., 494–496
Watanabe, Y., 494–496
Watson, B. D., 269–281
White, R. P., 131–145
Wilson, D. F., 500–501
Wisner, A., 100–111
Wolfe, L. S., 74–83
Woolworth, V., 237–247
Wu, K. K., 478–479

Xu, J., 282–295

Yadid, G., 485–487
Yao, J. K., 411–423
Yavin, E., 248–258
Yergey, J. A., 457–458, 497–499
Yoshidomi, M., 259–268
Yu, A. C. H., 237–247

Zaleska, M. M., 500–501